Frontiers of Biostatistical Methods and Applications in Clinical Oncology

Shigeyuki Matsui · John Crowley
Editors

Frontiers of Biostatistical Methods and Applications in Clinical Oncology

Springer

Editors
Shigeyuki Matsui
Graduate School of Medicine
Nagoya University
Nagoya, Aichi
Japan

John Crowley
Cancer Research and Biostatistics
Seattle, WA
USA

ISBN 978-981-10-0124-6 ISBN 978-981-10-0126-0 (eBook)
DOI 10.1007/978-981-10-0126-0

Library of Congress Control Number: 2017945240

Printed on acid-free paper

This Springer imprint is published by Springer Nature
The registered company is Springer Nature Singapore Pte Ltd.
The registered company address is: 152 Beach Road, #21-01/04 Gateway East, Singapore 189721, Singapore

Preface

The field of oncology is now in the midst of evolution owing to rapid advances in biotechnologies and cancer genomics that increasingly accelerate our understanding of cancer biology and the development of new diagnostics and therapeutics. This field is actually becoming one of the most promising disease fields in the shift toward precision medicine, involving the provision of a new paradigm of clinical trials based on molecular markers. Accordingly, many new statistical challenges have emerged in this field which warrant further progress in the methodology and practice of biostatistics. Importantly, biostatisticians have a critical role more than ever in the discovery of disease mechanisms/biomarkers and in the development of effective healthcare strategies for disease prevention, early detection, and treatment. Based on the accumulation of their experiences in these medical researches, biostatisticians will help establish the new framework of evidence-based medicine in the new era of precision medicine, with advanced statistical methodologies and tools.

This book presents state-of-the-art biostatistical methods and their applications in various stages of current cancer studies. Topics include molecular epidemiology, disease screening, complex clinical trials with drug combinations or predictive biomarkers, development of prognostic biomarkers/risk calculators, meta-analysis, and the analysis of large-scale omics and imaging data. Several chapters, providing general overviews on specific topics or fields in cancer research, would be beneficial for very wide audiences, including clinical investigators, translational scientists, and others who are involved in clinical studies. Several chapters provide nice methodological overviews for specialists and students in biostatistics and bioinformatics. On the other hand, as one of the unique features of this book, many chapters provide lush aspects in practical biostatistics that would be beneficial for practitioners and, also, methodologists and students in biostatistics.

Lastly, this book project was motivated by the first Pacific Rim Cancer Biostatistics Conference in Seattle in the summer of 2015 to establish an international network of biostatisticians in the oncology field. We sincerely express our thanks to all of the contributors to this project, who are leading experts in academia and government organizations for providing the "frontiers" of biostatistics in this field. We also thank a Grant-in-Aid for Scientific Research (16H06299) and JST-CREST (JPMJCR1412) from the Ministry of Education, Culture, Sports, Science and Technology of Japan for supporting the conference and book project.

Nagoya, Japan Shigeyuki Matsui
Seattle, USA John Crowley

Contents

Contributors

Donna Pauler Ankerst Department of Mathematics, Technical University Munich, Munich, Germany; Departments of Urology and Epidemiology/Biostatistics, University of Texas Health Science Center at San Antonio, San Antonio, TX, USA

Bart Barlogie Mt Sinai School of Medicine, New York, NY, USA

William E. Barlow Cancer Research and Biostatistics, Seattle, WA, USA

Yiyi Chen OHSU-PSU School of Public Health, Knight Cancer Institute, Oregon Health & Science University, Portland, OR, USA

Il Ju Choi Center for Gastric Cancer, National Cancer Center, Goyang, Korea

John Crowley Cancer Research and Biostatistics, Seattle, WA, USA

Racky Daffé Biostatistics, Knight Cancer Institute and School of Public Health, Oregon Heatlh & Science University, Portland, OR, USA

Sonja Grill Department of Mathematics, Technical University Munich, Munich, Germany

Satoshi Hattori Department of Integrated Medicine, Biomedical Statistics, Osaka University, Osaka, Japan

Rolando Herrero Prevention and Implementation Group, International Agency for Research on Cancer, Lyon, France

Akihiro Hirakawa Department of Biostatistics and Bioinformatics, Graduate School of Medicine, The University of Tokyo, Tokyo, Japan

Stephanie Page Hoskins Center for Quantitative Sciences, Vanderbilt University, Nashville, TN, USA

Atsushi Kawaguchi Center for Comprehensive Community Medicine, Faculty of Medicine, Saga University, Saga, Japan

Aya Kuchiba Biostatistics Division, Center for Research Administration and Support, National Cancer Center, Tokyo, Japan

Michael LeBlanc SWOG Statistical Center, Fred Hutchinson Cancer Research Center, Seattle, WA, USA

Ruitao Lin Department of Statistics and Actuarial Science, The University of Hong Kong, Hong Kong, Hong Kong

Xiaodong Luo Research and Development, Sanofi, Bridgewater, NJ, USA

Shigeyuki Matsui Department of Biostatistics, Nagoya University Graduate School of Medicine, Nagoya, Aichi, Japan

Stefan Michiels Service de Biostatistique et Epidémiologie, Gustave Roussy & INSERM CESP U1018 - OncoStat, Gustave Roussy Cancer Center, Université Paris Sud Saclay, Villejuif Cedex, France

Jess A. Millar Fariborz Maseeh Department of Mathematics and Statistics, Portland State University, Portland, OR, USA

Alan Mitchell Allergan, USA Inc, Seattle, WA, USA

Gareth Morgan Myeloma Institute, University of Arkansas for Medical Sciences, Little Rock, AR, USA

Motomi Mori Biostatistics, Knight Cancer Institute and School of Public Health, Oregon Heatlh & Science University, Portland, OR, USA

Byung-Ho Nam Department of Cancer Control and Policy, Graduate School of Cancer Science and Policy, National Cancer Center, Goyang, Korea; HERINGS, The Institute of Advanced Clinical and Biomedical Research, Seoul, Korea

Hisashi Noma Department of Data Science, The Institute of Statistical Mathematics, Tachikawa, Tokyo, Japan

Koji Oba Interfaculty Initiative in Information Studies, Graduate School of Interdisciplinary Information Studies & Department of Biostatistics, School of Public Health, Graduate School of Medicine, The University of Tokyo, Tokyo, Japan

Megan Othus Fred Hutchinson Cancer Research Center, Seattle, WA, USA

Xavier Paoletti Department of Biostatistics and Epidemiology, Gustave Roussy Cancer Center & INSERM U1018 CESP OncoStat, Villejuif Cedex, France

Byung S. Park Biostatistics, Knight Cancer Institute and School of Public Health, Oregon Heatlh & Science University, Portland, OR, USA

Jin Young Park Prevention and Implementation Group, International Agency for Research on Cancer, Lyon, France

Pingping Qu Cancer Research and Biostatistics, Seattle, WA, USA

Hiroyuki Sato Biostatistics Group, Office of New Drug V, Pharmaceuticals and Medical Devices Agency, Tokyo, Japan

Derek Shyr Department of Biostatistics, Harvard T.H. Chan School of Public Health, Boston, MA, USA

Yu Shyr Center for Quantitative Sciences, Vanderbilt University, Nashville, TN, USA

Noah Simon Department of Biostatistics, University of Washington, Seattle, WA, USA

Richard Simon R Simon Consulting, Potomac, MD, USA

Rajeshwari Sridhara Office of Biostatistics, Center of Drug Evaluation and Research, US Food and Drug Administration, Silver Spring, MD, USA

Andreas Strobl Department of Mathematics, Technical University Munich, Munich, Germany

Masataka Taguri Department of Biostatistics, Yokohama City University School of Medicine, Yokohama, Japan

Satoshi Teramukai Department of Biostatistics, Graduate School of Medical Science, Kyoto Prefectural University of Medicine, Kyoto, Japan

Erming Tian Myeloma Institute at University of Arkansas for Medical Sciences, Little Rock, AR, USA

Wei Yann Tsai Department of Biostatistics, Columbia University, New York, NY, USA

Jeffrey Tyner Knight Cancer Institute and Department of Cell, Developmental and Cancer Biology, Oregon Heatlh & Science University, Portland, OR, USA

Guosheng Yin Department of Statistics and Actuarial Science, The University of Hong Kong, Hong Kong, Hong Kong

Xiao-Hua Zhou HSR&D Center of Excellence, VA Puget Sound Health Care System, Seattle, USA; Department of Biostatistics, University of Washington, Seattle, WA, USA

Challenges for Biometry in 21st Century Oncology

Richard Simon

Abstract This chapter provides an overview of the current state of translational cancer research and a discussion of some of the opportunities for biostatisticians, bioinformaticians and computational biologists to accelerate progress in the efforts to reduce cancer mortality. We describe how advances in understanding of tumor genomics have changed the development of anti-cancer treatments and stimulated the development of new clinical trial designs. We propose that further progress will require the development of treatment focused systems-biology modeling that utilizes deep sequencing data and other new tumor and immunology characterization assays. The chapter urges biometricians to participate in trans-disciplinary collaboration and maximize the impact of their contributions by investing time to understand the biological subject matter and the therapeutic context of the problems they work on.

Keywords Translational research · Trans-disciplinary collaboration · Translational systems biology

1 Introduction

Many aspects of cancer research have changed dramatically as a result of the development of whole genome biotechnology platforms and advances in tumor genomics. Translating these developments into reduction in cancer mortality has been difficult, however. In this chapter I will provide a brief review of some of the traditional areas of translational research, highlighting some of the accomplishments and challenges in each area. I will then make some comments about challenges and opportunities that I see for accelerating progress in oncology using the tools of biostatistics, bioinformatics and biological modeling.

R. Simon (✉)
R Simon Consulting, 11920 Glen Mill Rd, Potomac, MD 20854, USA
e-mail: rmaceysimon@gmail.com
URL: http://rsimon.us

S. Matsui and J. Crowley (eds.), *Frontiers of Biostatistical Methods and Applications in Clinical Oncology*, DOI 10.1007/978-981-10-0126-0_1

2 Translational Cancer Research

2.1 *Cancer Cause and Prevention*

Many human cancers are caused by tobacco and alcohol use, exposure to ionizing and ultraviolet radiation, oncogenic viruses or industrial chemicals. Defining the specific molecular steps of carcinogenesis has been elusive for most kinds of cancer and the search for specific dietary and lifestyle factors that are associated with high penetrance risk has had limited success. Much of epidemiologic research in the past decade has been focused on finding inherited DNA polymorphisms associated with cancer risk. Although genome-wide association studies of thousands or tens of thousands of individuals have identified polymorphic sites associated with cancer risk, the effect size of these polymorphisms has generally been too small to be of value for clinical intervention or genetic counseling. Tomasetti and Vogelstein [1] have suggested that a large portion of human cancers are caused by mutations resulting from the thermodynamics of cell division. They showed that the estimated number of cell divisions in organ specific stem cells is correlated with organ specific cancer incidence rates. There are, however, geographic variations in cancer incidence that suggest that specific exposures or lifestyle factors also play a role.

The most successful cancer prevention program in the United States has been for reduction in tobacco use. The HPV vaccine for preventing cervical cancer is another success. Chemoprevention has been less successful because the agents identified as being effective have often had serious adverse effects which have limited their use. Radiation exposure is carefully regulated but programs for lifestyle reduction in alcohol exposure or dietary changes have not been successful.

2.2 *Early Cancer Detection*

Many kinds of human epithelial cancers are considered to have a pre-clinical course with an interval of many years from initiation to detection [2]. This long pre-clinical course should provide opportunities for early detection before the tumor has metastasized and could be cured by surgery. Early detection has been hampered by two main factors. One is technology for identifying early tumors and the other is identifying tumors which will become life threatening. New technologies for highly sensitive detection of circulating tumor DNA may help overcome the first limitation. However, because resection of the tumor can involve removal of a normal organ with serious adverse effects, the second factor is still limiting. What is needed is a better understanding of the steps of development for early tumors which will enable one to distinguish those which are likely to become life-threatening if not resected from those which are less likely to become clinically significant during the lifetime of the individual.

2.3 Cancer Treatment

Prior to 1990, curative drug treatments were developed for several types of cancer including pediatric leukemias, Wilms tumors, lymphomas and testicular cancer. The key principles employed in developing these curative regimens were (i) a given dose of drug kills a fixed proportion of the tumor cells, not a fixed number of cells; (ii) combinations of drugs can overcome resistant sub-populations of tumor cells existing at diagnosis and (iii) combining active drugs which do not have overlapping toxicity are often most effective. Unfortunately, these principles have not resulted in substantial cure rates when applied to advanced epithelial solid tumors of adults.

A new principle of drug treatment was developed following the identification of recurrent somatic mutations of oncogenes in tumors. For example, about half of metastatic melanomas contained an identical point mutation in the BRAF gene [3]. BRAF is a kinase which acts as a switch in translating signals received by membrane receptors to transcription factors which activate gene expression and cell proliferation. The mutation found in BRAF sets the switch to the "on" position even in the absence of a receptor signal. A drug, vemurafenib, was developed to interfere with the constituative activation of mutated BRAF and this drug was found to be very active, even as a single agent, against melanomas. Figure 1 shows the progression-free survival curves from the phase III trial comparing chemotherapy alone to vemurafenib in melanoma patients bearing the BRAF tumor mutations [4].

The development of crizotinib for patients with NSCLC bearing an ALK translocation followed a similar development path as that of vemurafenib for melanoma [5]. ALK translocations are found in about 4% of patients with NSCLC but because NSCLC is itself so common, it was possible to conduct a randomized pivotal clinical trial of crizotinib. ALK is also a kinase which is activated by the translocation.

The successes of drugs molecularly targeted to mutated kinase genes or over-expressed receptors established this approach as one of the two dominant strategies for drug development in oncology today. Drug development is driven by the recurrent somatic mutations in oncogenes found in large tumor sequencing studies [6]. The discovery of these recurrent somatic mutations has also had a strong influence on the kinds of clinical trials being conducted. Targeted "enrichment" randomized phase III trials in which patients are selected whose tumors carry the genomic alteration targeted by the new drug can require many fewer randomized patients than the usual broad eligibility clinical trial [7–9]. New "umbrella" trial designs consist of multiple targeted enrichment trials with a common infrastructure for sequencing the patients' tumors and triaging the patients to the trial appropriate for their identified genomic alteration [10]. Phase II "basket" clinical trials evaluate drugs approved for the subset of patients with a particular histologic type of tumor which carries a specific genomic alteration. Such a drug is evaluated in patients whose tumors are of a different histologic type but carry the same genomic alteration as that for which the drug was approved. These phase II basket trials are very popular [11].

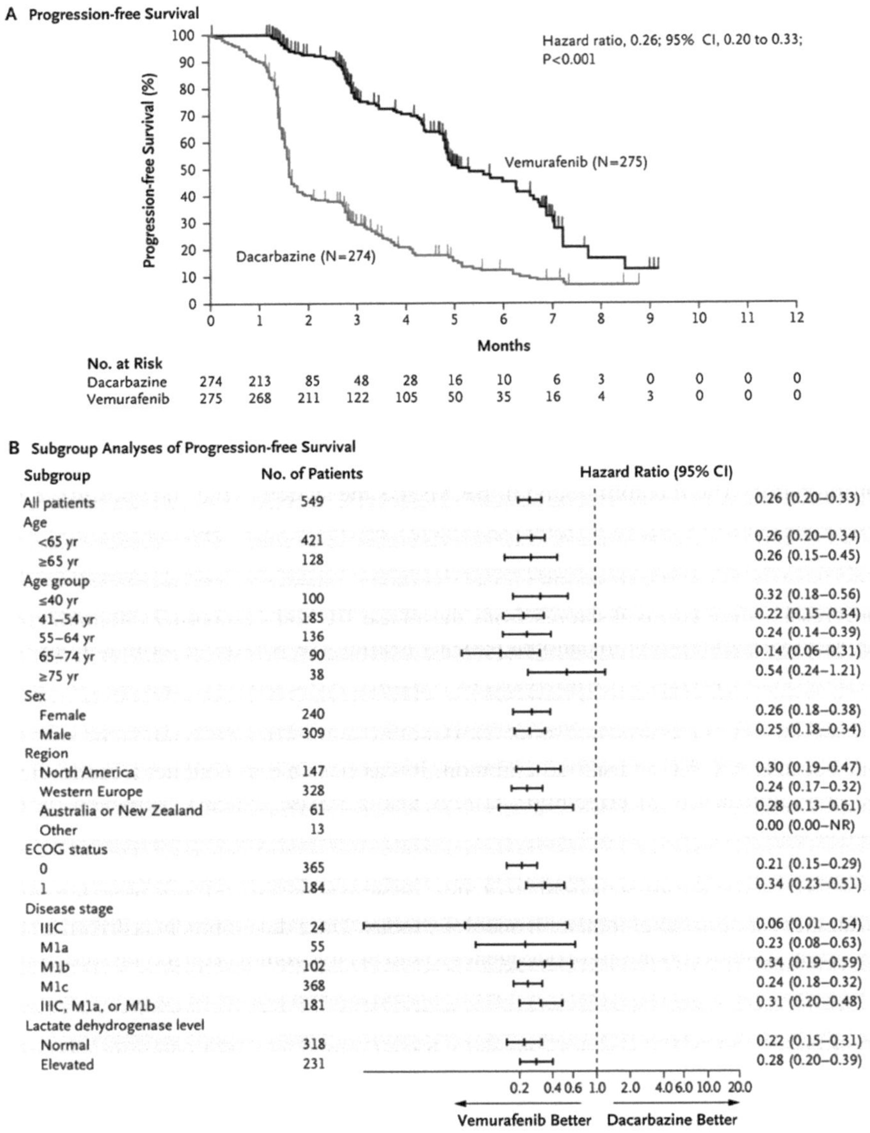

Fig. 1 Distribution of progression-free survival in a randomized clinical trial of vemurafenib versus decarbozine for patients with metastatic melanoma whose tumors contain the V600E BRAF mutation [4]

The second active area of cancer therapeutics today is immunotherapy. Although attempts to stimulate the immune system to attack human tumors had been attempted over many years, success has been limited by (i) difficulty in identifying good tumor-specific antigenic targets; and (ii) immune anergy in patients with cancer. It has now been determined that in many tumors there are actually tumor specific mutated neo-antigens presented on MHC molecules, but that the tumor plays an active role in down-regulating the immune response. One of the ways that tumors down-regulate the immune response is by secreting ligands which bind checkpoint receptors on the surface of effector T lymphocytes. These checkpoint receptors have evolved to limit the possibility of auto-immune responses but are used by tumors for other purposes. Inhibitors of the CTLA and PD-1 checkpoint receptors have been demonstrated to be able to cause sustained complete remissions of metastatic disease in several types of cancer [12]. The extension of these results to other types of cancer and other checkpoints is an active area of clinical research. Highly promising results have also been reported with transplantation of genetically engineered and expanded T lymphocytes.

3 Challenges for Biometry

I am using the term "biometry" in its traditional meaning as "the application of mathematical and statistical methods to the collection, analysis, and interpretation of biological data." Today, the application of such methods generally involves heavy use of computers and so we might view biometry as encompassing biostatistics, bioinformatics and computational biology.

3.1 Biostatistics

Biostatisticians have made major contributions to many areas of oncology research, particularly clinical oncology. The rise of genomics has introduced new problems involving high dimensional data analysis and challenges to the traditional clinical trial paradigm. The organ site based classification of cancer has been shown to be inaccurate in many cases; cancers of the same primary site are often different diseases with different causative mutations, different natural courses and different responses to treatment. Statisticians have for many years emphasized the importance of performing broad eligibility clinical trials to try and simulate the population of patients who might receive the test treatment in clinical practice. Such clinical trial designs are in some cases not appropriate for the newer molecularly targeted drugs which are very unlikely to be effective for patients whose tumors are not driven by de-regulation of the molecular target of the drug. Many of the clinical trial analysis procedures, such as the use of interaction tests, are also not appropriate for clinical trials in which a pre-specified subset hypothesis is part of the primary analysis plan. New classes of clinical trials such as enrichment designs [7–9] and adaptive enrichment designs [13–15], have been developed for such trials. There is increasing realization that even in clinical trials for which there is a statistically significant treatment effect for the eligible population, that population is not necessarily the best intended use population for the treatment. The treatment effect for the eligible population is often small because it is diluted by a substantial fraction of the eligible patients who do not benefit from the test treatment. Although such clinical trials may lead to regulatory approval of the test treatment, payers may refuse to pay for a drug with such a small average treatment effect. This accounts for some of the great interest in enrichment designs and in predictive biomarkers which identify patients most likely to benefit from a treatment. There is a growing recognition that a clinical trial has two major objectives; one to test whether a new treatment has any benefit relative to the control for the population as a whole, and the second to provide guidance for determining whom to treat with the new regimen. The second objective is not a hypothesis testing problem; it is one of determining a predictive classifier with good classification properties [16–18].

There has been relatively little research on "predictive classifiers". Instead, most of the biostatistics focus has been on developing "prognostic classifiers" when the number of candidate predictors is much greater than the number of cases. Unfortunately, prognostic classification studies are often performed in a manner which ignores the medical context and consequently have no impact. Prognostic classifiers can be medically useful if they help physicians identify the patients who need treatment, or who need more treatment than a standard control regimen, among patients in a medical context generally defined by stage and prior treatment history. Developing a classifier using a dataset of patients with a wide range of stages who have subsequently received a wide range of treatments is much less likely to produce a medically useful decision tool. Also, the question is often whether among patients with the same stage of disease who subsequently received no systemic treatment, is there a subset with such good prognosis that similar future patients do not need systemic treatment. That question is often not addressed; instead attention is focused on testing hypotheses about outcome differences for the risk groups.

Many "big data" problems that biostatisticians encounter involve genomic data and involve biological discovery or prediction rather than hypothesis testing. One of the main challenges for biostatistics in the future will be overcoming the viewpoint that their field is only about inference. Overcoming this will include overcoming the bias that proving theorems about asymptotic behavior is more valuable than development or application of novel tools for data analysis. Important contributions to specific fields of science must be highly valued. Departments should aim to train statistically knowledgeable scientific leaders, not just mathematical experts.

3.2 Bioinformatics

The advent of biotechnology platforms for whole genome characterization, particularly gene expression profiling and nucleic acid sequencing, has transformed biology and genetics research. These technologies have enabled new scientific questions to be addressed and old questions addressed in new ways. The generation of this data has necessitated the development of new methods for upstream and downstream analysis. It has also led to major growth in the fields of Bioinformatics and Computational Biology for development and use of these methods. Individuals from a wide variety of backgrounds have been attracted to the field and are needed in the field. I believe that a major challenge for bioinformatics is to develop a culture of trans-disciplinary collaboration and to do a better job of generating biologically meaningful knowledge. Although a project need not be hypothesis driven, good projects are usually motivated by clear scientific questions. Without a clear scientific question, it is not possible to design the appropriate experiment or to use the appropriate assay platform. A successful project obtains clear answers. To achieve this usually requires a closely working team of biological scientists and bioinformatics scientists. I headed a Computational and Systems Biology Branch at the National Cancer Institute and have focused on hiring computational biologists with strong biological backgrounds. We found that the development of innovative bioinformatics systems which permit biological scientists to directly perform detailed analyses of high dimensional data without computer programming can also be effective for enhancing discovery [19].

3.3 *Translationally Focused Systems Biology Modeling*

Somatic mutations have complex effects on tumor cell populations and on their interactions with surrounding tissue and the immune system. One might think that mathematical and computational modeling would have an important role in helping to understand these biological systems, but to date it has had limited impact on the development of improved prevention or treatment strategies. Too often the focus has been on characterizing general system properties rather than on elucidating actionable methods for system control. One of the problems with biological systems modeling is that we rarely know enough to model the system at a very detailed level. If we need to understand the system at that level, then we will have to perform many experiments and take many measurements. This is often beyond the scope of the modeler and beyond the interest of the experimentalist whose wants to develop treatments, not models. For the collaboration to be successful, the modeling process must be helpful in the development of effective interventions. It must be a stepwise approach at a level of detail chosen so that each step provides new clues about what kinds of interventions might be successful. Such modeling efforts need to be approached from a different perspective than the current standards in systems biology. Systems biology in therapeutics should have a clear objective. For example, a model of interaction of signaling pathways might have the objective of improving the development of combinations of molecularly targeted agents based on a tumor profile of genomic alterations. Similarly, a model of the interaction of a tumor with its stroma and the immune system might have the objective of improving the development of improved combinations of immunomodulating agents for eradicating tumors by T effector lymphocytes. Such models cannot be built based on public databases developed without focus on the particular objective. Experiments must be conducted to generate the data for the next stage of the process. This requires a close collaboration with the objective being not to develop the model per se, but to use the modeling process to discover new approaches for improved treatment. Although such systems modeling is challenging, therapeutics development, particularly improving response to immunotherapy regimens, is very complex and contains too many non-understood variables to be effectively pursued without some form of computational systems modeling.

4 Discussion

Progress in prevention, early detection and treatment of human cancers has in many cases been modest. More rapid progress may await a better understanding of the earliest stages of oncogenesis. Most of the experimental models of cancer are deficient in one form or other but the development of increasingly data rich whole genome assays provides the opportunity to more deeply probe and better understand human tumors. Translating this data into meaningful biological information, however, is very challenging and requires the involvement of biometric scientists. The pursuit of this area of research will continue to provide many opportunities for development of novel biostatistical methodology.

Major therapeutic advances in oncology are likely to require deeper understanding of cancer biology. The strategy of matching drugs to somatic mutations has been useful but has generally led to early drug resistance in treating patients with metastatic disease. Focused systems biology modeling and deep tumor sequencing studies are needed to elucidate the biology of tumors and the immune system and the interaction of signalling pathways to enable improved treatment regimens to be developed.

The randomized clinical trial will continue to play a very important role in therapeutics development. The genomic heterogeneity of tumors both between patients and within individual patients will, however, lead to new clinical trial designs which are more closely aligned with discoveries in tumor biology and immunology. There is sometimes a tension in the design and analysis of clinical trials which biostatisticians will continue to struggle with. No single clinical trial answers all the questions or produces the final treatment regimen. The appropriate analysis and interpretation of a clinical trial depends on the medical context, and on other available treatments. For a biostatistician involved in therapeutics development, the objective is to participate in a process that leads to more effective treatment for patients, not to just avoid type I errors. Cancer clinical trials are becoming based on stronger biological science with better tools for classifying the

tumors and for measuring treatment effect. As in the past, the effective use of these tools will open up new methodological problems whose solution will depend on the participation of talented and dedicated biostatisticians.

References

1. Tomasetti C, Vogelstein B. Variation in cancer risk among tissues can be explained by the number of stem cell divisions. Science. 2015;347:78–81.
2. Yachida S, Jones S, Bozic I, Anatal T, Leary R, et al. Metastasis occurs late during the genetic evolution of pancreatic cancer. Nature. 2010;467:1114–7.
3. Davies H, Bignell GR, Cox C, Stephens P, Edkins S, et al. Mutations of the BRAF gene in human cancer. Nature. 2002;417:949–54.
4. Sosman JA, Kim KB, Schuchter L, Gonzalez R, Pavlick AC, Weber JS, et al. Survival in BRAF V600-mutant advanced melanoma treated with vemurafenib. N Engl J Med. 2012;366:707–14.
5. Shaw AT, Kim SW, Nakagawa K, Seto T, Crino L, et al. Crizotinib versus chemotherapy in advanced ALK-positive lung cancer. N Engl J Med. 2013;368:2385–94.
6. Chin L, Andersen JN, Futreal PA, et al. Cancer genomics: from discovery science to personalized medicine. Nat Med. 2011;17:297–303.
7. Simon R, Maitournam A. Evaluating the efficiency of targeted designs for randomized clinical trials. Clin Cancer Res. 2004;10:6759–63.
8. Mandrekar SJ, Sargent DJ. Clinical trial designs for predictive biomarker validation: theoretical considerations and practical challenges. J Clin Oncol. 2009;27:4027–34.
9. Hoering A, LeBlanc M, Crowley JJ. Randomized phase III clinical trial designs for targeted agents. Clin Cancer Res. 2008;14:4358–67.
10. Simon R. Genomic alteration-driver clinical trial designs in oncology. Ann Intern Med. 2016;165:270–8.
11. Simon R, Geyer S, Subramanian J, Roychowdhury S. The Bayesian basket design for genomic variant-driven phase II trials. Semin Oncol. 2016;43:13–8.
12. Eggermont AMM, Maio M, Robert C. Immune checkpoint inhibitors in melanoma provide the cornerstones for curative therapies. Semin Oncol. 2015;42:429–35.
13. Wang SJ, Hung HMJ, O'Neill RT. Adaptive patient enrichment designs in therapeutic trials. Biometrical J. 2009;51:358–74.
14. Jennison C, Turnbull BW. Adaptive seamless designs: selection and prospective testing of hypotheses. J Biopharm Stat. 2007;17:1135–61.
15. Simon N. Adaptive enrichment designs: applications and challenges. Clin Invest. 2015;5:383–91.
16. Freidlin B, Simon R. Adpative signature design: an adaptive clinical trial design for generating and prospectively testing a gene expression signature for sensitive patients. Clin Cancer Res. 2005;11:7872–8.
17. Freidlin B, Jiang W, Simon R. The cross-validated adaptive signature design. Clin Cancer Res. 2010;16:691–8.
18. Matsui S, Simon R, Qu P, Shaughnessy JD, Barlogie B, Crowley J. Developing and validating continuous genomic signatures in randomized clinical trials for predictive medicine. Clin Cancer Res. 2012;18:6065–73.
19. Simon R, Lam A, Li MC, Ngan M, Menenzes S, Zhao Y. Analysis of gene expression data using BRB-array tools. Cancer Inform. 2007;3:11–7.

Statistical Challenges with the Advances in Cancer Therapies

Rajeshwari Sridhara

Abstract Statistical challenges in designing, analyzing and interpreting the data are being encountered with the recent development of new classes of drugs to treat cancer. The existing paradigm of drug development from Phase I to Phase III clinical trials is not optimal. New and innovative trial designs and statistical methods are needed to evaluate the new classes of drugs. In this chapter we present the regulatory considerations in the evaluation of drug products, the drug development paradigm in the last century and the current time, and the statistical challenges that need to be addressed.

keywords Regulations · Cancer drug development paradigm · Immunotherapies

1 Regulatory Considerations

With the signing into law of the Kefauver-Harris Drug Amendments to the Food and Drug Cosmetic Act in 1962, drug manufacturers were for the first time required to prove to the US FDA the effectiveness of their products before marketing them [1]. This amendment was intended to ensure both drug efficacy and safety, and gave a statistical framework for conducting clinical trials to prove the effectiveness of drug products. Section 505(d) of the Food and Drug Cosmetic Act [2, 3] as amended states that "…evidence consisting of adequate and well-controlled investigations, including clinical investigations, by qualified scientific experts, that proves the drug will have the effect claimed by its labeling …". This statement has been used as the regulatory standard for establishing evidence and interpreted to mean the following: the evidence should be reproduced in at least two independent studies, the probability of one-sided type I error should be controlled at a threshold of 0.025, a clinically meaningful treatment effect should in general be established

R. Sridhara (✉)
Office of Biostatistics, Center of Drug Evaluation and Research,
US Food and Drug Administration, Silver Spring, MD 20993, USA
e-mail: Rajeshwari.Sridhara@fda.hhs.gov

S. Matsui and J. Crowley (eds.), *Frontiers of Biostatistical Methods and Applications in Clinical Oncology*, DOI 10.1007/978-981-10-0126-0_2

even if the results are statistically significant, and the product should have an acceptable risk-benefit profile.

Two decades later, in 1981, the FDA and the Department of Health and Human Services revised the regulations for the protection of human subjects, detailing the contents of informed consent and widening the representation in institutional review boards. Another landmark in the history of the FDA was the publication of regulations in 1991 establishing a new path to accelerate the review of drugs for life-threatening diseases. Today we have two regulatory pathways for marketing approval of drug products: regular or traditional approval and accelerated approval.

The regular approval decision is based on demonstrated clinical benefit of the drug product, for example, improved overall survival in cancer patients compared to placebo, or on an outcome that clearly benefits a patient, such as an improvement in disease related symptoms. The accelerated approval decision is based on a surrogate endpoint reasonably likely to predict clinical benefit, such as objective tumor response rate, and the treatment effect should be better than available therapy. Products approved under the accelerated approval pathway are, however, required to subsequently establish improved clinical benefit by conducting a confirmatory clinical trial.

The statistical considerations in evaluating drug products include (1) quality and quantity of data, (2) design of the study, (3) method of analyses, and (4) interpretation of the results from the analyses. With respect to clinical trial design, the important considerations are whether the study is randomized or not, the presence or absence of adaptive features, whether a superiority or non-inferiority hypothesis is tested, the extent to which the overall false positive rate is controlled, and whether the results are replicated. Important considerations in the analyses include clear definition, measurement and validation of the outcome of interest; the statistic used to test the hypothesis and whether the data conform to the assumptions of the chosen analysis method; whether any subgroups were identified and pre-specified to be tested; imbalances between treatment groups in the subgroup; and finally whether multiple hypothesis testing was conducted.

2 The Drug Development Paradigm in the Last Century

The development of cytotoxic drugs, the predominant treatment of cancer in the last century, has generally been comprised of a step-wise approach with clearly defined phases of clinical trials: Phase I trials for dose finding, Phase II trials to determine drug activity, and Phase III trials for confirming efficacy. Phase I trials have been designed to find the maximum tolerated dose (MTD), commonly using an algorithmic design such as a 3 + 3 design or more recently a model-based design (for example, modified continual reassessment methodology). In these trials, the dose was continuously increased until dose limiting toxicity (DLT) was observed. A lower dose than the DLT dose was considered the maximum tolerated dose (MTD). The MTD was further evaluated in the next phases of the study to assess the efficacy and overall risk-benefit of the drug. In this cytotoxic paradigm a 'more is better' approach was used, because of the desire to kill the maximum number of cancer cells. For cytotoxic therapies, there were reasonably good preclinical models prior to conducting first-in-human Phase I studies, treatment was limited to a finite number of treatment cycles of 21–28 days, the dose given to a patient was based on body surface area, toxicities were observed in a short period of time, and the toxicities (hematologic, neurologic, etc.) were well characterized.

The Phase II single-arm trials evaluated activity of the drug using intermediate outcomes such as tumor response rate that could be observed in a relatively short time. Typically, these trials were designed using the Simon two-stage approach [4] as single-arm studies. In this approach, patients would be enrolled and treated in two stages. If the tumor response rate in the group of patients enrolled and treated at MTD in the first stage was less than a pre-specified threshold, the drug would not be studied any further; and if response rate was more than this threshold, an additional group of patients would be enrolled to the second stage. Only if the overall response rate was more than a desired threshold in the two groups of patients combined would the drug would be further evaluated in Phase III trials.

The confirmatory Phase III trials evaluating the efficacy and safety of the drug were randomized controlled trials comparing the investigational drug to the standard of care, with overall survival as the primary outcome of the clinical trial. Because the toxicities were well characterized for the cytotoxic products and the treatment was limited to a finite number of treatment cycles, the toxicities observed during the different phases of drug development formed an adequate basis to guide physicians in the management of patient treatment.

3 The Current Drug Development Paradigm

With the understanding of the biology of the disease and the development of non-cytotoxic drugs such has kinase inhibitors and immunotherapy, cancer treatment options have changed in the last two decades. In terms of both toxicity and activity/efficacy, these products are very different from cytotoxic products. There are few if any good pre-clinical models to predict the likely starting dose and toxicities in humans, although these products are in general better tolerated. Severe toxicities of these drugs are not always observed in a short duration of time, and treatment is not limited to a few cycles, but typically continued until disease progression is observed. Many of these products are taken orally and administered in fixed doses rather than based on body surface area. Often a long-term effect on overall survival is observed in the absence of objective tumor response rate (example: sorafenib, ipilimumab) [5, 6]. Thus, the cytotoxic paradigm fails in every phase of drug development for the current generation of drug products. The cytotoxicity-based definition of dose-limiting toxicity is no longer useful, because many of these products do not have the well characterized hematologic or non-hematologic toxicities. For example, the kinase inhibitor erlotinib has severe skin toxicity, which is not observed with typical cytotoxic drugs. Many of the toxicities do not occur within the short time of observation in the Phase I trials where more refractory patients with a shorter life expectancy are enrolled. Some of these drugs may not shrink tumors but rather stabilize the disease, resulting in poor response rates and requiring randomized Phase II studies to better understand the activity of the products with respect to other outcomes such as progression-free survival. Because of the unknown long-term toxicities of these drugs it is not uncommon to have dose interruptions and reductions in Phase III trials, with the result that when the confirmatory clinical trial is completed, recommended dose and monitoring guidelines for patient care are not always clear.

3.1 Biomarker-Based Clinical Trials

The patient population enrolled in a clinical trial is recognized to be heterogeneous, (for example with respect to age, race, gender, genetic markers, subgroups of the disease, etc.), despite stringent inclusion and exclusion criteria. Therefore, when confirmatory clinical trial results do not demonstrate efficacy of the investigational drug, it is common to hypothesize that the drug is likely to be effective in a subgroup of the population. However, the challenge is in finding the specific subgroup that may benefit from the investigational drug. It is important to recognize whether the subgroup is defined based on a prognostic or predictive biomarker or both.

A prognostic biomarker is a biomarker that is measured at baseline (prior to administration of a treatment) that correlates with the treatment outcome for a heterogeneous set of patients and is independent of the treatment (Fig. 1a). For example, stage of disease that is measured at baseline is a prognostic marker of the overall survival of a given patient irrespective of the treatment received. A predictive marker is a biomarker that is measured at baseline prior to administration of a treatment that predicts whether a particular treatment is likely to be beneficial and it is associated with outcome of a specific therapy (Fig. 1b). Based on the predictive marker status, it is expected that there would be a differential benefit of a given treatment. For example, patients with metastatic melanoma with BRAF mutations benefit from BRAF inhibitors such as vemurafenib [7] and dabrafenib [8], and on the contrary, patients whose tumor is BRAF-negative (i.e., the BRAF gene is not mutated, or wild type) do not benefit from these treatments. Thus in many cases the biomarker status may guide the treatment options.

Various adaptive designs have been used and reported in the literature to identify and evaluate prognostic and predictive biomarkers. An ideal design would be to use a biomarker-stratified, randomized design as shown in Fig. 2. An example of this design is the lung cancer MARVEL trial [9] in which the patients' tumors were assessed prior to randomization for epidermal growth factor receptor gene (EGFR) status as measured by fluorescent in situ hybridization (FISH). Randomization was stratified by the EGFR status, and patients are randomly assigned to receive either

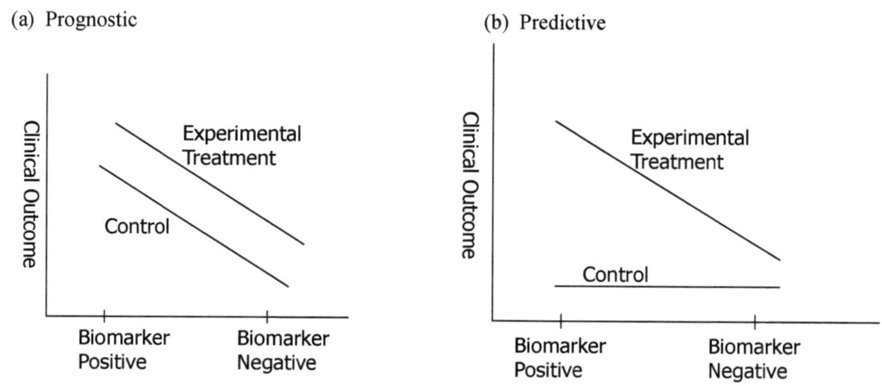

Fig. 1 Prognostic and predictive markers

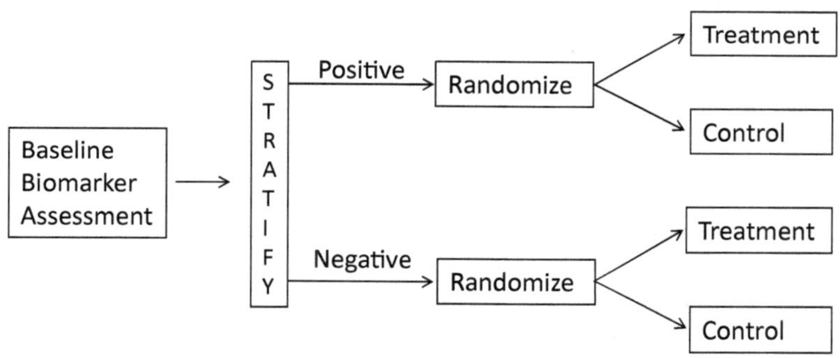

Fig. 2 Biomarker-stratified, randomized design

erlotinib or pemetrexed. In this design, the biomarker status is known for all randomized patients, and it can be evaluated as a prognostic and a predictive marker. On the other hand, if there is scientific evidence that given the mechanism of action of a particular drug it is unlikely that patients with biomarker-negative tumors would benefit from that drug, then an enrichment design (Fig. 3) is preferred as in the example of vemurafenib clinical trial where only patients whose tumor expressed BRAF mutation [7]. However, such a design assumes that the biomarker is predictive, and as such this design does not lend to evaluation of the biomarker as a prognostic or a predictive biomarker since marker-negative patients are not studied. Use of enrichment designs have increased with the development of targeted therapies. However designing such trials can be challenging as often the treatment effect of the standard of care in the enriched population may be unknown due to lack of information on the biomarker of interest in the historical control resulting in potentially underpowered Phase III studies, or the prevalence of the biomarker subgroup may be too small for a randomized clinical trial to be feasible.

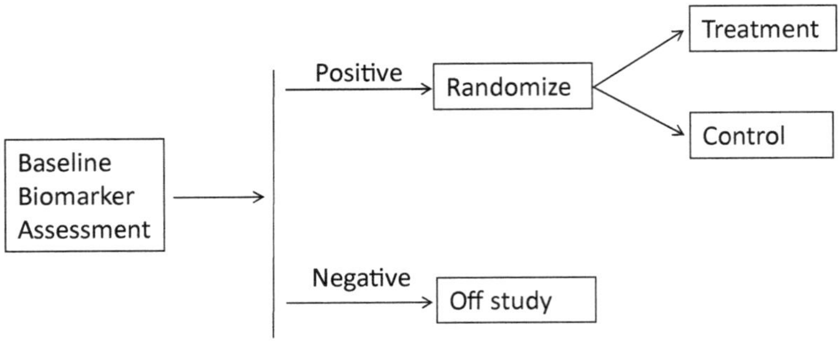

Fig. 3 Enrichment design

The ideal goal is to treat patients who benefit from a drug while not exposing patients who may not benefit and experience unwanted toxicity. However, due to the complex biology of the diseases not all characteristics that influence the outcome are measurable or known, and it is difficult to identify characteristics of patients who are likely to respond to a given treatment. Clinical trial designs have been proposed that evaluate predictive and prognostic molecular biomarkers and identify subgroups of patients who are likely to benefit from a given treatment after the clinical trial is completed in all patients [10–12].

More complex designs with adaptive enrichment strategies where enrichment occurs during the course of the clinical trial based on interim analysis of the data have also been suggested [13, 14]. Such designs with pre-planned decision criteria provide a scientific strategy to select the enriched population based on data accumulated in the initial stages of the clinical trial. Recently clinical trial designs [15–18] that can evaluate multiple diseases, multiple molecular biomarkers and/or multiple drugs (umbrella, platform, or basket trials) have been adopted in disease areas with unmet medical need. These trials typically have one umbrella or master protocol with a central governance structure, with adaptive features that allow adding and removing treatment arms, and are an efficient way of using patient resources. These clinical trials require adequate resources, coordination among different stakeholders and a trial network to conduct the studies. The approval of a new drug based on another trial while the current trial is ongoing, frequent adaptations to the design, multiple hypotheses testing, and overlapping characteristics of patients among two or more subgroups can pose challenges in execution and interpretation of the results of such clinical trials. Careful and detailed pre-planning, particularly in international studies, is essential.

Another component of the biomarker-based clinical trials is the companion or complementary diagnostics that are essential in defining the subgroups. Analytical validation of the biomarker assay based on performance (precision, accuracy, sensitivity and specificity), and quantitative and qualitative variability (e.g., differences in platforms, labs, technicians) are crucial in ensuring replication and interpretation of results. Because the use of a targeted drug is often tied to a diagnostic device in identifying the patient to be treated, there needs to be coordination between the drug and device manufacturing companies as well as co-development of drug and device during the course of the product development cycle [19]. Often clinical trials are conducted with an investigator- or site-based diagnostic. It can be a challenge in evaluating the drug-device product for regulatory approval if the investigator- or site-based diagnostic differs with respect to operating characteristics from the scaled up version that is manufactured at a device manufacturing company.

3.2 Clinical Trials Evaluating Immunotherapy

Unlike chemotherapy and other targeted therapies, immunotherapy activates the immune system and thus indirectly targets the malignant disease. Thus, the early assessment of activity of products using tumor-based endpoints such as objective tumor response rate may not be ideal. Table 1 lists the FDA-approved immunotherapy products for the treatment of patients with advanced metastatic disease. These products have been approved under both accelerated approval and

Table 1 Immunotherapy products USFDA approved in metastatic diseases

Ipilimumab	Pembrolizumab	Nivolumab
March 2011, RA Unresectable/metastatic melanoma	**September 2014, AA** Unresectable/metastatic melanoma after Ipilimumab and BRAF inhibitor when indicated	**December 2014, AA** Unresectable/metastatic melanoma after Ipilimumab and BRAF inhibitor where indicated
	October 2015, AA PD-L1 + metastatic NSCLC after platinum based chemo	**March 2015, RA** Metastatic squamous NSCLC after platinum based chemotherapy
	December 2015, RA Unresectable or metastatic melanoma	**September 2015, RA** as single agent in unresectable/metastatic melanoma with BRAF wild type tumor **January 2016, AA** combination with Ipilimumab in unresectable/metastatic melanoma **AA** in BRAF mutant unresectable/ metastatic melanoma
		October 2015, RA metastatic NSCLC after platinum based chemo
		November 2015, RA metastatic RCC after anti-angiogenic treatment

regular approval provisions. The observed objective response rates were not always large, although duration of response tended to be long among those who have a response, and there were no meaningful differences observed in progression-free survival despite significant differences in overall survival [20]. In the immunotherapy clinical trials, it is also common to observe non-proportionality of hazard function in the analysis of progression-free survival [21]. Although some of the clinical trials evaluating antibodies blocking programmed cell death receptor 1 (PD-1) appear to suggest that programmed death ligand 1 (PD-L1) expression may be a predictive marker, it has not been evaluated systematically and it is unclear what threshold or cut-off value for PD-L1 expression is optimal in identifying the subgroup that benefits from these products [22]. In general in the clinical trials for these products the treatment continued until disease progression was observed. Because of this design, it is not known if the treatment can be stopped after a finite number of cycles of therapy or whether continued use is necessary. Although the currently approved products have demonstrated a favorable benefit-to-risk ratio, these early approvals have relatively short follow-up, and the safety of long-term use of these products is unknown at this time.

In designing future studies, the challenges will be in selecting the optimal endpoints for evaluation of these types of products, both in early-phase clinical trials where the objective is to evaluate the activity of product using intermediate endpoints that can be observed in relatively short time, and in late-phase clinical trials where it may be difficult to demonstrate superiority with respect to overall survival compared to currently approved products due to switch-over of control to experimental treatment arm after disease progression.

4 Summary

Our current understanding of diseases at a molecular level, based in part on advances in genomics, has made it possible to further subdivide disease categories previously defined by site and histology, resulting in smaller populations to study new products. The current generation of products do not fit into the cytotoxic chemotherapy paradigm and require innovative thinking in designing, conducting and interpreting results from clinical trials. We must rethink the goal of each phase of clinical trials in the overall development of new drug products given the differing mechanisms of action and treatment effects of new targeted therapies. Future clinical trials are likely to be more complex and biomarker-based, with adaptive features. Simulation of such designs may become necessary to understand the operational complexities such that statistical properties such as type I error control and study power are not compromised. Further research is needed in identifying intermediate endpoints (for example, response criteria that would capture responses to immunotherapy) so that informative go-no-go decisions for further development of a product can be made.

Most of the clinical trials with time-to-event endpoints are designed assuming an exponential distribution of the outcome measure and a proportional hazard function. However it is not uncommon to observe that these assumptions are violated. Simulation of clinical trials where these assumptions do not hold may be useful in designing and planning such clinical trials. Ultimately, there should be a prospective statistical plan detailing alternative statistical methods for analyzing and summarizing the data should be in place if these assumptions do not hold true.

The selection of endpoints can become even more challenging if, for example, immunotherapy in combination with chemotherapy is being studied. A single intermediate endpoint in such circumstances may not capture the activity and effectiveness of both types of therapies. Careful consideration of the selection of endpoint, length of treatment and length of follow-up would be needed at the design stage.

The importance of timing and rigor in determining the analytic performance of the companion diagnostic test cannot be ignored with the advent of increasing number of targeted therapies. Understanding the statistical properties of the device such as sensitivity, specificity, positive and negative predictive values is essential.

Finally, with the limited number of patients and other resources, collaboration among pharmaceutical and device companies, academicians, government agencies including regulatory agencies, payers and patient advocacy groups is crucial in order to conduct future clinical trials that are informative as to the safe and effective use of a product. Statisticians are in a unique position to resolve the complexities inherent in the design of efficient and informative clinical trials.

References

1. Mile stones in U.S. Food and Drug law history. http://www.fda.gov/AboutFDA/WhatWeDo/History/Milestones/ucm128305.htm.
2. 21 Code of Federal Regulations, Part 314.126.
3. FDA Guidance for Industry: Providing Clinical Evidence of Effectiveness for Human Drugs and Biological Products. 1998.
4. Simon R. Optimal two-stage designs for phase II clinical trials. Control Clin Trials. 1989;10:1–10.
5. Kane RC, et al. Sorafenib for the treatment of advanced renal cell carcinoma. Clin Cancer Res. 2006;12:7271–8.
6. Hodi FS, et al. Improved survival with ipilimumab in patients with metastatic melanoma. N Engl J Med. 2010;363:711–23.
7. Chapman PB, et al. Improved survival with vemurafenib in melanoma with BRAF V600E mutation. N Engl J Med. 2011;364:2507–16.
8. Hauschild A, et al. Dabrafenib in BRAF-mutated metastatic melanoma: a multicentre, open-label, phase 3 randomised controlled trial. Lancet. 2012;380:358–65.
9. Wakelee H, et al. Cooperative group research efforts in lung cancer 2008: focus on advanced-stage non-small-cell lung cancer. Clin Lung Cancer. 2008;9:346–51.
10. Freidlin B, Simon R. Adaptive signature design: an adaptive clinical trial design for generating and prospectively testing a gene expression signature for sensitive patients. Clin Cancer Res. 2005;11:7872–8.

11. Freidlin B, et al. The cross-validated adaptive signature design. Clin Cancer Res. 2010;16:691–8.
12. Redman MW, Crowley JJ, Herbst RS, Hirsch FR, Gandara DR. Design of a phase III clinical trial with prospective biomarker validation: SWOG S0819. Clin Cancer Res. 2012; 18(15):4004–12.
13. Simon N, Simon R. Adaptive enrichment designs for clinical trials. Biostatistics. 2013;14:613–25.
14. Mehta C, et al. Biomarker driven population enrichment for adaptive oncology trials with time to event endpoints. Stat Med. 2014;33:4515–31.
15. Barker AD, et al. I-SPY 2: an adaptive breast cancer trial design in the setting of neoadjuvant chemotherapy. Clin Phamacol Ther. 2009;86:97–100.
16. Herbst RS, et al. Lung master protocol (Lung MAP)—a biomarker-driven protocol for accelerating development of therapies for squamous cell lung cancer: SWOG S1400. Clin Cancer Res. 2015;21:1514–24.
17. National Cancer Institute Press Release. NCI-MATCH trial will link targeted cancer drugs to gene abnormalities. 2015. http://www.cancer.gov/news-events/press-releases/2015/nci-match.
18. Sridhara R, et al. Current statistical challenges in oncology clinical trials in the era of targeted therapy. Stat Biopharm Res. 2015;7(4):348–56. doi:10.1080/19466315.2015.1094673.
19. In vitro companion diagnostic devices: Guidance to Industry and Food and Drug Administration Staff. 2014. http://www.fda.gov/downloads/MedicalDevices/DeviceRegulationandGuidance/GuidanceDocuments/UCM262327.pdf.
20. Kazandjian D, et al. FDA approval summary: Nivolumab for the treatment of metastatic non-small cell lung cancer with progression on or after platinum-based chemotherapy. Onclologist. 2016;21:634–42.
21. Pembrolizumab product label: Section 14.1, Figure 2. http://www.accessdata.fda.gov/drugsatfda_docs/label/2015/125514s004s006lbl.pdf.
22. Nivolumab product label: Section 14. http://www.accessdata.fda.gov/drugsatfda_docs/label/2015/125554s001lbl.pdf.

Random Walk and Parallel Crossing Bayesian Optimal Interval Design for Dose Finding with Combined Drugs

Ruitao Lin and Guosheng Yin

Abstract Interval designs have recently attracted enormous attention due to their simplicity, desirable properties, and superior performance. We study random-walk and parallel-crossing Bayesian optimal interval designs for dose finding in drug-combination trials. The entire dose-finding procedures of these two designs are nonparametric (or model-free), which are thus robust and also do not require the typical "nonparametric" prephase used in model-based designs for drug-combination trials. Simulation studies demonstrate the finite-sample performance of the proposed methods under various scenarios. Both designs are illustrated with a phase I two-agent dose-finding trial in prostate cancer.

Keywords Bayesian method · Dose finding · Drug combination · Interval design · Random walk

1 Introduction

Given a large number of approved agents for cancer treatment, it becomes commonplace to evaluate the joint effects when multiple drugs are used in combination. In general, combined therapies are expected to induce better patient response, but meanwhile they may lead to more severe adverse events and toxicity. Hence, the primary objective in a two-agent dose-finding trial is to find the maximum tolerated dose (MTD) combination that yields a prespecified target toxicity rate. However, dose finding for combined therapies is complicated since the joint toxicity order of paired doses is only partially known. For a single-agent trial, dose movement is along a line and the toxicity order is known due to the monotonic toxicity

R. Lin (✉) · G. Yin
Department of Statistics and Actuarial Science, The University of Hong Kong, Pokfulam Road, Hong Kong, Hong Kong
e-mail: ruitaolin@gmail.com

G. Yin
e-mail: gyin@hku.hk

S. Matsui and J. Crowley (eds.), *Frontiers of Biostatistical Methods and Applications in Clinical Oncology*, DOI 10.1007/978-981-10-0126-0_3

assumption. By contrast, there are up to eight adjacent dose combinations for the next dose movement in a two-agent combination trial, including diagonal and off-diagonal directions.

To find the MTD combination based on the partially known order, a common approach is to reduce the dimensionality of the dose searching space to a one-dimensional searching line [1]. Toward this goal, Yuan and Yin [2] introduced a simple design based on the partial orders of the joint toxicities, which is compatible with any single-agent dose-finding method. In contrast to dimension reduction approaches, numerous designs have been proposed by directly modeling the joint toxicity rates, which, in general, are extended from the conventional single-agent designs. Thall et al. [3] proposed an adaptive two-stage Bayesian design by considering a six-parameter joint toxicity rate model. Yin and Yuan [4] utilized a copula-type approach to linking the toxicity rates of two drugs in combination based on several viable conditions, which can be viewed as a generalized or two-dimensional version of the continual reassessment method (CRM) [10]. In a more general framework, Yin and Yuan [5] introduced a latent contingency table approach to two-agent dose finding. Wages et al. [6] developed a partial ordering CRM by laying out several selected orders for the joint toxicity rates. Shi and Yin [7] extended the method of escalation with overdose control by utilizing a four-parameter logistic regression model for drug combinations. For a comprehensive review on the model-based designs, see [8]. Most of the existing two-agent model-based designs often involve relatively more unknown parameters due to extra characterization of the joint toxicity action. Thus, estimation of these parameters can be unstable due to a limited sample size, especially at the beginning of a trial when decisions need to be made after even one or two cohorts of patients are treated. To address this issue, Hirakawa et al. [9] proposed a shrunken predictive approach to finding the MTD for drug-combination trials.

Often, a start-up phase using a certain algorithm is required prior to the initiation of a model-based method to ensure stable estimates at the beginning of a trial, while there is no universal rule for the prephase and it is unclear when the transition should be initiated. On the other hand, algorithm-based designs do not require such a start-up procedure because no parameter estimation is needed. Due to their model-free nature, algorithm-based designs can proceed to locate the MTD without imposing any parametric assumptions, and thus they are considered more robust than the model-based counterparts. Despite the advantages of algorithm-based designs, limited research has been conducted on nonparametric dose-finding methods for two agents. Conaway et al. [11] developed an isotonic design for two-agent dose-finding trials based on simple and partial orders. Ivanova and Wang [12] applied the Narayana design and bivariate isotonic regression to drug-combination trials. Huang et al. [13] introduced a two-agent "3 + 3" design by dividing the two-dimensional space into several dose zones. Fan et al. [14] proposed a three-stage "2 + 1 + 3" design, which allows for both one- and two-dimensional dose searching. Lee and Fan [15] made a further extension by considering the toxicity profile of each agent. The escalation rules in most of the existing nonparametric designs for two agents are rather ad hoc and do not have solid theoretical support, which cannot guarantee the convergence of the selected dose to the true MTD. Furthermore, some of these methods are not flexible enough to target any chosen toxicity rate.

To develop a more flexible nonparametric approach to two-agent dose finding, Lin and Yin [16] proposed a simple two-dimensional interval design by extending the Bayesian optimal interval (BOIN) design [17] to drug-combination trials. The strategy of interval designs is to guide the dose-finding procedure by comparing the observed toxicity rate with a prespecified toxicity tolerance interval. If the observed toxicity rate falls inside the interval, the current dose level should remain for the next cohort; otherwise, the dose level is either escalated or de-escalated, depending on whether the observed toxicity rate is below the lower bound or above the upper bound of the interval. Yuan and Chappell [18] suggested retaining the current dose level if the corresponding estimated toxicity rate is within (0.2, 0.4) when the target toxicity rate is 0.2. Gezmu and Flournoy [19] considered a similar approach to dose-finding trials, which is called the group up-and-down design. However, the treatment allocation rule for the next cohort is only based on the data from the current cohort of patients. To account for the cumulative information at the current dose including both the current and previous cohorts at the same dose level, Ivanova et al. [20] introduced a more formal cumulative cohort design. Interval designs, which are built upon a solid theoretical foundation, are extremely easy to implement in practice [21]. To choose an appropriate interval, Liu and Yuan [17] cast the design in a Bayesian decision-making framework. By minimizing the probability of incorrect dose allocation, an optimal tolerance interval can be derived that has desirable finite- and large-sample properties. We study two versions extended BOIN designs for two-agent dose-finding trials: the random walk BOIN (RW-BOIN) design and the parallel crossing BOIN (PC-BOIN) design. With ease of implementation, both can adaptively search for the MTD using the accrued information. We compare the two interval designs with existing model-based methods and show their comparative and stable operating characteristics.

The rest of the chapter is organized as follows. In Sect. 2, we review the single-agent BOIN design. Section 3 extends the BOIN design to two-dimensional dose-finding trials. In Sect. 4, we illustrate the RW-BOIN and PC-BOIN with a prostate cancer trial example. Simulation studies are conducted in Sect. 5 to examine the operating characteristics of the new designs. Section 6 concludes with some remarks.

2 Single-Agent Interval Design

In a single-agent interval design, let $p_1 < \cdots < p_J$ be the true toxicity probabilities of a set of J doses for the drug under consideration, and let ϕ denote the target toxicity rate specified by the investigator. Furthermore, let $\Delta_L > 0$ and $\Delta_U > 0$ denote the prespecified lower and upper cutoffs, satisfying $0 < \Delta_L < \Delta_U < 1$. Suppose the current cohort is treated at dose level j, and let $\hat{p}_j$ denote the estimated toxicity probability based on the cumulative data at level j. The decisions on the next dose assignment are described as follows:

- if $\Delta_L < \hat{p}_j < \Delta_U$, then the next cohort continues to be treated at the same dose level j;
- if $\hat{p} \leq \Delta_L$, escalate the dose level to $j+1$ for the next cohort;
- if $\hat{p} \geq \Delta_U$, de-escalate the dose level to $j-1$.

To determine Δ_L and Δ_U, we consider three hypotheses at dose level j [17],

$$H_{0j}; p_j = \phi, \quad H_{1j}; p_j = \phi_1, \quad H_{2j}; p_j = \phi_2,$$

where ϕ_1 denotes the highest toxicity probability that is deemed sub-therapeutic such that dose escalation should be pursued, and $\phi_2 (>\phi_1)$ denotes the lowest toxicity probability that is deemed overly toxic such that dose de-escalation is needed.

Let π_{ij} be the prior probability of the ith hypothesis being true, $i = 1, 2, 3$. For simplicity, we specify a noninformative prior probability for the three hypotheses, i.e., $\pi_{0j} = \pi_{1j} = \pi_{2j} = 1/3$. The probability of incorrect decisions can be formulated as

$$\begin{aligned}\Pr(\text{Incorrect}|y_j) &= \pi_{0j}\Pr(\mathbb{E}\text{ or }\mathbb{D}|H_{0j}) + \pi_{1j}\Pr(\mathbb{S}\text{ or }\mathbb{D}|H_{1j}) + \pi_{2j}\Pr(\mathbb{S}\text{ or }\mathbb{E}|H_{2j})\\ &= \pi_{0j}\Pr(\hat{p}_j \leq \Delta_L\text{ or }\hat{p}_j \geq \Delta_U|H_{0j}) + \pi_{1j}\Pr(\hat{p}_j > \Delta_L|H_{1j})\\ &\quad + \pi_{2j}\Pr(\hat{p}_j < \Delta_U|H_{2j}),\end{aligned}$$

where $\mathbb{E}$, $\mathbb{D}$ and $\mathbb{S}$ stand for "Escalation", "De-escalation" and "Stay", respectively. By minimizing the probability of incorrect decisions at each step, the lower and upper bounds of the optimal interval have closed forms,

$$\Delta_L = \frac{\log\left(\frac{1-\phi_1}{1-\phi}\right)}{\log\left\{\frac{\phi(1-\phi_1)}{\phi_1(1-\phi)}\right\}}, \quad \Delta_U = \frac{\log\left(\frac{1-\phi}{1-\phi_2}\right)}{\log\left\{\frac{\phi_2(1-\phi)}{\phi(1-\phi_2)}\right\}}. \tag{1}$$

The single-agent Bayesian optimal interval (BOIN) design is easy to implement and has comparable average performance with the existing dose-finding methods [17]. In practice, the choices of $\phi_1 \in [0.5\phi, 0.7\phi]$ and $\phi_2 \in [1.3\phi, 1.5\phi]$ are suitable for most trials. Moreover, one can also use varying ϕ_1 and ϕ_2 to take into consideration the accumulated sample size. For example, a smaller gap between ϕ_1 and ϕ_2 would accelerate the trial at the earlier stage, while a larger gap at the later stage of a trial tends to keep more patients treated at the MTD. We set $\phi_1 = 0.6\phi$ and $\phi_2 = 1.4\phi$ as the default values.

3 Double-Agent Interval Design

3.1 Random Walk BOIN

In a two-dimensional dose-finding study, let p_{jk} denote the toxicity probability of the two agents at dose combination (j, k), $j = 1, \ldots, J$, $k = 1, \ldots, K$. Suppose the current dose combination is (j, k), and let $\hat{p}_{jk}$ denote the estimated toxicity rate based on the accumulated information on dose combination (j, k), $\hat{p}_{jk} = y_{jk}/n_{jk}$, where y_{jk} and n_{jk} denote the number of toxicities and patients at dose combination (j, k), respectively. We define an admissible dose escalation set as $\mathscr{A}_E = \{(j+1,k),(j,k+1)\}$ and an admissible dose de-escalation set as $\mathscr{A}_D = \{(j-1,k),(j,k-1)\}$. The two-dimensional random walk BOIN (RW-BOIN) design proceeds as follows:

1. Treat the first cohort at the lowest dose combination (1, 1).
2. For the next cohort of patients:
   (a) If $\hat{p}_{jk} \leq \Delta_L$, we escalate to the dose combination that belongs to $\mathscr{A}_E$ and has the largest value of $\Pr\{p_{j'k'} \in (\Delta_L, \Delta_U)|y_{j'k'}\}$.
   (b) If $\hat{p}_{jk} \geq \Delta_U$, we de-escalate to the dose combination that belongs to $\mathscr{A}_D$ and has the largest value of $\Pr\{p_{j'k'} \in (\Delta_L, \Delta_U)|y_{j'k'}\}$.
   (c) Otherwise, if $\Delta_L < \hat{p}_{jk} < \Delta_U$, then the doses stay at the same combination (j, k).
3. This process continues until the total sample size is exhausted.

During dose escalation and de-escalation, if there are multiple optimal dose combinations in the sets of $\mathscr{A}_E$ and $\mathscr{A}_D$, we randomly choose one with equal probability. If no dose combinations exist in the sets of $\mathscr{A}_E$ and $\mathscr{A}_D$, we retain the current dose combination. We further consider the boundary cases. If $j = 1$ and $\hat{p}_{jk} \geq \Delta_U$, the next dose combination is $(j, k - 1)$, unless $(j, k) = (1, 1)$ for which the dose would remain at the same combination. If $j = J$ and $\hat{p}_{jk} \leq \Delta_L$, the next dose combination is $(j, k + 1)$, unless $(j, k) = (J, K)$ for which the current dose combination retains. Due to symmetry between j and k, the same rules also apply to k. To impose a non-informative prior distribution, we take the Jeffreys prior Beta (0.5, 0.5) for each p_{jk}, which corresponds to the information of one subject only.

3.2 Parallel Crossing BOIN

The major advantage of the RW-BOIN design is that it does not incorporate any model assumption of the two-dimensional toxicity surface and can be easily implemented. However, the RW-BOIN design aims at locating only one of the MTDs without conducting a more extensive exploration of other MTDs. To search for multiple MTDs, we propose a parallel crossing BOIN (PC-BOIN) design such

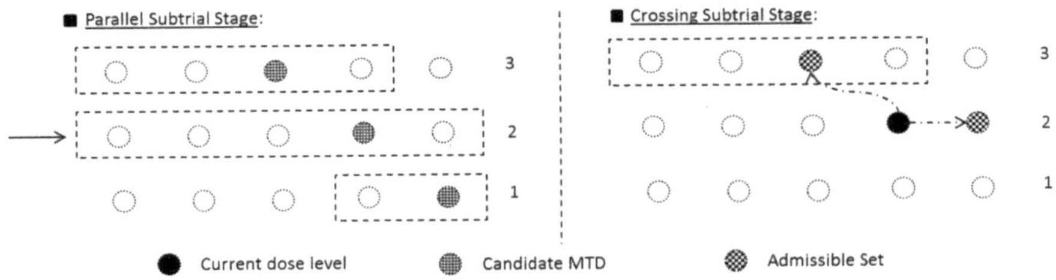

Fig. 1 Illustration of the PC-BOIN design with the parallel subtrial stage (*left panel*) and crossing subtrial stage (*right panel*)

that a broader spectrum of dose levels can be explored. The PC-BOIN design consists of two stages: Stage 1, named as the parallel subtrial stage, converts the two-dimensional dose-finding trial to a series of parallel one-dimensional subtrials by fixing the dose level of one drug. Several candidate MTDs can be identified from the one-dimensional subtrials based on the single-agent BOIN design. After pooling the information together from all the dose levels using the pool adjacent violators algorithm (PAVA), stage 2 starts from the candidate MTD that is closest to the target toxicity rate, and the corresponding subtrial is treated as the primary one-dimensional subtrial. If the accumulated data indicate that the primary subtrial does not contain the MTD, we adaptively switch the primary subtrial to another one. A key feature of stage 2 is to continuously validate the candidate MTD by crossing between the subtrials, and hence we name stage 2 as the crossing subtrial stage.

Without loss of generality, suppose $J < K$. We first divide the entire two-dimensional space into J parallel subtrials by fixing the dose level of drug A at j, $j = 1, \ldots, J$. In the parallel subtrial stage, we impose the sequential scheme [2], which is depicted in Fig. 1 (left panel) and described as follows.

Stage 1 (Parallel subtrials):

(1) Sequentially divide the J subtrials into groups of size 3, and thus we have ceiling(J/3) subgroups, where ceiling(x) rounds x to the next larger integer.
(2) Starting from the first group, sequentially conduct the subtrials in the following order:

    (i) First, run the intermediate-dose subtrial to find the candidate MTD, which is denoted as (j^*, k^*).
    (ii) Based on the candidate MTD of the intermediate-dose subtrial, shrink the dose searching ranges of the higher- and lower-dose subtrials. More specifically, the range of the higher-dose subtrial is from $(j^* + 1, 1)$ to $(j^* + 1, k^*)$ or $(j^* + 1, k^* - 1)$, depending on whether the estimated toxicity rate at dose level (j^*, k^*) is smaller or greater than ϕ. Similarly, the lower-dose subtrial is from $(j^* - 1, k^*)$ or $(j^* - 1, k^* + 1)$ to $(j^* - 1, K)$, depending on whether the estimated toxicity rate at dose level (j^*, k^*) is smaller or greater than ϕ.

(iii) Each subtrial is terminated if more than six patients have been treated at any dose level.

For additional rules to appropriately truncate the dose searching space, see [2]. If the cohort size is m, and the number of dose levels in the current subtrial is K' ($K' \leq K$), we assign mK' patients to that subtrial. Based on this allocation rule, the parallel subtrial stage can be viewed as the preliminary stage. By adaptively conducting the parallel subtrials, we can obtain J possible MTDs. For more accurate identification, the trial then enters into the second stage.

Stage 2 (Crossing subtrials):

(1) Based on the observed data, we perform two-dimensional PAVA to borrow all the information to estimate the dose–toxicity surface. The dose level (j^*, k^*), which belongs to the candidate MTD set as well as being closest to the target toxicity rate, is selected as the starting dose level for the crossing subtrial stage.
(2) Suppose the current dose level is (j, k), and we observe y_{jk} DTLs,

  (i) If $\hat{p}_{jk} \leq \Delta_L$ and no patient has been assigned to dose level (j, $k + 1$), we escalate the dose level to (j, $k + 1$). Otherwise, if dose level (j, $k + 1$) has been administrated before, we consider an admissible escalation set $\mathscr{A}_E = \{(j, k+1), (j+1, k')\}$, where ($j + 1$, k') is the dose level in the higher-dose subtrial with the isotonically estimated toxicity rate greater than that of the current level as well as being closest to ϕ. We then select the dose level from $\mathscr{A}_E$ whose toxicity rate is closer to ϕ.
  (ii) If $\hat{p}_{jk} \geq \Delta_U$, we define an admissible dose de-escalation set $\mathscr{A}_D = \{(j, k-1), (j-1, k')\}$, where ($j - 1$, k') is the dose level in the lowerer-dose subtrial with the isotonically estimated toxicity rate less than that of the current level as well as being closest to ϕ. We then select the dose level from $\mathscr{A}_D$ whose toxicity rate is closer to ϕ.
  (iii) Otherwise, we retain the same dose level (j, k) for the next cohort.

(3) This process continues until the total sample size is exhausted.

If there are multiple optimal dose levels, we randomly choose one with equal probability. Cautions should be taken at the boundaries of the dose searching space. Typically, we eliminate those levels outside of the dose range from the admissible escalation or de-escalation set. In addition, if no dose level lies in the admissible set, we retain the current dose level. By continually updating the information, the PC-BOIN design can switch among these subtrials and thus prevent the trial from being trapped in some suboptimal dose level.

For further safety, we implement extra rules for both RW-BOIN and PC-BOIN to exclude overly toxic dose combinations that satisfy $\Pr(p_{jk} > \phi | y_{jk}) \geq \lambda$, where λ is a prespecified threshold probability. In addition, the trial is terminated early if the dose combination (1, 1) is overly toxic, as noted by $\Pr(p_{11} > \phi | y_{11}) \geq \lambda$. By imposing these safety rules, we can avoid assigning a large number of patients to the overly toxic dose combinations.

Once the trial is completed, we perform the isotonic regression so that the estimated toxicity rates satisfy partial orders when fixing one drug at a certain dose level. Specifically, let $\tilde{p}_{jk}$ denote the bivariate isotonic regression estimator of the observed toxicity rate $\hat{p}_{jk}$ using the PAVA. The MTD $(j^{\dagger}, k^{\dagger})$ is finally selected as the dose level whose toxicity rate $\tilde{p}_{j^{\dagger}k^{\dagger}}$ is closest to the target ϕ:

$$(j^{\dagger}, k^{\dagger}) = \arg\min_{(j,k)\in\mathcal{N}} |\tilde{p}_{jk} - \phi|,$$

where the set $\mathcal{N} = \{(j, k) : n_{jk} > 0\}$ contains all the dose levels that have been administered. When there are ties for $\tilde{p}_{j^{\dagger}k^{\dagger}}$ on the same row or the same column, the highest dose combination satisfying $\tilde{p}_{j^{\dagger}k^{\dagger}} < \phi$, or the lowest dose combination satisfying $\tilde{p}_{j^{\dagger}k^{\dagger}} > \phi$, is selected as the MTD. However, when the ties lie on different rows or columns, e.g., $(j + 1, k - 1)$ and $(j - 1, k + 1)$, we select the one that has the largest value of $\Pr\{p_{j^{\dagger}k^{\dagger}} \in (\phi - \Delta_L, \phi + \Delta_U)|y_{j^{\dagger}k^{\dagger}}\}$, which is approximately equivalent to the dose tested with more patients.

4 Illustrative Example

4.1 *Prostate Cancer Trial*

For patients with metastatic hormone-refractory prostate cancer, mitoxantrone has been demonstrated to be an active agent, while its prostate-specific antigen response rate is low. Genasense is a phosphorothioate antisense oligonucleotide complementary to the bcl-2 mRNA open reading frame, which contributes to inhibiting expression of bcl-2, delaying androgen independence as well as enhancing chemosensitivity in prostate and other cancer models. As a result, a phase I dose-finding study of combined treatment with mitoxantrone and genasense is considered to meet the need for more effective treatment of prostate cancer [24]. The goal of the trial is to evaluate the safety and biological effect of the combination of genasense and mitoxantrone, and to determine the preliminary antitumor activity. Specifically, three doses (4, 8, and 12 mg/m^2) of mitoxantone and five doses (0.6, 1.2, 2.0, 3.1, 5.0 mg/kg) of genasense were investigated in this trial. To identify the MTD combination, the trial selectively chose seven ad hoc combined levels: (mitoxantone, genasense) = (4, 0.6), (4, 1.2), (4, 2.0), (4, 3.1), (8, 3.1), (12, 3.1), (12, 5.0), and applied the modified 3 + 3 dose escalation scheme. However, the chosen dose pairs from the two-dimensional space are arbitrary, so that the MTD might have already been excluded. In addition, using the 3 + 3 design, only one MTD can be identified in the trial, even though multiple MTDs may exist in the drug-combination space. The performance of the 3 + 3 design is known to be inferior to some existing model-based methods, which further demonstrates the need for a more effective as well as simple dose-finding design in drug-combination trials.

4.2 RW-BOIN Design

We applied the RW-BOIN design to the aforementioned prostate cancer trial for illustration. As described previously, the trial examined 3 dose levels of mitoxantrone and 5 dose levels of genasense, which results in a 3×5 drug-combination space. The target toxicity rate is $\phi = 0.3$, the cohort size is set as 3 and 20 cohorts are planned for the trial. Based on formula (1), the optimal interval is $(\Delta_L, \Delta_U) = (0.236, 0.358)$. In addition, we impose a safety rule by setting the threshold $\lambda = 0.95$. The first cohort of patients is treated at the lowest dose level (1, 1). Figure 2 (the top panel) shows the path of the dose assignments for the subsequent cohorts, from which we can see that the BOIN design can search the MTD adaptively and treat most of the patients at the right dose level. Specially, three dose-limiting toxicities (DLTs) are observed for the 8th cohort at dose level (3, 3), thus de-escalation should be made for the next cohort. The admissible de-escalation set is $\{(3, 2), (2, 3)\}$ while dose level (3, 2) has never been administrated before, so the RW-BOIN design selects dose level (3, 2) for the next assignment. In addition, dose-escalation for the 14th cohort is based on comparing the posterior probabilities $\Pr(p_{23} \in (\Delta_L, \Delta_U)|y_{23})$ and $\Pr(p_{32} \in (\Delta_L, \Delta_U)|y_{32})$, and chooses dose level (2, 3) due to its larger value of the posterior probability. At the end of the trial, the estimated toxicity probability matrix after implementing the two-dimensional PAVA is given by

$$\begin{bmatrix} - & 0.67 & 0.67 & - & - \\ - & 0.21 & 0.21 & \mathbf{0.28} & - \\ 0 & 0 & 0 & - & - \end{bmatrix},$$

where "–" represents the dose levels that have not been administered in the trial. Thus, dose level (2, 4) would finally be selected as the MTD.

4.3 PC-BOIN Design

Next, we consider the prostate cancer trial again using PC-BOIN. Since drug A (mitoxantrone) has 3 levels, we first divide the two-dimensional space into three subtrials. We start the trial at the lowest dose level (2, 1) of the intermediate-dose subtrial with 5 cohorts assigned. From Fig. 2 (the bottom panel), dose level (2, 3) is selected as the potential MTD at the end of the intermediate subtrial. The estimated toxicity probability at dose level (2, 3) is 0.17. As a result, we focus on the levels

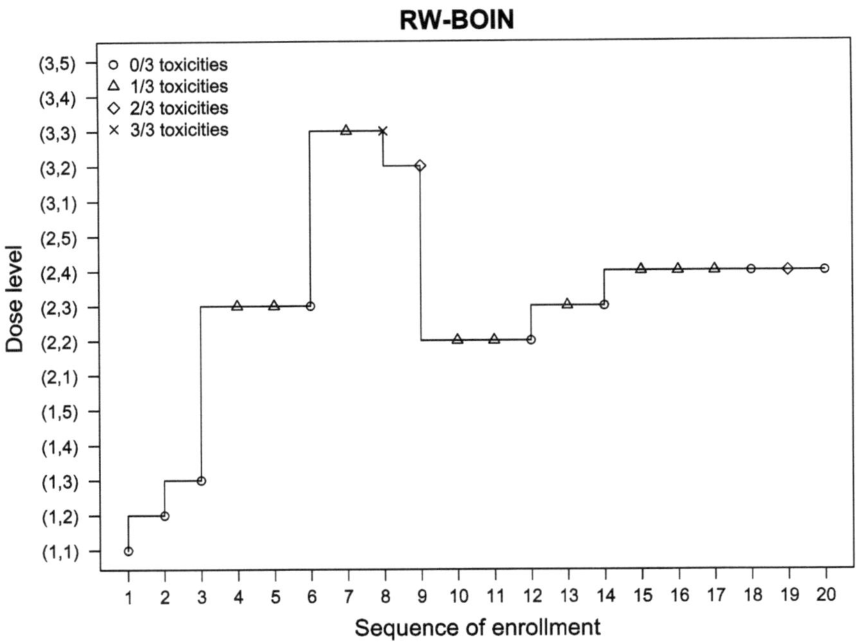
RW-BOIN
0/3 toxicities
1/3 toxicities
2/3 toxicities
3/3 toxicities
Dose level
(3,5)
(3,4)
(3,3)
(3,2)
(3,1)
(2,5)
(2,4)
(2,3)
(2,2)
(2,1)
(1,5)
(1,4)
(1,3)
(1,2)
(1,1)
1 2 3 4 5 6 7 8 9 10 11 12 13 14 15 16 17 18 19 20
Sequence of enrollment

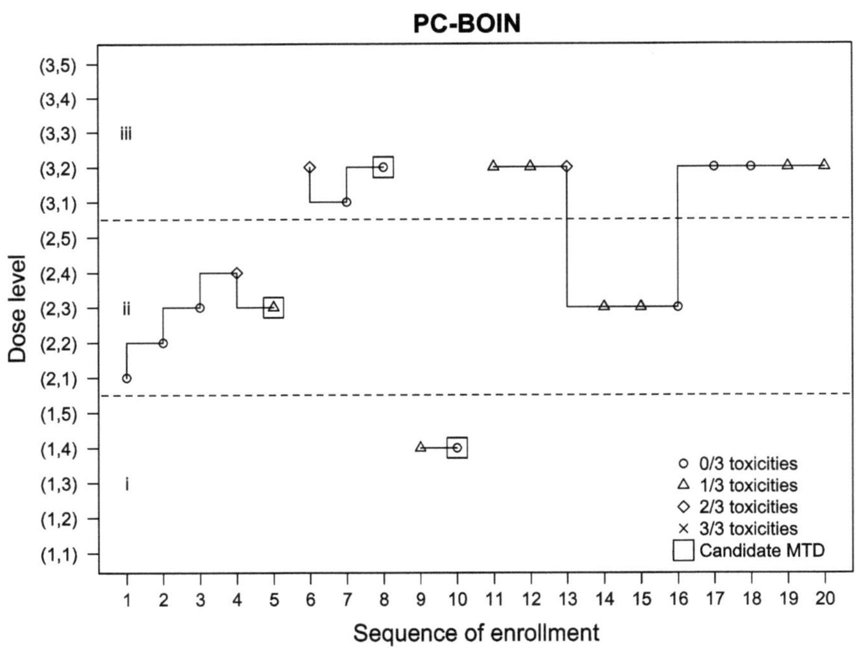
PC-BOIN
iii
ii
i
0/3 toxicities
1/3 toxicities
2/3 toxicities
3/3 toxicities
Candidate MTD
Dose level
(3,5)
(3,4)
(3,3)
(3,2)
(3,1)
(2,5)
(2,4)
(2,3)
(2,2)
(2,1)
(1,5)
(1,4)
(1,3)
(1,2)
(1,1)
1 2 3 4 5 6 7 8 9 10 11 12 13 14 15 16 17 18 19 20
Sequence of enrollment

◂**Fig. 2** Trial examples of RW-BOIN (*top panel*) and PC-BOIN (*bottom panel*). *Circles* represent patients without toxicity, *triangles* one toxicity, *diamonds* two toxicities, and *crosses* three toxicities. The candidate MTDs are inside the large *squares*

from (1, 4) to (1, 5) in the lower-dose subtrial, and (3, 1) to (3, 3) in the higher-dose subtrial. Both the two subtrials are terminated immediately when two cohorts are treated and the outcomes are collected. The parallel subtrial stage finally chooses dose levels (1, 4), (2, 3) and (3, 2) to be the candidate MTD set, among which (3, 2) is determined as the starting dose in the crossing subtrial stage since it has the estimated toxicity probability closest to the target. With the remaining ten cohorts of patients, the crossing subtrial stage continually assesses the subtrial: the trial crosses from the higher-dose subtrial to the intermediate-dose subtrial at the 13th cohort, and then crosses back at the 16th cohort. Based on all the available information at the end of the trial, the estimated toxicity matrix after isotonic regression is

$$\begin{bmatrix} 0 & \mathbf{0.33} & - & - & - \\ 0 & 0 & 0.17 & 0.67 & - \\ - & - & 0 & 0.17 & - \end{bmatrix},$$

which suggests that dose level (3, 2) should be chosen as the MTD.

5 Simulation Study

To assess the performances of the RW-BOIN and PC-BOIN designs for drug-combination trials, we make comparisons of their operating characteristics with two algorithm-based and two model-based methods: the up-and-down design (UD), the up-and-down design using the Student t test statistic (UDT), the partial ordering CRM (POCRM), and the copula-type regression using the Clayton copula function (CLAYTON). We examine the ten scenarios in Table 1, which involve various numbers and locations of the MTDs.

We take the maximum sample size to be 60 with a cohort size of 3, and the target toxicity probability ϕ is set at 0.3. For the RW-BOIN and PC-BOIN designs, we set $\phi_1 = 0.6\phi$ and $\phi_2 = 1.4\phi$, and thus the optimal interval is $(\phi - \Delta_L, \phi + \Delta_U) = (0.236, 0.359)$. In addition, we apply a safety rule for both interval designs: any dose combination satisfying $\Pr(p_{jk} > \phi | y_{jk}) \geq 0.95$ would be eliminated. For the POCRM, we utilize six default orderings, and assign an equal prior probability to them. The skeleton is chosen by the model calibration method of Lee and Cheung [22] using an indifference interval of 0.03 and an initial guess of the MTD position at 13 for each ordering. For the CLAYTON method, we set the dose escalation and de-escalation cutoffs to be 0.7 and 0.45, respectively [23]. We also take an even distribution from 0 to 0.3 for both skeletons: (0.06, 0.12, 0.18, 0.24, 0.3) and (0.1,

Table 1 Ten toxicity scenarios for two-drug combinations, with a target toxicity probability of 30% in boldface

Dose level		Agent 1									
		1	2	3	4	5	1	2	3	4	5
Agent 2		Scenario 1					Scenario 2				
	3	0.15	**0.30**	0.45	0.50	0.60	0.45	0.55	0.60	0.70	0.80
	2	0.10	0.15	**0.30**	0.45	0.55	**0.30**	0.45	0.50	0.60	0.75
	1	0.05	0.10	0.15	**0.30**	0.45	0.15	**0.30**	0.45	0.50	0.60
		Scenario 3					Scenario 4				
	3	0.10	0.15	**0.30**	0.45	0.55	0.50	0.60	0.70	0.80	0.90
	2	0.07	0.10	0.15	**0.30**	0.45	0.45	0.55	0.65	0.75	0.85
	1	0.02	0.07	0.10	0.15	**0.30**	**0.30**	0.45	0.60	0.70	0.80
		Scenario 5					Scenario 6				
	3	0.07	0.09	0.12	0.15	**0.30**	0.15	**0.30**	0.45	0.50	0.60
	2	0.03	0.05	0.10	0.13	0.15	0.09	0.12	0.15	**0.30**	0.45
	1	0.01	0.02	0.08	0.10	0.11	0.05	0.08	0.10	0.13	0.15
		Scenario 7					Scenario 8				
	3	**0.30**	0.50	0.60	0.65	0.75	0.08	0.15	0.45	0.60	0.80
	2	0.15	**0.30**	0.45	0.52	0.60	0.05	0.12	**0.30**	0.55	0.70
	1	0.07	0.10	0.12	0.15	**0.30**	0.02	0.10	0.15	0.50	0.60
		Scenario 9					Scenario 10				
	3	0.15	**0.30**	0.45	0.55	0.65	0.70	0.75	0.80	0.85	0.90
	2	0.02	0.05	0.08	0.12	0.15	0.45	0.50	0.60	0.65	0.70
	1	0.005	0.01	0.02	0.04	0.07	0.05	0.10	0.15	**0.30**	0.45

0.2, 0.3). The two model-based methods require a start-up phase to collect some preliminary data to gain stable estimates of the unknown parameters at the beginning of the trial, and the start-up schemes utilized in the simulation study correspond to those in the original papers [4, 6]. To ensure comparability across different methods, we do not impose the early stopping rule, so that we run the entire trial until exhaustion of the maximum sample size. We simulate 1000 replications for each scenario.

Figure 3 presents the percentages of MTD selections of our two interval designs in conjunction with those of existing algorithm- and model-based methods. Clearly, RW-BOIN and PC-BOIN perform much better than the algorithm-based UD and UDT methods with improvements between 5 and 35%, and on average, the interval designs tend to assign 6 more patients to the true MTDs. Scenarios 1–5 are typical examples of toxicity probabilities of different dose pairs. In scenario 4, the interval designs show the most striking superiority over other algorithm-based designs: The percentages of MTD selections are doubled and the numbers of patients treated at the MTDs are more than tripled. In comparison with the model-based methods, both RW-BOIN and PC-BOIN have comparable performance for these five scenarios. Scenarios 6 and 7 have irregular toxicity surfaces, for which RW-BOIN has the best

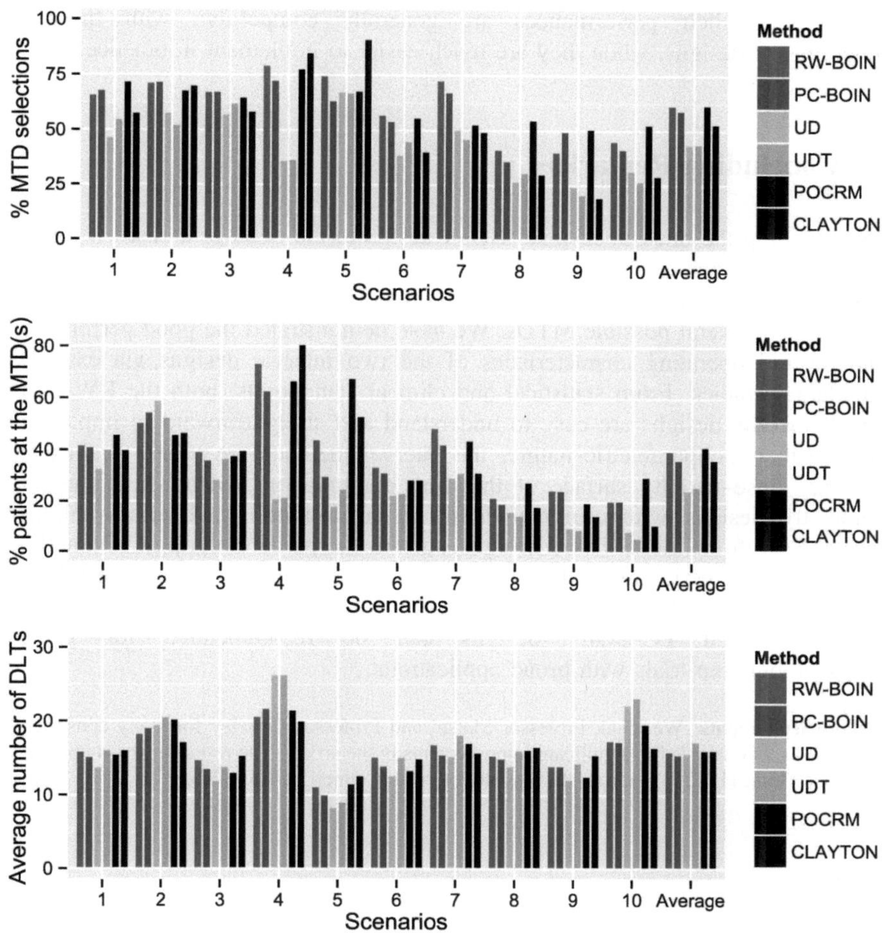

Fig. 3 Comparison of the RW-BOIN and PC-BOIN designs with existing algorithm- and model-based methods in terms of the percentage of MTD selections, the percentage of patients treated at the MTD(s), and the average number of DLTs based on ten scenarios with a target toxicity rate of 0.3

performance. In these cases, no models can fit the joint toxicity surfaces well and thus the model-based designs also lead to inferior performance. Under scenarios 8, 9 and 10 where only one MTD exists, RW-BOIN still ranks the second best among all the two-agent designs. On average, RW-BOIN performs slightly better than PC-BOIN in terms of the MTD selection and patient allocation percentages, and both perform superior to the CLAYTON method. With regard to the average number of DLTs, all six designs are comparable with each other. Overall, the simulation study demonstrates that both the RW-BOIN and PC-BOIN indeed offer substantial gains over the currently existing algorithm-based two-agent designs.

Furthermore, their performances are generally competitive with those of model-based designs, while they are much easier to implement in practice.

6 Concluding Remarks

By extending the one-dimensional BOIN design to the two-agent cases, we introduce two versions of the BOIN designs for drug-combination trials: RW-BOIN searches only one MTD in the entire two-dimensional space, while PC-BOIN can recommend several possible MTDs. We have demonstrated the good performance and desired operating characteristics of the two interval designs via extensive simulation studies. From statistical and clinical standpoints, both the RW-BOIN and PC-BOIN designs are easy to understand and straightforward to implement. Due to their nonparametric nature, the interval methods are robust against any arbitrary dose–toxicity surface of the drug combinations. Meanwhile, the nonparametric designs, without implementing a start-up phase, have comparable performance with the model-based designs, such as the partial ordering CRM and the copula-type regression method. Moreover, the two-dimensional interval designs can be modified for trials with more than two drugs in combination. In conclusion, the RW-BOIN and PC-BOIN designs can be recommended for general drug-combination trials with broad applications.

Acknowledgements We thank Professor Matsui and Professor Crowley for many constructive suggestions that have led to significant improvements in the article. The research was supported in part by a Grant (17125814) from the Research Grants Council of Hong Kong.

References

1. Kramar A, Lebecq A, Candalh E. Continual reassessment methods in phase I trials of the combination of two drugs in oncology. Stat Med. 1999;18:1849–64.
2. Yuan Y, Yin G. Sequential continual reassessment method for two-dimensional dose finding. Stat Med. 2008;27:5664–78.
3. Thall PF, Millikan RE, Müller P, et al. Dose-finding with two agents in phase I oncology trials. Biometrics. 2003;59:487–96.
4. Yin G, Yuan Y. Bayesian dose finding in oncology for drug combinations by copula regression. J R Stat Soc Ser C Appl Stat. 2009;61:211–24.
5. Yin G, Yuan Y. A latent contingency table approach to dose finding for combinations of two agents. Biometrics. 2009;65:866–75.
6. Wages NA, Conaway MR, O'Quigley J. Dose-finding design for multi-drug combinations. Clin Trials. 2011;8:380–9.
7. Shi Y, Yin G. Escalation with overdose control for phase I drug-combination trials. Stat Med. 2013;32:4400–12.
8. Harrington JA, Wheeler GM, Sweeting MJ, et al. Adaptive designs for dual-agent phase I dose-escalation studies. Nat Rev Clin Oncol. 2013;10:277–88.

9. Hirakawa A, Hamada C, Matsui S. A dose-finding approach based on shrunken predictive probability for combinations of two agents in phase I trials. Stat Med. 2013;32:4515–25.
10. O'Quigley J, Pepe M, Fisher L. Continual reassessment method: a practical design for phase 1 clinical trials in cancer. Biometrics. 1990;46:33–48.
11. Conaway MR, Dunbar S, Peddada SD. Designs for single- or multiple-agent phase I trials. Biometrics. 2004;60:661–9.
12. Ivanova A, Wang K. A nonparametric approach to the design and analysis of two-dimensional dose-finding trials. Stat Med. 2004;23:1861–70.
13. Huang X, Biswas S, Oki Y, et al. A parallel phase I/II clinical trial design for combination therapies. Biometrics. 2007;63:429–36.
14. Fan SK, Venook AP, Lu Y. Design issues in dose-finding phase I trials for combinations of two agents. J Biopharm Stat. 2009;19:509–23.
15. Lee BL, Fan SK. A two-dimensional search algorithm for dose-finding trials of two agents. J Biopharm Stat. 2012;22:802–18.
16. Lin R, Yin G. Bayesian optimal interval design for dose finding in drug-combination trials. Stat Methods Med Res. 2017; doi: 10.1177/0962280215594494.
17. Liu S, Yuan Y. Bayesian optimal interval designs for phase I clinical trials. J R Stat Soc Ser C Appl Stat. 2015;64:507–23.
18. Yuan Z, Chappell R. Isotonic designs for phase I cancer clinical trials with multiple risk groups. Clin Trials. 2004;1:499–508.
19. Gezmu M, Flournoy N. Group up-and-down designs for dose-finding. J Stat Plan Infer. 2006;136:1749–64.
20. Ivanova A, Flournoy N, Chung Y. Cumulative cohort design for dose finding. J Stat Plan Infer. 2007;137:2316–7.
21. Oron A, Azriel D, Hoff P. Dose-finding designs: the role of convergence properties. Int J Biostat. 2011. 7. Article 39.
22. Lee S, Cheung Y. Model calibration in the continual reassessment method. Clin Trials. 2009;6:227–38.
23. Yin G, Lin R. Comments on 'Competing designs for drug combination phase I dose-finding clinical trials' by M-K. Riviere, F. Dubois, S. Zohar. Stat Med. 2015;34:13–7.
24. Chi KN, Gleave ME, Klasa R, Murray N, Bryce C, de Menezes DEL, D'Aloisio S, Tolcher AW. A phase I dose-finding study of combined treatment with an antisense bcl-2 oligonucleotide (genasense) and mitoxantrone in patients with metastatic hormone-refractory prostate cancer. Clin Cancer Res. 2001;7:3920–7.

A Comparative Study of Model-Based Dose-Finding Methods for Two-Agent Combination Trials

Akihiro Hirakawa and Hiroyuki Sato

Abstract Little is known about the relative relationships of the operating characteristics for rival model-based dose-finding methods for two-agent combination phase I trials. In this chapter, we focus on the model-based dose-finding methods that have been recently developed. We compare the recommendation rates for true maximum tolerated dose combinations (MTDCs) and over dose combinations (ODCs) among these methods under 16 scenarios with 3×3, 4×4, 2×4, and 3×5 dose combination matrices through comprehensive simulation studies. We found that the operating characteristics of the dose-finding methods varied depending on (1) whether the dose combination matrix is square or not, (2) whether the true MTDCs exist within the same group consisting of the diagonals of the dose combination matrix, and (3) the number of true MTDCs. We also discuss the details of the operating characteristics and the advantages and disadvantages of the dose-finding methods compared.

Keywords Combination of two agents · Dose-finding design · Phase I trial · Oncology

1 Introduction

Phase I trials in oncology are conducted to identify the maximum tolerated dose (MTD), which is defined as the highest dose that can be administered to a population of subjects with acceptable toxicity. A model-based dose-finding approach is

A. Hirakawa (✉)
Department of Biostatistics and Bioinformatics, Graduate School of Medicine, The University of Tokyo, 7-3-1 Hongo, Bunkyo-Ku, Tokyo 113-8654, Japan
e-mail: hirakawa@m.u-tokoyo.ac.jp

H. Sato
Biostatistics Group, Office of New Drug V, Pharmaceuticals and Medical Devices Agency, 3-3-2 Kasumigaseki, Chiyoda-ku, Tokyo 100-0013, Japan
e-mail: sato-hiroyuki@pmda.go.jp

S. Matsui and J. Crowley (eds.), *Frontiers of Biostatistical Methods and Applications in Clinical Oncology*, DOI 10.1007/978-981-10-0126-0_4

efficient to estimate the MTD in phase I trials. The continual reassessment method (CRM) [2, 10] has provided a prototype for such an approach in single-agent phase I trials.

In two-agent combination phase I trials we need to capture the dose-toxicity relationship for combinations of two agents and to identify maximum tolerated dose combinations (MTDCs) of two agents. To accommodate these requirements many authors have developed dose-finding methods. Thall et al. [13] proposed a six-parameter model for the toxicity probabilities of the dose combinations and a toxicity equivalence contour for two-agent combinations. Conaway et al. [3] determined the simple and partial orderings of the toxicity probabilities by defining the nodal and non-nodal parameters. Wang and Ivanova [14] proposed a logistic-type regression for dose combinations that used the doses of the two agents as the covariates. Yin and Yuan developed a Bayesian adaptive design based on latent 2×2 tables [18] and a copula-type model [19] for two agents. Braun and Wang [1] proposed a hierarchical Bayesian model for the probability of toxicity for combinations of two agents. Wages et al. developed both Bayesian [15] and likelihood-based [16] designs based on the notion that there exist pairs of dose combinations for which the ordering of the probabilities of toxicity cannot be known a priori, resulting in a partial ordering. Hirakawa et al. [6] proposed a dose-finding method based on the shrunken predictive probability of toxicity for combinations of two agents. Recently, Riviere et al. [12] compared two algorithm-based and four model-based dose-finding methods using three evaluation indices under 10 scenarios of a 3×5 dose combination matrix. Among their conclusions was that the model-based methods performed better than algorithm-based ones such as the 3 + 3 method.

In this chapter, we compare the operating characteristics of the representative model-based dose-finding methods recently developed for two-agent combination phase I trials through the simulation studies under various toxicity scenarios. The existing methods can be roughly categorized into two groups: (1) those using a flexible (Bayesian) model with/without an interaction term of the two agents; and (2) those that extend CRM, taking into consideration the partial ordering of toxicity probabilities for dose combinations. As to the former methods, we focus on methods based on a copula-type model [19], termed the YYC methods. We also evaluate the method using a hierarchical Bayesian model [1], termed the BW method. Furthermore, we add the likelihood-based dose-finding method using a shrinkage logistic model [6], termed the HHM method. As to the latter method, we choose likelihood-based CRM with partial ordering (POCRM) [16], termed the WCO method. In the simulation studies, we compare the recommendation rates for true MTDCs and overdose combinations (ODCs) among these methods under the 16 scenarios with 3×3, 4×4, 2×4, and 3×5 dose combination matrices with different position and number of true MTDCs. Average number of patients allocated to true MTDCs, overall percentage of observed toxicities, average number of patients allocated to at a dose combination above the true MTDCs were also evaluated.

Table 1 Methodological characteristics of the 4 dose-finding methods we compared

Method	YYC	BW	WCO	HHM
Estimation theorem	Bayesian	Bayesian	Likelihood	Likelihood
Dose-toxicity model	Copula	Hierarchical	Power	Shrinkage logistic
Prior toxicity probability specification	Yes	Yes	Yes	No
Inclusion of interactive effect in the model	Yes	No	No	Yes
Cohort size used in the original paper	3	1	1	3
Restriction on skipping on dose levels	One dose level of change only and not allowing a simultaneous escalation or de-escalation of both agents	One dose level of change only but allowing a simultaneous escalation or de-escalation of both agents	No skipping restriction	Same as the YYC method

2 Dose-Finding Methods Compared

In this section we overview the four dose-finding methods for two-agent combination trials we compared. Their methodological characteristics are summarized in Table 1. The YYC and BW methods have been developed based on Bayesian inference, while the HHM and WCO methods are based on likelihood inference. The YYC and HHM methods model the interactive effect of two agents on the toxicity probability, but the BW method does not. The WCO method is based on the CRM and uses a class of under-parameterized working models based on a set of possible orderings for the true toxicity probabilities. In terms of the restriction on skipping dose levels, the BW method allows the simultaneous escalation or de-escalation of both agents, while the YYC and HHM methods do not. On the other hand, the WCO method allows a flexible movement of dose levels throughout the trial, and does not restrict movement to “neighbors” in the two-agent combination matrix.

In this section we introduce both the statistical model for capturing the dose-toxicity relationship and the dose-finding algorithm for exploring the MTDCs, because almost all of the dose-finding methods for two-agent combination trials have been often developed by improving or devising these components of the method. The other detailed design characteristics are not shown in this chapter. We considered a two-agent combination trial using agents A_j ($j = 1, \ldots, J$) and B_k ($k = 1, \ldots, K$) respectively, throughout. We denote the targeting toxicity probability specified by physicians by ϕ. The other symbols are independently defined by the dose-finding methods we compared.

2.1 Bayesian Approach Based on Copula-Type Model (YYC)

Yin and Yuan [19] introduced Bayesian dose-finding approaches using copula-type models. Let p_j and q_k be the pre-specified toxicity probability corresponding to A_j and B_k, respectively, and subsequently p_j^{α} and q_k^{β} be the modeled probabilities of toxicity for agent A and agent B, respectively, where $\alpha > 0$ and $\beta > 0$ are unknown parameters. Yin and Yuan [19] proposed to use a copula-type regression model in the form of

$$\pi_{jk} = 1 - \left\{ \left(1 - p_j^{\alpha}\right)^{-\gamma} + \left(1 - q_k^{\beta}\right)^{-\gamma} - 1 \right\}^{-1/\gamma},$$

where $\gamma > 0$ characterizes the interaction of two agents (i.e., the YYC method). Several authors have recently provided a more in-depth discussion on multiple binary regression models for dose-finding in combinations [4, 5, 20].

Using the data obtained at the time, the posterior distribution is obtained by

$$f(\alpha, \beta, \gamma|\text{Data}) \propto L(\alpha, \beta, \gamma|\text{Data})p(\alpha)p(\beta)p(\gamma),$$

where $L(\alpha, \beta, \gamma|\text{Data})$ is the likelihood function of the model and $p(\alpha)$, $p(\beta)$, and $p(\gamma)$ are prior distributions, respectively.

Let c_e and c_d be the fixed probability cut-offs for dose escalation and de-escalation, respectively. Patients are treated in cohorts of three. Dose escalation or de-escalation are restricted to one dose level of change only, while not allowing a translation along the diagonal direction (corresponding to simultaneous escalation or de-escalation of both agents). After adopting a start-up rule for stabilizing parameter estimation (not shown in this chapter), the dose-finding algorithm functions as follows: (1) If, at the current dose combination (A_j, B_k), $\Pr(\pi_{jk} < \phi) > c_e$, the dose is escalated to an adjacent dose combination with probability of toxicity higher than the current value and closest to ϕ. If the current dose combination is (A_J, B_K), the doses remain at the same levels. (2) If, at the current dose combination (A_j, B_k), $\Pr(\pi_{jk} > \phi) > c_d$, the dose is de-escalated to an adjacent dose combination with the probability of toxicity lower than the current value and closest to ϕ. If the current dose combination is (A_1, B_1), the trial is terminated. (3) Otherwise, the next cohort of patients continues to be treated at the current dose combination (doses staying at the same levels). (4) Once the maximum sample size $N_{\max}$ has been achieved, the dose combination that has the probability of toxicity that is closest to ϕ is selected as the MTDC.

2.2 A Hierarchical Bayesian Design (BW)

Braun and Wang [1] developed a novel hierarchical Bayesian design for two-agent combination phase I trials. Let a_j and b_k be the dose levels corresponding to A_j and B_k respectively, and the values of them will not be the actual clinical values of the doses, but will be "effective" dose values that will lend stability to their dose-toxicity model. It is assumed that each π_{jk} has a beta distribution with parameters α_{jk} and β_{jk}. Braun and Wang [1] proposed to model α_{jk} and β_{jk} using the parametric functions of a_j and b_k,

$$\log\{\alpha_{jk}(\boldsymbol{\theta})\} = \theta_0 + \theta_1 a_j + \theta_2 b_k \quad \text{and} \quad \log\{\beta_{jk}(\boldsymbol{\lambda})\} = \lambda_0 - \lambda_1 a_j - \lambda_2 b_k,$$

respectively, where $\boldsymbol{\theta} = \{\theta_0, \theta_1, \theta_2\}$ has a multivariate normal distribution with mean $\boldsymbol{\mu} = \{\mu_0, \mu_1, \mu_2\}$, $\boldsymbol{\lambda} = \{\lambda_0, \lambda_1, \lambda_2\}$ has a multivariate normal distribution with mean $\boldsymbol{\omega} = \{\omega_0, \omega_1, \omega_2\}$, and both $\boldsymbol{\theta}$ and $\boldsymbol{\lambda}$ have variance $\sigma^2 I_3$, in which I_3 is 3×3 identity matrix. The samples from the posterior distribution for $(\boldsymbol{\theta}, \boldsymbol{\lambda})$ are easily obtained using Markov chain Monte Carlo (MCMC) methods. These samples lead to posterior distributions for each element of $\boldsymbol{\theta}$ and $\boldsymbol{\lambda}$, which, in turn, lead to a posterior distribution for each π_{jk}. The corresponding posterior means $\bar{\pi}_{jk}$ are calculated.

The BW method necessitates careful elicitation of priors and effective dose values. Development of priors begins with the specification of p_{j1} and q_{1k}, which are a priori values for the $\mathrm{E}(\pi_{j1})$ and $\mathrm{E}(\pi_{1k})$. Braun and Wang [1] set the lowest dose of each agent to zero, that is, $a_1 = b_1 = 0$. Consequently, $\log(\alpha_{11}) = \theta_0$ and $\log(\beta_{11}) = \lambda_0$, so that θ_0 and λ_0 describe the expected number of DLTs for combination (A_1, B_1) and the remaining parameters in $\boldsymbol{\theta}$ and $\boldsymbol{\lambda}$ will describe how the expected DLTs for other combinations relate to (A_1, B_1). Braun and Wang [1] also used the fact that

$$\frac{Kp_{11}}{K(1-p_{11})} = \frac{\alpha_{11}}{\beta_{11}} = \frac{\exp\{\theta_0\}}{\exp\{\lambda_0\}} = \frac{\exp\{\mu_0\}}{\exp\{\omega_0\}}.$$

Then the prior values for μ_0 and ω_0 are obtained via $\mu_0 = \log(Kp_{11})$ and $\omega_0 = \log\{K(1-p_{11})\}$, where $K = 1000$ was chosen as a scaling factor to keep both hyperparameters sufficiently above 0. Further, Braun and Wang [1] select $\mu_1 = \mu_2 = \omega_1 = \omega_2 = 2\sqrt{\sigma^2}$ so that 97.5% of the prior distributions for θ_1, θ_2, λ_1, and λ_2 will lie above 0, depending upon the value of σ^2. The authors point out that a value in the interval [5, 10] is often sufficient in their settings for adequate operating characteristics, but each trial setting will require fine tuning of σ^2. Braun and Wang

[1] further define elicited odds ratios that can be approximated by $\tilde{\xi}_{j\cdot} = \exp\{(\mu_1 + \omega_1)a_j\}$ and $\tilde{\xi}_{\cdot k} = \exp\{(\mu_2 + \omega_2)b_k\}$ in which effective dose values are obtained by solving for a_j and b_k. All doses are rescaled to be proportional to log-odds ratios relative to the combination (A_1, B_1). The development of priors and effective dose values in BW are somewhat complex, and it is recommended to read the original paper of BW for further details.

The dose-finding algorithm is similar to that of the YYC method. Specifically, if a stopping rule for safety (not shown in this chapter) is not met, we extract the set of dose combinations, that is $S = \{(j,k)|j_{i-1} - 1 \le j \le j_{i-1} + 1, k_{i-1} - 1 \le k \le k_{i-1} + 1\}$, that contains combinations that are within one dose level of the corresponding doses in the combination assigned to the most recently enrolled patient (1, 2, …, (i − 1)), and we subsequently allocate the dose combination (A_{j^*}, B_{k^*}) in S as the one with smallest $|\bar{\pi}_{jk} - \phi|$ to the next patient i. We repeat these steps until the maximum sample size $N_{\max}$ is reached. Notably, the BW method allows for simultaneous dose escalations of both agents, and the cohort size of patients is 1.

2.3 *Partial Ordering Continual Reassessment Method (WCO)*

The CRM for partial orders is based on utilizing a class of working models that corresponds to possible orderings of the toxicity probabilities for the combinations. Specifically, suppose there are M possible orderings being considered which are indexed by m. For a particular ordering, Wages et al. [16] model the true probability of toxicity, π_{jk}, at combination (A_j, B_k) via a power model

$$\pi_{jk} \approx [p_{jk}(m)]^{\beta_m}; \quad m = 1, \ldots, M,$$

where the $p_{jk}(m)$ represent the skeleton of the model under ordering m. We let the plausibility of each ordering under consideration be described by a set of prior probabilities $\tau(m) = \{\tau(1), \ldots, \tau(M)\}$, where $\tau(m) \ge 0$ and $\sum_m \tau(m) = 1$. Using the accumulated data, Ω_n, from n patients, the maximum likelihood estimate (MLE) $\hat{\beta}_m$ of the parameter β_m can be computed for each of the M orderings, along with the value of the log-likelihood $\mathcal{L}_m(\hat{\beta}_m|\Omega_n)$ at $\hat{\beta}_m$. Wages et al. [15, 16] proposed an escalation method that first chooses the ordering with the largest maximized updated probability

$$\omega(m) = \frac{\exp\{\mathcal{L}_m(\hat{\beta}_m|\Omega_n)\}\tau(m)}{\sum_{m=1}^{M} \exp\{\mathcal{L}_m(\hat{\beta}_m|\Omega_n)\}\tau(m)}$$

before each patient inclusion. If we denote this ordering by m^*, the authors use the estimate $\hat{\beta}_{m^*}$ to estimate the toxicity probabilities for each combination under ordering m^*, so that $\hat{\pi}_{jk} \approx [p_{jk}(m^*)]^{\hat{\beta}_{m^*}}$.

The next entered patient is then allocated to the dose combination with estimated toxicity probability closest to the target toxicity rate ϕ. Within the framework of sequential likelihood estimation, an initial escalation scheme is needed, since the likelihood fails to have a solution on the interior of the parameter space unless some heterogeneity (i.e. at least one toxic and one non-toxic outcome) has been observed. The trial begins at the lowest combination (A_1, B_1) and, in the absence of toxicity, escalates to either (A_1, B_2) or (A_2, B_1). As long as no toxicities occur, the doses of each agent are escalated one at a time. This procedure continues until a toxicity is observed, at which time the second stage, based on the modeling described above, begins.

2.4 Approach Using a Shrinkage Logistic Model (HHM)

Hirakawa et al. [6] developed the dose-finding method based on a shrinkage logistic model. Hirakawa et al. [6] first model the joint toxicity probability π_i for patient i using an ordinary logistic regression model with a fixed intercept β_0, as follows:

$$\pi_i = \frac{\exp(\beta_0 + \beta_1 x_{i1} + \beta_2 x_{i2} + \beta_3 x_{i3})}{1 + \exp(\beta_0 + \beta_1 x_{i1} + \beta_2 x_{i2} + \beta_3 x_{i3})},$$

where x_{i1} and x_{i2} are the actual (or standardized) dose levels of agents A and B, respectively, and x_{i3} represents a variable of their interaction such that $x_{i3} = x_{i1} \times x_{i2}$ for patient i. Using MLEs for the parameters $\hat{\beta}_l$ (l = 1, 2, 3), Hirakawa et al. [6] proposed the shrunken predictive probability (SPP):

$$\tilde{\pi}_i = \frac{\exp\left(\beta_0 + (1-\delta_1)\hat{\beta}_1 x_{i1} + (1-\delta_2)\hat{\beta}_2 x_{i2} + (1-\delta_3)\hat{\beta}_3 x_{i3}\right)}{1 + \exp\left(\beta_0 + (1-\delta_1)\hat{\beta}_1 x_{i1} + (1-\delta_2)\hat{\beta}_2 x_{i2} + (1-\delta_3)\hat{\beta}_3 x_{i3}\right)},$$

where the shrinkage multiplier $1 - \delta_l$ (l = 1, 2, 3) is a number between 0 and 1. Hirakawa et al. [6] also developed an estimation method of the shrinkage multipliers.

Hirakawa et al. [6] invoke a rule-based dose allocation algorithm with the cohort size of 3 until the MLE for each parameter is obtained, although we do not show this rule in detail in this chapter. After obtaining the MLEs for the regression parameters, we calculate the SPP of toxicity for the current dose combination d_c. We adopt the same restriction on skipping dose levels proposed by the YYC method.

Let c_1 and c_2 be the allowable bands from the target toxicity limit ϕ as MTDCs. Hirakawa et al. [6] proposed the following dose-finding algorithm: if, at the current dose combination d_c, $\phi - c_1 \leq \tilde{\pi}(d_c) \leq \phi + c_2$, the next cohort of patients continues to be allocated to the current dose combination; otherwise, the next cohort of patients is allocated to the dose combination with the SPP closest to ϕ among the adjacent or current dose combinations; once the maximum sample size $N_{\max}$ is reached, the dose combination that should be assigned to the next cohort is selected as the MTDC. In addition, if we encounter the situation where $d_c = d_1$ and $\tilde{\pi}(d_c) > \phi + c_2$, we terminate the trial for safety.

3 Simulation Studies

3.1 Simulation Setting

We compare the operating characteristics among the 4 methods by simulating 16 scenarios with 3 × 3, 4 × 4, 2 × 4, and 3 × 5 dose combination matrices with different positions and number of true MTDCs, as shown in Table 2. The target toxicity probability that is clinically allowed, ϕ, is set to 0.3. The maximum sample size $N_{\max}$ is set to 30 throughout. Each simulation consisted of 1000 trials.

We used the C++ source program released at http://odin.mdacc.tmc.edu/~yyuan/index_code.html to perform the YYC method. The values of p_j are set to (0.15, 0.3) for J = 2, (0.1, 0.2, 0.3) for J = 3, (0.075, 0.15, 0.225, 0.3) for J = 4, and (0.06, 0.12, 0.18, 0.24, 0.3) for J = 5, respectively. The same setting are made for q_k. The fixed probability cut-offs for dose escalation and de-escalation are c_e = 0.80 and c_d = 0.45, respectively. As prior distribution for each parameter, we assumed gamma(2, 2) as the prior distribution for α and β and gamma(0.1, 0.1) as the prior distribution for γ.

We used the R code released at http://www-personal.umich.edu/~tombraun/BraunWang/ to perform the BW method. The variance parameter σ^2 is set to 3 in order to stabilize the implementation of the R package **rjags**. The prior probability of each dose combination is shown in Table 3.

For the WCO method, we utilized a subset of six possible dose-toxicity orderings, formulated according to the rows, columns, and diagonals of the drug combination matrix, as suggested by Wages and Conaway [17]. We placed a uniform prior $\tau(m) = 1/6$ on the orderings. The skeleton values, $p_{jk}(m)$, were generated according to the algorithm of Lee and Cheung [9] using the **getprior** function in **R** package **dfcrm**. Specifically, for 3 × 3 combinations, we used **getprior(0.05, 0.3, 4, 9)**; for 4 × 4 combinations, we used **getprior(0.05, 0.3, 7, 16)**; for 2 × 4 combinations, we used **getprior(0.05, 0.3, 4, 8)**; and for 3 × 5 combinations, we used **getprior(0.05, 0.3, 7, 15)**. The location of these skeleton values was adjusted to correspond to each of the six orderings using the **getwm** function in **R** package **pocrm**. All simulation results were carried out using the functions of **pocrm** with a cohort size of 1 in both stages.

Table 2 Sixteen scenarios for a two-agent combination trial (MTDCs are in boldface)

	A										
		1	2	3	4	5	1	2	3	4	5
B	Scenario 1						Scenario 2				
	3	**0.30**	0.40	0.50			0.50	0.70	0.80		
	2	0.20	**0.30**	0.40			**0.30**	0.60	0.70		
	1	0.10	0.20	**0.30**			0.05	**0.30**	0.50		
	Scenario 3						Scenario 4				
	3	0.40	0.60	0.80			0.15	0.40	0.60		
	2	**0.30**	0.50	0.70			0.05	**0.30**	0.40		
	1	0.05	0.10	0.40			0.01	0.05	0.15		
	Scenario 5						Scenario 6				
	4	**0.30**	0.50	0.65	0.70		**0.30**	0.50	0.60	0.70	
	3	0.10	**0.30**	0.60	0.65		0.15	0.40	0.50	0.60	
	2	0.05	0.10	**0.30**	0.50		0.10	**0.30**	0.40	0.50	
	1	0.01	0.05	0.10	**0.30**		0.05	0.10	0.15	**0.30**	
	Scenario 7						Scenario 8				
	4	0.40	0.45	0.60	0.85		0.15	0.60	0.75	0.80	
	3	0.15	**0.30**	0.55	0.60		0.10	0.45	0.70	0.75	
	2	0.08	0.15	0.23	**0.30**		0.04	**0.30**	0.45	0.60	
	1	0.01	0.02	0.03	0.04		0.02	0.10	0.15	0.40	
	Scenario 9						Scenario 10				
	2	0.10	0.20	**0.30**	0.40		**0.30**	0.40	0.50	0.60	
	1	0.05	0.10	0.20	**0.30**		0.01	0.10	0.20	**0.30**	
	Scenario 11						Scenario 12				
	2	0.15	**0.28**	**0.32**	**0.34**		0.50	0.60	0.70	0.80	
	1	0.10	0.15	**0.28**	**0.32**		0.10	0.20	**0.30**	0.40	
	Scenario 13						Scenario 14				
	3	0.25	**0.30**	0.40	0.50	0.70	0.20	0.45	0.50	0.60	0.75
	2	0.10	0.25	**0.30**	0.40	0.50	0.05	**0.30**	0.45	0.55	0.60
	1	0.05	0.10	0.25	**0.30**	0.40	0.01	0.05	0.15	**0.30**	0.50
	Scenario 15						Scenario 16				
	3	**0.30**	0.35	0.40	0.45	0.60	0.10	0.20	0.40	0.55	0.65
	2	0.05	0.20	**0.30**	0.40	0.45	0.05	0.10	**0.30**	0.50	0.60
	1	0.01	0.05	0.10	0.20	**0.30**	0.01	0.05	0.10	0.20	0.40

We performed the HHM method using the SAS/IML in SAS 9.3 (SAS Institute Inc., NC). The fixed intercept β_0 is set to be -3 throughout. c_1 and c_2 were commonly set to 0.05. We set $x_1 = \{1, 2, 3\}$ and $x_2 = \{1, 2, 3\}$ for 3×3 dose combinations, $x_1 = \{1, 2, 3, 4\}$ and $x_2 = \{1, 2, 3, 4\}$ for 4×4 dose combinations, $x_1 = \{1, 2\}$ and $x_2 = \{1, 2, 3, 4\}$ for 2×4 dose combinations, and $x_1 = \{1, 2, 3\}$ and $x_2 = \{1, 2, 3, 4, 5\}$ for 3×5 dose combinations, respectively.

Table 3 Prior toxicity probabilities we used in the simulation studies in the BW method

		A									
		1	2	3	4	5	1	2	3	4	5
		3 × 3					4 × 4				
B	4						0.30	0.375	0.45	0.525	
	3	0.30	0.40	0.50			0.225	0.30	0.375	0.45	
	2	0.20	0.30	0.40			0.15	0.225	0.30	0.375	
	1	0.10	0.20	0.30			0.075	0.15	0.225	0.30	
		2 × 4					3 × 5				
	3						0.30	0.35	0.40	0.45	0.50
	2	0.30	0.35	0.40	0.45		0.20	0.25	0.30	0.35	0.40
	1	0.15	0.20	0.25	0.30		0.10	0.15	0.20	0.25	0.30

3.2 Simulation Results

Table 4 shows the operating characteristics of the 4 methods under 16 scenarios. For scenarios 1 and 2 of 3 × 3 dose combination matrix where the underlying true MTDCs exist along with the diagonals of the dose-combination matrix, the WCO method showed higher recommendation rates for true MTDCs than the YYC, BW, and HHM methods by approximately 5–10%, while those were comparable among the YYC, BW, and HHM methods. The recommendation rates for true MTDCs were similar among all the methods under scenario 3. The recommendation rates of the BW and HHM methods were higher than the other 2 methods under scenario 4. The WCO method outperformed the other methods in scenarios 5 and 7, while the HHM method outperformed the other three methods in scenario 6. The recommendation rates for the ODCs of the HHM method were lower than or equal to the other methods under scenarios 1–8.

The recommendation rates for true MTDCs of the HHM and WCO methods in scenario 9, of the YYC, HHM, and WCO methods in scenario 10, of the BW and WCO methods in scenario 11, and of the WCO method in scenario 12 were higher than the remaining methods, respectively. The difference of the recommendation rates between the methods was approximately 10–15%. The WCO method performed as well or better than the other three methods under scenarios 9–12, and a similar tendency was observed under scenarios 13–16. The HHM method was competitive of the WCO method in scenarios 14 and 15. In terms of recommending the ODCs, the HHM method was lowest among the 4 methods under scenarios 9, 10, 12 and 13–16 scenarios.

Across the 16 scenarios, the YYC, BW, WCO, and HHM methods demonstrated average recommendations rates of 34, 40, 46, and 42% for true MTDCs, respectively. The YYC, BW, WCO, and HHM methods demonstrated average recommendations rates of 41, 33, 32, and 25% for ODCs, respectively. As to the other performance indices, the average number of patients allocated to true MTDCs of the YYC, BW, WCO, and HHM methods were 6, 9, 10, and 8, respectively.

Table 4 Summary of the operating characteristics of the 4 methods in all scenarios

Method	Scenarios																
	1	2	3	4	5	6	7	8	9	10	11	12	13	14	15	16	Average
Recommendation rates for true MTD dose combinations (%)																	
YYC	44	70	26	6	59	44	33	5	39	49	72	2	30	18	37	2	34
BW	50	66	24	36	58	37	28	24	39	38	83	29	38	33	33	20	40
WCO	56	73	32	31	77	40	37	23	49	48	86	36	39	44	41	26	46
HHM	45	66	28	38	64	49	31	29	47	46	70	22	30	44	42	20	42
Recommendation rates for overdose combinations (%)																	
YYC	23	23	54	70	27	32	42	55	26	40	n/a	47	25	41	49	54	41
BW	27	24	48	37	17	39	25	41	26	39	n/a	32	28	37	43	35	33
WCO	24	24	55	44	13	36	29	46	20	29	n/a	36	19	32	34	34	32
HHM	14	23	48	36	12	22	22	32	12	19	n/a	29	15	31	24	32	25
Average number of patients allocated to true MTD combinations																	
YYC	8	14	6	1	12	9	5	1	6	10	10	1	6	4	8	0	6
BW	11	14	5	9	12	8	6	6	10	8	23	5	8	8	6	4	9
WCO	14	16	7	7	16	10	7	5	11	12	21	8	8	10	9	5	10
HHM	11	14	6	6	9	8	3	5	8	9	15	5	5	7	7	3	8
Overall percentage of observed toxicities (%)																	
YYC	22	27	25	22	24	24	24	25	18	24	20	26	22	26	24	22	23
BW	30	34	32	29	31	31	29	31	27	31	27	33	31	32	30	30	30
WCO	28	35	33	27	26	27	23	28	25	29	26	32	26	28	26	24	28
HHM	22	33	28	19	15	18	15	19	17	24	21	29	18	20	17	13	20
Average number of patients allocated to at a dose combination above the true MTDCs																	
YYC	3	6	11	11	6	5	9	10	3	9	n/a	9	4	10	9	9	8
BW	9	10	15	11	8	12	9	12	8	12	n/a	12	10	13	14	12	11
WCO	7	9	16	11	4	9	6	12	5	9	n/a	11	6	9	9	8	9
HHM	3	11	14	7	0	3	3	6	2	6	n/a	9	1	5	3	2	5

The overall percentage of observed toxicities of the YYC, BW, WCO, and HHM methods averaged of 23, 30, 28, and 20%, respectively. The average number of patients allocated to at a dose combination above the true MTDCs of the YYC, BW, WCO, and HHM methods were 8, 11, 9, and 5, respectively.

3.3 Operating Characteristics for Each Representative Setting

According to the results of simulation studies, we found that the operating characteristics of the dose-finding methods varied depending on (1) whether the dose combination matrix is square or not, (2) whether the true MTDCs exist within the same group consisting of the diagonals of the dose combination matrix, and (3) the number of true MTDCs.

Table 5 shows the average recommendation rates for true MTDCs and ODCs of the four methods with respect to each type of the dose combination matrix, and position and number of true MTDCs. In the cases of the square dose combination matrix, the WCO method outperformed the YYC, BW, and HHM methods when the true MTDCs exist along with the diagonals of the dose-combination matrix and the number of true MTDCs is greater than or equal to 2. The HHM methods demonstrated the highest recommendation rates for true MTDCs when the true MTDCs do not exist along with the diagonals of the dose-combination matrix but the number of true MTDCs is greater than or equal to 2, or the number of true MTDCs is one. Next, in the cases of the rectangle dose combination matrix, the WCO method outperformed the other 3 methods when the true MTDCs exist along the diagonals of the dose-combination matrix and the number of true MTDCs is more greater or equal to 2, and when the number of true MTDCs is one, while the HHM and WCO methods outperformed when the true MTDCs do not exist along the diagonals of the dose-combination matrix but the number of true MTDCs is greater than or equal to 2. The HHM method demonstrated the lowest recommendation rates for the ODCs under all the configurations presented. The HHM method can be considered a more conservative method than the others evaluated in this work.

3.4 Some Possible Rationale for the Observed Performance Difference

The method in group (1) (i.e., YYC, BW, and HHM) showed the best performance with respect to recommendation for true MTDC(s) under five scenarios, while that in group (2) (i.e., WCO) did under ten scenarios. In Scenario 14, the WCO and HHM methods yielded nearly identical performance. Accordingly, the under-parameterized

Table 5 The recommendation rates for true MTDCs and ODCs on average with respect to each type of the dose combination matrix, and position and number of true MTDCs (the percentages for the best method are in bold)

Dose combination matrix	Position and number of true MTDCs	Scenario	Recommendation rates for true MTDCs (%)				Recommendation rates for ODCs (%)			
			YYC	BW	WCO	HHM	YYC	BW	WCO	HHM
Square (i.e., 3×3 and 4×4)	Diagonal and ≥ 2 true MTDCs	1, 2, 5	58	58	**69**	58	24	23	20	**16**
	Non-diagonal and ≥ 2 true MTDCs	6, 7	39	33	38	**40**	37	33	33	**22**
	1 True MTDC	3, 4, 8	12	28	28	**32**	60	42	48	**39**
Rectangle (i.e., 2×4 and 3×5)	Diagonal and ≥ 2 true MTDCs	9, 13	35	39	**44**	39	25	27	19	**14**
	Non-diagonal and ≥ 2 true MTDCs	10, 14, 15	35	35	**44**	**44**	44	40	32	**25**
	1 True MTDC	12, 16	2	24	**31**	21	51	34	35	**31**

approaches may be more efficient than the approaches using a flexible model with several parameters. This is because parameter estimation generally does not work well under the practical sample size of 30, irrespective of whether frequentist and Bayesian approaches are employed. Additionally, the cohort size of the trial may also impact the difference between the methods in groups (1) and (2). To further examine this, we ran YYC using cohorts of size 1, but the results were very similar on average. There were differences within particular scenarios, with size 3 doing better in some cases, and size 1 doing better in others. For instance, in Scenario 8, YYC with size 3 yielded a recommendation percentage for true MTDC's of 4.6%. Using cohorts of size 1 increased this to 8.4%. Conversely, decreasing the cohort size from 3 to 1 decreased the recommendation percentage in Scenario 6 from 44.3 to 38.4%. The average recommendation percentage for true MTDC across the 16 scenarios was 34% for size 3 and 35% for size 1. We also ran HHM using cohorts of size 1 and found that the average recommendation percentage for true MTDC across the 16 scenarios was 40% for size 1, and slightly smaller than that for size 3 (i.e., 42%). In the WCO method using cohort size of 1, once a DLT is observed in Stage 1, one can quickly move to the Stage 2 and obtain model-based estimates. This would be a very attractive feature for model-based dose-finding methods. Among the methods in group (1), the superiority in terms of recommending true MTDC(s) were HHM, BW, and YYC in that order. The shrinkage logistic model includes the model parameters for agents A and B, and its interaction, but does not need to specify the prior toxicity probability for each agent and hyper-parameter for prior distributions as in YYC and BW. Furthermore, YYC and BW commonly specify the prior toxicity probability for each agent, but the number of hyper-parameters for the prior distributions in BW (e.g., only σ^2) is smaller than that of YYC (e.g., α, β, γ). Thus, our simulation studies suggested that the degree of assumptions with regards to prior toxicity probability, hyper-parameters, and dose-toxicity model in the method may be associated with the average performance of selecting true MTDCs.

4 Discussion

In this chapter, we characterized the operating characteristics of the model-based dose-finding methods using the practical sample size of 30 under various toxicity scenarios. Although there are certain scenarios in which each of the methods performs well, and the operating characteristics between the methods are comparable, on average the WCO (46%) method yielded the largest recommendation rates for true MTDC's by at least 4% over the nearest competitor (HHM; 42%). These conclusions hold for patient allocation to true MTDC's as well. This average performance is across sixteen scenarios that encompass a wide variety of practical situations (i.e. dimension of combination matrix, location and number of true MTDC's, etc.). We also considered additional scenarios in which there was no "perfect" MTDC. That is, in each scenario, there are no combinations with true

DLT rate exactly equal to the target. In these scenarios, we evaluated the performance of each method in choosing, as the MTDC, combinations that have true DLT rates close to the target rate. The conclusions from the simulation studies above held, with WCO yielding the highest (37.1%) average recommendation percentage for combinations within 5% of the target rate (data not shown). Although we did not introduce them in this chapter, the dose-finding design based on order restricted inference proposed by Conaway et al. [3], termed the CDP method, and the Bayesian dose-finding method using standard logistic model proposed by Riviere et al. [11], termed the RYDZ method, are also useful. The average operating characteristics of the CDP and RYDZ methods were similar to that of the WCO method [7, 8].

There are no silver bullet designs to the two-agent dose-finding problem. The operating characteristics of model-based dose finding methods vary depending on prior toxicity probability, prior distributions, and cut-off probabilities for dose escalation and de-escalation. The simulation studies indicated that the performances in terms of recommending true MTDCs among the 4 methods may be associated with the degree of assumptions required in each method. Specifically, the uncertainty assumptions (e.g., prior toxicity probability, hyper-parameters, and specific dose-toxicity model) are less in order of WCO, HHM, BW, and YYC and the performances in terms of recommending true MTDCs were on average better in this order. This tendency was also found in the other performance indices. Although the operating characteristic of a dose-finding method is influenced by many methodological characteristics, this hypothetical consideration would be one of the reasons for the performance differences among the 4 methods.

Based on the results of simulation studies, we provide some recommendations in implementing each method in practice. The YYC and BW methods require specifications for both the toxicity probabilities of two agents and the hyper-parameters of prior distributions; therefore, these methods would be most useful in the cases where the toxicity data are available from a previous phase I monotherapy trial for each agent. We need to pay particular attention in using the YYC method because its operating characteristics were greatly impacted by the toxicity scenarios. The performance of the BW method was intermediate between the HHM and YYC methods. In implementing BW, the prior value of the variance should be fine-tuned, as the authors recommend. The HHM method can be employed without prior information on the two agents, but requires the MLE for the three parameters in the shrinkage logistic model. If investigators desire to be a bit more conservative, while still maintaining an adequate recommendation rate for true MTDCs, the HHM method can be recommended.

Acknowledgements The views expressed here are the result of independent work and do not represent the viewpoints or findings of the Pharmaceuticals and Medical Devices Agency. This work was partially supported by JSPS KAKENHI [Grant Number 15K15948] (Grant-in-Aid for Young Scientists B). This work was partially supported by JSPS KAKENHI [Grant Number 17K00045] (Grant-in-Aid for Scientific Research C).

References

1. Braun TM, Wang S. A hierarchical Bayesian design for phase I trials of novel combinations of cancer therapeutic agents. Biometrics. 2010;66:805–12.
2. Cheung YK. Dose-finding by the continual reassessment method. New York: Chapman and Hall/CRC Press; 2011. p. 57–62.
3. Conaway MR, Dunbar S, Peddada SD. Designs for single- or multiple-agent phase I trials. Biometrics. 2004;60:661–9.
4. Gasparini M, Bailey S, Neuenschwander B. Correspondence: Bayesian dose finding in oncology for drug combinations by copula regression. J R Stat Soc Ser C. 2010;59:543–6.
5. Gasparini M. General classes of multiple binary regression models in dose finding problems for combination therapies. J R Stat Soc Ser C. 2013;62:115–33.
6. Hirakawa A, Hamada C, Matsui S. A dose-finding approach based on shrunken predictive probability for combinations of two agents in phase I trials. Stat Med. 2013;32:4515–25.
7. Hirakawa A, Wages NA, Sato H, Matsui S. A comparative study of adaptive dose-finding designs for phase I oncology trials of combination therapies. Stat Med. 2015;34:3194–213.
8. Hirakawa A, Sato H. Authors' reply. Stat Med. 2016;35:479–80.
9. Lee SM, Cheung YK. Model calibration in the continual reassessment method. Clin Trials. 2009;6:227–38.
10. O'Quigley J, Pepe M, Fisher L. Continual reassessment method: a practical design for phase 1 clinical trials in cancer. Biometrics. 1990;46:33–48.
11. Riviere MK, Yuan Y, Dubois F, Zohar S. A Bayesian dose-finding design for drug combination clinical trials based on the logistic model. Pharm Stat. 2014;13:247–57.
12. Riviere MK, Dubois F, Zohar S. Competing designs for drug combination in phase I dose-finding clinical trials. Stat Med. 2015;34:1–12.
13. Thall PF, Millikan RE, Mueller P, Lee SJ. Dose finding with two agents in phase I oncology trials. Biometrics. 2003;59:487–96.
14. Wang K, Ivanova A. Two-dimensional finding in discrete dose space. Biometrics. 2005;61:217–22.
15. Wages NA, Conaway MR, O'Quigley J. Continual reassessment method for partial ordering. Biometrics. 2011;67:1555–63.
16. Wages NA, Conaway MR, O'Quigley J. Dose-finding design for multi-drug combinations. Clin Trials. 2011;8:380–9.
17. Wages NA, Conaway MR. Specifications of a continual reassessment method design for phase I trials of combined drugs. Pharm Stat. 2013;12:217–24.
18. Yin G, Yuan Y. A latent contingency table approach to dose-finding for combinations of two agents. Biometrics. 2009;65:866–75.
19. Yin G, Yuan Y. Bayesian dose finding in oncology for drug combinations by copula regression. J R Stat Soc Ser C. 2009;58:211–24.
20. Yin G, Yuan Y. Author's response: Bayesian dose-finding in oncology for drug combinations by copula regression. J R Stat Soc Ser C. 2010;59:544–6.

Evaluation of Safety in Biomarker Driven Multiple Agent Phase IB Trial

Motomi Mori, Racky Daffé, Byung S. Park and Jeffrey Tyner

Abstract Tyner and colleagues in the Center for Hematological Malignancies, Knight Cancer Institute, at the Oregon Health & Science University have recently developed a novel kinase-inhibitor assay and rapid mutation screening to identify molecularly targeted drugs to which patient leukemic cells are sensitive. As a proof of concept and feasibility trial, they proposed a phase IB trial focusing on feasibility and safety of an assay-based kinase-inhibitor treatment assignment in combination with the standard induction chemotherapy among newly diagnosed acute myeloid leukemia patients. Because each patient receives one of five kinase inhibitors in combination with standard chemotherapy, the sample size for each kinase inhibitor group is varied and limited. In addition, there is a different toxicity profile associated with each inhibitor, making safety assessment challenging. We will discuss a continuous toxicity monitoring plan in biomarker driven, multiple agent feasibility and safety trials, and evaluate its operating characteristics in a simulation study.

Keywords Phase I oncology trials · Early phase clinical trials · Continuous toxicity monitoring · Precision medicine · Safety evaluation · Multi-drug trials

M. Mori (✉) · R. Daffé · B.S. Park
Biostatistics, Knight Cancer Institute and School of Public Health,
Oregon Heatlh & Science University, 3181 SW Sam Jackson Park Road,
Portland, OR 97239-3098, USA
e-mail: morim@ohsu.edu

R. Daffé
e-mail: daffer@ohsu.edu

B.S. Park
e-mail: parkb@ohsu.edu

J. Tyner
Knight Cancer Institute and Department of Cell, Developmental
and Cancer Biology, Oregon Heatlh & Science University,
3181 SW Sam Jackson Park Road, Portland, OR 97239-3098, USA
e-mail: tynerj@ohsu.edu

S. Matsui and J. Crowley (eds.), *Frontiers of Biostatistical Methods and Applications in Clinical Oncology*, DOI 10.1007/978-981-10-0126-0_5

1 Introduction

Acute myeloid leukemia (AML) is the most common type of blood cancer in adults, with more than 50% of cases recorded in individuals over 65. The American Cancer Society estimates about 20,830 new cases in 2015 in the U.S. The disease is aggressive, with only 40–50% of patients that can be cured [1, 2]. Relapse is nearly always fatal [3]. The standard initial treatment for newly diagnosed AML consists of a combination chemotherapy with 7 days of continuous infusion of cytarabine and 3 days of anthracycline, referred to as the "7 + 3" treatment. It results in 70–80% complete response in patients, while 20–30% of patients are refractory and require re-induction. AML is considered a highly heterogeneous disease in terms of genetic and molecular characteristics, clinical presentation, response to treatment and overall prognosis [4], making it challenging to establish a successful, single-agent modality.

Tyner et al. [5] in the Knight Cancer Institute at Oregon Health & Science University developed a rapid, high-throughput kinase inhibitor screening assay to identify tyrosine kinase inhibitors to which patient's leukemic cells are sensitive. The assay is a 384-well plate format, containing eight different concentrations of 90 small-molecule kinase inhibitors (drugs) that are FDA approved or in clinical trials. Briefly a patient's primary leukemia sample (peripheral blood or bone marrow) is subject to in vitro cell viability assay, a dose-response curve is generated for each drug with the response being % of live leukemia cells at each concentration, and the IC50 ("half maximal inhibitor concentration") is determined for each drug (Fig. 1). IC50 is the dose that kills 50% of leukemia cells. To standardize the IC50s across all drugs, percent (%) median IC50 is computed by dividing the observed IC50 by

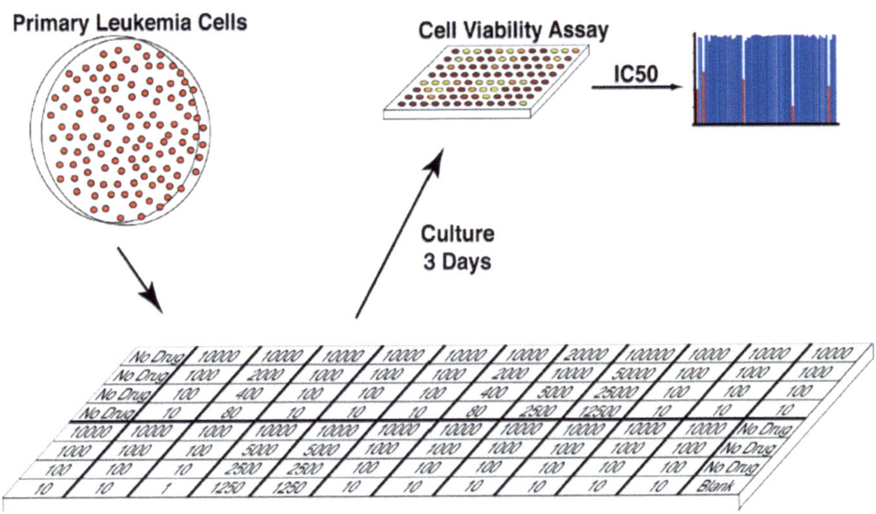

Fig. 1 Illustration of the kinase inhibitor assays and target drug identification

the median IC50 of the drug based on the past samples. A drug with the lowest % median IC50 is considered as the most sensitive drug for the patient.

The OHSU eIRB #11766 (NCT02779283) (PIs: Marc Loriaux, MD, PhD; Stephen Spurgeon, MD) is a phase IB trial to evaluate the feasibility and safety of the combination of a target kinase inhibitor and the standard chemotherapy regimen for newly diagnosed AML patients. In this trial, five FDA approved drugs are being studied: dasatinib, sorafenib, sunitinib, ponatinib, and nilotinib. A patient receives the standard chemotherapy plus the target drug. The inhibitor assay is used to determine a target drug by Day 7, which is administered on Day 8 (Fig. 2). Because the five kinase inhibitors have not been combined with the "7 + 3" regimen, safety assessment is considered critical; specifically, it was felt necessary to establish continuous toxicity monitoring.

2 Statistical Methods for Continuous Toxicity Monitoring

2.1 *Single-Stage, Single-Agent Trial*

Ivanova et al. [6] proposed a method for deriving a continuous stopping boundary for toxicity in a single-arm, single-stage phase II oncology trial. The boundary is derived based on Pocock [7] boundaries with K stages, where K is equal to the number of patients enrolled in a trial. A basic concept is presented below:

Notations:

N the sample size
Θ the probability of a dose limiting toxicity (DLT)
θ_0 the target DLT probability (i.e.the maximum acceptable DLT probability)
φ the probability of early termination when $\theta = \theta_0$
b_k the boundary for the kth subject

The goal is to construct a stopping boundary (b_k) based on the target DLT probability such that the probability of early stopping is at most φ if the DLT probability is equal to θ_0. In order to find a boundary, a set of pointwise probabilities $(\alpha_1, \ldots, \alpha_K)$ are chosen and b_k is then computed as the smallest integer such that Pr $(Y_k \geq b_k) \leq \alpha_k$, where Y_k denotes the cumulative DLT events among k patients and a binomial random variable with parameter k and θ_0. A Pocock boundary is obtained by setting $\alpha_1 = \cdots = \alpha_K = \alpha$ where α is such that if $\theta = \theta_0$ the probability of early stopping is as close as φ as possible. The solution for α is tabulated by Jennison and Turnbull [8]. Ivanova provides an online program to calculate a continuous stopping boundary for toxicity for a single-arm, single-stage trial: http://cancer.unc.edu/biostatistics/program/ivanova/ContinuosMonitoringForToxicity.aspx. For example, if $N = 40$ (sample size), $\theta_0 = 0.20$ (target DLT probability), and $\varphi = 0.05$ (probability of early termination when $\theta = \theta_0$), the program provides the boundary and the operating characteristics shown in Table 1.

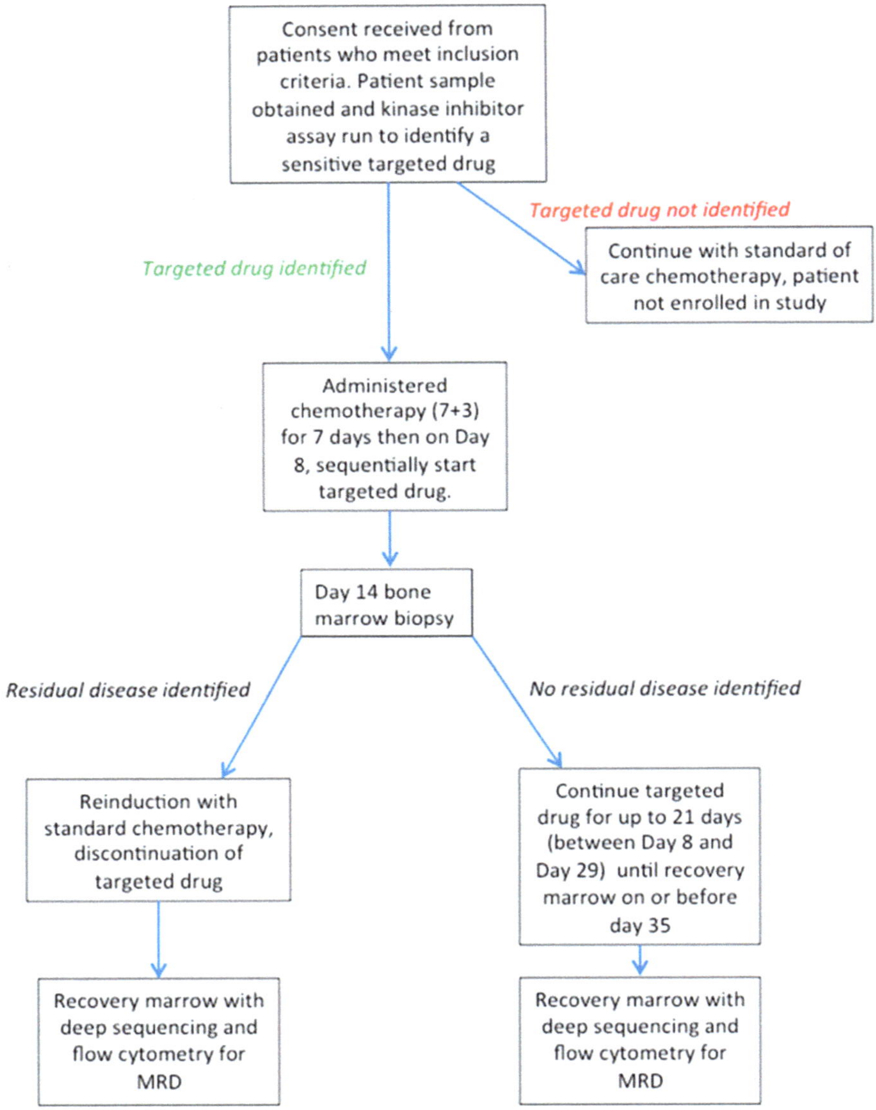

Fig. 2 Flowchart of OHSU eIRB #11766 (a combination of the "7+3" treatment and the targeted therapy). Note that MRD refers to minimal residual disease

2.2 *Extension to Assay-Guided Multiple Agents Trial*

Tang et al. [9] proposed an extension of a group sequential procedure to multiple endpoints. More recently Ye et al. [10] proposed a group sequential Holms procedure for multiple endpoints. However, these approaches are not intended for

Table 1 Pocock boundary and operating characteristics for 40 patients based on 5% probability of early termination when the DLT probability is 20%

k	1	2	3	4	5	6	7	8	9	10	11	12	13	14	15	16	17	18	19	20
Pocock boundary b_k	–	–	3	4	4	5	5	5	6	6	6	7	7	7	8	8	8	9	9	9
k	21	22	23	24	25	26	27	28	29	30	31	32	33	34	35	36	37	38	39	40
Pocock boundary b_k	9	10	10	10	11	11	11	11	12	12	12	13	13	13	13	14	14	14	15	15

This boundary is equivalent to testing the null hypothesis, after each patient, that the event rate is equal to 0.2, using a one-sided level 0.015124 test

θ	Actual probability of early stopping	Number of events expected values		Number of patients expected values			
	φ	E[Y]	SD[Y]	E[N]	SD[N]	E[Y/N]	SD[Y/N]
0.2	0.0495	0.0495	7.76	2.4	38.8	5.77	0.21
0.3	0.3521	9.83	2.74	32.77	11.7	0.35	0.17
0.4	0.7992	8.82	3.31	22.06	12.8	0.49	0.19
0.5	0.9789	6.72	2.78	13.43	9.03	0.61	0.19
0.6	0.9995	5.25	1.91	8.75	5.54	0.7	0.19
0.7	1	4.38	1.34	6.25	3.5	0.79	0.17
0.8	1	3.79	0.96	4.74	2.26	0.87	0.15
0.9	1	3.35	0.63	3.72	1.33	0.94	0.11
1	1	3	0	3	0	1	0

The output is obtained using the online software by Ivanova [6] at: http://cancer.unc.edu/biostatistics/program/ivanova/ContinuosMonitoringForToxicity.aspx
Y = the number of events, random, between 0 and N; N = the number of patients, random, between 1 and K; φ^* = the actual probability of early stopping (hitting the boundary); E[] = expected value (mean); SD[] = standard deviation

multiple agents. We will extend the approach of Ivanova et al. [6] to a biomarker driven trial where multiple agents are studied.

Let N be the total sample size, and p be the number of drugs under study. Let $(f_1,\ldots,f_p)$ denote a vector of frequencies of p target drugs. Let $(\theta_1,\ldots,\theta_p)$ denote the true DLT probability of each drug. The goal is to construct a continuous stopping boundary based on DLT events for the all drug groups combined as well as for each drug group separately such that the probability of early termination is at most φ if the toxicity rate is equal to θ_0. A rationale for having both types of stopping boundaries are: (a) to evaluate the safety of the assay-based drug assignment as a whole; (b) if one drug is associated with higher DLT, a drug-specific boundary will allow the drug group to stop, while allowing all other drug groups to continue, and; (c) since some drug groups have small sample sizes, combining all drug groups may provide more power in detecting excessive DLTs. We would like to protect patients from excessive DLT events, while evaluating the feasibility of the assay-guided approach.

Notations:

$(f_1,\ldots,f_p)$	the frequency of p target drugs
$(\theta_1,\ldots,\theta_p)$	the true toxicity rate of p drugs
$(N_1,\ldots,N_p)$	the number of patients in p drug groups
$(Y_1,\ldots,Y_p)$	the number of toxicity event in p drug groups
$N=\sum_{i=1}^{p} N_i$	the planned sample size
$Y=\sum_{i=1}^{p} Y_i$	the total number of DLT events
θ_0	the target DLT probability
φ	the probability of early termination when $\theta=\theta_0$

Conditional on $(N_1,\ldots,N_p)$, $(Y_1,\ldots,Y_p)$ is independently distributed as binomial (N_i,θ_i), and therefore the joint distribution is given by:

$$f(Y_1,\ldots,Y_p|N_1,\ldots,N_p)=\prod_i \binom{N_i}{Y_i}\theta_i^{Y_i}(1-\theta_i)^{N_i-Y_i}$$

The number of patients in each target drug group, $(N_1,\ldots,N_p)$, follows a multinomial distribution with the parameters $(f_1,\ldots,f_p)$. Therefore, a joint distribution of $(N_1,\ldots,N_p)$ and $(Y_1,\ldots,Y_p)$ is:

$$\begin{aligned} f(Y_1,\ldots,Y_p,N_1,\ldots,N_p) &= f(Y_1,\ldots,Y_p|N_1,\ldots,N_p)f(N_1,\ldots,N_p) \\ &= \prod_i \binom{N_i}{Y_i}\theta_i^{Y_i}(1-\theta_i)^{N_i-Y_i}\binom{N}{N_1\cdots N_p}f_1^{N_1}\cdots f_p^{N_p} \end{aligned}$$

The marginal distribution of $(Y_1,\ldots,Y_p)$ can be obtained by summing over all possible $(N_1,\ldots,N_p)$ configuration. Similarly conditional on $(N_1,\ldots,N_p)$, the distribution of the total number of DLT events, $Y=\sum_{i=1}^{p} Y_i$, is binomial $(N, \sum f_i\theta_i)$ given by:

$$f(Y|N_1,\ldots,N_p) = \binom{N}{Y}(\sum f_i\theta_i)^Y(1-(\sum f_i\theta_i))^{N-Y}$$

A joint distribution of $(N_1,\ldots,N_p)$ and Y is given by:

$$\begin{aligned} f(Y,N_1,\ldots,N_p) &= f(Y|N_1,\ldots,N_p)f(N_1,\ldots,N_p) \\ &= \binom{N}{Y}(\sum f_i\theta_i)^Y(1-(\sum f_i\theta_i))^{N-Y}\binom{N}{N_1\cdots N_p}f_1^{N_1}\cdots f_p^{N_p} \end{aligned}$$

To derive continuous toxicity boundaries, let's simplify a problem and assume first that N_i is fixed and equal to m, so that $N = mp$. This means that the trial continues until m patients are enrolled in each drug group. In this special setting, $(Y_1,\ldots,Y_p)$ is independently distributed as binomial (m,θ_i), and therefore the joint distribution is given by:

$$f(Y_1,\ldots,Y_p) = \prod_i \binom{m}{Y_i}\theta_i^{Y_i}(1-\theta_i)^{m-Y_i}$$

The Pocock type boundaries can be derived by finding a set of common b_k under $\theta_i = \theta_0$ for all $i = 1, \ldots, p$ such that b_k is the smallest integer to satisfy:

$$\Pr\left[\bigcup_i (Y_i \geq b_k)\right] = 1 - \prod_i [1 - \Pr(Y_i \geq b_k)] \leq 1 - (1-\alpha)^p \leq p * \alpha$$

where Y_i denotes a binomial random variable with parameter k and θ_0, and α is such that if $\theta = \theta_O$ the probability of early stopping is as close as φ as possible. Note that in general, regardless of independence or dependence, $\Pr\left[\bigcup_i (Y_i \geq b_k)\right]$ is equal to or less than α, providing the upper probability of the overall type I error rate for the multiple boundary problem.

In many cases, while the total sample size is fixed, the number of patients in each target drug group is a random variable. Deriving a continuous toxicity boundary is complex when $(N_1,\ldots,N_p)$ is a random vector with the multinomial distribution with the parameters $(f_1,\ldots,f_p)$. In theory, the boundaries can be constructed using the marginal distribution of $(Y_1,\ldots,Y_p)$ with the expected value and variance are given by:

$$\begin{aligned} E(Y_i) &= E[E(Y_i|N_i)] = E(N_i\theta_i) = Nf_i\theta_i \\ Var(Y_i) &= Var[E(Y_i|N_i)] + E(Var[(Y_i|N_i)]) = \theta_i^2 Nf_i(1-f_i) + Nf_i\theta_i(1-\theta_i) \end{aligned}$$

The term $\theta_i^2 Nf_i(1-f_i)$ reflects additional variance due to N_i being a random variable.

For the OHSU eIRB #11766 trial, there are six toxicity boundaries, one for the total number of DLT events, and five for DLT in each drug group. Each boundary was derived using $\alpha = 0.02$, so that the overall probability of early termination when $\theta = \theta_0$ for all drug groups is at most $p\alpha = 0.12$. However, because the number of subjects in each drug group is not fixed and can be regarded as a random variable, we evaluated the operating characteristics of the boundaries through a simulation study.

3 Evaluation of Operating Characteristics

3.1 Simulation Settings

Using Ivanova's online program, we derived a continuous toxicity boundary under the following specifications: (1) $N = 40$ patients; (2) the maximum acceptable DLT probability (θ_0) = 20%; (3) the probability of early termination when $\theta = \theta_0$ is 5%. The boundary is then applied to DLT events in each drug group as well as the total DLT events for all groups combined. The overall probability of early termination due to any of six boundaries is at most 30%.

We evaluated the stopping boundaries under the following eleven conditions (Table 2). The frequency of each of five drug groups is denoted by f_i, which are chosen to match with the expected frequency of each drug in the trial. Eleven toxicity profiles are assumed (Table 2) ranging from the case of uniform safety (Case 1), uniform moderate toxicity (Case 2) to high toxicity (Case 11). The overall toxicity represents a weighted average of the target drug frequency and DLT probability, $\theta = \sum_i f_i \theta_i$. A simulation was run 1000 times under each condition.

3.2 Simulation Results

Table 2 shows overall and drug-specific probabilities of early termination for eleven different DLT probability profiles. The expected number of patients in each drug group is based on the expected frequencies in the OHSU eIRB #11766 trial. Figure 3 shows the probability of early termination as a function of DLT probability by each drug group as well as all drug groups combined. When the DLT probability is uniformly low (10%), the probability of early termination is close to 0. In contrast, when the DLT probability is uniformly high (70–80%), the probability of early termination is high (100%). When the toxicity profile is heterogeneous, e.g., 10–80%, the probability of early termination depends on both DLT probability and the frequency of the target drug group, i.e., the number of subjects in each drug group. When the frequency of the target group is moderate (e.g., 30%, Drug A), a drug-specific boundary has a reasonable probability of early termination

Table 2 Probability of early termination under each eleven conditions

Drugs	f_i	θ_{i1}	θ_{i2}	θ_{i3}	θ_{i4}	θ_{i5}	θ_{i6}	θ_{i7}	θ_{i8}	θ_{i9}	θ_{i10}	θ_{i11}
Drug A	0.30	0.10	0.30	0.60	0.80	0.80	0.35	0.40	0.10	0.10	0.50	0.80
Drug B	0.29	0.10	0.30	0.10	0.10	0.60	0.35	0.40	0.10	0.10	0.50	0.70
Drug C	0.14	0.10	0.30	0.10	0.10	0.10	0.10	0.40	0.10	0.70	0.60	0.80
Drug D	0.24	0.10	0.30	0.10	0.10	0.20	0.10	0.40	0.10	0.10	0.50	0.80
Drug E	0.03	0.10	0.30	0.10	0.10	0.10	0.10	0.10	0.80	0.80	0.60	0.70
Overall		0.10	0.30	0.25	0.31	0.48	0.25	0.39	0.12	0.21	0.52	0.77
E(N)	P(ET) = Probability of early termination											
Drug A	12	0.000	0.019	0.545	0.901	0.926	0.070	0.111	0.000	0.000	0.303	0.904
Drug B	11	0.000	0.033	0.000	0.000	0.505	0.070	0.118	0.000	0.000	0.286	0.747
Drug C	6	0.000	0.005	0.000	0.000	0.000	0.000	0.025	0.000	0.237	0.106	0.358
Drug D	10	0.000	0.005	0.000	0.000	0.001	0.000	0.076	0.000	0.000	0.202	0.779
Drug E	1	0.000	0.000	0.000	0.000	0.000	0.000	0.000	0.001	0.004	0.000	0.000
Overall		0.001	0.337	0.142	0.398	0.973	0.158	0.773	0.003	0.054	0.990	1.000
Any boundaries		0.001	0.349	0.251	0.578	1	0.186	0.839	0.003	0.102	1	1.000

Probabilities of early termination after simulation of a 1000 trials using Pocock-type boundary that yields probability of early stopping of 0.05 when the true event probability is 0.20

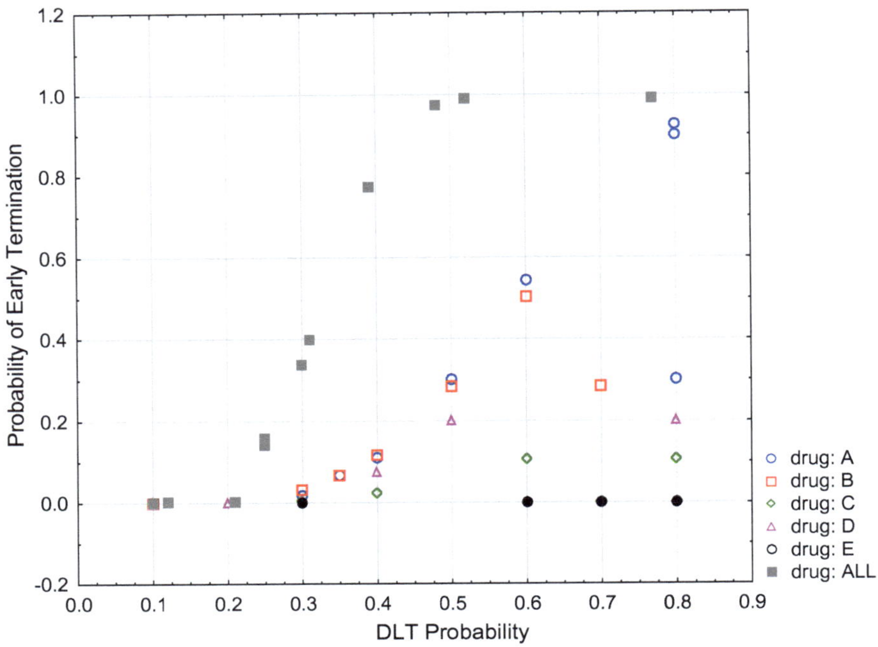

Fig. 3 Probability of early termination as a function of DLT probability by each drug group and all groups combined

in the presence of excess toxicity. Not surprisingly when the frequency of the target drug group is low (e.g., 3%, Drug E), the probability of early termination is low regardless of the DLT probability. In contrast, the boundary based on the total DLT events is more powerful and has a higher probability of termination than any of the drug-specific boundaries because of a larger sample size (Fig. 3). This benefit is evident in the 7th condition where DLT probabilities are 40% for Drugs A–D and 10% for Drug E; the boundary based on the total DLT events is clearly more powerful than drug-specific boundaries and is likely to be able to detect moderately higher DLT event rates in four drug groups. Note that presumably because the power is so low, a multiplicity problem is not apparent (i.e., an increased probability of early termination when the DLT probability is low).

4 Concluding Remarks

In early phase oncology clinical trials, it is common to have a continuous toxicity boundary in order to insure patient safety. We extended the method of Ivanova [6] to a biomarker driven, multiple agent trial, where the sample size for each drug is not fixed. We evaluated the operating characteristics of multiple toxicity boundaries through simulation. The results indicate that having both drug-specific and overall toxicity boundaries is beneficial in early phase trials, when the sample size is relatively small. Overall, however, the results point out that having a fixed sample size for each drug group is necessary if we would like to assess the safety of each drug group, even when the objective of the trial is to evaluate the assay-guided strategy rather than individual drug efficacy. The results also highlight the challenge of safety evaluation in precision medicine settings, when there are several drugs being evaluated in a single trial, and where the sample size for each drug may be very small.

In toxicity and safety monitoring, we are more interested in detecting any possible safety issues, and therefore the increased α level due to multiple boundaries may be acceptable. In the simulation the power is uniformly low when the sample size is small, which is typically the case in early phase oncology trials. Therefore, to achieve a reasonable power, we may need to accept a larger α level. In practice, crossing the toxicity boundary does not always result in the immediate early termination of the trial, but triggers a more rigorous safety evaluation including dose modification, dose schedule change, and reassessment of the eligibility criteria. In those instances, having both drug-specific and overall boundaries may be helpful, as well as setting the minimum sample size for each drug group to allow safety evaluation of each drug under study. Further research on this topic is encouraged, including Bayesian adaptive toxicity boundaries that leverage prior toxicity information as well as cumulative toxicity events across drug groups.

References

1. Jemal A, Thomas A, Murray T, Thun M. Cancer statistics. CA Cancer J Clin. 2002;52(1):23–47. Erratum in: CA Cancer J Clin. 2002;52(2):119. CA Cancer J Clin. 2002;52(3):181–2. (PubMed PMID: 11814064).
2. Breems DA, Van Putten WL, Huijgens PC, Ossenkoppele GJ, Verhoef GE, Verdonck LF, Vellenga E, De Greef GE, Jacky E, Van der Lelie J, Boogaerts MA, Löwenberg B. Prognostic index for adult patients with acute myeloid leukemia in first relapse. J Clin Oncol. 2005;23 (9):1969–78 Epub 2005 Jan 4 (PubMed PMID: 15632409).
3. Giles F, O'Brien S, Cortes J, Verstovsek S, Bueso-Ramos C, Shan J, Pierce S, Garcia-Manero G, Keating M, Kantarjian H. Outcome of patients with acute myelogenous leukemia after second salvage therapy. Cancer. 2005;104(3):547–54 (PubMed PMID: 15973664).
4. Khwaja A, Bjorkholm M, Gale RE, Levine RL, Jordan CT, Ehninger G, Bloomfield CD, Estey E, Burnett A, Cornelissen JJ, Scheinberg DA, Bouscary D, Linch DC. Acute myeloid leukaemia. Nat Rev Dis Primers. 2016;10(2):16010. doi:10.1038/nrdp.2016.10 (PubMed PMID: 27159408).
5. Maxson JE, Gotlib J, Pollyea DA, Fleischman AG, Agarwal A, Eide CA, Bottomly D, Wilmot B, McWeeney SK, Tognon CE, Pond JB, Collins RH, Goueli B, Oh ST, Deininger MW, Chang BH, Loriaux MM, Druker BJ, Tyner JW. Oncogenic CSF3R mutations in chronic neutrophilic leukemia and atypical CML. N Engl J Med. 2013;368(19):1781–90. doi:10.1056/NEJMoa1214514 (PubMedPMID:23656643; PubMedCentralPMCID: PMC3730275).
6. Ivanova A, Qaqish BF, Schell MJ. Continuous toxicity monitoring in phase II trials in oncology. Biometrics. 2005;61(2):540–5 (PubMed PMID: 16011702).

7. Pocock SJ. Group sequential methods in the design and analysis of clinical trials. Biometrika. 1977;64(2):191–9.
8. Jennison C, Turnbull BW. Group sequential methods with applications to clinical trials. Boca Raton: Chapman & Hall/CRC; 2000.
9. Tang D, Gnecco C, Geller NL. Design of group sequential clinical trials with multiple endpoints. J Am Stat Assoc. 1989;84(407):776–9.
10. Ye Y, Li A, Liu L, Yao B. A group sequential Holm procedure with multiple primary endpoints. Stat Med 2012; Stat Med. 2013;32(7):1112–24. doi:10.1002/sim.5700. Epub 2012 Dec 14. PMID: 23239078.

Bayesian Phase II Single-Arm Designs

Satoshi Teramukai

Abstract Phase II exploratory clinical trials in oncology are often designed as single-arm trials using a binary efficacy outcome with or without interim monitoring. This chapter focused on the Bayesian designs which considered both efficacy and safety outcomes associated with early stopping. In particular, we introduce a Bayesian adaptive design denoted as predictive sample size selection design (PSSD). The design allows for sample size selection following any planned interim analyses for early stopping of a trial, together with sample size determination. An extension of the PSSD to add continuous monitoring of safety is also described. We investigate the operating characteristics of the design through simulation studies.

Keywords Sample size determination · Analysis prior · Design prior · Prior predictive distributions · Sample size re-estimation · Bayesian adaptive design · Predictive sample size selection design · Beta priors · Bayesian conjugate analysis · Predictive probability criterion · Interim monitoring

1 Introduction

The aim of exploratory clinical trials in oncology is to determine whether an experimental treatment is promising for evaluation in confirmatory clinical trials. Phase II exploratory trials focus mainly on the evaluation of efficacy, and single-arm trials are designed to assess the clinical response related to anti-tumour activity as the primary endpoint. If such an efficacy-related clinical response is based on tumor shrinkage, the assessment will be made using the response evaluation criteria in solid tumors (RECIST), which is based on computed tomography scans of tumor size [1]. In this case, the response is categorised as progressive

S. Teramukai (✉)
Department of Biostatistics, Graduate School of Medical Science,
Kyoto Prefectural University of Medicine, 465 Kajii-cho, Kawaramachi-Hirokoji,
Kamigyo-ku, Kyoto 602-8566, Japan
e-mail: steramu@koto.kpu-m.ac.jp

S. Matsui and J. Crowley (eds.), *Frontiers of Biostatistical Methods and Applications in Clinical Oncology*, DOI 10.1007/978-981-10-0126-0_6

disease, stable disease, partial response, or complete response. This ordinal response is often further dichotomised as a binary response according to some threshold that defines the "success" or the "failure" of the treatment.

One of the most commonly-used designs for a phase II single-arm trial is Simon's two-stage group sequential design [2], in which the trial is terminated early if the clinical response rate is poor in the first stage. However, Zohar et al. [3] emphasised that Bayesian approaches are ideal for such exploratory clinical trials, as they take into account previous information about the quantity of interest as well as accumulated data during a trial. In this context various Bayesian designs have been proposed. For instance, Tan and Machin [4] developed a Bayesian two-stage design called the single threshold design (STD), and Mayo and Gajewski [5, 6] extended this proposition into a design incorporating informative prior distributions. Whitehead et al. [7] formulated a simple approach to sample size determination (SSD) in which they incorporate historical data in the Bayesian inference. Furthermore, Sambucini [8] proposed a predictive version of the STD (PSTD) using two kinds of prior distributions pursuing different aims: the 'analysis prior' used to compute posterior probabilities and the 'design prior' used to obtain prior predictive distributions. Indeed, according to Sambucini and Brutti [8, 9], the two-priors approach is useful when implementing the Bayesian SSD process and providing a general framework that incorporates frequentist SSD (corresponding to a non-informative analysis prior and a degenerate design prior) as a special case.

Sambucini [10] modified the PSTD and suggested a Bayesian adaptive two-stage design in which the sample size for the second stage depends on the results of the first stage. However, as these methods [4–6, 8, 10] focus on the two-stage design only, their application is somewhat restricted. Brutti et al. [11] proposed a Bayesian SSD with sample size re-estimation based on a two-priors approach; however their approach was based on approximately normally distributed outcomes and not directly on binary outcomes. Lee and Liu [12] proposed a Bayesian predictive probability approach for single-arm trials that combines SSD with multiple interim analyses. Recently, Teramukai et al. [13] proposed a Bayesian adaptive design for single-arm exploratory clinical trials with binary outcomes based on a two-priors approach and predictive probabilities. The design, denoted as predictive sample size selection design (PSSD), consists of SSD at the planning stage and sample size selection at any required stage following interim analyses during the course of the trial.

Such flexible designs seem attractive because they avoid the problem of continuing to treat patients enrolled in a trial with a futile treatment. However, in such a phase II trial toxicity data are also collected, since the toxicity information in its preceding phase I trial may not be reliable, as patients in the phase I trial typically differ from those in the phase II trial. Unfortunately, most of the commonly-used designs for phase II trials, including two-stage designs, do not explicitly utilize the toxicity data but rather separately impose arbitrary stopping rules for safety on the clinical trial protocol in case of excessive toxicity, rather than within the designs themselves. As a result, these imposed rules might obscure or even nullify the designs' operating characteristics. Some authors have proposed adaptive designs that model efficacy and toxicity data jointly. The first to propose such a group sequential design in a frequentist framework were Bryant and Day [14], who developed a method evaluating both clinical response and toxicity, similar in structure to Simon's two-stage designs. They were followed by Thall et al. [15], Conaway and Petroni [16], Stallard et al. [17], and Chen and Smith [18], who later proposed phase II designs jointly modelling toxicity and efficacy data using Bayesian inference. In this context, Teramukai et al. [19] proposed an integrative approach that takes into account both binary efficacy and toxicity data and that also provides sample size determination. It seems more ethical and informative to evaluate safety and efficacy according to interim monitoring for each endpoint. Safety monitoring may also be done more frequently than efficacy monitoring to avoid missing important signals regarding toxicity.

The outline of this chapter is as follows. Sect. 2 introduces some preliminaries on the Bayesian setting. In Sect. 3, we describe the basic concept of PSSD. We show the procedures and operating characteristics of the design in Sect. 4. We illustrate an extension of PSSD that considers both efficacy and safety, and we present the properties of the design through some simulations in Sect. 5, and an illustrative example in Sect. 6. Finally, we conclude with a discussion in Sect. 7.

2 Preliminaries

Suppose that n patients are treated in a trial. Let θ_{T} and θ_{R} denote the parameters representing the probabilities of toxicity and efficacy of the experimental treatment, respectively. Let $Y_{\mathrm{T,i}}$ denote the binary toxicity outcome for patient i for $i = 1,\ldots,n$, which takes a value of 1 with probability θ_{T} and 0 with probability $1-\theta_{\mathrm{T}}$, and similarly let $Y_{\mathrm{R,i}}$ denote the binary efficacy outcome for the same patient, which takes a value of 1 with probability θ_{R} and 0 with probability $1-\theta_{\mathrm{R}}$. Let T and S denote the random numbers of patients who experience toxicity and efficacy, respectively, such that $T = \sum_{i=1}^{n} Y_{\mathrm{T,i}}$ and $S = \sum_{i=1}^{n} Y_{\mathrm{R,i}}$. Then, T and S have the following marginal binomial distributions, respectively:

$$f_{\mathrm{n}}(t|\theta_{\mathrm{T}}) = \mathrm{Bin}(t;n,\theta_{\mathrm{T}}) \text{ for all } t = 0,\ldots,n, \text{ and}$$
$$f_{\mathrm{n}}(s|\theta_{\mathrm{R}}) = \mathrm{Bin}(s;n,\theta_{\mathrm{R}}) \text{ for all } s = 0,\ldots,n.$$

We assume the Beta priors for θ_{T} and θ_{R}, that is, respectively,

$$\pi(\theta_{\mathrm{T}}) = \mathrm{Beta}(\theta_{\mathrm{T}};a_{\mathrm{T}},b_{\mathrm{T}}) \text{ and } \pi(\theta_{\mathrm{R}}) = \mathrm{Beta}(\theta_{\mathrm{R}};a_{\mathrm{R}},b_{\mathrm{R}}), \tag{2.1}$$

where a_{T}, b_{T}, a_{R}, and b_{R} are hyper-parameters. In a Bayesian conjugate analysis, we obtain the following posterior distributions, respectively:

$$\pi_n(\theta_T|T=t) = \text{Beta}(\theta_T; a_T+t, b_T+n-t) \text{ and}$$
$$\pi_n(\theta_R|S=s) = \text{Beta}(\theta_R; a_R+s, b_R+n-s). \tag{2.2}$$

3 Basic Concept of the Predictive Sample-Size Selection Design (PSSD)

3.1 Sample Size Determination

The sample size determination method is based on the concept proposed by Sambucini [8], where a predictive probability criterion with two types of prior distributions, that is, a "design prior" used to obtain prior predictive distributions, and an "analysis prior" used to compute posterior probabilities, is adopted. As the sample size determination in the trial is usually based on the efficacy outcome, we consider the design and analysis priors for the efficacy probability parameter θ_R. Based on Eq. (2.1), these are represented with superscripts "D" and "A", respectively, as follows:

$$\pi^D(\theta_R) = \text{Beta}(\theta_R; a^D, b^D) \text{ and } \pi^A(\theta_R) = \text{Beta}(\theta_R; a^A, b^A), \tag{3.1}$$

where $a^D = n^D\pi_0^D + 1$, $b^D = n^D(1-\pi_0^D) + 1$, $a^A > 0$, and $b^A > 0$; π_0^D represents the prior mode, and n^D is a type of tuning parameter for the variance of $\pi^D(\theta_R)$; $a^A = b^A = 1$ if there is no prior information for efficacy. Let $\theta_{R,0}$ denote a fixed value that previous evidence suggests would be the efficacy probability with a control or standard treatment, and let δ represent a 'minimally clinically significant effect'. Therefore, $\theta_{R,0} + \delta$ is a pre-specified target value for the efficacy probability. In this connection, the prior mode π_0^D should be chosen such that $\pi_0^D > \theta_{R,0} + \delta$. In particular, when $n^D = \infty$, $\pi^D(\theta_R)$ is the degenerate distribution at π_0^D.

If S patients among n patients experience efficacy, the posterior distribution for the analysis prior $\pi^A(\theta_R)$ is obtained as $\pi_n^A(\theta_R|S)$ in the same manner as Eq. (2.2). Then, for $S = 1, \ldots, n$, the posterior probability that θ_R is greater than $\theta_{R,0} + \delta$, denoted as $p_n(S)$, can be represented as follows:

$$p_n(S) = \pi_n^A(\theta_R > \theta_{R,0} + \delta|S).$$

For a pre-specified probability threshold $\lambda \in (0,1)$, the treatment is declared efficacious if the observed number of successes s is such that

$$p_n(s) = \pi_n^A(\theta_R > \theta_{R,0} + \delta|S = s) \geq \lambda. \tag{3.2}$$

The predictive probability criterion is defined as follows [9]: for a pre-specified probability threshold $\gamma \in (0,1)$, the smallest n is selected as the sample size N, such that

$$\mathrm{P}^{\mathrm{D}}[p_{\mathrm{n}}(s) \geq \lambda] \geq \gamma,$$

where P^{D} is the probability measure associated with the prior predictive distribution on the design prior. The prior predictive distribution is given by

$$m^{\mathrm{D}}(s) = \int_0^1 f_{\mathrm{n}}(s|\theta_{\mathrm{R}})\pi^{\mathrm{D}}(\theta_{\mathrm{R}})\mathrm{d}\theta_{\mathrm{R}} \quad \text{for all} \quad s = 0, \ldots, n.$$

The prior predictive probability of the treatment being declared efficacious at the sample size N may therefore be rewritten as

$$\mathrm{P}^{\mathrm{D}}[p_{\mathrm{N}}(s) \geq \lambda] = \sum_{s=u_{\mathrm{N}}}^{N} m^{\mathrm{D}}(s), \tag{3.3}$$

where $u_{\mathrm{N}} = \min\{s \in \{0, \ldots, N\} : p_{\mathrm{N}}(s) \geq \lambda\}$.

In the PSSD, the above sample size N can be adaptively increased up to a maximum, denoted as $N_{\max}$, during the course of a trial, depending on some belief of the efficacy probability. A method for determining a maximum sample size $N_{\max}$ can be based on a 'sceptical' design prior $\pi^{\mathrm{D}}_{\mathrm{scept}}(\theta_{\mathrm{R}})$. This design prior has the same beta distribution as Eq. (3.1), but reflects a sceptical belief of the efficacy probability, such that

$$\pi^{\mathrm{D}}_{\mathrm{scept}}(\theta_{\mathrm{R}}) = \mathrm{Beta}(\theta_{\mathrm{R}}; n^{\mathrm{D}}\pi^{\mathrm{D}}_{0,\mathrm{scept}} + 1, n^{\mathrm{D}}(1 - \pi^{\mathrm{D}}_{0,\mathrm{scept}}) + 1),$$

where $\pi^{\mathrm{D}}_{0,\mathrm{scept}}$ represents the mode of $\pi^{\mathrm{D}}_{\mathrm{scept}}(\theta_{\mathrm{R}})$. But note that if it should be determined that $\theta_{\mathrm{R},0} + \delta < \pi^{\mathrm{D}}_{0,\mathrm{scept}} < \pi^{\mathrm{D}}_0$, although n^{D} is not changed in $\pi^{\mathrm{D}}(\theta_{\mathrm{R}})$, it results in $N < N_{\max}$. In the same manner as Eq. (3.3), the prior predictive probability on the sample size $N_{\max}$ is given by

$$\mathrm{P}^{\mathrm{D}}[p_{\mathrm{N}_{\max}}(s) \geq \lambda] = \sum_{s=u_{\mathrm{N}_{\max}}}^{N_{\max}} m^{\mathrm{D}}(s),$$

where $u_{\mathrm{N}_{\max}} = \min\{s \in \{0, \ldots, N_{\max}\} : p_{\mathrm{N}_{\max}}(s) \geq \lambda\}$.

Table 1 shows the required sample size N for different values of $\theta_{\mathrm{R},0} + \delta$, π^{D}_0, n^{D}, λ and γ ($\pi^{\mathrm{A}}(\theta_{\mathrm{R}}) = \mathrm{Beta}(1,1)$: non-informative). $n^{\mathrm{D}} = 100$ corresponds to approximately 0.20 for the range of the 95% credible interval. The larger λ or γ is relative to the other parameters, the greater the sample size. The choice of π^{D}_0 has some degree of impact on the sample size, and n^{D} has a large effect if π^{D}_0 is close to

Table 1 Sample size N for different criteria and values of $\theta_{R,0}+\delta$, π_0^D, n^D, λ and γ ($\pi^A(\theta_R) = \text{Beta}(1,1)$)

$\theta_{R,0}+\delta$	γ	π_0^D											
		$(\theta_{R,0}+\delta)+0.10$				$(\theta_{R,0}+\delta)+0.15$				$(\theta_{R,0}+\delta)+0.20$			
		n^D				n^D				n^D			
		100		∞		100		∞		100		∞	
		λ		λ		λ		λ		λ		λ	
		0.8	0.9	0.8	0.9	0.8	0.9	0.8	0.9	0.8	0.9	0.8	0.9
0.2	0.7	38	67	34 [48]	58 [72]	16	29	16 [26]	29 [38]	12	17	9 [17]	17 [22]
	0.8	65	107	51 [70]	84 [98]	29	42	25 [34]	41 [47]	16	25	16 [22]	22 [30]
	0.9	143	A	87 [102]	124 [135]	51	72	42 [48]	58 [68]	25	41	21 [30]	33 [42]
0.3	0.7	50	90	44 [57]	75 [88]	20	37	20 [27]	34 [41]	14	20	11 [18]	20 [24]
	0.8	93	154	68 [76]	105 [115]	32	57	29 [36]	48 [58]	20	31	17 [24]	28 [32]
	0.9	A	A	103 [119]	154 [162]	65	99	47 [57]	69 [79]	32	51	26 [33]	37 [44]
0.4	0.7	61	103	47 [62]	82 [97]	24	39	24 [26]	39 [45]	15	24	15 [16]	22 [29]
	0.8	106	185	75 [83]	117 [125]	40	66	33 [41]	48 [58]	22	33	16 [25]	28 [34]
	0.9	A	A	113 [126]	166 [179]	75	110	52 [55]	73 [83]	33	51	29 [34]	40 [49]

(continued)

Table 1 (continued)

$\theta_{R,0}+\delta$	γ	π_0^D											
		$(\theta_{R,0}+\delta)+0.10$				$(\theta_{R,0}+\delta)+0.15$				$(\theta_{R,0}+\delta)+0.20$			
		n^D				n^D				n^D			
		100		∞		100		∞		100		∞	
		λ		λ		λ		λ		λ		λ	
		0.8	0.9	0.8	0.9	0.8	0.9	0.8	0.9	0.8	0.9	0.8	0.9
0.5	0.7	61	110	53 [60]	89 [94]	27	43	25 [28]	41 [44]	14	25	14 [17]	23 [26]
	0.8	118	199	76 [83]	121 [126]	40	65	36 [41]	52 [57]	23	34	18 [24]	30 [33]
	0.9	A	A	118 [125]	167 [179]	76	112	53 [58]	76 [79]	36	52	29 [32]	41 [44]
0.6	0.7	59	110	51 [57]	80 [92]	26	44	23 [27]	38 [42]	15	23	15 [16]	20 [24]
	0.8	112	185	72 [76]	110 [119]	40	60	32 [35]	46 [53]	21	29	18 [22]	26 [30]
	0.9	A	A	112 [115]	155 [162]	67	102	48 [52]	69 [73]	32	46	26 [30]	38 [42]
0.7	0.7	58	93	47 [48]	75 [76]	20	36	20 [21]	32 [33]	13	20	13 [14]	15 [21]
	0.8	94	152	61 [70]	93 [102]	36	52	28 [29]	40 [45]	17	24	17 [18]	20 [25]
	0.9	A	A	94 [98]	134 [135]	54	78	39 [44]	56 [57]	24	36	20 [21]	28 [29]

Label A means $N > 200$. The numbers within brackets indicate sample sizes based on a binomial distribution using the frequentist approach with $\alpha = 1 - \lambda$ and $\beta = 1 - \gamma$

$\theta_{R,0} + \delta$. The two-priors approach is a general framework that incorporates the frequentist SSD method as a special case when $\pi^A(\theta_R)$ is non-informative and $\pi^D(\theta_R)$ is degenerate. The sample size for $n^D = \infty$ is slightly larger but almost the same as that obtained from the frequentist approach that corresponds to the hypothesis testing framework: null hypothesis $H_0 : \theta \le \theta_{R,0} + \delta$ and alternative hypothesis $H_1 : \theta \ge \pi_0^D$, $\alpha = 1 - \lambda$ and $\beta = 1 - \gamma$. The frequentist results are displayed in brackets in Table 1.

3.2 Sample Size Selection

To select the sample size, we specify the number of sample size selections, K. We recommend $K = 1$ because multiple sample size selections result in complicated switching between N and N_{max} during the course of a trial. Given a sample size N or N_{max} (see Sect. 3.1), suppose that we plan J interim observations or 'looks' for efficacy ($J \ge K$). Let n_j be the number of patients at interim observation j for $j = 1, 2, \ldots, J$, and let $S_j = \sum_{i=1}^{n_j} Y_{S,i}$ be the number of efficacies obtained at the interim observation of n_j patients. After observing s_j successes out of n_j patients, the posterior predictive distribution for S at interim observation j, denoted as $m(s)$, is given by the beta-binomial, since:

$$m(s) = \int_0^1 f_{r_j}(s|\theta_R)\pi_{n_j}(\theta_R|S_j = s_j)d\theta_R \quad \text{for all} \quad s = 0, \ldots, r_j, \tag{3.4}$$

where $r_j = N - n_j$ or $r_j = N_{max} - n_j$.

Then, we make a choice between N and N_{max} as the final sample size on the basis of the posterior predictive probabilities that are calculated based on Eq. (3.4) for N and N_{max}, that is, $\sum_{s=u_N-s_j}^{N-n_j} m(s)$ and $\sum_{s=u_{N_{max}}-s_j}^{N_{max}-n_j} m(s)$. If $\sum_{s=u_N-s_j}^{N-n_j} m(s)$ is greater than or equal to $\sum_{s=u_{N_{max}}-s_j}^{N_{max}-n_j} m(s)$, N is selected; otherwise, N_{max} is selected.

3.3 Interim Monitoring for Efficacy

Interim monitoring for efficacy should be based on predictive probability to be consistent with the sample size determination and selection process. As mentioned above, the predictive probability during the trial depends on the final sample size, N or N_{max}. The stopping rule for efficacy is as follows: let $\tau_R \in [0, 1]$ be pre-specified probability thresholds. If $\sum_{s=u_N-s_j}^{N-n_j} m(s) < \tau_R$ under the final sample size N or $\sum_{s=u_{N_{max}}-s_j}^{N_{max}-n_j} m(s) < \tau_R$ under the final sample size N_{max}(see Sect. 3.2), we will stop the trial for inefficacy; otherwise, the trial will be continued until the next interim observation or the final analysis.

4 Procedures and Operating Characteristics for PSSD

Before starting a trial

Step 1: Determine two sample sizes, N and $N_{\max}$.
Step 2: Specify an interim monitoring plan.
Step 3: Specify a sample size selection plan.

During the trial

Step 1: At the interim looks for efficacy, if the predictive probability for efficacy is low, stop the trial for inefficacy; otherwise, continue the trial.
Step 2: At the interim look with sample size selection, choose between N and $N_{\max}$ as the final sample size, based on the predictive probabilities.

4.1 Example

Suppose that the design parameters are specified as $\theta_{R,0} + \delta = 0.3$, $\pi_0^D = 0.50$, $\pi_{0,\text{scept}}^D = 0.45$, $n^D = \infty$, $\pi^A(\theta_R) = \text{Beta}(1,1)$, $\lambda = 0.9$ and $\gamma = 0.8$. In this case, the two sample sizes will be calculated as $N = 28$ and $N_{\max} = 48$. An interim analysis is planned after enrolling 10 patients and sample size selection is also planned at that

Table 2 Posterior mean and predictive probability at the first interim look, when $\theta_{R,0} + \delta = 0.3$, $\pi_0^D = 0.50$, $\pi_{0,\text{scept}}^D = 0.45$, $n^D = \infty$, $\pi^A(\theta_R) = \text{Beta}(1,1)$, $\lambda = 0.9$, $\gamma = 0.8$, $n_1 = 10$, $\tau_R = 0.1$

s_1	Posterior mean	Predictive probability	
		$N = 28$ ($u_N = 12$)	$N_{\max} = 48$ ($u_{N_{\max}} = 19$)
0	0.083	0.00035	0.00187
1	0.167	0.00710	0.02146
2	0.250	0.05347	0.10543
3	0.333	0.20806	**0.30009**
4	0.417	0.48631	**0.57091**
5	0.500	0.76962	**0.80789**
6	0.583	0.93489	**0.94059**
7	0.667	**0.98937**	0.98799
8	0.750	**0.99910**	0.99852
9	0.833	**0.99996**	0.99990
10	0.917	**1.00000**	0.99999

time. Suppose that the probability threshold for inefficacy stopping τ_R is 0.1. Table 2 shows the posterior mean and predictive probability for success number at the first interim look s_1 (=0,...,10). If s_1 is 2 or less, the predictive probability of trial success is smaller than 0.1 and the trial will be stopped for inefficacy. If s_1 is 3 or more, the trial will be continued until the final analysis, and the sample size will be selected by comparing the predictive probabilities. If s_1 is 3–6, the predictive probability under N_{max} is larger than that under N (*in boldface*), and thus N_{max} = 48 should be selected. If s_1 is 7 or more, the predictive probability under N is larger than that under N_{max} (*in boldface*), and thus N = 28 should be selected.

4.2 Operating Characteristics

We have compared the frequentist operating characteristics of the proposed design with those of fixed sample size designs based on 10,000 simulated trials. The data were generated from Bernoulli distributions. In the context of hypothesis testing, $H_0 : \theta \leq \theta_{R,0} + \delta$ versus $H_1 : \theta \geq \pi_0^D$, the evaluated properties are the probability of a type I error at $\theta = \theta_{R,0} + \delta$, the probability of type II errors at $\theta = \pi_0^D$ and $\theta = \pi_{0,scept}^D$, the probability of early termination (PET) and the expected sample size (ESS) at pre-specified design values. Table 3 shows the results when $\theta_{R,0} + \delta$ = 0.30, π_0^D = 0.50, $\pi_{0,scept}^D$ = 0.45, $n^D = \infty$, $\pi^A(\theta_R) = \text{Beta}(1, 1)$, λ = 0.9, γ = 0.8, N = 28, N_{max} = 48, τ_R = 0.1. As references, two fixed sample size designs (A: π_0^D = 0.50 and N = 28; B: π_0^D = 0.45 and N = 48) are considered.

As the number of interim looks increases, the probability of type I errors slightly decreases and that of type II errors increases. The type I error probabilities of the proposed PSSD are similar to those of the non-adaptive designs (nearly equal to $1 - \lambda$). In this case, as the fixed sample size design A or B without interim analysis is optimised at $\theta = \pi_0^D$ (=0.50) or $\theta = \pi_{0,scept}^D$ (=0.45), respectively, the type II error probabilities evaluated at these values are around 0.20 (equal to $1 - \gamma$). The type II error probabilities of the PSSD are between those of the two fixed sample size designs. The type II error probabilities in the PSSD are around 0.05 higher than that in fixed sample size design B. It was found that the PET increases and the ESS decreases as the number of interim looks increases. The ESS of the PSSD are between those of the two non-adaptive designs.

5 An Extension of the PSSD

The process of sample size determination and selection, and interim monitoring for efficacy for the extension of the PSSD is the same as that of the original PSSD. In this extension, we need to specify an interim monitoring plan for toxicity.

Table 3 Type I error, type II error, probability of early termination and expected sample size for various designs, when $\theta_{R,0} + \delta = 0.30$, $\pi_0^D = 0.50$, $\pi_{0,scept}^D = 0.45$, $n^D = \infty$, $\pi^A(\theta_R) = \text{Beta}(1, 1)$, $\lambda = 0.9$, $\gamma = 0.8$, $N = 28$, $N_{max} = 48$, $\tau_R = 0.1$

(Proposed design: $N = 28$, $N_{max} = 48$)		$\theta_R = 0.30$			$\theta_R = 0.45$			$\theta_R = 0.50$		
		Type I error	PET	ESS	Type II error	PET	ESS	Type II error	PET	ESS
P1	One interim analysis: $n_1 = 10$, and one sample size selection: $n_1 = 10$	0.094	0.386	33.1	0.252	0.105	42.0	0.106	0.060	42.4
P2	Two interim analyses: $n_1 = 10$, $n_2 = 20$, and one sample size selection: $n_2 = 10$	0.092	0.515	29.5	0.260	0.129	41.3	0.110	0.069	42.1
Fixed sample size design A: $N = 28$										
A0	No interim analysis:	0.100	–	–	0.346	–	–	0.182	–	–
A1	One interim analysis: $n_1 = 10$	0.096	0.384	21.1	0.367	0.096	26.3	0.205	0.058	27.0
A2	Two interim analyses: $n_1 = 10$, $n_2 = 20$	0.094	0.653	18.9	0.372	0.177	25.6	0.209	0.095	26.7
Fixed sample size design B: $N = 48$										
B0	No interim analysis:	0.097	–	–	0.189	–	–	0.054	–	–
B1	One interim analysis: $n_1 = 10$	0.095	0.148	42.4	0.201	0.025	47.1	0.062	0.012	47.5
B2	Two interim analyses: $n_1 = 10$, $n_2 = 20$	0.091	0.438	34.3	0.214	0.067	45.9	0.071	0.028	47.1

PET probability of early termination, *ESS* expected sample size

5.1 Interim Monitoring for Toxicity

In the following, suppose that we plan L interim observations or 'looks' for toxicity. We assume that the number of interim observations of toxicity, will be equal to or larger than that of interim observations of efficacy, J (see Sect. 3.3); $L \geq J$. Let n_l be the number of patients at interim observation l for $l = 1, 2, \ldots, L$; then $\{n_1, \ldots, n_\mathrm{J}\} \in \{n_1, \ldots, n_\mathrm{L}\}$, that is, the J efficacy analyses are a subset of the L safety analyses.

There are two types of options available for methods of safety monitoring: the posterior probability-based method and the predictive probability-based method.

Posterior probability-based method

Let $\theta_{\mathrm{T},0}$ denote a pre-specified maximum tolerated toxicity value, and let $T_\mathrm{l} = \sum_{i=1}^{n_\mathrm{l}} Y_{\mathrm{T,i}}$ be the number of toxicities obtained at the interim observation of n_l patients. At the lth interim observation, if t_l patients among n_l patients experience toxicity, then the posterior distribution is $\pi_{\mathrm{n_l}}(\theta_\mathrm{T}|T_\mathrm{l} = t_\mathrm{l})$ (see Eq. 2.2). The posterior probability that the toxicity probability θ_T is greater than $\theta_{\mathrm{T},0}$ is then

$$p_{\mathrm{n_l}}(T_\mathrm{l}) = \pi_{\mathrm{n_l}}(\theta_\mathrm{T} > \theta_{\mathrm{T},0}|T_\mathrm{l}).$$

For a pre-specified probability threshold $\omega_\mathrm{T} \in (0, 1)$, the trial will be stopped for safety if the observed number of toxicities t_l is such that $p_{\mathrm{n_l}}(t_\mathrm{l}) \geq \omega_\mathrm{T}$; otherwise, the trial will be continued until the next interim observation or the final analysis.

For a pre-specified probability threshold $M_{2i} \geq M_{1i}$, the trial will be stopped for safety if the observed number of toxicities *PFSr* is such that *PFS*; otherwise, the trial will be continued until the next interim observation or the final analysis.

Predictive probability-based method

Let the minimum number of toxicities for the treatment being declared toxic at sample size N and N_max be denoted $v_\mathrm{N} = \min\{t \in \{0, \ldots, N\}\}$ such that $p_\mathrm{N}(t) \geq \omega_\mathrm{T}$, and $v_{\mathrm{N_{max}}} = \min\{t \in \{0, \ldots, N_\mathrm{max}\}\}$ such that $p_{\mathrm{N_{max}}}(t) \geq \omega_\mathrm{T}$. At the lth interim observation, if t_l patients among n_l patients experience toxicity, the posterior predictive distribution for T at interim observation l, denoted as $m(t)$, is again given by beta-binomial, since:

$$m(t) = \int_0^1 f_{\mathrm{r_l}}(t|\theta_\mathrm{T})\pi_{\mathrm{n_l}}(\theta_\mathrm{T}|T_\mathrm{l} = t_\mathrm{l})\mathrm{d}\theta_\mathrm{T} \quad \text{for all} \quad t = 0, \ldots, r_\mathrm{l}, \tag{5.1}$$

where $r_l = N - n_l$ or $r_l = N_\mathrm{max} - n_l$. Based on Eq. (5.1), the posterior predictive probabilities for toxicity for N and N_max, are represented as $\sum_{t=v_\mathrm{N}-t_\mathrm{l}}^{N-n_\mathrm{l}} m(t)$ and $\sum_{t=v_{\mathrm{N_{max}}}-t_\mathrm{l}}^{N_\mathrm{max}-n_\mathrm{l}} m(t)$, respectively, in the same manner as those for efficacy. The stopping rule is as follows. Let $\tau_\mathrm{T} \in [0, 1]$ be the pre-specified probability thresholds. If $\sum_{t=v_\mathrm{N}-t_\mathrm{l}}^{N-n_\mathrm{l}} m(t) > \tau_\mathrm{T}$ under the final sample size N or $\sum_{t=v_{\mathrm{N_{max}}}-t_\mathrm{l}}^{N_\mathrm{max}-n_\mathrm{l}} m(t) > \tau_\mathrm{T}$ under the final sample size $N_{\max}$, the trial will be stopped for toxicity; otherwise, the trial will be continued until the next interim observation or the final analysis.

5.2 Simulation Study

Suppose that the design parameters are specified as $\theta_{R,0} + \delta = 0.3$, $\pi_0^D = 0.5$, $\pi_{0,\text{scept}}^D = 0.45$, $n^D = \infty$, $\pi^A(\theta_R) = \text{Beta}(1,1)$, $\lambda = 0.9$ and $\gamma = 0.8$. In this case, the two sample sizes are $N = 28$ and $N_{\max} = 48$. The interim observation for sample size selection is planned once after enrolling 10 patients, i.e., $K = 1$, and the interim observation for efficacy is planned twice after enrolling 10 and 20 patients, i.e., $J = 2$, with $\tau_R = 0.1$.

Suppose that the pre-specified maximum tolerated toxicity value $\theta_{T,0}$ is 0.2 and the two types of priors for toxicity probability with the same mode (0.2) are $\pi(\theta_T) = \text{Beta}(1.2, 1.8)$ and $\pi(\theta_T) = \text{Beta}(3,9)$, which represent a less informative case and a more informative case, respectively. In particular, the latter corresponds to the case in which data on toxicity from the previous phase I trials are available. For the safety monitoring plan, we will have eight interim analyses; that is $L = 8$ and $n_l = 10, 15, 20, 25, 30, 35, 40, 45$. We specify ω_T as 0.8 in the posterior probability-based method and both ω_T and τ_T as 0.8 in the predictive probability-based method.

Under the following six scenarios, we examined the operating characteristics, the probability of early termination (PET) and the expected sample size (ESS), of the proposed design based on 10,000 simulated trials.

Scenario 1: low response and low toxicity (true response $\theta_R^* = 0.3$ and true toxicity $\theta_T^* = 0.1$)
Scenario 2: low response and middle toxicity ($\theta_R^* = 0.3$ and $\theta_T^* = 0.2$)
Scenario 3: low response and high toxicity ($\theta_R^* = 0.3$ and $\theta_T^* = 0.3$)
Scenario 4: high response and low toxicity ($\theta_R^* = 0.5$ and $\theta_T^* = 0.1$)
Scenario 5: high response and middle toxicity ($\theta_R^* = 0.5$ and $\theta_T^* = 0.2$)
Scenario 6: high response and high toxicity ($\theta_R^* = 0.5$ and $\theta_T^* = 0.3$)

To incorporate the correlation ρ between efficacy and toxicity into the simulations, the joint probability θ_{RT}^* is transformed into a correlation through the following relationship [20]:

$$\rho = \frac{\theta_{RT}^* - \theta_R^* \theta_T^*}{\sqrt{\theta_R^*(1-\theta_R^*)\theta_T^*(1-\theta_T^*)}}.$$

The range of the correlation is limited by the joint probability. When $\theta_{RT}^* = 0$, the correlation will be the smallest at

Table 4 Stopping boundaries for safety monitoring

Prior: $\pi(\theta_T)$	Methods for safety monitoring	n_1							
		10	15	20	25	30	35	40	45
Beta(1.2, 1.8)	*Posterior probability-based*	3	5	6	7	8	9	10	11
	Predictive probability-based								
	$N = 28$	4	5	7	8	–	–	–	–
	$N_{max} = 48$	4	5	6	8	9	10	11	12
Beta(3, 9)	*Posterior probability-based*	4	5	6	7	8	9	11	12
	Predictive probability-based								
	$N = 28$	5	6	7	8	–	–	–	–
	$N_{max} = 48$	4	6	7	8	9	10	11	12

$$\frac{-\theta_R^*\theta_T^*}{\sqrt{\theta_R^*(1-\theta_R^*)\theta_T^*(1-\theta_T^*)}}.$$

Conversely, when $\theta_{RT}^* = \min(\theta_R^*, \theta_T^*)$, the correlation will be the largest value. We conducted simulations for each scenario under three possible correlations: minimum/negative, none/zero, and maximum/positive.

Table 4 shows the safety stopping boundaries according to different priors and methods to monitor safety. In this setting, the prior for toxicity has little impact on the stopping boundary. The posterior-based method has a more stringent stopping boundary for toxicity than the predictive-based method.

In Table 5, we show the simulation results when $\pi(\theta_T) = \text{Beta}(1.2, 1.8)$ using the two types of methods of safety monitoring, compared with the results of using efficacy monitoring alone as references. In each cell, the maximum value and the minimum value as a range under the three possible correlations are shown. Both methods have similar operating characteristics under all the scenarios. When the response is low (scenario 1–3), the probability of positive results is 0.087 under the reference case, which corresponds to a type I error rate, i.e., $1 - \lambda = 0.1$. The higher the true toxicity, the lower are the probabilities of positive results, the PET for inefficacy, and the ESS. By contrast, the PET for toxicity dramatically increases according to the true toxicity probability. If toxicity is high (scenario 3), then the trial will stop for toxicity with probability of 0.45–0.6. If response is high (scenarios 4–6), the probability of positive results will be 0.893, which corresponds to the power. The higher the true toxicity, the lower are the probability of positive results and the ESS. However, the PET for inefficacy remains unchanged. In particular, if toxicity is low (scenario 4), the probability of positive results (the power) is still greater than 0.8. If toxicity is high (scenario 6), the trial will stop for toxicity with probability of 0.7–0.85. The posterior probability-based method has a higher PET for toxicity due to the stringent stopping boundary. The simulation results for $\pi(\theta_T) = \text{Beta}(3, 9)$ show less PET for toxicity than for $\pi(\theta_T) = \text{Beta}(1.2, 1.8)$, reflecting the less stringent stopping boundaries.

Table 5 Probability of positive results, probability of early termination and expected sample size under various scenarios when $\pi(\theta_T) = \text{Beta}(1.2, 1.8)$

Methods and scenarios		Probability of positive results	PET for inefficacy	PET for toxicity	ESS
Posterior probability based method for safety monitoring					
Efficacy monitoring only		0.087	0.511	–	29.7
Efficacy and safety monitoring					
Low response ($\theta_R^* = 0.3$)	1. Low toxicity ($\theta_T^* = 0.1$)	0.065–0.083	0.503	0.031–0.083	27.0–28.8
	2. Middle toxicity ($\theta_T^* = 0.2$)	0.008–0.061	0.464–0.469	0.234–0.402	17.3–23.7
	3. High toxicity ($\theta_T^* = 0.3$)	0.000–0.023	0.381–0.426	0.513–0.619	10.0–16.0
Efficacy monitoring only		0.893	0.065	–	42.1
Efficacy and safety monitoring					
High response ($\theta_R^* = 0.5$)	4. Low toxicity ($\theta_T^* = 0.1$)	0.812–0.832	0.064–0.065	0.068–0.084	39.5–39.8
	5. Middle toxicity ($\theta_T^* = 0.2$)	0.425–0.498	0.059–0.064	0.433–0.480	28.9–29.1
	6. High toxicity ($\theta_T^* = 0.3$)	0.056–0.146	0.057–0.063	0.797–0.868	16.7–17.5
Predictive probability based method for safety monitoring					
Efficacy monitoring only		0.087	0.511	–	29.7
Efficacy and safety monitoring					
Low response ($\theta_R^* = 0.3$)	1. Low toxicity ($\theta_T^* = 0.1$)	0.078–0.086	0.508–0.510	0.007–0.026	28.9–29.5
	2. Middle toxicity ($\theta_T^* = 0.2$)	0.017–0.072	0.485–0.501	0.145–0.273	21.6–26.3
	3. High toxicity ($\theta_T^* = 0.3$)	0.000–0.037	0.436–0.466	0.445–0.534	12.0–19.1
Efficacy monitoring only		0.893	0.065	–	42.1
Efficacy and safety monitoring					
High response ($\theta_R^* = 0.5$)	4. Low toxicity ($\theta_T^* = 0.1$)	0.868–0.875	0.065	0.022–0.026	41.4–41.5
	5. Middle toxicity ($\theta_T^* = 0.2$)	0.586–0.645	0.061–0.065	0.278–0.312	34.0–34.5
	6. High toxicity ($\theta_T^* = 0.3$)	0.127–0.236	0.058–0.065	0.706–0.787	21.3–21.7

PET probability of early termination, *ESS* expected sample size

6 An Illustrative Example

Marlin et al. [21] conducted a single-arm trial for assessing success rates in children of achieving optimal hematopoietic progenitor cells harvest after mobilization with 300 μg/kg of pegfilgrastim. The success was defined as achieving at least 5×10^6

CD34+ cells/kg during the first standard apheresis (less than 3 blood volumes processed). There was no planned sample size, with a target success rate of 30%. After 26 inclusions, the final success rate was 61.5% (16/26). Out of the first 10, 20, and 26 enrolled patients, successes were observed in 7, 10, and 16 patients, respectively. In this trial, no drug-related adverse events (AE) of grade >3 occurred.

For illustration of the proposed approach, we hypothetically specified the design parameters such that $\theta_{R,0} + \delta = 0.3$, $\pi_0^D = 0.5$, $\pi_{0,\text{scept}}^D = 0.45$, $n^D = \infty$, $\pi^A(\theta_R) = \text{Beta}(1, 1)$, $\lambda = 0.8$, $\gamma = 0.9$. From these parameters, the two sample sizes were calculated as $N = 26$ ($u_N = 10$) and $N_{\max} = 47$ ($u_{N_{\max}} = 17$). Suppose that two efficacy interim analyses were planned after enrolling the first 10 and 20 patients ($n_1 = 10$, $n_2 = 20$), and sample size selection was planned at the first interim analysis, i.e., $J = 2$ and $K = 1$. Suppose that the probability threshold for inefficacy stopping τ_R was 0.1. For safety monitoring, suppose that $\theta_{T,0} = 0.2$, $\pi(\theta_T) = \text{Beta}(1.2, 1.8)$, $L = 8$ and $n_l = 10, 15, 20, 25, 30, 35, 40, 45$. If we specify ω_T as 0.8 in the posterior probability-based method, the stopping boundary for safety monitoring was shown in the first row of Table 4.

In the case of low toxicity such that the observed AE would be under the stopping boundary, at the first interim analysis for efficacy, the success rate was 70% (7/10) and the predictive probability $\sum_{s=N-7}^{N-10} m^A(s)$ was 0.998, and $\sum_{s=N_{\max}-7}^{N_{\max}-10} m^A(s)$ was 0.995. Because the former value was over 0.10, the trial had not been stopped for inefficacy. For the sample size selection, as the predictive probability based on N was larger than that based on $N_{\max}$, N should be selected as the re-determined sample size. At the second interim analysis for efficacy, the success rate was 50% (10/20). As the predictive probability $\sum_{s=N-10}^{N-20} m^A(s)$ was 1, the trial had been continued until 26 patients were enrolled. Because the final success rate was 61.5% (16/26), the posterior mean was 60.7% (95% credible interval: 42.4–77.6%) and the posterior probability that the success probability was greater than the target value was as follows:

$$\pi_{26}^A(\theta_R > 0.3 | S = 16) = 0.9996$$

Accordingly, we would conclude that a single injection of pegfilgrastim in the haematological steady state is an efficient and well-tolerated method in children with solid malignancies, as also concluded in the original report. By contrast, in the case of high toxicity such that the observed AE would be over the stopping boundary, the trial could be stopped for safety before reaching the determined sample size.

7 Conclusion Remarks

The PSSD is a coherent Bayesian adaptive design in the sense that we only use predictive probabilities for determining sample sizes, monitoring efficacy outcomes, and selecting a final sample size. At the design stage, we recommend that an analysis prior $\pi^{A}(\theta)$ should be objectively determined based on prior information such as reliable historical or external data. In practice, Biswas et al. [22] have reported that they have used 20% or less as a discount factor for historical information. As a result, if it is difficult to take existing information into consideration, since the amount of available data can be limited and there can be some uncertainty about the treatment effect in most exploratory clinical trials, a uniform non-informative analysis prior Beta$(1, 1)$ may be appropriate. Robust Bayesian SSD [9] considers a class of plausible analysis priors instead of a single analysis prior in order to incorporate the uncertainty of prior information into SSD. However, it should be emphasised that uncertainty in a design prior is more important for SSD, where the inference could be based on subjective information about the quantity of interest. To consider the uncertainty of prior information, we employ n^{D} (a tuning parameter for the variance of design priors) and two kinds of design priors. The elicitation and determination of design parameters, including $\theta_{R,0}$, δ, $\pi^{A}(\theta_{R})$, $\pi^{D}(\theta_{R})$ and $\pi^{D}_{scept}(\theta_{R})$, are essential aspects of designing clinical trials.

In the PSSD, the sample size determination is based on the approach of Sambucini [8] and Brutti et al. [9]. On the other hand, the interim monitoring based on predictive probability is based on the method of Lee et al. [12]. As they emphasised, the predictive probability approach for interim monitoring is a consistent, efficient and flexible method that more closely resembles the clinical decision making process. Unlike the approach by Lee et al. [12], the PSSD does not require intensive computation for sample size searching due to the separation of the interim monitoring procedure from the SSD procedure. Instead, comprehensive simulations may be required at the design phase to evaluate the operating characteristics (including type I and type II error probabilities) from the frequentist point of view. The adaptive predictive single threshold design (APSTD) by Sambucini [10] is an adaptive design that allows additional sample size while keeping the 'Bayesian power' based on updated information, i.e., updated analysis priors and updated design priors. In the APSTD, the consistency of design parameters between SSD at the first stage and sample size re-estimation at the second stage (adaptive stage) seems not clear, and early stopping for efficacy is inevitably incorporated into the procedure. In contrast, our design provides two fixed sample sizes (N and N_{max}), mainly for practical reasons, and it selects an optimal sample size by comparing the 'Bayesian power' between the two sample sizes at the interim stage. The difference in 'Bayesian power' may be very small (at most 0.10 as shown in the example of Table 2). By applying sample size selection, however, type II error probabilities are reduced by 0.10–0.12 while type I error probabilities remain unchanged, as shown in Table 3.

We also proposed an extension of the PSSD to monitor efficacy with sample size adaptation, and add continuous monitoring of safety. In the design, we considered two types of methods to monitor safety: the posterior-based method and the predictive-based method. From the simulation results using the same threshold values ($\omega_{T} = \tau_{T} = 0.8$), the probability of early termination for toxicity with the posterior-based method is higher than that with the predictive-based method. This is due to the way the stopping boundaries are determined, so that the boundaries of the posterior-based method are similar to but slightly more stringent than that of the predictive-based method. As a result, we recommend the posterior probability based-method to monitor safety, because in general posterior probabilities are easier to calculate and interpret than predictive probabilities. To determine priors of toxicity probabilities, we may use toxicity data from previous phase I trials. However, if the prior is too informative, the prior will dominate stopping boundaries over data from current trials. Therefore, we propose the less informative prior for toxicity, for example, $\pi(\theta_{\mathrm{T}}) = \mathrm{Beta}(\theta_{\mathrm{T}}; a_{\mathrm{T}}, b_{\mathrm{T}})$ with hyperparameters $a_{\mathrm{T}} = p_{\mathrm{T}} + 1$ and $b_{\mathrm{T}} = (1 - p_{\mathrm{T}}) + 1$, where p_{T} is an average toxicity probability estimated from the previous studies. Thall et al. [15] and Brutti et al. [23] assumed the Dirichlet-multinomial model which took into account the association between the toxicity and efficacy outcomes, in order to allow us to monitor both of them. The former provided an approach for multi-stage or continuous monitoring for multiple outcomes but not a sample size determination. Two stopping boundaries of this approach were substantially constructed on the basis of the beta-binomial models, the so-called marginal models, for the toxicity and efficacy outcomes. The latter developed a sample size determination scheme in the context of two-stage monitoring. Its stopping boundaries were based on the joint probability of simultaneously experiencing efficacy and no toxicity and on the marginal probability of experiencing toxicity. On the other hand, we combined both ideas and give a compromise proposal. Consequently, our proposed design has the following advantages: (1) frequent, multi-stage, or continuous monitoring for the toxicity and efficacy outcomes like Thall et al.'s approach, (2) sample size determination at the planning stage of a trial like Brutti et al.'s design, plus the sample size selection during a course of the trial, and (3) much easier design parameter specification and computational procedure for the marginal model than counterparts for the joint model. For the first advantage, being able to have a close monitoring of the tolerance without penalising the efficacy monitoring is more ethical for patients, as in early phase clinical trials the safety of a new drug or combination is still uncertain. Particularly, the designs based on the joint model would, if anything, intend to simultaneously monitor both safety and efficacy at any interim observation. Unless both types of monitoring are completed, the joint probability of simultaneously experiencing efficacy and no toxicity cannot be obtained at the interim observation. For the second advantage, the sample size required for a trial from a viewpoint of efficacy can be not only determined in advance but also increased as necessary in our proposed design. However, the third advantage, to put it the other way around, leads to some limitation of our design that cannot explicitly consider the association between toxicity and efficacy outcomes. It will be possible to further extend the design to single-arm trials with multinomial endpoints with the use of the Dirichlet-multinomial model, as such a model has some advantages in terms of flexibility with respect to types of endpoints and their associations, although it may be more complicated. The design could be also extended to multi-arm trials, other types of endpoints, and other types of outcome measures including odds ratios or relative risks through more appropriate Bayesian modelling.

Acknowledgements This work was supported in part by Grant-in Aid for Scientific Research (26330037) from Japan Society for the Promotion of Science, Japan. The author is grateful to Dr. Takashi Daimon, Hyogo College of Medicine, Hyogo, Japan, and Dr. Sarah Zohar, INSERM, U1138 team 22, Paris, France, for their contributions to this research.

References

1. Therasse P, Arbuck SG, Eisenhauer EA, Wanders J, Kaplan RS, Rubinstein L, Verweij J, Van Glabbeke M, van Oosterom AT, Christian MC, Gwyther SG. New guidelines to evaluate the response to treatment in solid tumors. European Organization for Research and Treatment of Cancer, National Cancer Institute of the United States, National Cancer Institute of Canada. J Natl Cancer Inst. 2000;92:205–16. doi:10.1093/jnci/92.3.205.
2. Simon R. Optimal two-stage designs for phase II clinical trials. Control Clin Trials. 1989;10:1–10. doi:10.1016/0197-2456(89)90015-9.
3. Zohar S, Teramukai S, Zhou Y. Bayesian design and conduct of phase II single-arm clinical trials with binary outcomes: a tutorial. Contemp Clin Trials. 2008;29:608–16. doi:10.1016/j.cct.2007.11.005.
4. Tan SB, Machin D. Bayesian two-stage designs for phase II clinical trials. Stat Med. 2002;21:1991–2012. doi:10.1002/sim.1176.
5. Mayo MS, Gajewski BJ. Bayesian sample size calculations in phase II clinical trials using informative conjugate priors. Control Clin Trials. 2004;25:157–67. doi:10.1016/j.cct.2003.11.006.
6. Gajewski BJ, Mayo MS. Bayesian sample size calculations in phase II clinical trials using a mixture of informative priors. Stat Med. 2006;25:2554–66. doi:10.1002/sim.2450.
7. Whitehead J, Valdés-Márquez E, Johnson P, Graham G. Bayesian sample size for exploratory clinical trials incorporating historical data. Stat Med. 2008;27:2307–27. doi:10.1002/sim.3140.
8. Sambucini V. A Bayesian predictive two-stage design for phase II clinical trials. Stat Med. 2008;27:1199–224. doi:10.1002/sim.3021.
9. Brutti P, De Santis F, Gubbiotti S. Robust Bayesian sample size determination in clinical trials. Stat Med. 2008;27:2290–306. doi:10.1002/sim.3175.
10. Sambucini V. A Bayesian predictive strategy for an adaptive two-stage design in phase II clinical trials. Stat Med. 2010;29:1430–42. doi:10.1002/sim.3800.
11. Brutti P, De Santis F, Gubbiotti S. Mixtures of prior distributions for predictive Bayesian sample size calculations in clinical trials. Stat Med. 2009;28:2185–201. doi:10.1002/sim.3609.
12. Lee JJ, Liu DD. A predictive probability design for phase II cancer clinical trials. Clin Trials. 2008;5:93–106. doi:10.1177/1740774508089279.
13. Teramukai S, Daimon T, Zohar S. A Bayesian predictive sample size selection design for single-arm exploratory clinical trials. Stat Med. 2012;31:4243–54. doi:10.1002/sim.5505.
14. Bryant J, Day R. Incorporating toxicity considerations into the design of two-stage phase II clinical trials. Biometrics. 1995;51:1372–83.
15. Thall PF, Simon R, Estey EH. Bayesian sequential monitoring designs for single-arm clinical trials with multiple outcomes. Stat Med. 1995;14:357–79. doi:10.1002/sim.4780140404.
16. Conaway MR, Petroni GR. Designs for phase II trials allowing for a trade-off between response and toxicity. Biometrics. 1996;52:1375–86.
17. Stallard N, Thall PF, Whitehead J. Decision theoretic designs for phase II clinical trials with multiple outcomes. Biometrics. 1999;55:971–7. doi:10.1111/j.0006-341X.1999.00971.x.
18. Chen Y, Smith BJ. Adaptive group sequential design for phase II clinical trials: a Bayesian decision theoretic approach. Stat Med. 2009;28:3347–62. doi:10.1002/sim.3711.
19. Teramukai S, Daimon T, Zohar S. An extension of Bayesian predictive sample size selection designs for monitoring efficacy and safety. Stat Med. 2015;34:3029–39. doi:10.1002/sim.6550.

20. Ray HE, Rai SN. Flexible bivariate phase II clinical trial design incorporating toxicity and response on different schedules. Stat Med. 2013;32:470–85. doi:10.1002/sim.5671.
21. Marlin E, Zohar S, Jérôme C, Veyrat-Masson R, Marceau G, Paillard C, Auvringnon A, Le Moine P, Gandemer V, Sapin V, Halle P, Boiret-Dupré N, Chevret S, Deméocq F, Dubray C, Kanold J. Hematopoietic progenitor cell mobilization and harvesting in children with malignancies: do the advantages of pegfilgrastim really translate into clinical benefit? Bone Marrow Transplant. 2009;43:919–25. doi:10.1038/bmt.2008.412.
22. Biswas S, Liu DD, Lee JJ, Berry DA. Bayesian clinical trials at the University of Texas M. D. Anderson Cancer Center. Clin Trials. 2009;6:205–16. doi:10.1177/1740774509104992.
23. Brutti P, Gubbiotti S, Sambucini V. An extension of the single threshold design for monitoring efficacy and safety in phase II clinical trials. Stat Med. 2011;30:1648–64. doi:10.1002/sim.4229.

Phase III Clinical Trial Designs Incorporating Predictive Biomarkers: An Overview

Shigeyuki Matsui

Abstract Advances in biotechnology have revolutionized clinical trials in oncology, shifting the emphasis to co-development of molecularly targeted drugs and companion predictive biomarkers. However, the difficulty in developing and validating biomarkers in the early phases of clinical development complicates the design and analysis of definitive phase III trials that aim to establish the clinical utility of new treatments with the aid of predictive markers. This chapter provides an overview of several designs for phase III trials that incorporate predictive markers at various levels of development and credibility, the latter in terms of these markers' abilities to predict treatment responsiveness at the initiation of phase III trials. We first discuss the enrichment design and marker-stratified all-comers designs with a single binary marker. For the marker-stratified designs, multi-stage analyses for sequential testing across the subgroups and adaptive subgroup selection are provided. We also discuss other adaptive designs, including the adaptive threshold design and the adaptive signature design with some variants, in cases where the threshold for marker positivity is unclear or a single marker for use in evaluating treatment efficacy is not available at the initiation of phase III trials. Lastly, we introduce the prospective-retrospective approach that allows for the evaluation of treatment efficacy in a marker subgroup based on external evidence.

Keywords Clinical trial designs · Phase III trials · Predictive biomarkers · Genomic signatures

S. Matsui (✉)
Department of Biostatistics, Nagoya University Graduate School of Medicine,
65 Tsurumai-cho, Showa-ku, Nagoya, Aichi 466-8550, Japan
e-mail: smatsui@med.nagoya-u.ac.jp

S. Matsui and J. Crowley (eds.), *Frontiers of Biostatistical Methods and Applications in Clinical Oncology*, DOI 10.1007/978-981-10-0126-0_7

1 Introduction

Recent advances in biotechnology have revealed that the biology of human cancers is highly complex, and is heterogeneous among histologically defined cancers. With better understanding of cancer biology, treatment has shifted to the use of molecularly targeted drugs that inhibit specific targeted molecules related to carcinogenesis and tumor growth.

The anti-cancer effects of many molecularly targeted drugs are likely to be restricted to a subgroup of patients in whom alterations in the drug target are driving the growth of the cancer. Hence the traditional randomized clinical trial design, which evaluates an average treatment effect in a broad patient population, is no longer effective for this type of drug. The chance of overlooking effective drugs may increase due to the dilution of the treatment effect by enrolling non-responsive patients. This may lead to an under-treatment problem as a result of missed opportunities to treat future responsive patients using effective drugs. On the other hand, even if the overall effect of a molecularly targeted drug is significant, this does not necessarily mean that the treatment will be efficacious in all patients. This may raise concerns regarding over-treatment of future non-responsive patients when using this drug.

The way to address the above fundamental problems of the traditional design of randomized clinical trials is to incorporate a *predictive biomarker* to capture the heterogeneity in drug responsiveness or to identify a subgroup of patients who benefit from the treatment. One example of a predictive marker is the V600E *BRAF* point mutation when using the *BRAF* enzyme inhibitor vemurafenib in melanoma patients [1]. Another but more complex example with graded or continuous markers is the use of the overexpression of the *HER2* protein or amplification of the *HER2* gene when using a monoclonal antibody, trastuzumab, in metastatic breast cancer patients [2, 3].

Assays for predictive markers need to be analytically validated to confirm that they accurately measure the status of binary markers (e.g., the presence or absence of a point mutation) and that they are robust and reproducible when measuring levels of ordered or continuous markers (e.g., gene amplification or gene/protein expressions) [4, 5]. For the latter type of markers, it is often unclear how to determine marker positivity precisely when used in defining the subgroup of patients who are deemed to benefit from the treatment, and thus a threshold for marker positivity should be identified in earlier phase I and II trials.

In addition to being analytically validated, a predictive marker should be clinically validated to assess its ability to predict treatment responsiveness in a patient population [4, 6]. The clinical validity of a candidate predictive marker is typically assessed on the basis of short-term endpoints in earlier clinical trials (e.g., pharmacodynamic endpoints in proof-of-concept trials or tumor shrinkage/progression-free survival endpoints in phase II trials). The actual predictive accuracy may also reflect the analytical accuracy of the marker. However, the clinical utility of the predictive marker ultimately needs to be evaluated in a confirmatory phase III trial to demonstrate that it is actionable in clinical practice and that its use results in improved patient outcomes (in terms of clinical endpoints) [4, 6].

One approach to designing phase III trials to establish the clinical utility of a predictive marker is to randomize patients either to the use or non-use of the marker in determining treatments [7, 8]. However, such a marker-strategy design is generally inefficient because patients in both the marker-based and non-marker-based arms may receive the same treatment. For example, in a setting in which patients in the marker-based arm receive an experimental treatment if they are marker-positive and a standard treatment if they are marker-negative, and those in the non-marker-based arm receive the same standard treatment regardless of whether they are marker positive or negative, the treatment effect for comparing the two strategy arms may reduce to the treatment effect in the marker-positive subgroup multiplied by the prevalence of marker-positive patients in the trial population [9]. When the marker prevalence is very low (or there is substantial overlap in the number of patients receiving the standard treatment in both strategy-based arms), the inefficiency of such a strategy-based design becomes a serious problem. The enrichment or marker-stratified all-comers designs are generally more efficient than the marker-strategy design because they can directly evaluate treatment efficacy in a marker-positive subgroup [9–12]. These designs demonstrate the clinical utility of a treatment with the aid of a marker (through evaluating the efficacy of the treatment across marker-defined subgroups), instead of demonstrating the clinical utility of using the marker itself (through evaluating the efficacy of using a marker-based strategy in the entire patient population).

In this chapter, we provide an overview of the enrichment and various all-comers designs for phase III trials to establish the clinical utility of new treatments with the aid of predictive markers. As we have seen so far, the process needed for marker development and validation complicates the clinical development of new treatments. At the design stage of confirmatory phase III trials, the status of marker development and validation may vary widely, and candidate markers may have differing levels of credibility. This means that such phase III designs may be more complicated than traditional phase III designs that do not involve assessment of predictive markers.

We first consider situations where a single binary marker is available at the launch of phase III trials. We discuss the enrichment design in Sect. 2 and marker-stratified all-comers designs in Sect. 3. For the marker-stratified all-comers designs, we discuss various multiple hypothesis tests across the marker subgroups, depending on assumptions regarding the ability of the marker to predict treatment responsiveness. We also discuss multi-stage analyses for sequential testing across the subgroups and adaptive subgroup selection. In Sect. 4, we discuss other adaptive designs for marker development and validation in cases where the threshold for positivity is unclear, or a single marker for use in evaluating treatment efficacy is not available when initiating phase III trials; these designs include the adaptive threshold design and the adaptive signature design, with some variants. In Sect. 5, we introduce the prospective-retrospective approach to evaluating treatment efficacy in a marker subgroup based on external evidence. Lastly, concluding remarks are provided in Sect. 6.

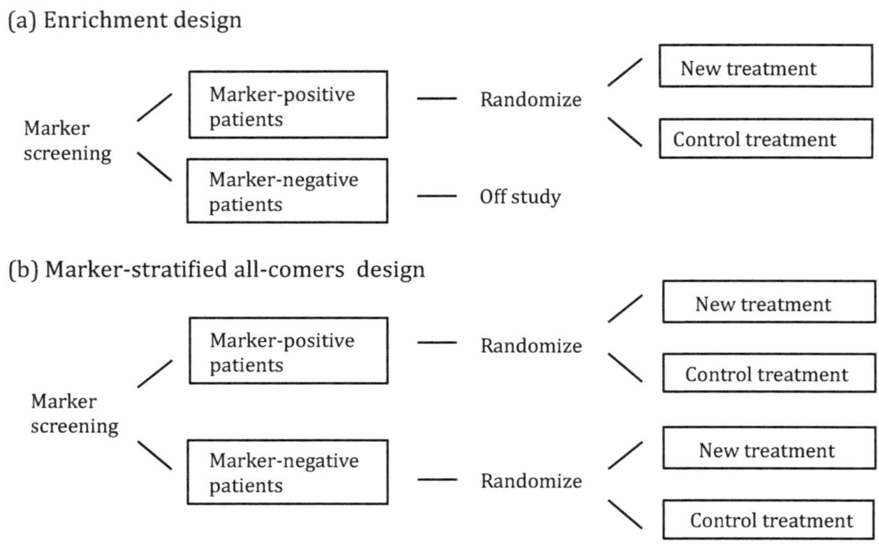

Fig. 1 Enrichment and marker-stratified all-comers designs

2 Enrichment Designs

When a binary marker that is analytically and clinically validated is available and there are compelling biologic or early trial data that support the assumption, called Marker-Assumption (I), that the benefit of the new treatment is only limited to marker-positive patients, it is best to consider an enrichment or targeted design that limits the eligibility for treatment randomization to these patients [9–14] (see Fig. 1a). The enrichment design is more efficient than the traditional all-comers design (which does not measure the marker) in terms of the number of randomized patients, especially under the condition that the prevalence of marker-positive individuals in the general population is small (e.g., <0.5) and the treatment is relatively ineffective in marker-negative patients [15]. If this condition is satisfied, enrichment trials can be fairly small in size because relatively large treatment effects can be expected for marker-positive patients. This attractive feature, however, does not necessarily imply a small number of patients for marker screening or a short study duration. In particular, when the marker prevalence is low, a substantial number of patients might have to undergo marker screening until the required number of marker-positive patients is enrolled to ensure treatment randomization [16].

A major drawback to the enrichment design relates to correctness of the strong Marker-Assumption (I) that only marker-positive patients benefit from the treatment. Possible factors that can threaten this assumption include imperfections in measuring the molecular target, such as misclassification errors, possible alternative threshold points that could better define marker-positives (especially for graded or continuous markers), and possible off-target effects of the treatment [9, 14]. When information regarding these factors is limited at the design stage of a phase III trial, we cannot rule out the possibility that the remaining marker-negative patients might also benefit from the treatment. The major limitation of the enrichment design is that it does not provide data to evaluate treatment efficacy in marker-negatives to check Marker-Assumption (I) in the confirmatory phase of clinical development.

To address this issue, some authors have proposed a sequential enrichment approach that conducts a second trial for marker-negative patients when an initial trial for marker-positive patients demonstrates treatment efficacy [17, 18]. It is believed that this approach allows for quicker assessment of the treatment for the patient population that is considered to most likely benefit from it [17]. This tandem approach, however, could require a long period of clinical development as a whole. Also, the sequential subgroup assessment is not necessarily efficient when treatment effects are relatively homogeneous across marker subgroups [16].

3 Marker-Stratified All-Comers Designs

Another approach to situations where a binary marker is available when planning phase III trials is the concurrent assessment of both marker-positive and marker-negative patients using a marker-stratified, randomize-all or all-comers design (see Fig. 1b). The stratification ensures observation of the marker status for all randomized patients and can also incorporate possible prognostic effects of the marker. When planning a marker-stratified trial, it is natural to make a more general assumption than Marker-Assumption (I), namely, that the treatment is more effective in marker-positives than in marker-negatives; this will be referred to as Marker-Assumption (II). However, this assumption may complicate the statistical analysis of treatment efficacy within marker subgroups and also in the overall population. Recently, various hierarchical or split-alpha multiple testing procedures have been proposed for marker-stratified trials with single and multiple stages of analysis. In what follows, we suppose a two-arm phase III trial to compare a new treatment with its control treatment using one-sided statistical tests to spend the study-wise alpha (or type I error) rate of $\alpha = 0.025$.

3.1 Single-Stage Designs

Under Marker-Assumption (II), when there is relatively strong evidence on the marker that a treatment is efficacious in marker-positive patients, a fixed-sequence procedure that first tests treatment efficacy in marker-positives would be reasonable. If this test is significant at a level of $\alpha = 0.025$, then the treatment effect is also tested in marker-negatives at the same significance level α. This procedure was employed in a randomized phase III trial of panitumumab with infusional fluorouracil, leucovorin, and oxaliplatin (FOLFOX) versus FOLFOX alone for untreated metastatic colorectal cancer [19]. The treatment arms were first compared regarding progression-free survival in patients with wild-type *KRAS* tumors, and treatment comparison in patients with mutant *KRAS* tumors was conditional on a significant difference in the first test for the wild-type *KRAS* subgroup. The power of the fixed-sequence procedure is determined by the (first) test for the marker-positive subgroup, like in the enrichment and sequential enrichment designs. Accordingly, the fixed-sequence procedure is expected to perform well when there is a fairly large treatment effect in marker-positives [20]. This might be the case where the marker accuracy in predicting treatment responsiveness is excellent, such that a *qualitative* treatment-by-marker interaction holds, where there is a large treatment effect in the marker-positive subgroup, but null (or clinically meaningless) effects in the marker-negative subgroup.

In more common cases where there is no strong evidence on the marker, it is reasonable to consider split-alpha procedures that allocate some portion of alpha to the possibility that the treatment is also efficacious in the marker-negative subgroup; that is, the treatment is efficacious in the overall population under Marker-Assumption (II). A simple procedure for this "co-primary" analysis is to apply the Bonferroni approach. For example, in the SATURN trial [21] to assess the use of erlotinib as maintenance therapy in patients with non-progressive disease following first-line platinum-doublet chemotherapy, progression-free survival after randomization was tested in all patients at a significance level of 0.015, and at a level of 0.01 in patients whose tumors had *EGFR* protein overexpression. We can improve the efficiency of the co-primary approach using less stringent significance levels that incorporate the correlation between the overall and subgroup tests [22, 23]. Another more efficient split-alpha procedure is guided by a test on treatment-by-marker interaction to determine whether treatment efficacy is tested in the marker-positive subgroup or in the overall population [20]. The interaction test can also serve as a definitive analysis for clinical validation of the predictive marker, if it is appropriately sized and powered under a qualitative interaction of clinical importance. For a full comparison of the hierarchical and split-alpha procedures, see [20].

The important feature of the aforementioned multiple testing procedures is that they can make either of two kinds of assertions regarding treatment efficacy, one for the overall population and the other for the marker-positive subpopulation of patients. However, a caveat for the co-primary analysis approach is that treatment efficacy in the overall population can be demonstrated even when there is a large treatment effect in the marker-positive subgroup, but no effect in the marker-negative subgroup [20]. This is problematic because it could lead to over-assertion of treatment efficacy in marker-negative patients who are in fact not treatment responsive. An additional assessment on treatment efficacy in the marker-negative subgroup is therefore warranted, outside of the primary analysis, to protect future marker-negative patients from over-treatment [20, 24, 25].

It can be argued that this issue reflects a failure in incorporating Marker-Assumption (II) in the co-primary analysis approach to test null hypotheses $H_0^{(o)}$ and $H_0^{(+)}$ (and their intersection $H_0^{(o)} \cap H_0^{(+)}$). Here $H_0^{(o)}$ and $H_0^{(+)}$ represent a null effect in the overall population and that in the marker-positive subgroup, respectively. In contrast, in a subgroup-specific analysis, e.g., the fixed-sequence procedure, the two null hypotheses $H_0^{(+)}$ and $H_0^{(-)}$ are tested, where the latter represents a null effect in the marker-negative subgroup. Marker-Assumption (II) restricts to the two possible null effect scenarios, (1) true $H_0^{(+)}$ and true $H_0^{(-)}$, called the *global null hypothesis*, and (2) false $H_0^{(+)}$ and true $H_0^{(-)}$. The fixed-sequence procedure strictly controls the study-wise type I error rate for both null scenarios. On the other hand, the co-primary analysis approach does not control for it (in testing $H_0^{(o)}$ and $H_0^{(o)} \cap H_0^{(+)}$) for the second null scenario. This represents a failure in incorporating Marker-Assumption (II), a source of possible over-assertion of treatment efficacy for marker-negative patients in the co-primary analysis approach.

One approach to addressing this issue is to modify the split-alpha procedures for a strict control of both null scenarios, i.e., *strong control* [26]. A hybrid of the fixed-sequence and alpha-split procedures was recently proposed [27]. Another possibly more practical approach is to separate the inspection of the marker-negatives from the primary analysis to test treatment efficacy across the populations, given a strict control of the study-wise alpha under the global null hypothesis, i.e., *weak control* [20]. Here, the global null hypothesis can be tested using a procedure to test the intersection hypothesis, $H_0^{(o)} \cap H_0^{(+)}$, in the co-primary analysis approach or using a stratified test that assumes constant effects across marker subgroups in the subgroup-specific analysis. The second approach allows for various degrees of alpha control, probably less stringent for the second null scenario (i.e., false $H_0^{(+)}$ and true $H_0^{(-)}$) on a case-by-case basis, given strict alpha control under the global null hypothesis. In determining the alpha level for the second null scenario, many external factors could be incorporated, probably involving the analytical performance of the marker, marker prevalence, possible adverse effects, prognosis of the disease, availability of other treatments, treatment costs, etc. [20]. For example, given a demonstration of a very large treatment effect in the marker-positive subgroup, it could be worthwhile to consider a less stringent or even informal control for testing $H_0^{(-)}$ for advanced diseases with no established treatments. This is similar to the approach that separates the demonstration of treatment efficacy and consideration of an *indication classifier* to identify the marker-based characteristics of the patients for whom the new treatment should be used [24]. Here the former component is accomplished by a significant result with strict alpha control under the global null hypothesis.

3.2 Multi-stage Designs

Generally, interim analysis is warranted to fulfill ethical requirements for the safety and benefit of the patients enrolled in a clinical trial, as well as for other patients who will be treated in the future. An appropriate early stopping guideline may allow patients enrolled in the trial to make earlier decisions about treatment changes, as well as help provide future patients with more timely information regarding better treatments. In marker-stratified trials, owing to Marker-Assumption (II), an interim analysis for non-efficacy or futility would be particularly warranted for marker-negative patients with presumably limited treatment efficacy to protect them from unnecessary treatments and follow-ups [6]. On the other hand, an interim analysis for efficacy or superiority could be worthwhile for marker-positive patients with presumably high treatment efficacy in order to quickly deliver superior treatment to these patients. Another aim of interim analysis relates to improving the efficiency of clinical development with a marker-stratified trial. In particular, the statistical power in detecting treatment effects could be enhanced by adaptively narrowing the patient population down to a patient subgroup that could benefit from the treatment, based on interim clinical trial data.

For time-to-event endpoints typically evaluated in the primary analysis of phase III oncology trials, however, flexible interim adaptations are generally precluded due to the specific difficulty in assuring the independence of an adaptation from any subsidiary information derived from censored cases who have not experienced an event at the time of the interim analysis [28]. For possible techniques to address this difficulty, see [29, 30]. In many cases, the adaptation rule, including the information fraction at the interim analysis, may be pre-specified based on the primary test statistic on the time-to-event endpoint. This is essentially equivalent to the traditional group sequential analysis.

Brannath et al. [31] considered a futility stopping rule for marker-negative patients to determine which of the overall or only marker-positive patients are followed up and analyzed at the end of the trial (Fig. 2a). Treatment efficacy is tested in both overall and marker-positive patients using a closed testing procedure that incorporates possible early futility stopping in the marker-negative subgroup based on multiple stage combination tests, such as those with inverse normal combination functions. In this design, a combination of the conditional error function and the split-alpha approach can improve the efficiency in testing the intersection hypothesis, $H_0^{(o)} \cap H_0^{(+)}$, in the closed testing procedure [32].

In the framework of group sequential analysis, Magnusson and Turnbull [33] proposed a group sequential enrichment design incorporating subgroup selection, which may also be applicable to clinical trials with time-to-event endpoints. Taking into account the complicated nature of interim monitoring across subgroups under possible marker assumptions, Redman et al. [34] considered subgroup-focused interim monitoring in evaluating the efficacy of cetuximab for advanced non-small cell lung cancer. The interim monitoring plan specifies interim evaluations of both efficacy and futility in the marker-positive (*EGFR* FISH-positive) subgroup alone. The futility-monitoring plan to determine early stopping in the marker-negative subgroup is based on evaluation within both marker-positive and -negative subgroups and the entire study population.

More recently, Matsui and Crowley [16] proposed a simple but flexible subgroup-focused design that allows for both sequential assessment across the

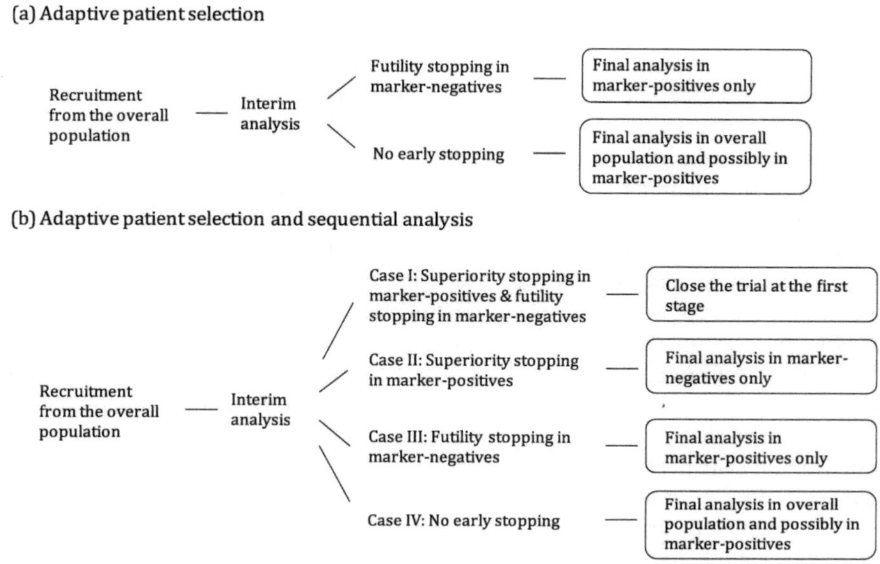

Fig. 2 Two-stage marker-stratified designs with adaptive patient selection

subgroups as well as adaptive subgroup selection, while retaining assessment using the entire patient data at the final analysis stage. The scheme of a two-stage design in this approach is shown in Fig. 2b. This can be viewed as a concurrent subgroup-focused design with a futility stopping rule in the marker-negative subgroup and a superiority stopping rule in the marker-positive subgroup. It involves sequential testing across the subgroups as in the sequential enrichment design (Case II in Fig. 2b), and adaptive patient selection (Cases III–IV). In Case IV with no early stopping in either subgroup, the subgroup data are combined for the final analysis, possibly using the established marker-based multiple testing procedures described in Sect. 3.1. See [16] for an assessment of the impact of introducing the within-subgroup interim analyses on the number of randomized patients, the number undergoing marker screening, and the study duration in a marker-stratified design, as well as a comparison among various marker-based designs.

Another subgroup-focused design is proposed in the framework of Bayesian inference using a family of priors for four-points (combination of two levels of treatment effect, a null and an effect of clinical importance, and a binary marker) to represent the degree of a priori confidence in the predictive marker [35]. This design involves interim analysis to stop accrual of marker-negative patients or accrual of all patients. Although this design intends to provide a rigorous testing of the global null hypothesis, it also provides a useful tool for determining the treatment indication across marker subgroups. The combination of a frequentist inference for testing treatment efficacy and a Bayesian inference for deriving a tool for decision on treatment indication would be an interesting area for future research.

3.3 Sample Size Determination

We have seen so far that marker-stratified all-comers trials test multiple hypotheses on treatment efficacy across different patient populations. In determining sample sizes of such trials, it is natural to introduce the total power P_{total}, defined as the probability of obtaining a statistically significant result for any hypotheses on treatment efficacy across all the tests (in single or multi-stage designs) planned in the trial under some scenario of non-null treatment effects across marker-subgroups. For the statistical analysis plans described in Sects. 3.1 and 3.2, P_{total} may correspond to the probability of asserting treatment efficacy for either the overall population or the marker-positive subpopulation [20]. Specifically, it can be decomposed into two components, one asserting treatment efficacy for the overall population, $P_{overall}$, and the other relevant to the marker-positive subpopulation, $P_{subgroup}$, such that $P_{total} = P_{overall} + P_{subgroup}$, based on the individual hypotheses tested in the statistical analysis plan [20]. P_{total} can also be interpreted as asserting treatment efficacy *at least* for the marker-positive subpopulation.

The component probabilities $P_{overall}$ and $P_{subgroup}$ may be particularly useful when the multiple tests are used not only for testing treatment efficacy but also for making a decision on whether treatment efficacy should be asserted on the overall population or the marker-positive subpopulation. For example, under a scenario with qualitative treatment-by-marker interaction (with a large treatment effect in marker-positives, but no or clinically meaningless effect in marker-negatives), one may try to ensure a high level of $P_{subgroup}$, but a small level of $P_{overall}$ to reduce the chance of over-treatment for marker-negatives. On the other hand, under a scenario where the treatment has effects of clinical importance in both marker-positive and -negative subgroups (i.e., constant effects or quantitative interactions), one may desire to have a high level of $P_{overall}$, but a small level of $P_{subgroup}$ to protect marker-negatives from under-treatment. See [20] for evaluation of P_{total}, $P_{overall}$, and $P_{subgroup}$ for various analysis plans in single-stage designs.

In many marker-stratified trials, the researchers may consider testing all the patient populations, so that they are adequately sized. However, there may be some exceptions. For example, in a subgroup-specific analysis using the fixed-sequence procedure, one may consider sizing the marker-positive subgroup only, because the first test on that subgroup determines P_{total}. In this case, one could also consider an additional criterion on the size of the marker-negative subgroup to ensure a relatively high level of $P_{overall}$ for the same level of P_{total}. When the marker prevalence in the general population is known to be relatively small, say 0.2, where a large number of patients has to be screened for the marker to enroll the targeted number of marker-positives, this additional criterion could help prevent enrolling extra marker-negatives (with presumably limited treatment efficacy). On the other hand, when the marker prevalence is fairly large (>0.5), this criterion for sizing the marker-negative subgroup might not be pursued because it could entail an extension of patient accrual for this subgroup after the targeted number of marker-positives is recruited.

In determining sample sizes of marker-stratified all-comers trials, possible profiles of treatment effects across subgroups under Marker-Assumption (II), particularly qualitative and quantitative treatment-by-marker interactions, need to be accommodated. Practically, a sensitivity analysis assuming a plausible range of treatment effect profiles should be conducted.

4 Unstratified All-Comers Designs with Marker Development and Validation

When the biology of the molecular target of a new treatment is not well understood because of the complexity of disease biology, it is quite common that a completely specified predictive marker is not available before initiating the definitive phase III trial. In one scenario, a single marker may be available but no threshold for marker positivity is defined before the phase III trial. In another scenario, a single marker for use in evaluating treatment efficacy is not available, but data on several candidate markers or even tens of thousands of genomic markers are measured for pre-treatment tissue specimens before the trial or are scheduled to be measured during the trial. In the latter situation with high-dimensional genomic marker data, there are no a priori credentials for predictive markers from among the large number of genomic markers. One approach to these situations is to prospectively design and analyze the randomized trial in such a way that both developing a predictive marker (or signature) and testing treatment efficacy based on the developed marker are conducted in a valid manner.

Unlike a marker-stratified trial with a prespecified binary marker as described in Sect. 3, all-comers trials in this approach may not be stratified by any markers. Unstratified randomization does not diminish the validity of inference regarding treatment efficacy within marker-defined subgroups with moderate-to-large sizes. Under unstratified randomization, marker measurements can be delayed until the time of analysis. This strategy may permit situations where an analytically validated marker is not available at the start of the trial but will be available by the time of analysis [6, 9]. However, careful consideration of missing marker data is needed to ensure collection of sufficient numbers of patients with observed marker status and also to prevent selection bias, i.e., dependence of missing measurements on the treatment assignment and other clinical variables.

As the marker for evaluating treatment efficacy is not available at the initiation of the trial, the analysis for marker development and validation would be positioned as a fallback option that spends a small portion of the study-wise alpha, α^*, say 0.005 (of $\alpha = 0.025$), and it is conducted only when a test of treatment efficacy in the overall population that spends the main portion of the study-wise alpha, $\alpha - \alpha^*$, say 0.02, is not significant. The outstanding features of this approach are the application of an optimization or prediction algorithm to develop a marker (or signature) to identify an appropriate marker-positive subgroup in the development stage and the implementation of a *single* test on treatment efficacy within an identified "marker-positive" subgroup based on the developed marker in the validation stage. The latter feature is in contrast to the traditional exploratory subgroup analysis with multiple tests across subgroups. All the elements in the analysis for marker development and validation must be prospectively defined and specified in the statistical analysis plan.

4.1 Adaptive Threshold Design

The adaptive threshold design [36] is for settings where a single marker is available but no threshold of positivity for the marker is predefined. The basic idea is that for a set of candidate threshold values (b_1, ..., b_K) one searches for an optimal threshold value by maximizing a log likelihood ratio statistic for testing treatment efficacy in the patient subgroup with marker value $\geq b_k$ over possible threshold values ($k = 1$, ..., K). The maximum log likelihood ratio (at the optimal threshold value) T is used as the test statistic for testing treatment efficacy. Its null distribution under the global null hypothesis that the new treatment is no better than control for any marker-determined subgroup is approximated by repeating the whole analysis after randomly permuting treatment levels several thousand times. The P value to reject the global null hypothesis is obtained as an upper percentile for the observed value of T in the null permutation distribution. A confidence interval of the chosen threshold can be constructed based on a non-parametric bootstrap method. For a given value of the marker, the empirical distribution of the chosen threshold across bootstrap samples can provide an estimate of the probability that the true threshold level is less than that value, possibly interpreted as the probability that a patient with given marker value will benefit from the treatment in the absence of overall treatment effect.

4.2 Adaptive Signature Design

The adaptive signature design develops a predictor or predictive signature using a set of covariates x, possibly high-dimensional genomic markers [37]. In the marker development and validation stage, the full set of patients in the clinical trial is partitioned into a training set and a validation set by the split-sample method. A pre-specified algorithmic analysis plan is applied to the training set to generate a predictor. This is a function of x and predicts whether a given patient with a particular covariate value x is responsive or non-responsive to the new treatment. Specifically, using a training dataset, we develop a signature score $U(x; A$, training data) for a given covariate value x based on a pre-specified scoring algorithm A. For example, such a score can be derived as a linear predictor in the logistic or Cox proportional hazard models, possibly using penalized regression techniques to handle high-dimensional data [38–40]. Typically, a patient with covariate value x will be predicted as "responsive" to the new treatment, if $U(x) > c$, and "non-responsive" otherwise, using a threshold point c on U. The predictor developed using the training data is used to make a prediction for each patient in the validation set. Then, the treatment efficacy is tested in the subset of patients who are predicted to be responsive to the treatment in the validation set.

4.3 Cross-Validated Adaptive Signature Design and Its Variant

The efficiency of the adaptive signature design can be enhanced by applying a cross-validation method rather than the split-sample method in Sect. 4.2 [41]. In a K-fold cross-validation, the entire patient population is split into K roughly equally sized, non-overlapping subsamples based on a prospectively defined rule. Accordingly, the full dataset, D, in the trial is split into K subsets, such that $D = (D_1, \ldots, D_K)$. The kth training dataset consists of the full dataset except for the kth dataset, $T_k = D - D_k$ ($k = 1, \ldots, K$).

In the kth round of cross-validation, we apply all aspects of the signature development, including feature selection, from scratch to the training dataset T_k to obtain a prediction score function $U_k(x; A, T_k)$. When the feature selection is optimized based on a cross-validated predictive accuracy, a nested inner loop of K-fold cross-validation should be applied for the training dataset T_k [42, 43]. The threshold point c_k on U_k can be pre-specified or tuned based on predictive accuracy using the nested inner loop of cross-validation. Then, the score function $U_k(x; A, T_k)$ and the threshold c_k are applied to make a prediction for each patient in the remaining dataset, D_k, i.e., the validation set.

At the end of the cross-validation, each of the study patients is predicted to be either responsive or non-responsive to the new treatment. The former now constitute a "marker-positive" subgroup. The treatment efficacy in this subgroup can be tested using a standard test statistic (e.g., a log-rank statistic) to compare the outcomes on the primary endpoint between the two treatment arms. However, since the marker-positive subgroup is data-driven, i.e., obtained via cross-validation of the entire study sample, the standard asymptotic distribution does not apply to the test statistic. As in the adaptive threshold design, a permutation method is applied to test the global null hypothesis or a sharp null hypothesis of no treatment effects in any patients. In this method, the whole process of the analysis to obtain the test statistic is re-performed for each dataset generated by permuting treatment levels.

A variant of this design, called continuous cross-validated adaptive signature design, is proposed to provide a continuous function of the underlying treatment effects across patients as a more relevant diagnostic tool, rather than qualitatively classifying patients (using a threshold point c_k) as members of the responsive subgroup or not [44].

In the kth round of cross-validation, the prediction scoring function $U_k(x; A, T_k)$ built in the training set is directly used to obtain a predicted score for each patient in the validation set. Specifically, using an empirical cumulative distribution $F_k(u)$ of $U_k(x; A, T_k)$ in the training set, we obtain a quantile score for a patient with covariate x^* in the validation set as $S_k(x^*) = F_k(U_k(x^*; A, T_k)) \in (0, 1)$. Of note, this score can be interpreted as a *pre-validation* score, which will be used for modeling using clinical variables [45].

At the end of the cross-validation, the cross-validated prediction score, S, which is essentially continuous, is used to model treatment responsiveness using the entire patient population. For example, for a time-to-event endpoint, we assume the multivariate Cox proportional hazards model,

$$\log\{h_i(t; r_i, s_i)/h_0(t)\} = \beta_1 r_i + f_2(s_i) + r_i f_3(s_i),$$

where r_i is the treatment assignment indicator such that $r_i = 1$ if patient i is assigned to the new treatment and $r_i = 0$ otherwise, and S_i is the prediction score for patient i ($i = 1, \ldots, n$). The functions f_2 and f_3 capture the main effect of S and the interaction between S and r, respectively. From this model, we can derive the treatment effects function,

$$\Psi(s) = \beta_1 + f_3(s),$$

which represents the log hazard for a patient with the prediction score s when receiving the new treatment minus that when receiving the control treatment, where negative values of Ψ represents better outcomes when receiving the new treatment rather than the control treatment. Figure 3 is an estimated treatment effects function [44] using a fractional polynomial [46] for f_3 that was obtained using microarray gene expression data from pre-treatment plasma cells in a randomized clinical trial with multiple myeloma [47, 48].

Based on an estimated function, we can define a marker-positive subgroup Ω, such that $\Omega = \{s : \widehat{\Psi}(s) < c\}$, where c is set as zero or the minimum size of clinically meaningful effects. Like in the original cross-validated adaptive signature design, we can test treatment efficacy in the marker-derived subgroup using an average treatment effect in that subgroup based on the estimated function as a test statistic:

$$T = \int_{s \in \Omega} \widehat{\Psi}(s) ds.$$

Again, its null distribution under the strong null hypothesis can be derived using the permutation method, where the P value is obtained as the proportion of permutations when the values of T are equal to or less than the observed value of T. In the multiple myeloma example, using the threshold of $c = 0$ for defining marker-positives, the P-value obtained from 2000 permutations was 0.019 [44]. Lastly, in this estimation framework, we can develop signature-based, patient-level

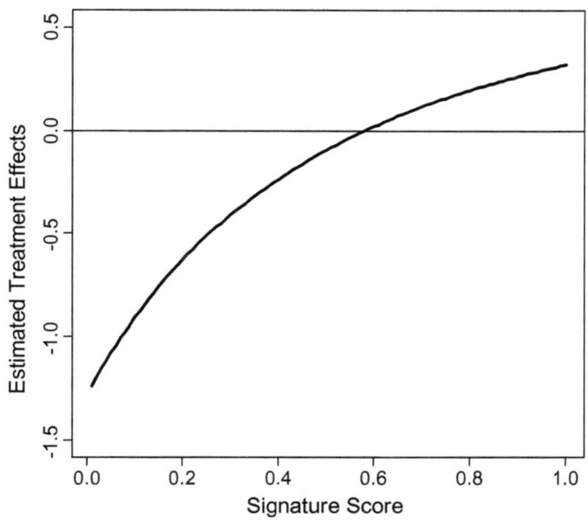

Fig. 3 An estimate of the treatment effects function Ψ for the predicted signature score, *S*, in terms of logarithm of hazard ratio in a randomized clinical trial with microarray gene expression data from pre-treatment plasma cells in multiple myeloma. The score *S* was derived via a 5-fold cross-validation with a compound covariate predictor based on a test statistic on treatment-by-gene interaction. A fractional polynomials function was used for modelling the effect of *S* on survival outcomes (see [44] for more detail of the analysis)

survival curves to predict survival distributions of future individual patients, through incorporating a cross-validated prognostic score, as well as the cross-validated predictive score *S* [44].

5 Prospective-Retrospective Approach

Another approach to the situations where no single promising predictive marker has been identified by the time of initiation of the phase III trial is to delay the evaluation of treatment efficacy within a marker-based subgroup until the time when external evidence on the predictive marker(s) becomes available [49]. With this approach, one could reserve a small portion of the total alpha for a single test of treatment effect in the subgroup to be determined in the future [9]. This approach is only applicable to clinical trials that archive pre-treatment specimens for marker evaluation. At the time of evaluating a new marker in the future, the analysis plan will be prospectively specified for retrospectively utilizing and analyzing the archived specimens.

Typically, accumulating biological evidence can identify an appropriate predictive marker. For example, a marker of *KRAS* mutation status was identified to be useful for predicting responsiveness to an anti-*EGFR* (epidermal growth factor receptor) antibody, cetuximab, for colorectal cancer [50]. Actually, the prospective-retrospective approach could limit the indication for the treatment to a subgroup of patients with *KRAS* wild-type tumors after demonstrating treatment efficacy in the overall population [50]. Another possibility is the development of a new predictive signature using the data-driven approach using external clinical trial data, as in the development of predictors or signatures in the adaptive signature designs.

Simon et al. [49] proposed several conditions for appropriately conducting the prospective-retrospective approach to establish the clinical utility of a treatment with the aid of a companion marker. In summary,

(1) Archived specimens, adequate for a successful assay, must be available from a sufficient large number of patients to permit appropriately powered analyses in the pivotal trial and to ensure that the patients included in the marker evaluation are representative of the patients in the trial.
(2) Substantial data on the analytical validity of the marker must exist to ensure that results obtained from the archived specimens will closely resemble those that would have been obtained from analysis of specimens collected in real time. Assays should be conducted blinded to the clinical data.
(3) The analysis plan for the marker evaluation must be completely developed before the performance of the marker assays. The analysis should focus on a single diagnostic marker that is completely defined and specified. The analysis should not be exploratory, and practices that might lead to a false-positive conclusion (e.g., multiple analyses of different candidate markers based on the archived specimens from the same trial) should be avoided.
(4) The results must be validated in at least one or more similarly designed studies using the same assay techniques.

6 Concluding Remarks

A deeper understanding of the molecular heterogeneity of histologically defined cancers has led to a paradigm shift in the clinical development of cancer treatments toward precision or predictive medicine, with the co-development of molecularly targeted drugs and companion predictive markers. Confronted with this paradigm shift, statistical methodologies for design and analysis of clinical trials have to evolve, involving the integration of statistical inference and prediction analysis.

On the other hand, the clinical development of new treatments becomes more complicated, compared with the traditional paradigm of clinical development without the use of predictive markers. The critical role of biostatisticians is to appropriately inform clinical investigators of the effectiveness and limitations of the new statistical methodologies and to practice them appropriately. The ultimate goal should not just be to achieve reconciliation with the new paradigm of predictive medicine, but to play an active role in implementing its concepts.

Acknowledgements This research was supported by CREST, JST and a Grant-in-Aid for Scientific Research (24240042 and 16H06299) from the Ministry of Education, Culture, Sports, Science and Technology of Japan.

References

1. Chapman PB, Hauschild A, Robert C, Haanen JB, Ascierto P, Larkin J, et al. Improved survival with vemurafenib in melanoma with BRAF V600E mutation. N Engl J Med. 2011;364:2507–16.
2. Slamon DJ, Leyland-Jones B, Shak S, Fuchs H, Paton V, Bajamonde A, et al. Use of chemotherapy plus a monoclonal antibody against HER2 for metastatic breast cancer that overexpresses HER2. N Engl J Med. 2001;344:783–92.
3. Wolff AC, Hammond ME, Hicks DG, Dowsett M, McShane LM, Allison KH, et al. Recommendations for human epidermal growth factor receptor 2 testing in breast cancer: American Society of Clinical Oncology/College of American Pathologists clinical practice guideline update. J Clin Oncol. 2013;31(31):3997–4013.
4. Hunter DJ, Khoury KJ, Drazen JM. Letting the out of the bottle—will we get our wish? N Engl J Med. 2008;358(2):105–7.
5. McShane LM, Cavenagh MM, Lively TG, Eberhard DA, Bigbee WL, Williams PM, et al. Criteria for the use of omics-based predictors in clinical trials: explanation and elaboration. BMC Med. 2013;11:220.
6. Simon R. Clinical trial designs for evaluating the medical of prognostic and predictive biomarkers in oncology. Pers Med. 2010;7(1):33–47.
7. Cobo M, Isla D, Massuti B, Montes A, Sanchez JM, Provencio M, et al. Customizing cisplatin based on quantitative excision repair cross-complementing 1 mRNA expression: a phase III trial in non-small-cell lung cancer. J Clin Oncol. 2007;25(19):2747–54.
8. Cree IA, Kurbacher CM, Lamont A, Hindley AC, Love S, TCA Ovarian Cancer Trial Group. A prospective randomized controlled trial of tumour assay directed chemotherapy versus physician's choice in patients with recurrent platinum-resistant ovarian cancer. Anticancer Drugs. 2007;18(9):1093–101.
9. Simon R, Matsui S, Buyse M. Clinical trials for predictive medicine: new paradigms and challenges. In: Matsui S, Buyse M, Simon R, editors. Design and analysis of clinical trials for predictive medicine. Boca Raton, FL: Chapman and Hall/CRC Press; 2015. p. 3–10.
10. Hoering A, Leblanc M, Crowley JJ. Randomized phase III clinical trial designs for targeted agents. Clin Cancer Res. 2008;14(14):4358–67.
11. Mandrekar SJ, Sargent DJ. Clinical trial designs for predictive biomarker validation: theoretical considerations and practical challenges. J Clin Oncol. 2009;27(24):4027–34.
12. Freidlin B, McShane LM, Korn EL. Randomized clinical trials with biomarkers: design issues. J Natl Cancer Inst. 2010;102(3):152–60.
13. Buyse M, Michiels S, Sargent DJ, Grothey A, Matheson A, de Gramont A. Integrating biomarkers in clinical trials. Expert Rev Mol Diagn. 2011;11(2):171–82.
14. Freidlin B, Korn EL. Biomarker enrichment strategies: matching trial design to biomarker credentials. Nat Rev Clin Oncol. 2014;11(2):81–90.
15. Simon R, Maitournam A. Evaluating the efficiency of targeted designs for randomized clinical trials. Clin Cancer Res. 2004;10(20):6759–63.
16. Matsui S, Crowley J. Biomarker-stratified phase III clinical trials: enhancement with a subgroup-focused sequential design. Clin Cancer Res (In press).
17. Fridlyand J, Simon RM, Walrath JC, Roach N, Buller R, Schenkein DP, et al. Considerations for the successful co-development of targeted cancer therapies and companion diagnostics. Nat Rev Drug Discov. 2013;12(10):743–55.

18. Liu A, Liu C, Li Q, Yu KF, Yuan VW. A threshold sample-enrichment approach in a clinical trial with heterogeneous subpopulations. Clin Trials. 2010;7(5):537–45.
19. Douillard JY, Siena S, Cassidy J, Tabernero J, Burkes R, Barugel M, et al. Randomized, phase III trial of panitumumab with infusional fluorouracil, leucovorin, and oxaliplatin (FOLFOX4) versus FOLFOX4 alone as first-line treatment in patients with previously untreated metastatic colorectal cancer: the PRIME study. J Clin Oncol. 2010;28(31): 4697–705.
20. Matsui S, Choai Y, Nonaka T. Comparison of statistical analysis plans in randomize-all phase III trials with a predictive biomarker. Clin Cancer Res. 2014;20(11):2820–30.
21. Cappuzzo F, Ciuleanu T, Stelmakh L, Cicenas S, Szczésna A, Juhász E, et al. Erlotinib as maintenance treatment in advanced non-small-cell lung cancer: a multicentre, randomised, placebo-controlled phase 3 study. Lancet Oncol. 2010;11(6):521–9.
22. Song Y, Chi GY. A method for testing a prespecified subgroup in clinical trials. Stat Med. 2007;26(19):3535–49.
23. Spiessens B, Debois M. Adjusted significance levels for subgroup analyses in clinical trials. Contemp Clin Trials. 2010;31(6):647–56.
24. Simon RM. Genomic clinical trials and predictive medicine. Cambridge: Cambridge University Press; 2013.
25. Millen BA, Dmitrienko A, Song G. Bayesian assessment of the influence and interaction conditions in multipopulation tailoring clinical trials. J Biopharm Stat. 2014;24(1):94–109.
26. Rothmann MD, Zhang JJ, Lu L, Fleming TR. Testing in a prespecified subgroup and the intent-to-treat population. Drug Inf J. 2012;46(2):175–9.
27. Freidlin B, Korn EL, Gray R. Marker Sequential Test (MaST) design. Clin Trials. 2014;11 (1):19–27.
28. Bauer P, Posch M. Letter to the editor: Modification of the sample size and the schedule of interim analyses in survival trials based on data inspections, by H. Schäfer and H.-H. Müller. Stat Med 2001; 20: 3741–51. Stat Med. 2004; 23(8): 1333–4.
29. Jenkins M, Stone A, Jennison C. An adaptive seamless phase II/III design for oncology trials with subpopulation selection using correlated survival endpoints. Pharm Stat. 2011;10 (4):347–56.
30. Mehta C, Schäfer H, Daniel H, Irle S. Biomarker driven population enrichment for adaptive oncology trials with time to event endpoints. Stat Med. 2014;33(26):4515–31.
31. Brannath W, Zuber E, Branson M, Bretz F, Gallo P, Posch M, Racine-Poon A. Confirmatory adaptive designs with Bayesian decision tools for a targeted therapy in oncology. Stat Med. 2009;28(10):1445–63.
32. Friede T, Parsons N, Stallard N. A conditional error function approach for subgroup selection in adaptive clinical trials. Stat Med. 2012;31(30):4309–20.
33. Magnusson BP, Turnbull BW. Group sequential enrichment design incorporating subgroup selection. Stat Med. 2013;32(16):2695–714.
34. Redman MW, Crowley JJ, Herbst RS, Hirsch FR, Gandara DR. Design of a phase III clinical trial with prospective biomarker validation: SWOG S0819. Clin Cancer Res. 2012;18 (15):4004–12.
35. Karuri S, Simon R. A two-stage Bayesian design for co-development of new drugs and companion diagnostics. Stat Med. 2012;31(10):901–14.
36. Jiang W, Freidlin B, Simon R. Biomarker adaptive threshold design: a procedure for evaluating treatment with possible biomarker-defined subset effect. J Natl Cancer Inst. 2007;99(13):1036–43.
37. Freidlin B, Simon R. Adaptive signature design: an adaptive clinical trial design for generating and prospectively testing a gene expression signature for sensitive patients. Clin Cancer Res. 2005;11(21):7872–8.
38. Hastie T, Tibshirani R, Friedman J. The elements of statistical learning. 2nd ed. New York: Springer; 2009.
39. Witten DM, Tibshirani R. Survival analysis with high-dimensional covariates. Stat Methods Med Res. 2010;19(1):29–51.

40. Tian L, Alizadeh AA, Gentles AJ, Tibshirani R. A simple method for estimating interactions between a treatment and a large number of covariates. J Am Stat Assoc. 2014;109(508):1517–32.
41. Freidlin B, Jiang W, Simon R. The cross-validated adaptive signature design. Clin Cancer Res. 2010;16(2):691–8.
42. Dudoit S, Fridlyand J. Classification in microarray experiments. In: Speed TP, editor. Statistical analysis of gene expression microarray data. Boca Raton: Chapman & Hall/CRC; 2003. p. 93–158.
43. Varma S, Simon R. Bias in error estimation when using cross-validation for model selection. BMC Bioinform. 2006;7:91.
44. Matsui S, Simon R, Qu P, Shaughnessy JD, Barlogie B, Crowley J. Developing and validating continuous genomic signatures in randomized clinical trials for predictive medicine. Clin Cancer Res. 2012;18(21):6065–73.
45. Tibshirani RJ, Efron B. Pre-validation and inference in microarrays. Stat Appl Genet Mol Biol. 2002;1.
46. Royston P, Altman DG. Regression using fractional polynomials of continuous covariates: parsimonious parametric modelling (with discussion). Appl Stat. 1994;43(3):429–67.
47. Barlogie B, Tricot G, Anaissie E, Shaughnessy J, Rasmussen E, van Rhee F, et al. Thalidomide and hematopoietic-cell transplantation for multiple myeloma. N Engl J Med. 2006;354(10):1021–30.
48. Barlogie B, Anaissie E, van Rhee F, Shaughnessy J, Szymonifka J, Hoering A, et al. Reiterative survival analyses of total therapy 2 for multiple myeloma elucidate follow-up time dependency of prognostic variables and treatment arms. J Clin Oncol. 2010;28(18):3023–7.
49. Simon RM, Paik S, Hayes DF. Use of archived specimens in evaluation of prognostic and predictive biomarkers. J Natl Cancer Inst. 2009;101(21):1446–52.
50. Karapetis CS, Khambata-Ford S, Jonker DJ, O'Callaghan CJ, Tu D, Tebbutt NC, et al. K-ras mutations and benefit from cetuximab in advanced colorectal cancer. N Engl J Med. 2008;359 (17):1757–65.

Bayesian, Utility-Based, Adaptive Enrichment Designs with Frequentist Error Control

Noah Simon

Abstract Our improving understanding of the biology underlying various diseases has reinforced the idea that many diseases previously considered homogeneous are in fact heterogeneous collections with different prognoses, pathologies, and causal mechanisms. To this end, the biomedical field has begun to focus on developing targeted therapies: therapies aimed at treating only a subset of the population with a given disease (often derived by the molecular pathology of the disease). However, characterizing these subsets has been a challenge: Hundreds of patients may be required to effectively characterize these subsets. Often information on this many patients is not available until well into large-scale trials. In this chapter we discuss adaptive enrichment designs: clinical trial designs that allow the simultaneous construction and use of biomarkers, during an ongoing trial. We first detail common scenarios where adaptive enrichment designs could be fruitfully applied to gain efficiency over classical designs. We then discuss two classes of adaptive enrichment strategies: Adaptation based on prespecified covariate-based stratification, and adaptation based on modeling response as a potentially more complex function of covariates. We will contrast these strategies with more classical non-enriched biomarker strategies (based on post hoc modeling/testing). Finally, we will discuss and address a number of potential issues and concerns with adaptive enrichment designs.

Keywords Clinical Trial · Adaptive Enrichment · Biomarker · Bayesian

1 Introduction

Therapies have classically been developed with the intent to treat an entire population with a given disease; and with the hope that the majority of that population will benefit from treatment. This has been successful in the past: prednisone and immune-suppressants successfully control many autoimmune diseases; broad

N. Simon (✉)
Department of Biostatistics, University of Washington, Seattle, WA, USA
e-mail: nrsimon@uw.edu

S. Matsui and J. Crowley (eds.), *Frontiers of Biostatistical Methods and Applications in Clinical Oncology*, DOI 10.1007/978-981-10-0126-0_8

spectrum antibiotics are effective for bacterial infections; and chemotherapy/radiotherapy have been key for treating many cancers.

However, in many cases, this approach has not been successful. As our understanding of biomolecular pathology of disease grows, we see that many/most diseases are actually very heterogenous. Where we once considered cases of a disease to have near identical underlying biology, we now understand that most "diseases" are a heterogeneous collection that manifests in phenotypically similar ways, but with different causal mechanisms and different protective mutations. Given this, we cannot hope to successfully treat all patients with the same therapy.

We have begun to create targeted therapeutics, molecules that inhibit particular pathways dysregulated in a subset of the diseased population. These molecules can only be expected to effectively treat those patients whose disease is driven by that target pathway. Thus, there is significant interest in using clinical and genomic information to develop *predictive biomarkers* that indicate those patients with such dysregulation, who will benefit from the targeted therapy over standard of care. Targeting has several success stories: trastuzumab [19, 33]/tamoxifen [22] for HER-2/ER positive breast cancer; vemurafenib [8] for melanoma with certain B-Raf mutations; cetuximab [1, 2, 7] for colon cancer without mutant KRAS; and immune checkpoint inhibitors for cancers with activated immune checkpoints [9], among others [5, 20, 23, 30].

In evaluating *targeted* therapeutics there is an additional challenge: One needs to determine the intent-to-treat (ITT) population. For non-targeted therapies this is generally everyone with the disease (perhaps restricted by disease severity, or simple clinical features). For a targeted therapy we require a strong characterization of the *target population* (those patients for whom the molecular pathology of their disease indicates they will benefit from the new treatment). In particular, we need a reproducible assay, and a rule based on this assay, that we can use to determine who we believe will benefit from treatment. Potential biomarkers include, but are not limited to, disease histology, mutation status, expression of various genes or proteins, or epigenetic abnormalities. In some cases a strong characterization of the target population is available before phase III, in which case one should employ an enrichment design [11, 16, 24]. Rather than enrolling all diseased patients into the trial (provided they meet the usual broad enrollment criteria; e.g. sick enough but not too sick… etc.), we instead assay potential patients, and enroll only those our biomarker indicates will benefit. By choosing not to enroll patients who will clearly not benefit we improve our trial in two ways: (1) we estimate efficacy of treatment for only our intended treatment population, and (2) we run a more effective clinical trial. Enrolling patients who clearly will not benefit would decrease our effective sample-size and add additional noise to our estimates [27].

Unfortunately, we often only have a broadly characterized target population entering phase III trials. We may have a biological rationale and some experimental evidence for a candidate biomarker; however we generally do not have strong evidence of its predictive strength in humans. In addition, even if we have an assay which is clearly related to the effectiveness of treatment, there are often still questions: For multivariate assays (e.g. mutations at multiple sites), one needs to identify how to combine measurements; even for univariate continuous assays, one must determine an optimal cut-point for characterizing patients as biomarker positive. In these cases, restricting enrollment at the onset of the trial may be premature. However, as the trial progresses, we may be able to leverage new patient information to address these questions and improve our characterization of the target population. As we better understand which patients to target we may wish to use that knowledge to change our enrollment criteria and enrich that target population in our trial. We call designs of this nature, that outcome-adaptively update enrollment criteria to enrich an in-progress trial, *Adaptive Enrichment Designs*.

2 Adaptive Enrichment for 3 Scenarios

We will consider 3 scenarios in which one might employ an adaptive enrichment design: Developing a biomarker for a treatment based on

1. A single categorical assay: This could be binary (e.g. mutation status at a single position); based on simple combinations of binary markers (e.g. HER2 vs ER +/PR + vs TN breast cancer); ordered categorical (e.g. gene copy number) or based on an ordered categorical breakdown of a continuous assay (e.g. protein expression in tumor microenvironment measured via IHC, though there is a natural ordering here that one can leverage). This scenario becomes more difficult as the number of categories increases (especially for unordered categories).
2. A single continuous assay: This is often seen with expression of a single candidate gene or protein (either in the tumor, or in peripheral blood), but can also be based on other serum/plasma level measurements (e.g. testosterone level).
3. A combination of several assays: This could be multiple candidates for measuring the same underlying biology (e.g. HER2 expression via IHC vs HER2 copy number for trastuzumab); or multiple candidate drivers in the same pathway (e.g. EGFR expression vs RAS mutations vs BRAF mutation, for cetuximab [6, 15, 25]); or even multiple candidates from various pathways. We would caution against using a large number of candidate assays in an adaptive enrichment design. While in theory this could be employed with genome-wide technologies, we recommend restricting those technologies to more uniformly exploratory designs (rather than the combination exploratory/confirmatory nature of an adaptive enrichment design).

In addition we will touch on two classes of adaptive enrichment designs. The first are designs wherein we have prespecified strata in which we evaluate treatment effect separately, and may drop at interim points during the trial. The second are *stratification free* designs, wherein we do not need to prespecify strata: During the trial we build/update models linking outcome, treatment, and candidate biomarker-features to block-sequentially update our enrollment criteria. In these stratification-free designs, though we use models to aid in decision-making, the validity of our null-hypothesis test does not depend on correct specification of our models.

2.1 Single Categorical Biomarker

There are a number of biomarkers that are naturally categorical: Disease histology, mutation status in a pathway of interest, status of several candidate mutations [14, 31]. The levels of this categorical variable define natural strata. A stratification-based adaptive enrichment design is natural in this setting. The main strategy here is to run a group sequential trial, and to potentially drop strata at interim analyses: as treatment reveals itself to be ineffective in certain strata, patients from those strata are no longer recruited for the trial [17, 26, 32, 35, 36].

2.2 Single Continuous Biomarker with Unknown Cutpoint

There are many examples of single continuous candidate biomarkers: expression of surface receptors (e.g. HER2, EGFR), protein expression in tumor microenvironment (e.g. PDL-1) or peripheral blood (e.g. inflammatory cytokines), immune-response to candidate antigens (e.g. as measured by ELISA or ELISPOT assays). In this scenario one could create strata based on ranges of the continuous assay; from here one could use designs developed for the categorical biomarkers of Sect. 2.1. However this ignores the natural ordering of the strata—which in practice can be quite important for efficient cutpoint evaluation. In addition it can lead to difficult decisions: Suppose we expect higher expression levels to benefit more from treatment; if we observe a very significant effect in the medium expression stratum and a more marginal effect in the high expression stratum, we might like to incorporate our prior expectation and reject both; however an analysis based on simple stratification which ignores ordering will not.

2.3 Combination of Assays/Biomarkers

In this final scenario, we aim to combine multiple sources of information into a single rule that characterizes the target population. These sources might be the expression of multiple genes [13, 18, 29] or proteins; we might also combine different data-types like mutation status and epigenetic features (e.g. transcription factor binding or methylation in a nearby genetic region). Though the term "Biomarker" is often used to refer to each individual source of information, we will use it here to refer to the "rule" which combines them all. This is the most general scenario, and in many ways the most difficult.

3 Flexible Adaptive Enrichment

In this chapter we discuss a general framework for adaptive enrichment. This framework can accommodate all of the scenarios above; it can be used with stratification, without stratification (where we build models connecting treatment, features and outcome), for single markers, or for combining multiple markers. This framework is built around work discussed in [34]. There are several important points we will touch on in this chapter but would like to quickly outline below:

- In this framework, a single null hypothesis will be tested. This will be a frequentist test and will not be dependent on any modeling assumptions.
- Intermediate decisions (about who to enroll) may be made using models (and potentially Bayesian methods).
- Estimation of various quantities for a *successful trial* (based on our assumption-free frequentist null hypothesis test) may involve the use of models/ Bayesian methods. This includes characterizing the "biomarker-positive" subpopulation and evaluating treatment-effect in that subpopulation.

In addition we note that the designs we outline in this chapter are not solely concerned with statistical optimality (as is often the case in statistical literature). We try to balance statistical performance, administrative burden, robustness to departures from assumptions, and parsimony.

3.1 Framework

We give an overview of the framework here. Suppose we have a single new treatment we are comparing to control. We randomize each patient that we accrue with equal probability to one of the two arms. Let x_i ($\in \mathcal{X} \subset \mathbb{R}^p$) denote a vector of covariates measured on patient i. Let y_i be the outcome for patient i where $y_i = 1$ for response and $y_i = 0$ for non-response, and let z_i be the treatment assignment (1 for treatment, 0 for control). Note, we illustrate the framework with binary response, but it could just as easily be used with continuous, or time-to-event outcome (though with time-to-event, a short term surrogate outcome might be required within block). Suppose we accrue patients sequentially in K blocks. In the kth block we accrue $2n_k$ patients with n_k randomized to treatment and n_k to control. Assume that we observe the responses (y_i) for patients on the k th block before accruing patients for block $k+1$.

Further, assume we have some rule, which for each block (k) takes in all the data from previous blocks (covariates, assignments, and outcomes) and creates a decision function/indication classifier D_k, with $D_k(x) \in \{0, 1\}$ for all covariate vectors x. For each block we admit only patients with $D_k(x_i) = 1$.

More formally, let X_k, y_k, z_k be the X, y and z values for block k, let $\mathbb{D}_k = [X_1, y_1, z_1, \ldots, X_k, y_k, z_k]$. We define our "rule" $\mathscr{D}$ as a function which takes in $\mathbb{D}$ and returns an enrollment criteria $\mathscr{D}(\mathbb{D}_k) \in \{D | D : \mathscr{X} \to [0,1]\}$.

We conduct our trial as follows:

1. Prespecify K, $n_1, \ldots, n_k$, and $\mathscr{D}$.
2. For the first block use $D_1(x) = 1$ for all x. Enroll (without restriction) and randomize $2n_1$ patients for this block.
3. For blocks $k = 2, \ldots, K$ repeat:
    (a) Calculate $D_k = \mathscr{D}(\mathbb{D}_{k-1})$ based on previous patients outcomes.
    (b) Enroll $2n_k$ new patients with $D_k(x) = 1$, and randomize treatment assignment.
4. At the final analysis a single significance test is performed using as test statistic

$$z = \frac{1}{\sqrt{n/2}} \sum_{k \le K} \sqrt{n_k/2} \left(\frac{\hat{p}_{T(k)} - \hat{p}_{C(k)}}{2\sqrt{\hat{p}_{pool(k)}\left(1 - \hat{p}_{pool(k)}\right)/n_k}} \right)$$

where $\hat{p}_{T(k)}$ and $\hat{p}_{C(k)}$ are the response proportions for the treatment and control arms in block k, $\hat{p}_{pool(k)} = \left(\hat{p}_{T(k)} + \hat{p}_{C(k)}\right)/2$, and $n = \sum_{k \le K} n_k$.

Our statistic here, z, is the usual inverse normal combination test statistic that has been widely used in adaptive trial designs [4]. Comparing this statistic to the tails of a standard Gaussian distribution provides a test which asymptotically controls type 1 error essentially regardless of how we construct the D_k. The power of this test and its ability to identify the subset that benefits from treatment, however, strongly depend on that construction. This tests the strong null hypothesis H_0 : $p_T(x) \le p_C(x)$ for all covariates x, where $p_T(x)$ and $p_C(x)$ are the true response probabilities on the test treatment and control for a patient with covariate vector x. This test preserves the type I error regardless of the method used for making enrichment decisions and regardless of (possibly data dependent) time trends in the characteristics (measured or not) of the patients. One might consider using a rerandomization test; however, as discussed in [34], simple rerandomization tests which are nominally level 0.05 can have type I error in excess of 0.2.

There is a useful alternative formulation of the strong null hypothesis. If we let $\Theta \equiv \{x | p_T(x) > p_C(x)\}$ be the set of feature-values for which treatment outperforms control, then our strong null is equivalently testing if Ω is empty.

For time-to-event data there is potential concern about bias due to followup of censored observations in subsequent blocks [3]. In this framework there is no bias so long as, in the final analysis, observations are included in the block in which they were recruited. This is because there is no sample-size re-estimation, the number of blocks is fixed in advance, and (under H_0) statistics within each block are $N(0, 1)$.

The design above still leaves several open questions: How do we choose $\mathscr{D}$? At the conclusion of a successful trial how do we determine treatment indication?

And how do we estimate the treatment effect-size in the indicated population? In contrast to our model-free method for testing the null hypothesis, these decisions will be based on working models for $p_T(x)$ and $p_C(x)$. In particular we discuss a Bayesian formalism which provides justified choices for all of these questions.

4 A Bayesian Framework for Adaptation

As mentioned above, we propose the use of working models to assist with the various decisions one needs to make both during the trial, and at its termination (excluding hypothesis testing). In particular one must estimate $p_T(x)$ and $p_C(x)$. These estimates need to be updated after each block of patient accrual. In addition one needs to assess the uncertainty of these estimated models for each x. We believe that this is simplest to do using the Bayesian paradigm as: (1) the likelihood principle implies that the sampling distribution of the x's need not be considered in evaluating the uncertainty of our estimates; and (2) decisions can be made to maximize a posterior predictive utility. To apply Bayesian ideas to this process we require specification of 2 things before the trial:

1. A model class for p_T and p_C (the functions indicating response probability on new treatment and standard of care/control as a function of our candidate features); as well as a prior distribution, Π, on that model class. Choices for the model-class and prior are discussed further in Sect. 5.
2. A measure of *utility*, U, for a trial: Trials that successfully reject the null hypothesis should be of higher utility than those do not. *Utility* should also take into account operating characteristics of the "discovered" biomarker (e.g. sensitivity/specificity), accrual time, among other things. This is also discussed in more detail in Sect. 5.

From here one can specify an *optimal* decision rule (given the prior, Π) for the specified utility measure, U. That is the rule that maximizes the expected utility of the trial: $\mathscr{D}^* = \text{argmin}_{\mathscr{D}} E_{\Pi}[U(\text{trial}_{\mathscr{D}})]$. In practice finding the optimal decision rule over all potential decision rules is computationally intractable, so we optimize over a more restricted class. As our prior, Π is generally only a rough estimate of the truth; we worry less about optimality for that prior, and more about balancing good performance under our prior with parsimony and computational tractability. These restrictions are discussed further in Sect. 4.1.

Operationally, our procedure which optimizes over these decision functions will look like:

1. Choose a prior for (p_T, p_c), and a utility measure U for the trial.
2. Enroll the first block of patients without restriction.
3. Update our prior based on the observed treatments, outcomes, and covariates of enrolled patients to get a posterior.

4. Using the posterior, simulate the rest of the trial (many times) to find an "optimal" enrollment decision rule (with respect to our utility) for enrolling patients in the next block.
5. Enroll a new block of patients using our "optimal" rule.
6. Repeat steps 2–4 for each additional block.

We still have several decisions to make: we need a prior distribution for (p_T, p_c), as well as a utility function. To make things computationally tractable, a few simplifications will be employed in developing an "optimal" enrollment decision rule. These will be discussed further, in Sect. 5.

4.1 Utility-Based Enrollment Criteria

Our decision function gives us a rule for determining eligibility at each stage of our trial. As mentioned in Sect. 4, given a utility, model-space, and prior distribution, there is an optimal decision rule for maximizing the expected utility of the trial: $U(trial)$. More formally, for an enrollment rule $\mathscr{D}$ our expected utility is

$$\mathrm{E}[U(trial)] = \int \mathrm{E}[U(trial)|\mathscr{D}, (p_T, p_C)] d\Pi(p_T, p_C), \tag{1}$$

where $trial|\mathscr{D}, (p_T, p_C)$ is a random trial generated with true response probabilities $p_T(x)$ and $p_C(x)$, run using rule $\mathscr{D}$. Unfortunately, maximizing the quantity in (1) involves a functional maximization over an infinite dimensional space, and to our knowledge the solution in general is computationally intractable.

We instead propose optimizing the utility over a restricted class of decision functions. To make this optimization tractable we suggest considering only a finite number of candidates. One tractable and relatively flexible option is to use rules of the form:

$$\mathscr{D}(\mathbb{D}_{k-1})(x) = D_k(x) = \begin{cases} 1: & \Pi(p_T(x) > p_C(x) + \varepsilon|\mathbb{D}_{k-1}) > \eta_k(\mathbb{D}_{k-1}) \\ 0: & else \end{cases} \tag{2}$$

where $\varepsilon \geq 0$ is a prespecified minimum relevant treatment efficacy, and $\eta_k(\mathbb{D}_{k-1})$ is a single parameter per block over which we optimize (from a discrete set of prespecified candidate values). Here we only allow decisions to be made based on the posterior probability that a patient has a higher response rate on the new treatment than standard of care. This functional of the data effectively combines information about the expectation and variability of $p_T(x) - p_C(x)|\mathbb{D}_{k-1}$, though other functionals may also work well. Also note, η_k is written as $\eta_k(\mathbb{D}_{k-1})$ to make clear that it is a function of the previous data—this allows one to be more conservative or liberal in our enrollment, based on the quality of information attained so far in the trial. In addition, we note that by using a discrete set of candidate models, optimization over this class be done by brute force: simulating a large number of trials under each potential rule, and choosing the decision function for which those simulations had the highest average utility.

We should note that we are *not* just enrolling patients in each block who are in our current best estimate of Θ: At intermediate stages of the trial we need to take into account both (a) *if we expect a given patient to benefit* and (b) *how likely that expectation is to change given additional data*. Thus our enrollment criteria is a bit broader than what our estimated indication would be if the trial terminated at that stage: In addition to enrolling patients whom we expect to benefit, we would also like to enroll patients whom we do not have enough information on to make a well informed decision. While a criterion based on (2) contains a happy medium of information from (a) and (b), there are many other options to use instead e.g. a pre-specified quantile of the distribution of $(p_T(x) - p_C(x)|\mathbb{D}_{k-1})$, or a 2 dimensional statistic like $\mathrm{E}[p_T(x) - p_C(x)|\mathbb{D}_{k-1}]$ and $\mathrm{var}(p_T(x) - p_C(x)|\mathbb{D}_{k-1})$—though this increases the size of the search space.

One might wonder at the cost of using this restricted optimal rule, rather than the unrestricted optimal rule. While this is hard to assess, one might believe the cost is minimal (if there is a cost at all). The unrestricted rule is only "optimal" in so far as the model class and prior for p_T and p_C are correctly specified. In practice we never believe this specification (especially of the prior) is perfect; and thus do not worry overly about optimality—we use the Bayesian framework as a principled way to choose a good rule, rather than a dogma forcing us to choose the "optimal" rule.

4.2 Estimates for Labeling

At the termination of a successful trial we are left with two important labeling questions. *For whom should the treatment be indicated*? And *what is the effect size of treatment in that indicated population*? We discuss two options for answering these questions. As we move forward we will let $\Omega \subset \mathscr{X}$ denote our treatment indication.

Model-Free Approach: The first approach uses the enrollment criteria for the final period as our treatment indication: i.e.

$$\Omega \leftarrow \{x|D_K(x) = 1\}.$$

We can estimate treatment-effect in that indicated population by just the difference in sample means from our final period:

$$\hat{\delta} = \hat{p}_{T(K)} - \hat{p}_{C(K)}.$$

The upside of this approach is that, as with our hypothesis test, the validity of these estimates does not require correct specification of our models or priors. The downside is two fold: (1) we only get to use a subset of our data in estimating treatment effect. While this estimate is unbiased, it may be high variance, and this approach may result in a negative effect-size estimate for a trial which in-fact rejects the null hypothesis; and (2) using utility-based enrollment, for many utility choices, enrollment in the final block may not be optimized towards enrolling *only* those patients whom we believe benefit from treatment—there may still be patients enrolled for whom there is uncertainty leading into the final block (but perhaps not uncertainty after that block). We would like to use that information from the final block to further refine our classifier.

Model-Based Approach: The second approach leverages the models $p_T(x)$, and $p_C(x)$ to determine our indication and evaluate treatment-effect. At the end of the trial, we can base our indication on our posterior expectation for both models using:

$$\Omega \leftarrow \{x|\mathrm{E}[p_T(x) - p_C(x)|\mathbb{D}_K] \geq \varepsilon\},$$

where $\varepsilon \geq 0$ is some minimal relevant effect-size (possibly 0). This is just the set of patients for whom we expect posterior benefit. In practice this could be a complicated set (likely not characterized by a simple linear rule). Using the posterior distribution affords the ability to consider things like the optimal linear rule:

$$\Omega \leftarrow \left\{x|x^\top a(\mathbb{D}_K) \geq a_0(\mathbb{D}_K)\right\}$$

where

$$(a, a_0)(\mathbb{D}_K) \leftarrow \mathrm{argmax}_{a,a_0} \int_x \mathrm{E}[p_T(x) - p_C(x)]I\left\{a^\top x > a_0\right\}dG(x)$$

with $dG(x)$ the density of our covariate(s), x. Regardless of the rule we use, estimating average treatment is straightforward in these scenarios: We just use the posterior estimate

$$\hat{\delta} = \frac{1}{G(\Omega)} \int_{x\in\Omega} \mathrm{E}[p_T(x) - p_C(x)|\mathbb{D}_K]dG(x).$$

In the Bayesian framework, our effect-size estimates do not have selection bias (even though we use our models to select the subset over which we average). Here, the prior provides natural shrinkage.

Estimating the Distribution of Covariates: In estimating effect-size (or choosing the optimal linear rule) we need an estimate of the distribution of our covariates. One possibility is to use the empirical distribution of covariates in the first block of the trial. Unfortunately, using the unmodified empirical distribution from future blocks of the trial will lead to a bias because the changing enrollment criteria (based on adaptive enrichment) will lead to biased covariate distribution. However, in practice, while not all patients will be enrolled in the trial, in every block, all candidate patients who apply to the trial will need to have their covariate values measured (to check their eligibility). If these measurements are saved, then we can use the empirical distribution of all those measurements for $\hat{dG}$.

4.3 Benefit-Based Stratification

Rather than only characterizing the subpopulation of patients believed to benefit from treatment over control, one may want to stratify patients into more subgroups; e.g. perhaps 3 subgroups: those likely to benefit, those unlikely to benefit, and those for whom there is no clear indication either way. One way to develop these subgroups is based on a statistic that combines posterior expected benefit, and posterior variance, e.g.:

$$T(x) = \frac{\mathrm{E}[p_T(x) - p_C(x)]}{\sqrt{\mathrm{var}(p_T(x) - p_C(x))}}.$$

For some prespecified cutpoint $c > 0$, we can define

$$\begin{aligned} \Omega_{unlikely} &= \{x | T(x) < -c\} \\ \Omega_{uncertain} &= \{x | -c \leq T(x) \leq c\} \\ \Omega_{likely} &= \{x | T(x) > c\}. \end{aligned}$$

However, these sets may have complicated boundaries in x which are highly non-linear.

Instead we may consider the linear combination, $x^\top a$, from our optimal linear rule. Here we can find cutoffs a_{low} and a_{high} based on this linear combo; with

$$\begin{aligned} \Omega_{unlikely} &= \left\{x | x^\top a < a_{low}\right\} \\ \Omega_{uncertain} &= \left\{x | a_{low} \leq x^\top a \leq a_{high}\right\} \\ \Omega_{likely} &= \left\{x | x^\top a > a_{high}\right\}. \end{aligned}$$

Here, a_{low} and a_{high} might be selected based on quantiles of $x^\top a$. Or they could be selected based on

$$T(x; a_{min}, a_{max}) \equiv \int_{a_{min} < x^\top a < a_{max}} (p_T(x) - p_C(x)) dG(x)$$

where a_{high} is selected to be the minimum value such that

$$\frac{\mathrm{E}\left[T\left(x; a_{high}, \infty\right)\right] - \varepsilon}{\sqrt{\mathrm{var}\left(T\left(x; a_{high}, \infty\right)\right)}} > c$$

and a_{low} is selected to be the maximum value such that

$$\frac{\mathrm{E}[T(x;\infty,a_{low})]-\varepsilon}{\sqrt{\mathrm{var}(T(x;\infty,a_{low}))}}<-c$$

This is one of many potential options that considers both the expected treatment effect and the variability of that treatment effect.

5 Choosing Utility, Models, and Priors

As mentioned in Sect. 4, to run an adaptive enrichment trial under this framework one must choose a utility, and model classes with a joint prior for response as a function of covariates under treatment and control. We discuss these choices below, and give recommendations under various scenarios.

5.1 Choice of Utility

There are many possibilities for codifying utility. One noteworthy aspect here is that utility is not solely a function of trial success/power (and enrollment time) as it might be in a classical biomarker-free trial. Power is generally maximized by choosing only a very small subset of patients—rather than enrolling all patients who would likely benefit from treatment, instead, power is increased by including only those who will receive very large benefit from treatment. However, this is at odds with our goal of characterizing and enrolling all those patients who would benefit from the new treatment over control. The utility we choose should reflect this, combining power to reject the global null, with sensitivity of the developed biomarker. One can directly combine these with something like

$$U(trial)=\alpha\underbrace{I\{rejectH_0\}}_{\text{trial success}}+(1-\alpha)\underbrace{\int\left[\frac{\int I\{x\in\Omega(\mathbb{D}_K)\}I[p_T(x)-p_C(x)>0]dG(x)}{\int I[p_T(x)-p_C(x)>0]dG(x)}\right]d\Pi(p_T,p_C|\mathbb{D}_K)}_{\text{average biomarker sensitivity}},$$

where $0\leq\alpha\leq 1$ is a prespecified weight, and $\Omega(\mathbb{D}_K)$ is our subpopulation indicated for treatment at the end of the trial. Other utilities might also be used. One strong candidate is what we term *expected future patient outcome penalized by accrual time*:

$$U(trial)=(\text{expected future patient outcome})-\gamma(\text{Accrual Time}),$$

where *expected future patient outcome* (EFPO) is

$$\text{EFPO} = \begin{cases} \int_{\mathcal{X}} (I\{x \in \Omega(\mathbb{D}_K)\}\mathrm{E}[p_T(x)|\mathbb{D}_K] \\ \quad + I\{x \notin \Omega(\mathbb{D}_K)\}\mathrm{E}[p_C(x)|\mathbb{D}_K])dGx & : \text{if we reject } H_0 \\ \int_{\mathcal{X}} \mathrm{E}[p_C(x)|\mathbb{D}_K]dG(x) & : \text{if we fail to reject } H_0 \end{cases}$$

and γ is some prespecified parameter that trades off between future patient benefit and accrual time. Note, if our indicated subpopulation is just the subpopulation with posterior expected benefit, i.e.

$$\Omega \leftarrow \{x|\mathrm{E}[p_T(x) - p_C(x)|\mathbb{D}_K] \geq 0\},$$

then for a successful trial, our utility becomes

$$\int_{\mathcal{X}} \max\{\mathrm{E}[p_T(x)|\mathbb{D}_K], \mathrm{E}[p_C(x)|\mathbb{D}_K]\}dG(x).$$

This utility naturally balances accrual time, power, and sensitivity:

Accrual Time: Penalizing by accrual time means we will not run too lengthy a trial (often in practice, even trials with $\gamma = 0$ are not too long).
Power: Because we only allow the treatment to be used for future patients if we successfully reject H_0, this criterion attempts to increase power.
Sensitivity: As we better characterize our biomarker + subgroup, we gain value from using $I\{x \in \Omega(\mathbb{D}_K)\}\mathrm{E}[p_T(x)|\mathbb{D}_K] + I\{x \notin \Omega(\mathbb{D}_K)\}\mathrm{E}[p_C(x)|\mathbb{D}_K]$ in our utility.

We also note that this utility optimizes for future patient outcome *using the rule we plan to develop during the trial*, i.e. if we use an *optimal linear rule* then future patient outcome is based on the optimal linear rule.

5.2 *Modeling Outcome as a Function of Treatment and Covariates*

As discussed earlier, we propose the use of working models to assist with the various decisions one needs to make both during the trial, and at its termination (excluding hypothesis testing). In particular one must estimate $p_T(x)$ and $p_C(x)$. Here, we will discuss modeling strategies for the 3 scenarios from Sect. 2.

5.2.1 Unordered Categorical Biomarker

Here we suppose our assay takes on one of M values: $x \in \{v_1, \ldots, v_M\}$. This is the simplest scenario. Without biomarker-specific apriori knowledge, one might use

$$p_T(v_m) \sim \text{Beta}(\alpha_T, \beta_T) \qquad p_C(v_m) \sim \text{Beta}(\alpha_C, \beta_C) \qquad \text{for each } m$$

where α_C, β_C are chosen based on historical response rates, and α_T, β_T are based on early clinical or preclinical data. If insufficient data are available for selecting α_T, β_T one can use $\alpha_T = \alpha_C, \beta_T = \beta_C$. One should note that choosing α_T, β_T such that $E[p_T(\cdot)] > > E[p_C(\cdot)]$ actually leads to more conservative adaptation (as it encourages us to believe that treatment is generally beneficial across levels of the biomarker). In addition, our final hypothesis test is completely frequentist and does not incorporate the prior, so this does not lead to anti-conservatism. This is in contrast to a trial with a Bayesian hypothesis test, where choosing a prior with a large treatment effect will lead to inflated type-1 error.

In situations where more information is known about the prognostic value of the biomarker, but no information is available on treatment, one might use

$$p_T(v_m) \sim \text{Beta}(\alpha_m, \beta_m) \qquad p_C(v_m) \sim \text{Beta}(\alpha_m, \beta_m) \qquad \text{for each } m,$$

where α_m, β_m are chosen based on biomarker-level specific historical response rates. This can be extended via hierarchical Bayesian modeling [12].

5.2.2 Univariate Continuous Biomarker

Here, for ease of notation we will assume our assay, x, takes on values in $[0, 1]$. One simple approach is to use separate logistic models for response on treatment and control:

$$\text{logit}(p_T(x)) = \beta_0 + \beta x \qquad \text{logit}(p_C(x)) = \alpha_0 + \alpha x.$$

This is equivalent to a single model with interactions

$$p(y = 1|x, treatment) = \gamma_0 + \gamma_1 I\{treatment = T\} + \gamma_2 x + \gamma_3 x I\{treatment = T\}$$

with $\gamma_0 = \alpha_0$, $\gamma_1 = \beta_0 - \alpha_0$, $\gamma_2 = \alpha$, and $\gamma_3 = \beta - \alpha$. One could extend this to a more flexible estimate using a basis expansion: Let $\psi_1, \ldots, \psi_M$ be pre-specified functions. One might consider the model

$$\text{logit}(p_T(x)) = \beta_0 + \sum_{m=1}^{M} \beta_m \psi_m(x) \qquad \text{logit}(p_C(x)) = \alpha_0 + \sum_{m=1}^{M} \alpha_m \psi_m(x)$$

Some potential choices for $\{\psi_m\}_{m=1}^{M}$ are polynomial basis functions or a spline functions with prespecified knots. In particular, using 0-th order splines (i.e. $\psi_m(x) = I\{x \geq t_m\}$ where t_m is a prespecified knot) is equivalent to discretizing our continuous marker into a categorical marker. If we specifying priors for $\alpha_0, \ldots, \beta_0, \ldots$ then these become Bayesian models. Those priors can encode known information about directionality of an effect. For example suppose we were designing an adaptive enrichment trial to test the efficacy of trastuzumab vs chemotherapy, and were using HER2 expression in the tumor as a candidate biomarker. Our prior belief is that increased HER2 expression is a negative prognostic factor on chemotherapy; but likely correlated with increased effectiveness of trastuzumab. In this case one would want a joint prior on all the parameters such that: (a) there is little (or no) prior weight on any parameter-vectors with $\alpha_m > 0$ for any $m = 1, \ldots, M$; and (b) there is little (or no) prior weight on any parameter-vectors with $\beta_m - \alpha_m < 0$ for any m.

This approach with 0-th order splines can also be applied in the case of ordered categorical variables (with prior information on directionality). Here we assume categorical variables are coded as $1, \ldots, M$, and we can use $\psi_m(x) = I\{x \geq m\}$.

5.2.3 Multivariate Biomarker

Here we are interested in combining a number of features (potentially a combination of continuous and categorical features): $x_1, \ldots, x_p$. For ease of exposition we assume that any categorical features are encoded as dummy-variables in the preceding representation. One simple but generally effective strategy is to use linear-logistic models

$$\text{logit}(p_T(x)) = \beta_0 + \sum_j \beta_j x_j \qquad \text{logit}(p_C(x)) = \alpha_0 + \sum_j \alpha_j x_j.$$

This would assume monotonicity of effects and an additive-only structure. This approach can be made more flexible by including interactions and/or basis expansions of the features (as discussed in Sect. 5.2.2). Complex models however require many observations to fit: it is recommended here to restrict attention to those features for which there is strong biological rationale and limit additional complexity due to interactions/basis expansions. Recall that these models are used at intermediate stages to assist in the decision making process, but validity of the global null hypothesis test does not hinge on correct model specification. Furthermore there is no potential for confounding as patients on the trial are randomized to treatment arms. This relieves many of the modeling concerns that might push us towards more complex models. As with our other scenarios, these models, by specifying a joint prior for $\alpha_0, \ldots, \beta_0, \ldots$ we create Bayesian models. Informed prior specification for these joint models can be difficult—we recommend in most cases using very diffuse priors. A more in depth discussion of Bayesian multivariate logistic modeling can be found in [28].

6 Discussion

There are a number of additional philosophical and practical issues one might have about this framework for adaptive enrichment. We address some of these below.

6.1 *Bayesian Versus Frequentist Enrichment*

The framework detailed in this chapter uses the Bayesian paradigm for enrichment decisions, and the frequentist paradigm for testing. One might instead consider using a Bayesian test or frequentist models for enrichment decisions. We give our rationale for our choices below.

Making choices about adaptation is a decision theory problem. The Bayesian paradigm has simple, straightforward machinery for formalizing and optimizing decision theory problems. In addition updating our models after each block of patients is most easily done as a Bayesian. The likelihood principle implies that we need not concern ourselves with how covariate values are selected in calculating posterior model distributions. In contrast, as a frequentist, in finite samples the variability of our estimated model is not easily tractable: the x-values we see in future blocks are informative for the outcomes seen in previous blocks. Thus the maximum likelihood estimate conditional on our x-values is not our usual MLE. Finally, in estimating effect size the Bayesian framework allows natural shrinkage through the choice of prior distribution (though this may not be a simple choice). It is not clear how one might employ principled shrinkage in the frequentist formulation.

For ensuring that trial-wise type I error is controlled at a specified level, we believe the frequentist paradigm is more robust. For a Bayesian test to be valid we need valid models for $p_T(x)$ and $p_C(x)$, and we would need to demonstrate that the repeated sampling properties of the design are robust for a wide range of priors different from the ones used in the trial. Our frequentist test requires no modeling or parametric assumptions, and relies only very lightly on asymptotics. For pivotal regulatory clinical trials strong emphasis is placed on stringent control of the study-wise type I error in a manner not heavily dependent on model assumptions. However, in phase II trials where our covariates define a small number of pre-specified strata, a Bayesian test could be appropriate.

6.2 *The Strong Null Hypothesis*

In this chapter, we have discussed trial designs that test the *strong* null hypothesis: $H_0 : p_T(x) \leq p_C(x)$ for all $x \in \mathscr{X}$, where $p_T(x)$ and $p_C(x)$ are the response probabilities for a patient with covariate vector x under treatment and control respectively. This protects the study-wise type I error, but does not ensure that treatment is effective for the subpopulation indicated at the end of the trial. We do not believe this discrepancy is a common occurrence—one should only have additional power (over 0.05) to reject H_0 when our enrollment algorithm is actually enrolling patients for whom treatment is effective.

In addition a somewhat symmetric criticism can be applied to classical designs. There we test for overall treatment efficacy ignoring any potential biomarkers. When we do find a significant treatment effect, this is often driven by a small subset of patients for whom treatment is effective. In a classical trial however, we haven't characterized that subset, so rather than trying to target treatment at all, we indicate it for the entire population, incorrectly treating many patients! At least with these adaptive designs we give ourselves the opportunity to characterize the subpopulation. That said, this criticism is slightly less severe as in a traditional trial we have a formal statistical test showing that on average treatment benefits our indicated population (in that case the entire diseased population). In our adaptive design, though there is strong evidence for this, a formal statistical test was not run on that hypothesis.

In addition there is a literature on seamless phase II/III trials [10, 21] that takes another approach to this problem: They use a closed testing procedure in a two block design to reject the specific hypothesis selected in the second stage. We do not take this approach because (1) it requires prespecification of strata; the framework here is developed for a potentially continuous covariate space without the need to stratify; (2) if there are many strata, then the closed testing procedure will require one to test many intersection hypotheses. However, for problems with a small number of discrete covariates (with few levels) this closed testing approach could be a fruitful alternative.

6.3 Conclusion

In this chapter we have discussed a framework for adaptive enrichment trials. This framework formalizes the choices one needs to make (in terms of utility, prior response rates, a decision functional, and potential cutpoints) in an adaptive trial and carries through Bayesian machinery to make effective decisions. This chapter gives suggestions for these choices. In addition, a recipe is given for carrying out a complete adaptive enrichment clinical trial. The recipe uses a frequentist test to control the type 1 error, and this type 1 error control is valid regardless of unknown time-trends in the data. When the global null hypothesis is rejected, Bayesian methods are used to effectively find a subset of patients who will benefit from treatment and to estimate the average treatment effect in that subset. This may serve to reduce the over-treatment of the patient population that takes place in many clinical trials that use the initial eligibility criteria as the basis for defining the intended use population.

References

1. Amado RG, Wolf M, Peeters M, Van Cutsem E, Siena S, Freeman DJ, Juan T, Sikorski R, Suggs S, Radinsky R, et al. Wild-type KRAS is required for panitumumab efficacy in patients with metastatic colorectal cancer. J Clin Oncol. 2008;26(10):1626–34.
2. Andreyev HJN, Norman AR, Cunningham D, Oates J, Dix BR, Iacopetta BJ, Young J, Walsh T, Ward R, Hawkins N, et al. Kirsten ras mutations in patients with colorectal cancer: the 'RASCAL II' study. Br J Cancer. 2001;85(5):692.
3. Bauer P, Posch M. Modification of the sample size and the schedule of interim analyses in survival trials based on data inspections by H. Schäfer and H.-H. Müller, statistics in medicine 2001; 20: 3741–3751. Stat Med. 2004;23(8):1333–4.
4. Bauer P, Bretz F, Dragalin V, König F, Wassmer G. Twenty-five years of confirmatory adaptive designs: opportunities and pitfalls. Stat Med. 2016;35(3):325–47.
5. Bennett M, Dent CL, Ma Q, Dastrala S, Grenier F, Workman R, Syed H, Ali S, Barasch J, Devarajan P. Urine NGAL predicts severity of acute kidney injury after cardiac surgery: a prospective study. Clin J Am Soc Nephrol. 2008;3(3):665–73.
6. Bokemeyer C, Bondarenko I, Makhson A, Hartmann JT, Aparicio J, de Braud F, Donea S, Ludwig H, Schuch G, Stroh C, et al. Fluorouracil, leucovorin, and oxaliplatin with and without cetuximab in the first-line treatment of metastatic colorectal cancer. J Clin Oncol. 2009;27(5):663–71.
7. Bokemeyer C, Van Cutsem E, Rougier P, Ciardiello F, Heeger S, Schlichting M, Celik I, Köhne C-H. Addition of cetuximab to chemotherapy as first-line treatment for KRAS wild-type metastatic colorectal cancer: pooled analysis of the crystal and opus randomised clinical trials. Eur J Cancer. 2012;48(10):1466–75.
8. Bollag G, Hirth P, Tsai J, Zhang J, Ibrahim PN, Cho H, Spevak W, Zhang C, Zhang Y, Habets G, et al. Clinical efficacy of a RAF inhibitor needs broad target blockade in BRAF-mutant melanoma. Nature. 2010;467(7315):596–9.
9. Brahmer JR, Tykodi SS, Chow LQ, Hwu W-J, Topalian SL, Hwu P, Drake CG, Camacho LH, Kauh J, Odunsi K, et al. Safety and activity of anti-pd-l1 antibody in patients with advanced cancer. N Engl J Med. 2012;366(26):2455–65.
10. Bretz F, Schmidli H, König F, Racine A, Maurer W. Confirmatory seamless phase II/III clinical trials with hypotheses selection at interim: general concepts. Biom J. 2006;48(4): 623–34.
11. Cai T, Tian L, Wong PH, Wei LJ. Analysis of randomized comparative clinical trial data for personalized treatment selections. Biostatistics. 2011;12(2):270–82.
12. Chen BE, Jiang W, Tu D. A hierarchical Bayes model for biomarker subset effects in clinical trials. Comput Stat Data Anal. 2014;71:324–34.
13. Cobleigh MA, Bitterman P, Baker J, Cronin M, Liu ML, Borchik R, Tabesh B, Mosquera JM, Walker MG, Shak S. Tumor gene expression predicts distant disease-free survival (DDFS) in breast cancer patients with 10 or more positive nodes: high throughput RT-PCR assay of paraffin-embedded tumor tissues. In: Proc Am Soc Clin Oncol, vol 22; 2003.
14. Di Nicolantonio F, Martini M, Molinari F, Sartore-Bianchi A, Arena S, Saletti P, De Dosso S, Mazzucchelli L, Frattini M, Siena S, et al. Wild-type braf is required for response to panitumumab or cetuximab in metastatic colorectal cancer. J Clin Oncol. 2008;26(35): 5705–12.
15. Douillard J-Y, Oliner KS, Siena S, Tabernero J, Burkes R, Barugel M, Humblet Y, Bodoky G, Cunningham D, Jassem J, et al. Panitumumab–FOLFOX4 treatment and RAS mutations in colorectal cancer. N Engl J Med. 2013;369(11):1023–34.
16. Freidlin B, Korn EL. Biomarker enrichment strategies: matching trial design to biomarker credentials. Nat Rev Clin Oncol. 2014;11(2):81–90.
17. Friede T, Parsons N, Stallard N. A conditional error function approach for subgroup selection in adaptive clinical trials. Stat Med. 2012;31(30):4309–20.

18. Habel LA, Shak S, Jacobs MK, Capra A, Alexander C, Pho M, Baker J, Walker M, Watson D, Hackett J, et al. A population-based study of tumor gene expression and risk of breast cancer death among lymph node-negative patients. Breast Cancer Res. 2006;8(3):1.
19. Hudis CA. Trastuzumab—mechanism of action and use in clinical practice. N Engl J Med. 2007;357(1):39–51.
20. James CR, Quinn JE, Mullan PB, Johnston PG, Harkin DP. BRCA1, a potential predictive biomarker in the treatment of breast cancer. Oncologist. 2007;12(2):142–50.
21. Jennison C, Turnbull BW. Adaptive seamless designs: selection and prospective testing of hypotheses. J Biopharm Stat. 2007;17(6):1135–61.
22. Jordan VC. A current view of tamoxifen for the treatment and prevention of breast cancer. Br J Pharmacol. 1993;110(2):507–17.
23. Kidd EA, Siegel BA, Dehdashti F, Grigsby PW. The standardized uptake value for F-18 fluorodeoxyglucose is a sensitive predictive biomarker for cervical cancer treatment response and survival. Cancer. 2007;110(8):1738–44.
24. Li J, Zhao L, Tian L, Cai T, Claggett B, Callegaro A, Dizier B, Spiessens B, Ulloa-Montoya F, Wei L-J. A predictive enrichment procedure to identify potential responders to a new therapy for randomized, comparative controlled clinical studies. Biometrics. 2015;72:877–87.
25. Lievre A, Bachet J-B, Le Corre D, Boige V, Landi B, Emile J-F, Côté J-F, Tomasic G, Penna C, Ducreux M, et al. KRAS mutation status is predictive of response to cetuximab therapy in colorectal cancer. Can Res. 2006;66(8):3992–5.
26. Magnusson BP, Turnbull BW. Group sequential enrichment design incorporating subgroup selection. Stat Med. 2013;32(16):2695–714.
27. Mehta CR, Gao P. Population enrichment designs: case study of a large multinational trial. J Biopharm Stat. 2011;21(4):831–45.
28. O'brien SM, Dunson DB. Bayesian multivariate logistic regression. Biometrics. 2004;60(3): 739–46.
29. Paik S, Tang G, Shak S, Kim C, Baker J, Kim W, Cronin M, Baehner FL, Watson D, Bryant J, et al. Gene expression and benefit of chemotherapy in women with node-negative, estrogen receptor–positive breast cancer. J Clin Oncol. 2006;24(23):3726–34.
30. Penna G, Mondaini N, Amuchastegui S, Innocenti SD, Carini M, Giubilei G, Fibbi B, Colli E, Maggi M, Adorini L. Seminal plasma cytokines and chemokines in prostate inflammation: interleukin 8 as a predictive biomarker in chronic prostatitis/chronic pelvic pain syndrome and benign prostatic hyperplasia. Eur Urol. 2007;51(2):524–33.
31. Rajagopalan H, Bardelli A, Lengauer C, Kinzler KW, Vogelstein B, Velculescu VE. Tumorigenesis: RAF/RAS oncogenes and mismatch-repair status. Nature. 2002;418(6901): 934.
32. Rosenblum M, van der Laan MJ. Optimizing randomized trial designs to distinguish which subpopulations benefit from treatment. Biometrika. 2011;98(4):845–60.
33. Ross JS, Slodkowska EA, Symmans WF, Pusztai L, Ravdin PM, Hortobagyi GN. The HER-2 receptor and breast cancer: ten years of targeted anti-HER-2 therapy and personalized medicine. Oncologist. 2009;14(4):320–68.
34. Simon N, Simon R. Adaptive enrichment designs for clinical trials. Biostatistics. 2013;14 (4):613–25.
35. Wang S-J, James Hung HM, O'Neill RT. Adaptive patient enrichment designs in therapeutic trials. Biom J. 2009;51(2):358–74.
36. Wang S-J, O'Neill RT, Hung HM. Approaches to evaluation of treatment effect in randomized clinical trials with genomic subset. Pharm Stat. 2007;6(3):227–44.

Evaluating Personalized Medicine in Multi-marker Multi-treatment Clinical Trials: Accounting for Heterogeneity

Xavier Paoletti and Stefan Michiels

Abstract The assessment of the added value when matching the right treatment to the right population based on a molecular profile raises numerous statistical issues. Due to the low prevalence of potential molecular predictive factors of response to treatment as well as of the existence of many types of histology in oncology, it is often impossible to carry out a separate trial for each histology and molecular profile combination. Instead, several contemporary randomized clinical trials investigate the efficacy of algorithms that combine multiple treatments with multiple molecular markers. Some of them focus on a single histology, whereas other are histology-agnostic and test whether selecting the treatment based on biology is superior to selecting the treatment based on histology. Several important sources of variability are induced by these types of trials. When this variability also concerns the treatment effect, the statistical properties of the design may be strongly compromised. In this chapter, using the randomized SHIVA trial evaluating personalized medicine in patients with advanced cancers as example, we present strengths and pitfalls of designs and various analysis tools. In particular, we illustrate the lack of power in the case of an algorithm being partially erroneous, the necessity to use randomized trials compared to designs where the patient is his or (her) own control, and propose a modeling approach to account for heterogeneity in treatment effects at the analysis step.

Keywords Treatment algorithm · PFS ratio · Randomized mixed effect model

X. Paoletti (✉) · S. Michiels
Service de Biostatistique et Epidémiologie, Gustave Roussy & INSERM CESP U1018 - OncoStat, Gustave Roussy Cancer Center, Université Paris Sud Saclay, 114 Rue Ed Vaillant, 94805 Villejuif Cedex, France
e-mail: xavier.paoletti@gustaveroussy.fr

S. Michiels
e-mail: stefan.michiels@gustaveroussy.fr

S. Matsui and J. Crowley (eds.), *Frontiers of Biostatistical Methods and Applications in Clinical Oncology*, DOI 10.1007/978-981-10-0126-0_9

1 Introduction

Building on recent advances in biology and biotechnology, most new agents in oncology are designed to target molecular alterations or immunologic specificities involved in carcinogenesis. Anti-tumor activity is expected only in the presence of the matching molecular alterations or markers, which play the role of predictive factors of increased treatment benefit. Tumour genetics is increasingly being claimed as the main source of variability in the treatment effect compared to histology. Nevertheless, molecularly targeted agents (MTAs) have been assessed to date according to tumor location and histology before considering the molecular target. For instance, trastuzumab was first developed in breast cancer patients over-expressing HER2 before anti-tumor activity in advanced/metastatic stomach cancers with the same target was demonstrated [2]. This approach, that allows a fine description of the activity of new agents in every combination of histology and molecular marker, is rapidly limited by the sample sizes required for clinical trials: the combination of the low prevalence of some markers as well as low prevalence of specific tumor types transforms several subgroups into rare diseases. The classical sequential development of a MTA by tumor type with the same molecular abnormality is thus unrealistic in most cases. Therefore, there is strong interest in the possibility to investigate several tumors with common biological characteristics or markers matching several treatments in the same trial. Besides clinical trials, numerous companies or academic programs propose patients with refractory diseases to derive their molecular profiles and to apply an algorithm in order to select the most appropriate off-label regimen (Caris, Foundation Medicine, Myriad Genetics among others). So far, a convincing demonstration of the clinical utility of these algorithms on patients outcomes has not been made.

The integration of biomarkers in the design and analysis of clinical trials is a vast field of research. It includes the identification of the target population that may benefit from a treatment, the validation of a prognostic or predictive biomarker to treat patients, and the investigation of complex algorithms to select the adequate treatment among a set of agents in a single or in multiple diseases. Readers interested in the statistical designs tailored for the investigation of biomarkers in a single disease and for a single treatment are referred to several high-quality contributions that provide a comprehensive review of various approaches [4, 5, 26].

In this chapter, we focus on the issue of designing and analyzing trials with multiple tumour types and/or multiple treatments to assess the added value of a pre-defined algorithm. So far, the major successes of using molecular abnormalities rather than histology to drive treatment comes from non-randomized trials or cohorts. A recent meta-analysis of phase I trials compared the outcomes within phase I trials that selected patients based on the molecular abnormality versus those who did not. The authors concluded that there was a benefit of selecting treatment for refractory cancer based solely on the tumor biology [30, 35]. A pilot study by Von Hoff evaluated a multi-treatment multi-histology algorithm by comparing for each patient the progression-free survival (PFS) obtained with the targeted strategy to the PFS obtained during the previous line of treatment [37]. This is the so-called PFS ratio or tumor growth modulation index. However, the lack of randomization *vs* standard of care in these studies did not allow for drawing definitive conclusions [6]. Recently, several randomized trials assessing the added value of personalized medicine have been carried out [16] or are ongoing. The aim of these studies is no longer to investigate a unique biomarker but to study whether an algorithm, that is a combination of agents and rules to allocate the agents to patients, would be more efficient than the standard approach based on histology. These trials raise numerous issues at both the design and the analysis level. One of the common roots to these issues is the heterogeneity in the population characteristics and in the intervention (several agents, several targets). This heterogeneity is con-substantial of these trials that aim at demonstrating a global personalized approach.

To illustrate the various methodological questions we need to address to set up a trial in this context, we use the SHIVA trial [15] as running example. Multiple treatments were investigated in patients with any solid tumor cancers refractory to approved treatments for their disease.

Briefly, the SHIVA trial was designed to evaluate whether tumor biology is a more important driver for treating cancer patients than tumor location and histology in advanced, refractory cancers. The concept appeared particularly attractive for less common or rare tumor types for which dedicated randomized trials of MTAs are usually not carried out, which supported the idea to include all solid tumor types. This randomized trial compared MTAs approved at the time of the trial (outside of their approved indications) based on metastasis molecular profiling versus chemotherapy (or best supportive care) at investigators' choice. Eleven MTAs were available in the investigation arm.

It is important to remind that the preliminary step before engaging in such scientific questions, is to assess the validity of the measure of the marker [18]. It must be shown to have the properties of a solid diagnostic test, which includes the reproducibility of the assay, the metronomic quality of the measures, a high sensibility and specificity. This topic is beyond the scope of this chapter and the reader is encourage to refer to the evaluation of genomic applications in practice and prevention initiative (EGAPP) that proposes very rigorous means to evaluate the validity of proposed biomarkers; they include criteria for preliminary ranking of topics, hierarchies of data sources and study designs for the components of evaluation, criteria for assessing internal validity [32]. These recommendations apply to all diseases as there is no reason why oncology should develop its own (and weaker) set of rules. Many assays remain experimental and, if used, one should be certain that they will not be modified during the course of the trial, which would considerably limit the interpretation of the final results. We will assume that this is available, even if in many situations, including the trial used as example, we might lack this level of evidence.

We first introduce the rationale for the design, the choice of algorithm and endpoints of the trial (Sect. 2), and we discuss the type of conclusions we can draw, and specificities and limits due to this type of clinical question. In Sect. 2.5, we investigate the (lack of) power of randomized trials in case only part of the algorithm would be efficient, that is if only some MTAs actually work in the presence of the selected target while others do not. In Sect. 3, we then present a statistical analysis framework to evaluate the treatment effect in the overall study population, while estimating the treatment effect within patient groups defined by different markers with low prevalence. In the last Sect. 4, we review the PFS ratio as an endpoint and investigate its properties and distribution in a simulation study mimicking the SHIVA trial.

2 Design and Characteristics of Multi-marker Multi-treatment Trials

As recalled by EGAPP, a randomized clinical trial is mandatory to obtain high level of evidence of the clinical utility of omic-based classifiers to guide patients treatment compared to standard approaches [32]. Although the tumor biology, the mechanisms of drug resistance, and the role of the tumor environment are expected to be crucial to accurately predict patient outcomes, they remain largely unknown, making it necessary to have a comparator [29]. Furthermore, the prognosis of the highly selected patients (those whose tumors have a set of pre-defined molecular markers) enrolled in such trials is not well-known and may vary across molecular profiles. Only an intent-to-treat analysis that makes full use of the randomization is the most appropriate way to evaluate the efficacy.

To refine the context, consider that the primary objective is to compare the overall efficacy (global effect) of molecularly targeted therapy based on molecular profiling versus conventional therapy in patients with solid tumors refractory to standard treatments. Secondary efficacy objectives include the investigation of variations in the treatment effect according to the altered pathway (interaction tests or subgroup analyses). The primary endpoint is PFS.

2.1 Flowchart

Figure 1 describes the flowchart of the SHIVA trial. The molecular profile obtained from a mandatory biopsy/resection of a metastasis of a patient is analyzed. A short delay between biopsy and treatment recommendation is needed in order to not delay patients' treatment. It was set to be less than four weeks in SHIVA, and even as short as two weeks in the M-PACT trial (NCT01827384) that is introduced in the next subsection. If one or several molecular alterations are identified, a pre-defined algorithm is applied to select the MTA. Patients are then randomized between receiving the selected MTA or receiving a conventional therapy.

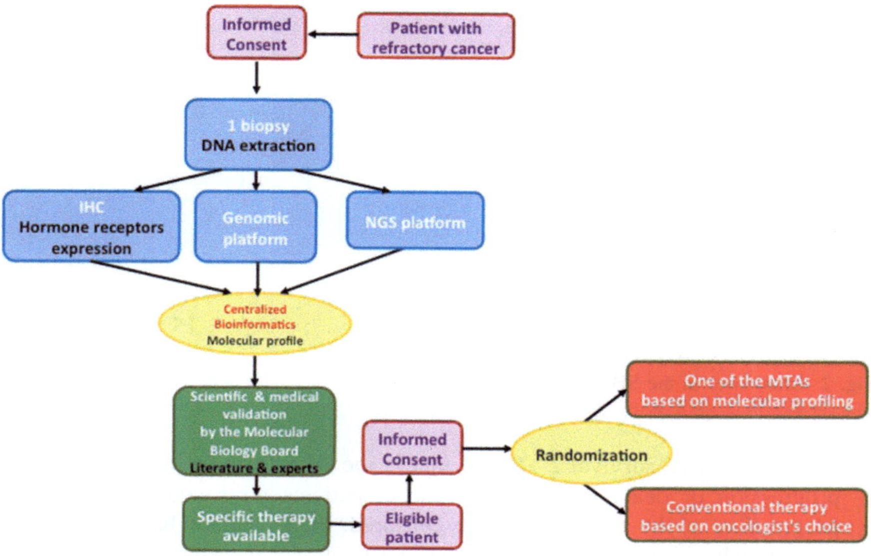

Fig. 1 Simplified flow chart of the multi-marker trials Shiva trial; IHC stands for immuno histo chemistry; MTAs for molecular targeted agents; NGS for next generation sequenting

Sample size computation is delicate due to the large number of unknown quantities. In the SHIVA trial, the expected PFS of this population in the control arm could be derived from the one reported in phase I clinical trials of cytotoxic agents that have eventually been approved: the 6-month PFS in this patient population was around 15% [11]. Under the hypothesis that doubling the 6-month PFS probability from 15 to 30% was clinically relevant (i.e. a hazard ratio of 0.63), a total of 142 events was required to detect a statistically significant difference in PFS between the randomized arms with a two-sided type I error of 5% and a power of 80%. To observe these events after an accrual time of 18 months and a minimum individual follow-up of six months, about 200 patients were randomized onto this trial. A total of 780 patients were eventually enrolled for molecular screening to end up with 195 randomized patients.

Patients were treated until progression. At progression, patients initially randomized in the intervention group were then allowed to receive conventional chemotherapy based on their tumor type, and patients in the control arm were allowed to receive the MTA matching the molecular alteration identified on the biopsy performed at inclusion, provided all eligibility criteria were still fulfilled at the time of progression. Those patients were then followed-up to the second progression or death. Several endpoints illustrated in Fig. 2, are determined:

- Progression free survival 1 (PFS_1) that is the time from randomization to first progression or death whatever the cause. Patients alive and free of progression at the cut-off date are censored. This was the primary endpoint.

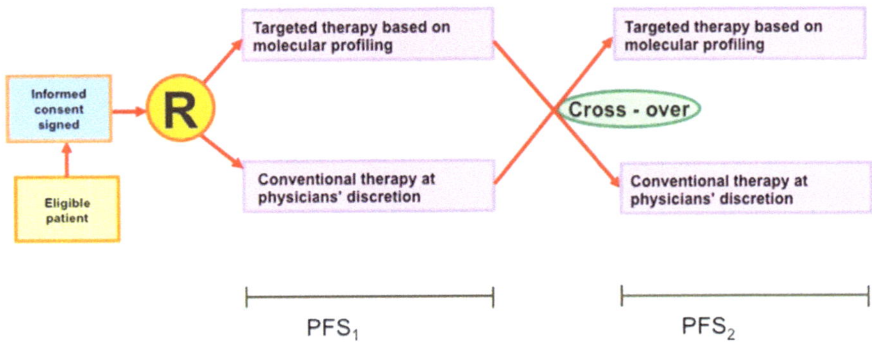

Fig. 2 Cross-over in the SHIVA trial

- Progression free survival 2 (PFS_2) that is the time from cross-over to second progression or death whatever the cause. Patients alive and free of second progression at the cut-off date are censored. PFS_2 cannot be computed for patients who do not progress after the first treatment (censored PFS_1).

Of note, for the patients going into the second period, PFS_1 is in fact time to progression (TTP_1) as patients dying before before progression 1 is observed do not receive second treatment. We will use PFS_1 for clarity in the following. This type of cross-over gave an opportunity to compare both therapeutic strategies in the same patients using each patient as his (her) own control but this raises specific design and analysis difficulties that are reviewed in Sect. 4.

2.2 *Definition of the Algorithm*

This complex intervention combines two aspects: the treatment effect and the choice of the putative matching marker. Therefore, the resulting efficacy can be related to either of the two and the final interpretation is the evaluation of the whole strategy compared to another strategy (standard therapy based on histology). As in any scientific experiment, the algorithm to select patients must be duly described, reproducible and applicable to all participants [17]. An example coming from the SHIVA trial is provided in Table 1. It includes the choice of treatments as well as a the set of rules to match treatments and targets. In particular in the case multiple molecular alteration would be detected in a patient, prioritization should be explicit. Algorithm rapidly gets quite complex as several levels can be considered that include the altered pathway, the number and type of abnormalities, the specific mutations.

Table 1 Algorithm for agent selection in the SHIVA trial

Targets	Molecular alterations	MTAs
ER, PR	Protein expression >10% IHC	Tamoxifen or Letrozole
AR	Protein expression >10% IHC	Abiraterone
PI3KCA, AKT1	Mutation − Amplification	
AKT2/3, mTOR, RICTOR, RAPTOR	Amplification	Everolimus
PTEN	Homozygous deletion, Heterozygous deletion + mutation or IHC	
STK11	Homozygous deletion, Heterozygous deletion + mutation	
INPP4B	Homozygous deletion	
BRAF	Mutation − Amplification	Vemurafenib
KIT, ABL1/2, RET	Mutation − Amplification	Imatinib
PDGFRA/B, FLT3	Mutation − Amplification	Sorafenib
EGFR	Mutation − Amplification	Erlotinib
HER-2	Mutation − Amplification	Lapatinib + Trastuzumab
SRC	Mutation − Amplification	Dasatinib
EPHA2, LCK, YES1	Amplification	

ER, PR and AR stand for Estrogen, Progesterone and Androgen receptors respectively; IHC stands for immuno histochemistry; MTA for molecularly targeted agents

2.2.1 Approved versus experimental agents

A very large set of MTAs is on the market or under development [1], with various levels of evidence of activity depending on the stage of development. For SHIVA, approved MTAs in France had been chosen as such activity and safety profile were well known. The relative treatment effect against standard of care had been demonstrated and quantified in at least one histology, which in turn provided us with reasonable hypotheses on the expected effect in other histologies. Eleven different targeted treatments have been administered based on 22 targets characterized by several dozens molecular alterations (see Table 1 from [17]). Those targets corresponded to three main biological pathways on which the randomization and analysis were stratified: (1) the hormone receptors pathway, (2) the PI3 K/AKT/mTOR pathway, and (3) the MAP kinase pathway.

Conversely some other trials, such as the MD Anderson program [30], tested new agents that had not fully demonstrated their efficacy in pivotal trials at the time of trial initiation. New molecules may have greater promises regarding the predictive value of the targeted molecular alterations, but the treatments activities are largely unknown, introducing another source of variability.

Defining the treatment algorithm is challenging as the knowledge regarding the biology of the tumors and the high-throughput platforms evolve quickly over time. Initial biological assumptions may become outdated during the course of the trial. Platforms should ideally use the same protocol throughout the trial. Likewise, all bioinformatics analyses have to be centralized and applied to all patients regardless of recruitment center. Finally, the algorithm should be applied to all patients enrolled in the trial in the same way. Any modification (new marker, new thresholds to define amplification etc.) induces extra variability in the overall experiment and hence in the data. This is crucial as any research must be self-explanatory and reproducible. A treatment algorithm that relies only on unstated experts opinion would not be applicable outside of the center and conclusions would not be applicable and generalizable to other samples. This is a key condition to be able to scientifically evaluate the overall efficacy of the intervention. A black box approach might initially lead to impressive results, but they may be difficult to reproduce.

2.2.2 Treatments, biomarkers and algorithm effect

The treatment algorithm is expected to have a prognostic impact; for instance HER2 amplification is associated with poor prognosis in breast cancer, but randomization should allow for controling this source of heterogeneity. An important question that will not be addressed in this type of trial is the independent effect of the matching algorithm. If a given MTA is active irrespective of the measure of the target, we would draw the same conclusions as if the treatment worked due to the adequate selection of the patients. The US National Cancer Institute sponsored M-PACT trial (NCT01827384) has been designed to specifically address the question of the added value of the algorithm independently of the treatment effects. M-PACT focuses on four MTAs. Patients whose tumor expresses molecular alterations are randomized between the MTA matching the detected molecular alteration versus one of three other non-matching therapy arms. In the latter case, the MTA is randomly allocated. Only the added value of the algorithm is tested. Conversely, the control arm used in the M-PACT trial does not correspond to any standard of care and the trial will not be able to conclude whether the global strategy is superior to the standard of care. Both types of trials are therefore quite complementary.

2.3 *Tumor Diversity*

Eligible patients in SHIVA had heterogeneous tumor types and had received various number of previous lines of treatment, which could be associated with various levels of prognosis. In clinical trials open to all tumour types, the distribution of cancer types depends strongly on the prevalence of the various cancers and the specific expertise of the participating centers. Yet, less common tumour types with frequent molecular abnormalities are of particular interest. To limit the risk that most patients have the same tumour type, which might reduce the applicability of the results, heterogeneity in the tumour-type may be increased by the design.

Quotas for tumor types can be set up to avoid over-representation of more frequent tumor types such as breast, lung or colorectal cancers. The obvious consequence is to increase the potential variability in treatment effects and to induce a risk of a cohort effect if patients with common histologies are included first and patients with rare histology are included later in the trial. In order to control for patient heterogeneity from differences in prognosis, randomization was stratified according to the signaling pathway relevant for the choice of the MTA and on the patient prognosis based on the two categories of the Royal Marsden Hospital (RMH) score for oncology phase I trials [21]. The randomization and the planned primary analysis were then stratified on six strata (three pathways and two prognostic levels).

2.4 *Blinding*

Blinding to the molecular profile is requested as the expectations of the physicians and of the patients in omic-based algorithms to select MTAs are high; there is a risk of bias in the follow-up as well as in the measure and interpretation of the primary outcome that may favor the intervention arm. Ideally, a double blind trial should be designed, which is delicate when several formulations, schedules, agents are tested in the same trial. Practically speaking even blinding the molecular profile is difficult to achieve as a large fraction of patients with advanced disease have participated to other profiling programs and the profile is nowadays often part of the medical records.

2.5 *Interpretation and Limits*

Several sources of variability related to the complexity of the intervention may contribute to the final results of the experiment. A non exhaustive list includes the tumor histology, the activity of MTAs and the validity of the various assays to define an altered pathway. The diversity of the tumor types in the SHIVA trial was increased in the hope of drawing conclusions that would be broadly applicable.

If randomization guarantees that the two groups of patients have comparable characteristics and the same overall prognosis, each prognostic factor may also be a predictive factor of response to MTA, also called treatment modifier, and hence impact the power of the experiment.

2.5.1 Power and Predictive Factors

A fundamental assumption behind the design is that the intervention has similar effects (or absence of effects) in all strata, whatever the allocated treatment and whatever the molecular alteration used to select the treatment. This is the homogeneity assumption. Statistically, lack of homogeneity corresponds to an interaction between the MTA effect and patients characteristics. In other words, the algorithm to select the right treatment would be efficient for some molecular alterations (or equivalently for some MTAs) and not for others. For instance, in the SHIVA trial suppose that the MTA selected to match an alteration on the PI3 K/AKT/mTOR pathway is not active in this subset of patients; this would reduce the power of the primary analysis.

To illustrate this aspect, let's consider the following framework. The outcome is a binary endpoint, e.g. PFS rate at six months assuming no censored observations before 6 months. Six strata of equal prevalence are considered. The trial is designed to demonstrate an increase in the 6-month PFS rate from 15 to 33%, that is an odds ratio (OR) of 2.67. As reported in [23], the power of the experiment in presence of heterogeneity across strata would be lower than the planned 80%. In the forest plots in Fig. 3, each line represents the expected MTA effect in a different stratum as measured with an odds ratio (OR) for the binary outcome considered here. In panel A, we have homogeneity of the MTA effect across all strata: whatever the signaling pathway and the prognostic group, the odds ratio for PFS is 2.67. Conversely, in panel B, the MTA has no effect in one of the strata and the overall power of the primary stratified analysis is reduced from 80 to 66%. The magnitude of the power loss depends on the number of strata where the MTA is not active, as shown in Table 2. The power calculation can be done through simulations or exact calculations [12]. The size of each stratum has also a direct impact on the power (results not shown). Homogeneity tests (or interaction tests) are notoriously underpowered as shown in Table 2 and a strong heterogeneity may remain statistically undetected at the 5% significance level.

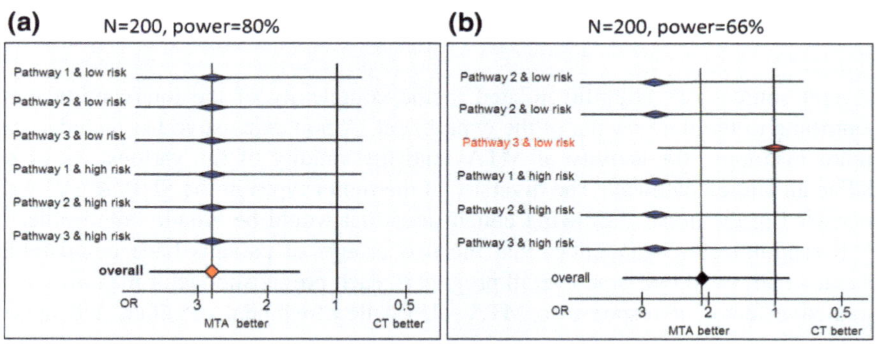

Fig. 3 Impact of heterogeneity in the treatment effect related to the algorithm assuming balanced prevalence for the six different strata and the same follow-up for all patients censored at the cut-off date. High and low risk denote the risk group; Pathway 1, 2, 3 correspond to the grouping of the different targets; MTA stands for molecularly targeted agent; CT stands for control treatment; *N* is the total sample size; OR stands for odds ratio; Point estimates and 95% confidence intervals (horizontal lines) are provided. *Panel A* Homogeneous benefit of the targeted treatment selected based on molecular alterations in all strata (OR = 2.67); *Panel B* benefit of the targeted treatment selected based on molecular alterations in all but one stratum

Table 2 Power of a randomized comparative trial of size $N = 200$ to detect an overall increase in the 6-month PFS rate from 15 to 33% in case of heterogeneity assuming balanced prevalence of signaling pathways and Royal Marsden Hospital risk groups

Number of strata in which MTA is better	Power for the comparative test (%)	Power for heterogenity test (%)
6	83	–
5	66	25
4	49	36
3	32	38
2	17	34

In strata where MTA selected on the target is not better than standard chemotherapy
Homogeneity is tested using Woolfs test
Heterogeneity = test for different OR accross the strata

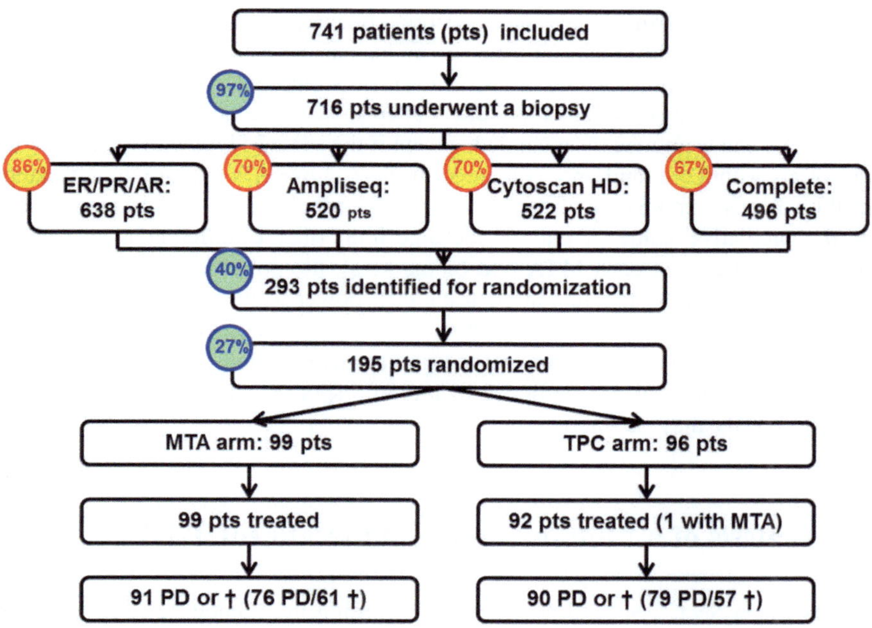

Fig. 4 Flowhchart in the SHIVA trial before cross-over; HD stands for high definition; PD for Progressive disease; CT for chemotherapy; MTA for Molecular targeted agents; † symbolizes death

2.5.2 Inclusion Criteria and Generalizations

As shown in the Consort flowchart of the SHIVA trial (Fig. 4), only about 33% of the included patients were eventually randomized. The main cause of failure was the inability to obtain a molecular profile of the patients due to insufficient tumor cells in the sample or failures of the high throughput platform analyses. An analysis of prognostic factors of a successful biopsy on 228 patients from the SHIVA study showed that success of biopsy was less frequent with chemotherapy guidance than with surgical or palpation-guided biopsy and was higher in soft tissues and lymph nodes than that in visceral metastasis; ongoing chemotherapy decreased tumor cell content and consequently the success of the biopsy samples for molecular profiling [7].

2.6 Summary

In summary, randomized designs allow for comparing two complex strategies on a valid clinical endpoint, while controlling for numerous confounding factors, including the prognostic value of the algorithm. A statistically significant difference between the two arms would be appropriately interpreted as the superiority of treating patients with MTAs based on molecular alterations and a pre-defined treatment algorithm compared to the conventional approach. However, treatment effect of the MTAs as well as biomarkers effects per se are not a principal result of such trials and cannot be disentangled, except if the same MTAs with or without the use of algorithm are randomly compared. In Sect. 3, we will explore the estimation of the various components of the algorithm. Nevertheless, in case of heterogeneity of the predictive value of part of the algorithm (that is different magnitude of interactions between each MTA and biomarkers), the power of the overall test is strongly reduced. As medium-sized trials lack power to detect interactions, interpretation of the final results is difficult in such setting. A non-significant global test of the efficacy of the algorithm may cover various situations; MTAs may lack of activity irrespective of the predictive factors of response to treatment or part of the algorithm only may be valid.

3 Analysis of a Multi-marker Multi-treatment Trial

As shown in Sect. 2 several assumptions regarding the homogeneity of treatment effects of the targeted therapies and the predictive value of the matched markers are made in trials evaluating algorithms to select the best treatment based on markers. If mutations in cancer cells are all predictive of enhanced benefit from different MTAs, that is if the treatment effect is homogeneous across mutations, the semi-parametric Cox model adjusting for mutation effect as well as for overall treatment effect would be a valid tool for analysis. But, if the homogeneity assumption does not hold, random effects models [8] could be used to estimate the overall treatment effect of the marker-based strategy and the treatment effect within patient groups defined by different markers; some of the subgroups may even correspond to rare diseases. Suppose that we observe censored time-to-event data from a study with L mutations and n_ℓ subjects per mutations ($\ell = 1, \ldots, L$), so that

$N = \sum_{\ell=1}^{L} n_\ell$ is the total sample size. How to incorporate the mutation effects into the analysis when the homogeneity assumption may not hold and when the number of events may be too low to adjust for all possible mutations per treatment combinations?

3.1 Random Effects Models

Let us consider the mixed effects Cox model where the hazard $h(t)$ is proportional to the baseline hazard $h_0(t)$ through the fixed effects of the design matrix X as well as of the random effects b for the design matrix Z:

$$h(t) = h_0(t)\exp(X\beta + Zb)$$

where b is classically assumed to follow a normal distribution.

This general formulation allows for introducing M_ℓ the ℓth marker and E the group of therapy (experimental or control). A random effect can be introduced at various levels depending on the objectives of the trial. If the interest focuses on both the prognostic effect of markers and the treatment, while accounting for treatment variations across subgroups defined by markers, then marker by treatment interactions can be seen as random and be included in the Z matrix.

$$h(t; E, M|\delta) = h_0(t)\exp(\beta E + \sum_{\ell=2}^{L} \gamma_\ell M_\ell + \sum_{\ell=1}^{L} \delta_\ell M_\ell E) \tag{1}$$

where γ_ℓ, the fixed prognostic effects of the markers are part of X and δ_j are random effects drawn from a normal distribution whose variances capture the variations of the treatment effect on the six subgroups defined by the markers.

When the prognostic effect of mutations is of no interest per se, a semi-parametric model stratified on the markers could estimate the treatment effect adjusted for the various components with a smaller number of degrees of freedom.

$$h(t; E, M|\delta) = h_{0j}(t)\exp(\beta E + \sum_{\ell=1}^{L} \delta_\ell M_\ell E) \tag{2}$$

Stratification may however negatively impact the power of the trial as the number of markers (and hence the number of strata) increases and may also run into convergence problems if the number of events in particular strata is small. The various strata may then be replaced by a semi-parametric model where the prognostic values of the markers γ_ℓ are also included in the Z matrix.

4 Using the Patient as His/Her Own Control: Time to Progression Ratio

In the SHIVA trial, patients were afforded the possibility to cross-over and to receive the alternative treatment. While it was primarily intended to give the possibility to patients from the controlled arm to eventually receive the targeted treatment, it provided additional information for evaluation of the treatment effect.

4.1 Background

As displayed in Fig. 2, two PFS variables (PFS_1, PFS_2) were measured for patients who progressed and were eligible to the cross-over. While the analysis of cross-over experiments with survival endpoints can be performed in the same way as with binary or continuous endpoints [31], that is estimating the treatment effect using survival models for correlated outcomes controlling for the period effect, Von Hoff [36] proposed to consider the ratio of the two progression free survival $(PFSr)$. The fundamental idea was that the tumor growth in metastatic patients gets faster as the disease gets more advanced. In other words, the natural history of the cancer should lead to PFS_2 being shorter than PFS_1 and hence the period effect can be considered to be known. If PFS_2 is in fact longer than PFS_1 (or equivalently the ratio greater than 1) then it should reflect the superiority of the treatment administered during the second period over the one administered in the first period. Several trials have proposed to use the patient as his or her own control [10, 28]. It can be noted that this approach has lot in common with the "preferences"' approach proposed by France et al. [9] for survival data where the preference for each patient is obtained by comparing the two outcomes at the two periods of time. Nevertheless, France et al. continued to defend the need for a randomized trial to control for the period effect. The statistical power of the analysis of $PFSr$ might theoretically be higher than the one comparing the treatment efficacy between the two parallel groups as it enables control for the various sources of patients-related heterogeneity such as the natural history of the disease (the tumor location and histology), the history of previous treatments etc. The underlying hypothesis is expressed statistically as the existence of a strong correlation between the PFS of the two consecutive lines of treatment. The stronger the correlation, the more powerful the statistical analysis would be [6, 19].

In the pilot study by Von Hoff [37], the observed PFS was compared to the PFS from the previous line of treatment. That latter one was collected retrospectively from medical records. The ratio was compared to a cut-off value of 1.33 to derive a binary variable (success or failure).

In addition to the underlying assumption of a natural history of cancer that would be known for each individual, another limit is the assessment of PFS_1 based on retrospective data; progression may be defined differently for both measures.

Conversely, in the SHIVA trial, both PFS_1 and PFS_2 were evaluated prospectively following the same protocol and the same RECIST v1.1 definition. Furthermore, cross-over was proposed to all randomized patients: the experimental design was much closer to a real cross-over design. Nevertheless, as shown in the flow chart 4, only one third of the patients switched from MTA to chemotherapy, introducting a high risk of selection bias and making any comparisons between the two sequences difficult to interpret.

4.2 Estimation and Testing Procedure

As patients typically do not start a second line of treatment before progression has been documented, PFS_1 is not censored and observed on all patients included in the analysis. That means that PFS_1 is in fact a time to progression measure. Conversely, PFS_2 can be censored at the time of analysis raising additional difficulty. The ratio can thus be seen as a continuous positive and censored value.

4.2.1 Uncensored *PFSr*

Let us denote this ratio $PFSr = \frac{PFS_2}{PFS_1}$ where PFS_2 is the outcome of the investigational strategy. In absence of censored observation, the distribution is straightforward to estimate. Von Hoff [37] considered that a patient for whom PFS_2 is 33% longer than PFS_1 benefited from the treatment.

Mick et al. [19] have proposed a testing framework that can serve to design the trial in terms of sample size if the expected correlation is known. The sample size is computed to detect a ratio between paired *PFS* of magnitude γ_0, which describes the expected ratio under which the investigational strategy is inefficient: $PFSr \leq \gamma_0$ (the null hypothesis is typically 1 or 0.7) against some alternative; power is calculated under some value γ_1 that would reflect a clinically significant increase (i.e. $\gamma_1 = 1.33$). Suppose that most of the observations are not censored, we can use a paired signed rank test [19]. Using their notation, for the ith patient, let r_i be equal to

$$+1 \text{ if } \log(PFS_2) > \log(PFS_1) + \log(\gamma_0)$$
$$-1 \text{ if } \log(PFS_2) \leq \log(PFS_1) + \log(\gamma_0) \text{ and } PFS_2 \text{ is uncensored}$$

The test statistic (equivalent to a sign test statistic) is

$$K = \left(\sum_i r_i\right)^2 / \sum_i r_i^2$$

has a χ^2 distribution with 1 degree of freedom as there is one pair by patient. This test formulation can easily be inverted to provide sample size calculation when the true correlation is known. For instance, for a type I error of 0.05, an 80% power, and a 50% expected correlation between the two consecutive *PFS* (adjusted for treatment effect), the sample size will be roughly reduced by a factor 4 as compared to the number of patients needed to carry out a randomized parallel arms trial.

4.2.2 Censored *PFSr*

In case of censored ratio (that is censored PFS_2), the Kaplan-Meier approach provides an estimate of the probability to exceed some threshold values $\gamma = 1.3$ and its variance. A Gehan-Wilcoxon test [13] can also be derived. Under the log-linear model for correlated failure times used by Mick et al. [19], the proposed rank test is unbaised in case of censored PFS_2; the pair does not contribute to the test statistics.

Another non-parametric test approach uses the ranks of each pair (PFS_1, PFS_2) [14]. Ranks of censored PFS_2 can be estimated by midranks. For each patient *i*, an interval (L_{2i}, R_{2i}) for PFS_{2i} is built as follows. If PFS_2 is uncensored, the interval is squeezed to the point $[PFS_{2i}, PFS_{2i}]$ otherwise it is $[PFS_{2i}, +\infty)$. The midranks M_{2i} are computed using the minimum and the maximum ranks calculated over the $2n$ values of R_{2i} and L_{2i} with $i = 1, \ldots, n$ and n the number of patients (or pairs). The minimum and maximum ranks are the ranks of L_{2i} and R_{2i} that minimize:

$$\min_{2i} : R_{2(1)} \leq R_{2(2)} \leq \cdots \leq R_{2(\min_i - 1)} \leq L_{2i} \leq R_{2(\min_i)} \leq \cdots \leq R_{2(2n)}$$
$$\max_{2i} : L_{2(1)} \leq L_{2(2)} \leq \cdots \leq L_{2(\max_i - 1)} \leq R_{2i} \leq L_{2(\max_i)} \leq \cdots \leq L_{2(2n)}$$

$$M_{2i} = \frac{\min_{2i} + \max_{2i}}{2}$$

To estimate the distribution function at value $\gamma, S(\gamma), PFS_1$ is replaced by $PFS'_1 = PFS_1 \times \gamma$ as done previously, the midranks of (PFS'_1, PFS_2) in turns provide the probability of interest:

$$\hat{S}(\gamma) = \frac{1}{n} \sum_{i=1}^{n} \mathbf{1}(M_{2i} \geq M_{1i})$$

where the indicator function **1** takes value 1 if $M_{2i} \geq M_{1i}$ and 0 otherwise.

Alternatively, Kovalchik et al. [14] followed by Texier et al. [33] proposed parametric methods to estimate the *PFSr*. In advanced diseases, a Weibull distribution commonly provides satisfactory goodness-of-fit on *PFS* data. As the dependence between PFS_1, PFS_2 is due to patients' characteristics that are then shared by the two time-to-event variables, it can be modeled in a very natural way via shared frailty models. Applied to Weibull marginal distributions for

PFS_1, PFS_2, with common shape parameter k and common frailty u_i for patient i, we can write the density f_j of PFS_j where j takes values 1 or 2 as

$$f_j(x; k, \lambda_j | u_i) = k(u_i \lambda_j)^{-k} x^{k-1} \exp^{\left(-\frac{x}{u_i \lambda_j}\right)^k}$$

Kovalchnik proposed to approximate the density of the ratio by a lognormal distribution. Owen has previously shown that in this setting the ratio follows a log-logistic distribution [22]:

$$f(\gamma; k, \lambda) = k\lambda^k \gamma^{k-1} (1 + (\gamma\lambda)^k)^{-2}$$

where $\lambda = \lambda_1 / \lambda_2$ and $\delta \geq 0$. The function f does not depend on the shared frailty u_i anymore. Texier et al. [33] proposed maximum likelihood estimates of the distribution parameters $(\hat{k}, \hat{\lambda})$ and we directly derive the probability of interest from the survival function

$$S(\gamma; \hat{k}, \hat{\lambda}) = \left(1 + (\gamma\hat{\lambda})^{\hat{k}}\right)^{-1}.$$

4.3 Application to the SHIVA Trial

The flow chart of the SHIVA trial after cross-over is illustrated in Fig. 5: among the 197 patients randomized, 95 crossed over, including 70 patients from the standard chemotherapy arm to the MTA arm and 25 patients from the MTA to the standard chemotherapy arm. Two additional patients without disease progression (PFS_1

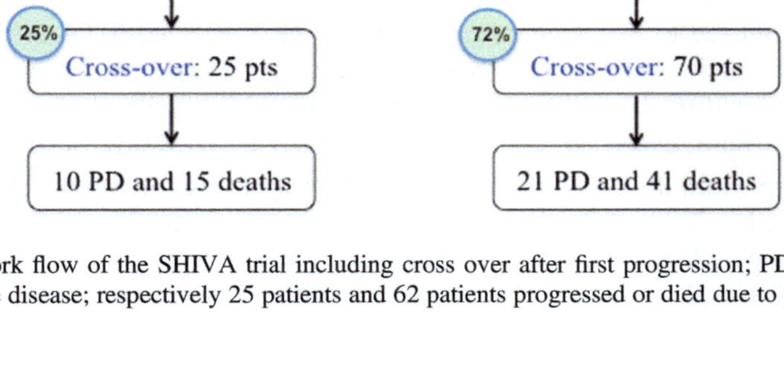

Fig. 5 Work flow of the SHIVA trial including cross over after first progression; PD stands for progressive disease; respectively 25 patients and 62 patients progressed or died due to progression

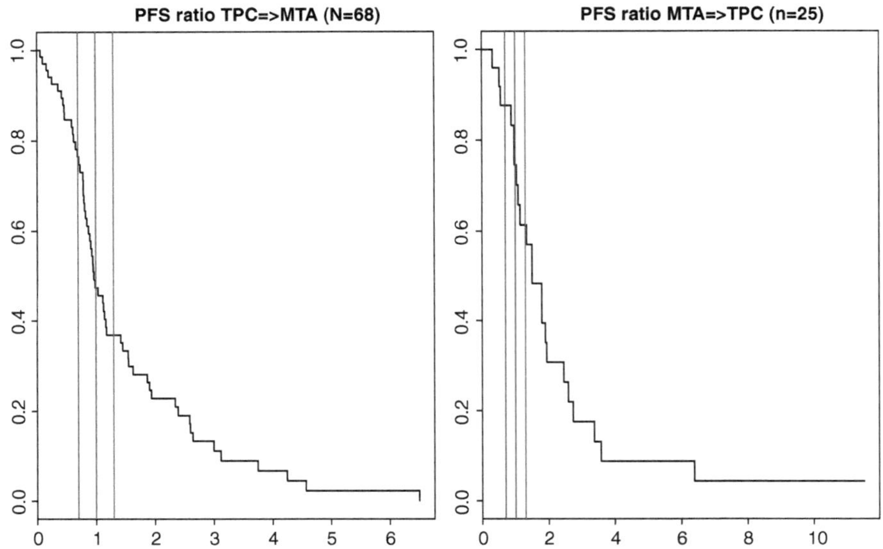

Fig. 6 Kaplan-Meier estimates of progression-free survival ratio ($PFSr$) on (*left*) 68 patients who crossed-over from CT to the MTA, and on (*right*) the 25 patients who crossed over from MTA to CT. MTA stands for Molecularly targeted agents and CT for chemotherapy. *Vertical lines* correspond to the thresholds 0.7, 1 and 1.3

censored) crossed over in the standard chemotherapy arm and were excluded. Patients dying without progression documented radiologically after cross-over were assumed to have died from their disease as it was very unlikely that they died from an unrelated cause. For clarity, the measurement under MTA will always be in the numerator. The PFS ratio is $\frac{PFS_{MTA}}{PFS_{CT}}$. In patients who switched over from chemotherapy to MTA, $PFSr$ corresponds to PFS_2/PFS_1, where PFS_2 denotes the PFS at the second period. For the other arm, this is equal to PFS_1/PFS_2.

Patients who did cross-over had a better prognosis at baseline as measured by the Royal Marsden prognostic score than patients who did not [3]. This selection bias makes any comparison between the two randomized arms (the two sequences) potentially biased; the complete cross-over design analysis cannot benefit from the randomization. Each arm is thus reported separately. Median follow-up at the time of the analysis was 14 months [range 0–32] in both arms. In the 70 patients who were randomized to the standard chemotherapy and received MTA at cross-over, median PFS under MTA in second period, denoted PFS_{MTA} was 2.1 months [95% CI 2.0–3.8] and median PFS_{CT} in first period was 2.0 months [95% CI 1.9–2.4]. The $\frac{PFS_{MTA}}{PFS_{CT}}$ ratio exceeded 1.3 in 37% ([95% CI 26–52%]) of patients who crossed-over from the chemotherapy to the MTA arm (Fig. 6). Some cut-off values are provided in Table 3. In the group of 25 patients who received MTA and then chemotherapy, PFS_{MTA} was longer than $PFS_{CT} \times 1.3$ in 61% [95% CI 44–85 of patients (Table 3), including 31% of patients with a ratio exceeding 2.

Table 3 Selected values of the ratio of the PFS_{MTA} over PFS_{CT} in patients who received chemotherapy and crossed over to receive MTA

PFSr	Sequence	<0.7	0.7–1.0	1.0–1.3	≥ 1.3	≥ 2
Cumulative probability	CT → MTA	0.24	0.29	0.10	0.37	0.23
	MTA → CT	0.12	0.13	0.13	0.61	0.31

The ratio was comprised between 1 and 1.3, 0.7 and 1.0, and was below 0.7 in 13, 13, and 12% of patients, respectively.

Von Hoff [37], in his pilot study, reported that 27% of the patients had ratio greater than 1.3, which suggests that the results in the SHIVA trial are also promising. In absence of fair comparisons, interpretation of these results is delicate. Have we identified a group of patients who benefited from the overall strategy of treatment selection based on the molecular profile? In other words, can we conclude to the algorithm superiority? As for any comparison to an historical control, the specifications of the null and the alternative hypotheses are central. In our context, PFS_2 greater than 1.3 was set up as promising without the support of scientific data in similar populations; careful examination of the distribution is reported in the next paragraph.

4.4 Calibration

4.4.1 Correlation on the Shiva data

In the SHIVA trial, the distribution of PFS_1 and PFS_2 were best fitted with log-normal distributions: mean $\ln(\mu) = 4.35$ and scale $\sigma = 0.7$ for PFS_1 and $\ln(\mu) = 4.34$ and scale $\sigma = 0.84$ for PFS_2. Using the 87 uncensored measures of *PFSr*, the Spearman rank and Kendall's tau correlations were approximated using a simple non parametric estimator. The rank correlation was 0.35, while Kendall's tau was 0.25. The rank correlation is in the range of the values reported in several other trials [19]. Alternatively, a Clayton copula approach assuming log-normal marginal distributions was fitted on all data. The resulting Kendall's tau was similar (0.22) quantifying a moderate correlation between PFS_1 and PFS_2. Going back to the power curves of Mick et al., using the patient as his (her) own control would not have increased strongly the power of the experiment compared to parallel randomized design in the setting of multi-histology trials due to the moderate correlation.

This moderate correlation together with the known large variability of lognormal distribution raise the concern of the correct calibration of a clinically significant ratio. We explored the distribution of the PFS ratio using simulations. Were survival endpoints to follow Weibull distributions with common shape parameters, we could have used the results of Owen [22] that the ratio follows a log-logistic distribution.

4.4.2 Simulation setting

Contrary to Mick et al. [19] who generated data using proportional exponential distributions, we carried out simulations mimicking the context of the Shiva trial using the Clayton copula model to generate pairs of correlated PFS_1, PFS_2. The Kendall's tau correlation was fixed at 0.25. Lognormal distributions $(\ln(\mu) = 4.35, \sigma = 0.7)$, corresponding to the observed distribution of PFS_1 in the SHIVA trial, were used as margins in the Clayton copula. We had the treatment effect vary from no effect $(\ln(\mu_1) = \ln(\mu 2))$ for PFS_1 and PFS_2) to a doubling of median survival time $(\ln(\mu_2) - \ln(\mu_1) = 0.65)$. It is worth noticing that there is no straightforward link between lognormal parameters and *PFSr*. A median *PFSr* of 0.7 corresponds to $\ln(\mu_2) = 3.99$.

We generated data for 5000 subjects from the copula model under the null hypothesis of no treatment effect and under the alternative hypothesis, and we derived the empirical distribution of *PFSr*. In all scenarios, administrative censoring was generated by setting a cut-off length of follow-up $(PFS_1 + PFS_2)$ in order to have about 10% of censored PFS ratios as in the SHIVA trial. Therefore, the cut-off delay was increased when the treatment effect was increased. Of note, the censoring process is not completely independent of the *PFSr* distribution as earlier cut-off point may be associated with excess of censored data in long PFS_1.

4.4.3 Simulation results

Under the null hypothesis of two correlated similar lognormal survival distributions (no treatment effect), the *PFSr* distribution was quite similar to the one obtained in the SHIVA trial as illustrated in Table 4. The mean value of the ratio was 1.2. If there is no period effect (time to progression is not shorter between the two consecutive treatment lines) and if the survival times are drawn from lognormal distributions, we should expect a large proportion of patients who display ratio greater than 1.

When increasing the treatment effect, the probabilities of *PFSr* greater than 1.3 and 2 increased up to .72 and 0.49 respectively (see Fig. 7), suggesting that careful calibration of the null hypothesis and of the clinically relevant cut-off to declare a treatment successful in a patient are requested. A simple description of the patients who have "success" as defined by *PFSr* greater than 1.3 may not allow for drawing any robust conclusions. A test should be carried out.

Table 4 Scenario 2 simulations under the null hypothesis: distribution of *PFSr* for selected values

PFSr	<0.7	0.7–1.0	1.0–1.3	>1.3	>2
Cumulative probability	0.32	0.18	0.13	0.37	0.20

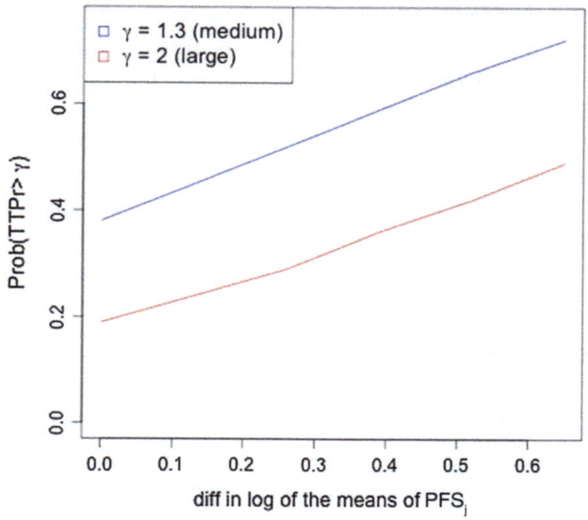

Fig. 7 Probability to exceed two *PFSr* values as a function of the true treatment effect

4.4.4 Some general remarks

To date there are few studies that have investigated this aspect and the correlation between consecutive progression free survival times is probably dependent upon the tumour type. For instance, strong correlation in GIST tumors treated with imatinib [38] and low correlations in colo-rectal trials [34] have been reported. They are on line with the largest review done so far by Mick et al. [19] but an update based on more recent trials may be useful.

PFSr can be computed using either retrospective assessment of PFS_1 or prospective assessment of PFS_1. In the first case and in absence of randomized control sequence (true cross-over), estimation of the treatment effect based on the ratio is expected to be unbiased under two conditions: (i) PFS_1 can be measured with the same criteria and on the same lesions as PFS_2, which is uncommon as criteria measured in clinical trials are typically not used for standard care; (ii) natural history of the disease is homogeneously regular, i.e. for all patients, the successive lines of treatment are associated with shorter and shorter PFS in absence of treatment effect.

In the second case, one should also bear in mind the intrinsic selection bias related to the *PFSr* if only patients who progressed after the initial treatment are included in the analysis. Therefore, a shared frailty model would be strongly recommended for inference. Instead of excluding patients dying or censored before the first progression is duly documented, those patients contributes to the estimate of PFS_1.

Finally, an important drawback of allowing cross-over is to most often compromise the analysis of the overall survival. Due to the uncertainty on the correlation between PFS_1 and PFS_2 in patients with multiple histologies and the huge variability of the ratio, this endpoint should preferably be used in the framework of a "complete" cross-over design (where the 2 sequences are proposed). It then gains high power due to the cross-over design while it maintains the benefit or randomization. The main limitation is then ethical. In the SHIVA trial, after failure of the targeted agents, should patients eligible for subsequent treatment receive systematically conventional therapies that have not demonstrated activity in advanced patients, or be proposed to enter in another trial? The set of trials that are currently designed based on $PFSr$ will bring valuable information on the appropriate calibration of the ratio and the observed intra-patient correlation that will serve to design future trials.

5 Discussion

More than 900 MTAs are currently under development [24] and many subgroups based on molecular markers represent less than 15% of the cancer patients with a tumor type. Several randomized trials have been set up to investigate which of tumor biology or tumor location and histology is the most important to select treatment in patients with cancer refractory to the standard of care. Interpretation of the results of such trials are complicated by the complexity of the algorithm, but only randomized trials can disentangle the consequence of prognostic factors in these highly selected patients from the intervention effect and enable to control for confounding factors in order to allow reliable conclusions [4]. The heterogeneity in the population will be balanced between the two treatment arms and thus should not induce spurious association, but heterogeneity in the treatment effect may dilute the benefit of the intervention. The standardization of the process to identify druggable molecular alterations and the matching MTA, as well as the blinding of the results are key elements in such trials. The same principles as those applied for the development of diagnostic tools should be implemented [27]. However, the assumption of an homogeneous treatment effect in all subgroups defined by biomarkers is central. As shown, violation of this assumption has major consequences on the statistical properties of the design and cannot be completely salvaged at the analysis time using mixed effect or random effects Cox models.

There is clearly a need for more sensible endpoints to evaluate such complex interventions. PFS is mildly sensitive to treatment variations and interaction tests to identify differential effects according to the matching between treatment and target are not powerful with 200 patients. Using the patient as his (her) own control requires more investigations as the variability induced by the ratio of two skewed distributions is quite large in multi-histology samples. Pharmacodynamic endpoints such as functional imaging or biomarkers are promising to detect early treatment failure but none have been yet validated. Overall, cancer biology is at the heart of this type of histology-agnostic trial. Current knowledge of tumor biology does not enable us to systematically predict the final outcome as shown by the disappointing efficacy obtained with vemurafenib in BRAF mutated colon cancer [25], or those obtained with crizotinib in neuroblastoma (that has common ALK-alterations) [20]. Taking into account the presence or absence of several molecular alterations might improve the accuracy of the treatment algorithms using systems biology approaches. However, any treatment algorithm should be clearly defined and rigorously evaluated in randomized trials. In addition, the tumor environment is likely an important factor of success of a therapeutic approach, as illustrated with the recent approval of immunotherapeutics. Nevertheless, the question of how to account for the multiple sources of variability in medium-sized trials samples is crucial for the validity of the research. Currently the risk of type I or type II errors is weakly controlled.

Acknowledgements The authors thank Matthieu Texier (Gustave Roussy/INSERM CESP-OncoStat) and Lisa Belin (Institut Curie) for sharing unpublished results. They are indebted to Pr Christophe Le Tourneau for initiating and conducting the SHIVA trial.

References

1. Abramson RG. Overview of targeted therapies for cancer. 2016. https://www.mycancergenome.org/content/molecular-medicine/overview-of-targeted-therapies-for-cancer/. Accessed 11 Oct 2016.
2. Bang Y-J, Van Cutsem E, Feyereislova A, Chung HC, Shen L, Sawaki A, Lordick F, Ohtsu A, Omuro Y, Satoh T, Aprile G, Kulikov E, Hill J, Lehle M, Rüschoff J, Kang Y-K. Trastuzumab in combination with chemotherapy versus chemotherapy alone for treatment of HER2-positive advanced gastric or gastro-oesophageal junction cancer (ToGA): a phase 3, open-label, randomised controlled trial. Lancet. 2010;376(9742):687–97.
3. Belin L, Kamal M, Mauborgne C, Plancher C, Mulot F, Delord J-P, Goncalves A, Gavoille C, Dubot C, Isambert N, Campone M, Tredan O, Ricci F, Alt M, Loirat D, Sablin M-P, Paoletti X, Servois V, Le Tourneau C. Shiva: randomized phase ii trial comparing molecularly targeted therapy based on tumor molecular profiling versus conventional therapy in patients with refractory cancer—pfs ratio from patients who crossed-over. Ann Oncol (34), 2016.
4. Buyse M, Michiels S. Omics-based clinical trial designs. Curr Opin Oncol. 2013;25(3): 289–95.
5. Buyse M, Michiels S, Sargent DJ, Grothey A, Matheson A, de Gramont A. Integrating biomarkers in clinical trials. Expert Rev Mol Diagn. 2011;11(2):171–82.
6. Buyse M, Quinaux E, Hendlisz A, Golfinopoulos V, Tournigand C, Mick R. Progression-free survival ratio as end point for phase II trials in advanced solid tumors. J Clin Oncol. 2011;29 (15):451–2.
7. Desportes E, Wagner M, Kamal M, Vincent-Salomon A, Deniziaut G, Pierron G, Rouleau E, Jouffroy T, Le Tourneau C, Paoletti X, Servois V. Prognostic factors of successful on-purpose tumor biopsies in metastatic cancer patients included in the SHIVA prospective clinical trial. OncoTargets. 2016;8(1):1760–73.
8. Duchateau L, Janssen P. The frailty model. New York: Springer; 2008.
9. France LA, Lewis JA, Kay R. The analysis of failure time data in crossover studies. Stat Med. 1991;10(7):1099–113.
10. Hollebecque A, Massard C, Soria J-C. Implementing precision medicine initiatives in the clinic: a new paradigm in drug development. Curr Opin Oncol. 2014;26(3):340–6.

11. Horstmann E, McCabe MS, Grochow L, Yamamoto S, Rubinstein L, Budd T, Shoemaker D, Emanuel EJ, Grady C. Risks and benefits of phase 1 oncology trials, 1991 through 2002. N Engl J Med. 2005;352(9):895–904.
12. Jung S-H. Stratified Fisher's exact test and its sample size calculation. Biom J. 2014;56 (1):129–40.
13. Jung SH. Rank tests for matched survival data. Lifetime Data Anal. 1999;5(1):67–73.
14. Kovalchik S, Mietlowski W. Statistical methods for a phase II oncology trial with a growth modulation index (GMI) endpoint. Comtemp Clin Trials. 2011;32(1):99–107.
15. Le Tourneau C, Delord J-P, Gonçalves A, Gavoille C, Dubot C, Isambert N, Campone M, Trédan O, Massiani M-A, Mauborgne C, Armanet S, Servant N, Bièche I, Bernard V, Gentien D, Jezequel P, Attignon V, Boyault S, Vincent-Salomon A, Servois V, Sablin M-P, Kamal M, Paoletti X. Molecularly targeted therapy based on tumour molecular profiling versus conventional therapy for advanced cancer (SHIVA): a multicentre, open-label, proof-of-concept, randomised, controlled phase 2 trial. Lancet Oncol 2015;1–11.
16. Le Tourneau C, Kamal M, Trédan O, Delord J-P, Campone M, Goncalves A, Isambert N, Conroy T, Gentien D, Vincent-Salomon A, Pouliquen A-L, Servant N, Stern MH, Le Corroller A-G, Armanet S, Rio Frio T, Paoletti X. Designs and challenges for personalized medicine studies in oncology: Focus on the SHIVA trial. Target Oncol. 2012;7(4):253–65.
17. Le Tourneau C, Kamal M, Tsimberidou M-M, Bedard P, Pierron G, Callens C, Rouleau E, Vincent-Salomon A, Servant N, Alt M, Rouzier R, Paoletti X, Delattre O, Bièche I. Treatment algorithms based on tumor molecular profiling: the essence of precision medicine trials. J Natl Cancer Inst. 2016;108(4):1–10.
18. McShane LM, Cavenagh MM, Lively TG, Eberhard DA, Bigbee WL, Williams PM, Mesirov JP, Polley M-YC, Kim KY, Tricoli JV, Taylor JMG, Shuman DJ, Simon RM, Doroshow JH, Conley BA. Criteria for the use of omics-based predictors in clinical trials. Nature. 2013;502(7471):317–20.
19. Mick R, Crowley JJ, Carroll RJ. Phase II clinical trial design for noncytotoxic anticancer agents for which time to disease progression is the primary endpoint. Control Clin Trials. 2000;21(4):343–59.
20. Mossé YP, Lim MS, Voss SD, Wilner K, Ruffner K, Laliberte J, Rolland D, Balis FM, Maris JM, Weigel BJ, Ingle AM, Ahern C, Adamson PC, Blaney SM. Safety and activity of crizotinib for paediatric patients with refractory solid tumours or anaplastic large-cell lymphoma: a Children's Oncology Group phase 1 consortium study. Lancet Oncol. 2013;14 (6):472–80.
21. Olmos D, Ahern RP, Marsoni S, Morales R, Gomez-Roca C, Verweij J, Voest EE, Schöffski P, Ang JE, Penel N, Schellens JH, Del Conte G, Brunetto AT, Evans TRJ, Wilson R, Gallerani E, Plummer R, Tabernero J, Soria J-C, Kaye SB. Patient selection for oncology phase I trials: a multi-institutional study of prognostic factors. J Clin Oncol. 2012;30(9):996–1004.
22. Owen WJ. A power analysis of tests for paired lifetime data. Lifetime Data Anal. 2005;11 (2):233–43.
23. Paoletti X, Asselain B, Kamal M, Servant N, Huppé P, Bieche I, Le Tourneau C. Design and statistical principles of the SHIVA trial. Chin Clin Oncol 2015;3(4).
24. PhRMA. Medicine in development for cancer: a report on cancer.
25. Prahallad A, Sun C, Huang S, Di Nicolantonio F, Salazar R, Zecchin D, Beijersbergen RL, Bardelli A, Bernards R. Unresponsiveness of colon cancer to BRAF(V600E) inhibition through feedback activation of EGFR. Nature. 2012;483(7387):100–3.
26. Renfro LA, Mallick H, An MW, Sargent DJ, Mandrekar SJ. Clinical trial designs incorporating predictive biomarkers. Cancer Treat Rev. 2016;43:74–82.
27. Rennie D. Improving reports of studies of diagnostic tests: the STARD initiative. JAMA. 2003;289(1):89–90.
28. Rodon J, Soria J-C, Berger R, Batist G, Tsimberidou A, Bresson C, Lee JJ, Rubin E, Onn A, Schilsky RL, Miller WH, Eggermont AM, Mendelsohn J, Lazar V, Kurzrock R. Challenges in

initiating and conducting personalized cancer therapy trials: perspectives from WINTHER, a Worldwide Innovative Network (WIN) Consortium trial. Ann Oncol. 2015;10(14):4645–51.
29. Saad E, Paoletti X, Burzykowski T, Buyse M. Precision medicine needs randomized clinical trials. Nat Rev Clin Oncol 2017; advanced online publication.
30. Schwaederle M, Zhao M, Lee JJ, Lazar V, Leyland-Jones B, Schilsky RL, Mendelsohn J, Kurzrock R. Association of biomarker-based treatment strategies with response rates and progression-free survival in refractory malignant neoplasms. JAMA Oncol. 2016;0658 (0658):1–8.
31. Senn S. Cross-over trials in clinical research. 2nd ed. Chicester: Wiley; 2002.
32. Teutsch SM, Bradley LA, Palomaki GE, Haddow JE, Piper M, Calonge N, Dotson WD, Douglas MP, Berg AO. The evaluation of genomic applications in practice and prevention (EGAPP) initiative: methods of the EGAPP Working Group. Genet Med. 2009;11(1):3–14.
33. Texier M, Rotolo F, Ducreux M, Bouch O, Pignon J-P, Michiels S. Evaluation of treatment effect with paired failure times in a single-arm phase II trial in oncology. Technical report, INSERM CESP, Oct 2016.
34. Tournigand C, André T, Achille E, Lledo G, Flesh M, Mery-Mignard D, Quinaux E, Couteau C, Buyse M, Ganem G, Landi B, Colin P, Louvet C, de Gramont A. FOLFIRI followed by FOLFOX6 or the reverse sequence in advanced colorectal cancer: a randomized GERCOR study. J Clin Oncol. 2004;22(2):229–37.
35. Tsimberidou A-M, Wen S, Hong DS, Wheler JJ, Falchook GS, Fu D, Piha-Paul S, Naing A, Janku F, Aldape K, Ye Y, Kurzrock R, Berry D. Personalized medicine for patients with advanced cancer in the phase I program at MD Anderson: validation and landmark analyses. Clin Cancer Res. 2014;20(18):4827–36.
36. Von Hoff DD. There are no bad anticancer agents, only bad clinical trial designs–twenty-first Richard and Hinda Rosenthal Foundation Award Lecture. Clin Cancer Res. 1998;4(5): 1079–86.
37. Von Hoff DD, Stephenson JJ, Rosen P, Loesch DM, Borad MJ, Anthony S, Jameson G, Brown S, Cantafio N, Richards DA, Fitch TR, Wasserman E, Fernandez C, Green S, Sutherland W, Bittner M, Alarcon A, Mallery D, Penny R. Pilot study using molecular profiling of patients' tumors to find potential targets and select treatments for their refractory cancers. J Clin Oncol. 2010;28(33):4877–83.
38. Zalcberg JR, Verweij J, Casali PG, Le Cesne A, Reichardt P, Blay J-Y, Schlemmer M, Van Glabbeke M, Brown M, Judson IR. Outcome of patients with advanced gastro-intestinal stromal tumours crossing over to a daily imatinib dose of 800 mg after progression on 400 mg. Eur J Cancer. 2005;41(12):1751–7.

The Probability of Being in Response Function and Its Applications

Wei Yann Tsai, Xiaodong Luo and John Crowley

Abstract Cancer clinical trials usually have two or more types of related clinical events (i.e. response, progression and relapse). Hence, to compare treatments, efficacy is often measured using composite endpoints. Temkin (Biometrics 34: 571–580, [18]) prosed the probability of being in response as a function of time (PBRF) to analyze composite endpoints. The PBRF is a measure which considers the response rate and the duration of response jointly. In this article, we develop, study and propose estimators of PBRF based on multi-state survival data.

Keywords Probability of being in response function · Nonparametric estimation

1 Introduction

The past decade has witnessed the introduction of multiple new therapies for the treatment of cancer patients, supported by evidence from clinical trials. Cancer clinical trials usually have composite endpoints. Patients with cancer typically experience different states of health as the disease advances or retreats, often as a result of treatment. For example, patients with solid tumors may experience a response (shrinkage of the tumor by a defined amount) after treatment, or instead a progression of disease (enlargement of the tumor). Patients in response may also eventually progress. Hence, to compare treatments, efficacy is often measured using multiple outcome variables. The fraction of responding patients and the duration of response in

W.Y. Tsai (✉)
Department of Biostatistics, Columbia University, New York, NY 10032, USA
e-mail: wt5@columbia.edu

X. Luo
Research and Development, Sanofi, Bridgewater, NJ 08807, USA
e-mail: xiaodong.luo@sanofi.com

J. Crowley
Cancer Research and Biostatistics, Seattle, WA 98101, USA
e-mail: johnc@crab.org

S. Matsui and J. Crowley (eds.), *Frontiers of Biostatistical Methods and Applications in Clinical Oncology*, DOI 10.1007/978-981-10-0126-0_10

responding patients are widely evaluated in cancer clinical trials, and both measures are considered clinically important determinants of therapeutic value by oncologists. Besides response rate and duration of response, many clinical trials use a primary composite endpoint such as disease-free survival or progression-free survival for measuring treatment efficacy. The analysis focuses on the time to first event such as time to progression or time to response for responders; Kaplan–Meier or cumulative incidence estimates, log-rank tests and Cox proportional hazards modeling are used to produce graphical comparisons, p values and hazard ratios of the time to first event. Although the use of the primary composite endpoint causes no difficulty, it is not uncommon for different endpoints to indicate different results. As demonstrated by Temkin [18], the trial of two chemotherapeutic agents against testicular cancer (denoted by A and ABV) completed by the Eastern Cooperative Oncology Group is one such case. Treatment ABV had a significantly higher response rate, but once response is achieved, treatment A had a significantly longer median duration of response.

In order to provide an objective measure which considers multiple endpoints to assist in the choice of therapy, some endpoints/measures have been developed. Gelber and Goldhirsch [6] and Gelber et al. [7] developed a quality-of-life-oriented endpoint which is time without symptoms of disease and toxicity of treatment (TWiST). Gelber et al. [8] applied TWiST to assess the benefit of treatment for cancer patients.

There are also other composite endpoints in many other types of clinical trials. For example, in cardiovascular (CV) trials, the endpoint of interest is often a composite of two or more types of related clinical events such as a composite of hospitalization and death. Pocock et al. [15] pointed out that the analysis of the time to first event has an inherent limitation. Hence Pocock et al. [15] proposed an alternative method, the win ratio, to analyze composite endpoints. Since hospitalization is of lesser concern than death, Pocock et al. [15] first compared the death times of two patients. If the death times cannot be compared due to censoring, then they compared the hospitalization times. Luo et al. [11] established a statistical theory for this win ratio approach.

Temkin [18] proposed as a summary measure the probability of being in response state as a function of time (PBRF), and suggested a method for its estimation. In an attempt to combine both the response rate of the treatment and the duration of response in responders, Ellis et al. [5] generalized the PBRF to define the expected duration of response (EDOR) for the entire sample. Ellis et al. [5] formally compared treatments using the EDOR by assuming that the time to response, time to relapse and duration of response all follow exponential distributions. It can be easily seen that the area under the PBRF, if available to infinity, is identical to EDOR. Hence, the PBRF (and functions of the PBRF) can be used to compare treatment efficacy in cancer clinical trials. The PBRF is an excellent measures which consider the response rate and the duration of response simultaneously. In particular, other composite endpoints may give contradictory results.

After the introduction of the PBRF by Temkin [18], Begg and Larson [2] studied the properties of the PBRF under exponential assumptions. Voelkel and Crowley [19] provided for nonparametric inference for the PBRF for a class of semi-Markov models. Tsai [16] and Pepe [13] proposed and studied nonparametric estimations of the PBRF, without any parametric or semi-parametric assumptors. However, though the PBRF was introduced and studied three decades ago, there have been few clinical trials using the PBRF. As pointed out by Perez et al. [14] that there were no statistical tests for comparison of two samples associated with the PBRF method, let alone K-sample testing procedures and statistical inference based on regression models which relates covariates to the PBRF. In this article, we establish the asymptotic properties of the estimator of the PBRF proposed by Temkin [18] under fully nonparametric assumptions. The statistical methods developed in this article extend and generalize the Kaplan–Meier estimator to multiple endpoints with censoring in survival analysis.

2 Methods

2.1 Introduction and Background

In clinical trials, the time that patients enter a specific illness state and the length of time the patient stays in that state are often of interest. Each patient may respond (RP) to a given treatment, may progress (PG) without responding, or may show no change (NC). Each patient who responds may then relapse (RL). Several models have been proposed for multistate survival analysis. Lagakos [9, 10] proposed a homogeneous Markov model in which the times of transition from one state to another are exponential random variables. Temkin [18] suggested a nonhomogeneous Markov model to describe the history of each patient. Voelkel and Crowley (1982) proposed a semi-Markov model.

According to the Eastern Cooperative Oncology Group (ECOG) criteria, the clinical criteria for entry into the PG state and the RL state are identical. Hence, we will borrow the concept of bivariate random variables introduced in Tsai's Ph.D. thesis to use the time T^0 to represent the progression time or the relapse time. Let T^0, X^0 and C be random variables, respectively, representing the time (relapse time or progression time), the response time, and the censoring time of the patient. We assume the patients cannot respond after relapse or progrssion. We assume that C and (T^0, X^0) are independent. As usual we cannot observe (T^0, X^0, C) completely, instead we observe $T = \min(T^0, C), X = \min(T^0, X^0, C), \delta_T = I(T = T^0)$ and $\delta_X = I(X = X^0)$, where $I(\cdot)$ is the indicator function. If $\delta_X = 1$, then X is the response time, T is the relapse time when $\delta_T = 1$, or T is the censoring time when $\delta_T = 0$. If $\delta_X = 0$ then T is the progression time when $\delta_T = 1$ (progression before response) or $T = X$ is the censoring time when $\delta_T = 0$ (censored before response and progression). The data has a special censoring pattern. In the region $\{(t, x)|x < t\}$ only the time T^0 may be censored, which is represented by right arrows in Fig. 1. In the diagonal line $\{(t, x)|t = x\}$ either the response time may be censored (represented by up arrow in Fig. 1), or both the response time and

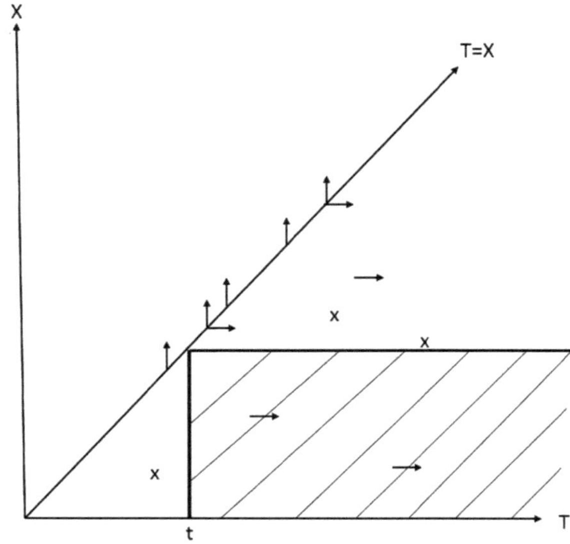

Fig. 1 Censoring pattern and PBRF

progression time may be censored. The probability of the shaded region in Fig. 1 is the PBRF at time t.

2.2 Nonparametric Estimators of the PBRF

Let $R(t)$ be the PBRF at time t, which is defined as

$$R(t) = Pr\left(X^0 \leq t \leq T^0\right).$$

Respectively, the marginal survival functions S_T, S_C and S_Y of random variables T^0, C and $Y^0 = \min(T^0, X^0)$ can be defined as

$$\begin{aligned} S_T &= Pr\left(T^0 \geq t\right), \\ S_C &= Pr(C \geq t) \end{aligned}$$

and

$$S_Y = Pr\left(Y^0 \geq t\right).$$

It is easy to see that

$$R(t) = S_T(t) - S_Y(t) \quad \text{and} \quad R(t) = \frac{R_o(t)}{S_C(t)},$$

where $R_o(t) = P(X \le t < T)$. Let $(T_i, X_i, \delta_{T_i}, \delta_{X_i}),\quad i = 1, \ldots, n$ are the observed random samples. Tsai [16] proposed following two nonparametric estimators of $R(t)$ as

$$\begin{aligned}\hat{R}_1(t) =& \hat{S}_T(t) - \hat{S}_Y(t)\\ \hat{R}_2(t) =& \frac{R_o^e(t)}{\hat{S}_C(t)},\end{aligned}$$

where

$$\begin{aligned}\hat{S}_T(t) &= \prod_{T_i < t}\left(1 - \frac{\delta_{T_i}}{N_T(T_i)}\right),\\ \hat{S}_Y(t) &= \prod_{Y_i < t}\left(1 - \frac{\delta_{Y_i}}{N_Y(Y_i)}\right),\\ \hat{S}_C(t) &= \prod_{T_i < t}\left(1 - \frac{(1 - \delta_{T_i})}{N_T(T_i)}\right),\\ R_o^e(t) &= \sum_{i=1}^{n} I(X_i \le t < T_i)/n,\\ N_T(t) &= \sum_{i=1}^{n} I(T_i \ge t),\\ N_Y(t) &= \sum_{i=1}^{n} I(Y_i \ge t),\\ Y_i &= \min(X_i, T_i) \quad \text{and}\\ \delta_{Y_i} &= 1 - (1 - \delta_{T_i})(1 - \delta_{X_i}).\end{aligned}$$

It easy to see that $\hat{S}_T, \hat{S}_Y$ and $\hat{S}_C$ are, respectively, the K-M estimator of S_T, S_Y and S_C.

Under the nonhomogeneous Markov model assumption, Temkin [18] proposed an estimator $\hat{R}_3(t)$, which maximized the likelihood, and is defined as

$$\hat{R}_3(t) = \sum_{X_i < t} \frac{\delta_{X_i}\hat{S}_Y(X_i)\tilde{S}_T(t)}{N_Y(X_i)\tilde{S}_T(X_i)},$$

where

$$\tilde{S}_T(t) = \prod_{T_i < t} \left(1 - \frac{\delta_{T_i}\delta_{X_i}}{N_T^*(T_i)}\right), \quad \text{and} \quad N_T^*(t) = \sum_{i=1}^n I(X_i \le t \le T_i).$$

$\tilde{S}$ is also a Product-Limit [17] estimator based on left truncated and right censored data (T_i, X_i, δ_{T_i}) with $T_i > X_i$.

Although the estimator $\hat{R}_1(t)$ is a nonparametric estimator, it is possible that $\hat{R}_1(t) < 0$. The estimator $\hat{R}_3(t)$ is properly bounded, that is $0 \le \hat{R}_3(t) \le 1$ However Temkin [18] proposed an estimator of variance of $\hat{R}_3(t)$ which was obtained from large sample properties of MLEs under the nonhomogeneous Markov model and assumptions that response times, progression time and relapse times are discrete and finite. However the calculation of the variance estimator requires inverting a large size matrix.

2.3 Asymptotic Properties

In this section, we establish the consistency and asymptotic normality of $\hat{R}_3(t)$. The asypmtotic properties of $\hat{R}_1(t)$ and $\hat{R}_2(t)$ have been studied by Tsai [16] and Pepe [13]. In Tsai's thesis, he showed by simulation that the performance of these 3 estimators are very similar even when the nonhomogeneous Markov model assumption fails. Also, without censoring, all three estimators $\hat{R}_i(t),\ i = 1, 2, 3$, will reduce to the estimator $R_o^e(t)$, which is the empirical estimator of $R(t)$. It is expected that the estimator $\hat{R}_3(t)$ will be consistent even without nonhomogeneous Markov model assumption. The estimator $\tilde{S}_T(t)$ in the definition of $\hat{R}_3(t)$ is the product-limit estimator of the survival function of T^0 under random left truncation and right censoring, so the conditions of asymptotic properties of the product-limit estimator should also be applied here (see [17, 20]). We have following two theorems about the asymptotic properties of $\hat{R}_3(t)$:

Theorem 1 (Consistency) *If there exists a positive* ϵ *such that* $R(t) > \epsilon$ *for* $a \le t \le b$ *and* $S_T(a) = 1$ *then* $\hat{R}_3(t)$ *is consistent for* $t \le b$ *even when the nonhomogeneous Markov assumption fails.*

Theorem 2 (Asymptotic Normality) *Under same conditions of Theorem* 1, $\sqrt{n}\big(\hat{R}_3(t) - R(t)\big)$ *converges weakly to a mean zero Gaussian process* $\Re_3(t)$ *as* $n \to \infty$ *with the variance covariance matrix* $Cov(\Re_3(s), \Re_3(t))$ *that can be consistently estimated by*

$$n^{-1}\sum_{i=1}^{n}[\hat{e}_{31i}(s)-\hat{e}_{32i}(s)+\hat{e}_{33i}(s)][\hat{e}_{31i}(t)-\hat{e}_{32i}(t)+\hat{e}_{33i}(t)]$$

where

$$\begin{aligned}
\hat{e}_{31i}(t) &= \frac{\delta_{Xi}I(X_i\le t)\tilde{S}_T(t)}{\tilde{S}_T(X_i)\hat{S}_C(X_i)}-\hat{R}_3(t)\\
\hat{e}_{32i}(t) &= \frac{\delta_{Xi}\delta_{Ti}I(T_i\le t)\tilde{S}_T(t)\hat{R}_3(T_i)}{\tilde{S}_T(T_i)R_o^e(T_i)}\\
&\quad - n^{-1}\sum_{j=1}^{n}\frac{\delta_{Xj}\delta_{Tj}\tilde{S}_T(t)\hat{R}_3(T_j)I(\delta_{Xi}=1,X_i\le T_j\le T_i\wedge t)}{\tilde{S}_T(T_j)\left(R_o^e\right)^2(T_j)}\\
\hat{e}_{33i}(t) &= \frac{\tilde{S}_T(t)}{N_T(T_i)/n}\left\{\frac{\hat{R}_3(t)}{\tilde{S}_T(t)}-\frac{\hat{R}_3(T_i)}{\tilde{S}_T(T_i)}\right\}I(\delta_{Ti}=0,T_i\le t)\\
&\quad - n^{-1}\sum_{j=1}^{n}\frac{\tilde{S}_T(t)}{\{N_T(T_j)/n\}^2}\left\{\frac{\hat{R}_3(t)}{\tilde{S}_T(t)}-\frac{\hat{R}_3(T_j)}{\tilde{S}_T(T_j)}\right\}I\left(\delta_{Tj}=0,T_j\le t\right).
\end{aligned}$$

The detailed proofs of Theorems 1–2 are provided in the appendix.

3 Simulation and Real Data Analysis

3.1 *Simulation*

We have performed limited simulations. Sample sizes of 1000 and 1000 simulations were performed. The progression time, the response time and the censoring times were simulated from Weibull distributions with $(\alpha,\lambda)=(2.0,0.04)$, $(\alpha,\lambda)=(1.5,0.05)$ and $(\alpha,\lambda)=(1.5,0.06)$ respectively; with the joint distribution of the progression time and the response time being a bivariate normal copula with mean zero, variance one and correlation coefficient −0.7. Figure 2 plots sample simulation variance and bias over time t for the three PBRF estimators $\hat{R}_i(t), i=1,2,3$.

The simulation sample variance and estimated variance (based on Theorem 2) of $\hat{R}_3(t)$ were plotted in Fig. 3.

3.2 *Real Data Analysis*

We apply the three estimators for the following two data sets.

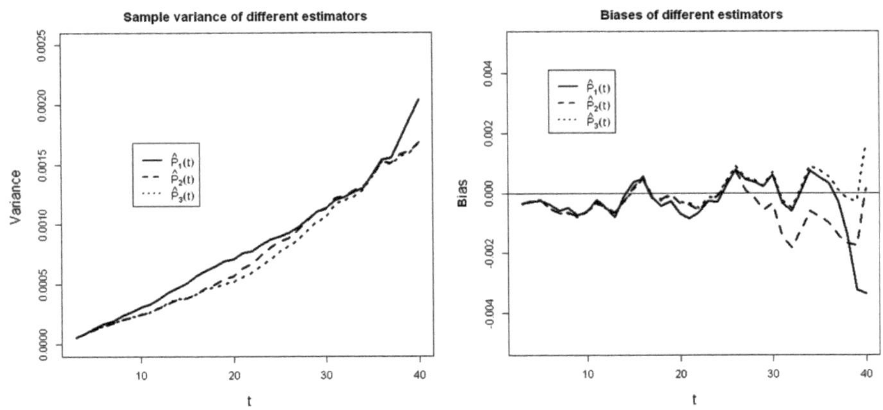

Fig. 2 Sample variance and bias of the three estimators where the *solid lines* are for $\hat{R}_1(t)$, the *dashed lines* are for $\hat{R}_2(t)$ and the *dotted lines* are for $\hat{R}_3(t)$

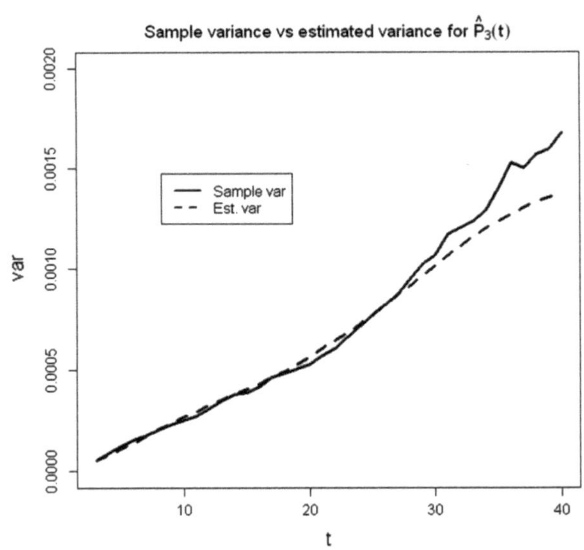

Fig. 3 Sample variance versus estimated variance of $\hat{R}_3(t)$

I. Data from the Stanford heart transplant study illustrate another possible application. Accepted patients can only receive a heart only if a suitable donor heart becomes available. Some patients may die or may be censored before suitable donor hearts become available. Other patients may die or be censored after the transplant operation. In this setting, the random variable X^0 represents the waiting time (time from entry to transplant operation) for the heart

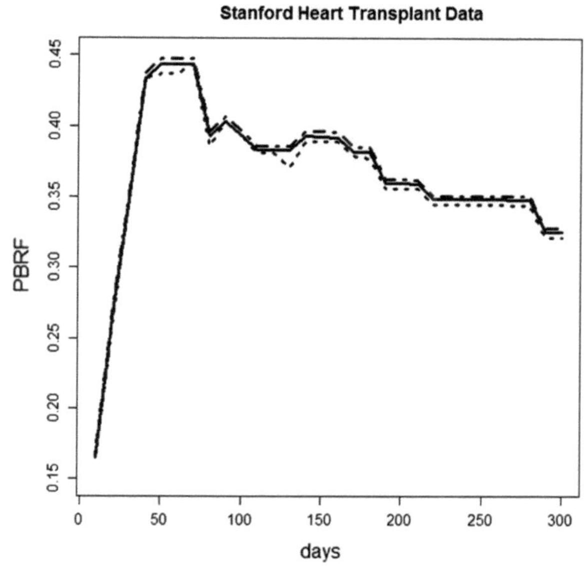

Fig. 4 The estimates of PBRF for the Standford heart transplant data, where the *solid lines* are for $\hat{R}_1(t)$, the *dotted lines* are for $\hat{R}_2(t)$ and the *dot-dashed lines* are for $\hat{R}_3(t)$

transplant patients and the random variable T^0 represents the death time from acceptance. The function $R(t)$ is the probability of being alive with a transplanted heart at time t after acceptance. The waiting times and death times and event indicators of the first 103 patients were reported in Crowley and Hu [4]. Figure 4 shows the three estimates of $R(t)$.

II. A randomized trial of two treatments (standard treatment and standard treatment plus Thalidomde) for patients with myeloma was conducted by the Myeloma Institute for Research and Therapy (MIRT). There were 334 patients in the control arm and 323 in treatment arm; among these patients, at the time of publication [1], 157 in control and 133 in treatment had died after partial response, 104 in control and 142 in treatment partially responded without yet dying, 56 in control and 33 in treatment died without partial response and 28 in control and 15 in treatment had not yet died nor responded. The three estimates of $R(t)$ for the combined sample are plotted in Fig. 5.

Figure 6 shows the estimates $\hat{R}_3(t)$ for the control arm and treatment arm based on MIRT data, and the difference of two PBRF estimates along the 95% confidence interval calculated based on the variance formula of Theorem 2.

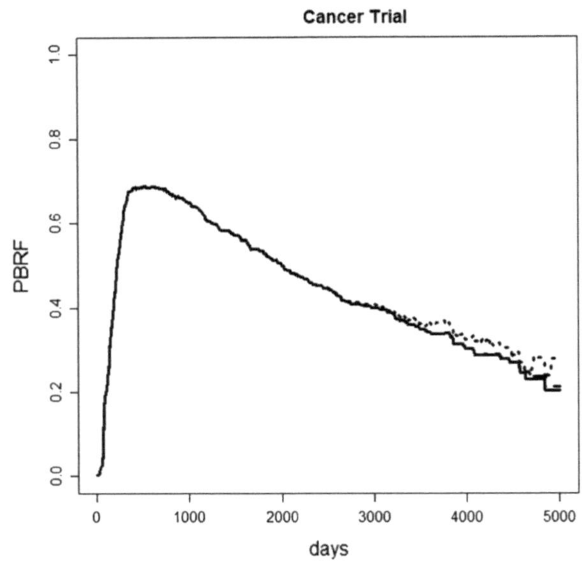

Fig. 5 The estimates of PBRF for the cancer trial data respectively, where the *solid lines* are for $\hat{R}_1(t)$, the *dotted lines* are for $\hat{R}_2(t)$ and the *dot-dashed lines* are for $\hat{R}_3(t)$

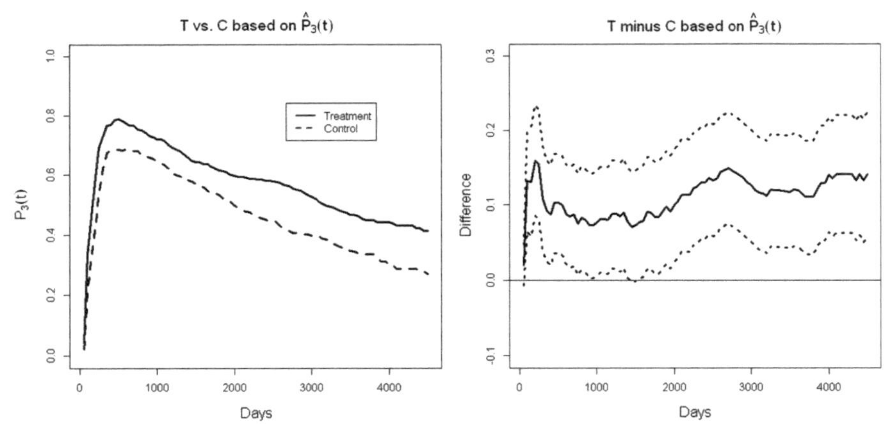

Fig. 6 Comparison of PBRFs in the treatment arm and control arm in the cancer trial based on $\hat{R}_3(t)$, where the *dotted lines* are the 95% point-wise confidence intervals for the difference

4 Discussion

In this article, we have proved the asymptotic properties of the estimator $\hat{R}_3$ which was proposed by Temkin [18]. We have proved that $\hat{R}_3$ is consistent and converges to a Gaussian process even when the nonhomogeneous Markov assumption doesn't hold. From the asymptotic normality, we may construct a 95% confidence interval of the PBRF. Based on our simulation studies, the variance estimator is unbiased and consistent. The methodologies developed here are useful additions to the statistical methods and theories in cancer research in the presence of censoring in survival analysis. In the near future, we plan to propose and to study statistics which are functional forms of the PBRFs and can be used to compare two or more PBBRFs. The ultimate goal is to generalize the Cox proportional hazards model to a proportional Log PBRF model and to study inference based on this generalization model.

Appendix

Proof of Theorem 1 (Consistency) Let the joint probability functions (pdf) of (T^0, X^0) be $f(t, x)$. Define the two sub-marginal functions $f_1(t)$ and $f_2(x)$, respectively, as

$$f_1(t) = \int_0^t f(t,x)dx$$

and

$$f_2(x) = \int_x^\infty f(t,x)dt.$$

Using the method which is similar to Tsai et al. [17], we may prove that $\tilde{S}_T(t)$ converges almost surly to

$$S_T^*(t) = \exp\left\{ - \int_0^t \frac{f_1(s)S_C(s)}{R_o(s)} ds \right\} = \exp\left\{ - \int_0^t \frac{f_1(s)}{R(s)} ds \right\}.$$

The Kaplan–Meier estimator $\hat{S}_Y(x)$ will converges almost surely to $S_Y(x)$. Combining these and the properties of empirical cumulative distribution function, we can show that $\hat{R}_3(t)$ will converge almost surely to

$$R_3(t) = S_T^*(t) \int_0^t \frac{f_2(x)}{S_T^*(x)} dx.$$

However, one may easily verify that

$$\left(\frac{R(t)}{S_T^*(t)}\right)' = \frac{f_2(t)}{S_T^*(t)},$$

which implies that

$$R(t) = S_T^*(t)\int_0^t \frac{f_2(x)}{S_T^*(x)}dx$$

and the consistency result follows.

Proof of Theorem 2 (Asymptotic Normality)
By Taylor expansion,

$$\sqrt{n}\big(\hat{R}_3(t) - R(t)\big) = \sqrt{n}A_1(t) + \sqrt{n}A_2(t) + \sqrt{n}A_3(t) + o_p(1),$$

where $A_1(t) = n^{-1}\sum_{i=1}^n e_{31i}(t), A_2(t) = n^{-1}\sum_{i=1}^n e_{32i}(t), A_3(t) = n^{-1}\sum_{i=1}^n e_{33i}(t)$ and for $i = 1, \ldots, n$

$$\begin{aligned}
e_{31i}(t) =& \frac{\delta_{Xi} I(X_i \le t) S_T^*(t)}{S_T^*(X_i) S_C(X_i)} - R(t), \\
e_{32i}(t) =& \frac{\delta_{Xi}\delta_{Ti} I(T_i \le t) S_T^*(t) R_3(T_i)}{S_T^*(T_i) r_o^e(T_i)} - \int_0^t \frac{S_T^*(t) R(s) I(X_i \le s \le T_i) f_{11}(s) ds}{S_T^*(s)\left[r_o^e(s)\right]^2} \\
e_{33i}(t) =& \frac{S_T^*(t)}{n_T(T_i)}\left\{\frac{R(t)}{S_T^*(t)} - \frac{R_3(T_i)}{S_T^*(T_i)}\right\} I(\delta_{Ti} = 0, T_i \le t) \\
& - \int_0^t \frac{S_T^*(t)}{n_T^2(s)}\left\{\frac{R(t)}{S_T^*(t)} - \frac{R(s)}{S_T^*(s)}\right\} f_2(s) ds \\
n_T(t) =& E\{N_T(t)\}/n \\
f_{11}(s) =& \text{pr}(X \le T = s, \delta_X = 1, \delta_T = 1) \\
f_2(s) =& \text{pr}(T = s, \delta_T = 0)
\end{aligned}$$

Since $A_j(t)$, $j = 1, 2, 3$ are all sum of i.i.d. random variables, $A_1(t) + A_2(t) + A_3(t)$ will converge to a mean zero Gaussian process $\Re_3(t)$ as $n \to \infty$ with the variance covariance matrix $Cov(\Re_3(s), \Re_3(t))$ that can be consistently estimated by

$$n^{-1}\sum_{i=1}^n [\hat{e}_{31i}(s) - \hat{e}_{32i}(s) + \hat{e}_{33i}(s)][\hat{e}_{31i}(t) - \hat{e}_{32i}(t) + \hat{e}_{33i}(t)],$$

where $\hat{e}_{3ji}(t)$ is the estimate of the $e_{3ji}(t)$ when the unknown functions are substituted by their estimates, $j = 1, 2, 3$.

References

1. Barlogie B, Tricot G, Anaissie E, Shaughnessy J, Rasmussen E, van Rhee F, Fassas A, Zangari M, Hollmig K, Pineda-Roman M, Lee C, Talamo G, Thertulien R, Kiwan E, Krishna S, Fox M, Crowley J. Thalidomide and hematopoietic-cell transplantation for multiple myeloma. N Engl J Med. 2006;354(10):1021–30.
2. Begg CB, Larson M. A study of the use of the probability-of-being-in-response function as a summary of tumor response data. Biometrics. 1982;38(1):59–66.
3. Cox DR. Regression models and life-tables. J R Stat Soc Ser B (Methodol). 1972;34(2):187–220.
4. Crowley J, Hu M. Covariance analysis of heart transplant survival data. J Am Stat Assoc. 1977;72(357):27–36.
5. Ellis S, Carroll KJ, Pemberton K. Analysis of duration of response in oncology trials. Contemp Clin Trials. 2008;29(4):456–65.
6. Gelber RD, Goldhirsch A. A new endpoint for the assessment of adjuvant therapy in postmenopausal women with operable breast cancer. J Clin Oncol. 1986;4(12):1772–9.
7. Gelber RD, Goldhirsch A, Castiglione M, Price K, Isley M, Coates A, Ludwig Breast Cancer Study Group. Time without symptoms and toxicity (TWiST): a quality-of-life-oriented endpoint to evaluate adjuvant therapy. Adjuvant Ther Cancer. 1987;5(1):455–65.
8. Gelber RD, Gelman RS, Goldhirsch A. A quality-of-life-oriented endpoint for comparing therapies. Biometrics. 1989;45(3):781–95.
9. Lagakos SW. A stochastic model for censored survival data in the presence of an auxiliary variable. Biometrics. 1976;32(3):551.
10. Lagakos SW. Using auxiliary variables for improved estimates of survival time. Biometrics. 1977;33(2):399–404.
11. Luo X, Tian H, Mohanty S, Tsai WY. An alternative approach to confidence interval estimation for the win ratio statistic. Biometrics. 2015;71(1):139–45.
12. Morgan TM. Analysis of duration of response: a problem of oncology trials. Control Clin Trials. 1988;9(1):11–8.
13. Pepe MS. Inference for events with dependent risks in multiple endpoint studies. J Am Stat Assoc. 1991;86(415):770–8.
14. Perez CA, Pajak T, Emami B, Hornback NB, Tupchong L, Rubin P. Randomized phase III study comparing irradiation and hyperthermia with irradiation alone in superficial measurable tumors: final report by the Radiation Therapy Oncology Group. Am J Clin Oncol. 1991;14(2):133–41.
15. Pocock SJ, Ariti CA, Collier TJ, Wang D. The win ratio: a new approach to the analysis of composite endpoints in clinical trials based on clinical priorities. Eur Heart J. 2012;33(2):176–82.
16. Tsai WY. Bivariate survival time and censoring. Unpublished Ph.D. dissertation. Madison: University of Wisconsin; 1982.
17. Tsai WY, Jewell NP, Wang MC. A note on the product-limit estimator under right censoring and left truncation. Biometrika. 1987;74(4):883–6.
18. Temkin NR. An analysis for transient states with application to tumor shrinkage. Biometrics. 1978;34(4):571–80.

19. Voelkel JG, Crowley J. Nonparametric inference for a class of semi-Markov processes with censored observations. Ann Stat. 1984;12(1):142–60.
20. Wang MC, Jewell NP, Tsai WY. Asymptotic properties of the product limit estimate under random truncation. Ann Stat. 1986;14(4):1597–605.

Cure-Rate Survival Models and Their Application to Cancer Clinical Trials

Megan Othus, Alan Mitchell, Bart Barlogie, Gareth Morgan and John Crowley

Abstract Many patients with cancer can be long-term survivors of their disease and cure models can be a useful tool to analyze and describe cancer clinical trial survival data. This goal of this chapter is to: (i) review what a cure model is, (ii) explain when it can be appropriate to use cure models, and (iii) use cure models to describe multiple myeloma survival trends, including analyses that account for competing risks. This chapter will show that by using cure models, in addition to the standard Cox proportional hazards model, we can evaluate whether there is evidence that some myeloma therapies induce a proportion of patients to be long-term survivors.

Keywords Cure model · Survival analysis · Regression model · Clinical trials

M. Othus (✉)
Fred Hutchinson Cancer Research Center, Seattle, WA, USA
e-mail: mothus@fredhutch.org

A. Mitchell
Allergan, USA Inc, Seattle, WA, USA
e-mail: alannmitchell@gmail.com

B. Barlogie
Mt Sinai School of Medicine, New York, NY, USA
e-mail: bart.barlogie@mssm.edu

G. Morgan
Myeloma Institute at University of Arkansas for Medical Sciences, Little Rock, AR, USA
e-mail: GJMorgan@uams.edu

J. Crowley
Cancer Research and Biostatistics, Seattle, WA, USA
e-mail: johnc@crab.org

S. Matsui and J. Crowley (eds.), *Frontiers of Biostatistical Methods and Applications in Clinical Oncology*, DOI 10.1007/978-981-10-0126-0_11

1 Introduction

Advances in therapy have made cure a possibility for some cancers. For example, multiple myeloma (MM) is generally considered an incurable disease [16], but recent research suggests that some MM patients could be cured. Investigators at the University of Arkansas for Medical Sciences (UAMS) have developed an approach called Total Therapy that has recently been shown to cure up to 30% of MM patients [14].

The most common regression model for survival data, the proportional hazards (PH) model [13], does not explicitly allow for inference on heterogeneous populations. When a population is a mixture of patients with very poor and very good outcomes, cure models can be useful in describing the different subgroups.

Cure models can also be useful for applications in which patients are not "cured" but rather there is a proportion of patients who will not fail during the finite follow-up of the study. These patients can be referred to as long-term survivors rather than cured. In this case the "cured" proportion provides an estimate of the proportion of patients who will not fail during follow-up.

Patients who have been cured of cancer will still eventually die of other causes, which complicates the implementation of many cure models to describe overall survival in datasets with long follow-up. Alternative cure models that incorporate cause of death data in competing risks models are needed to make appropriate inference for these populations.

This chapter is organized as follows: Sect. 3 reviews the general classes of cure models; Sect. 4 summarizes important assumptions common to cure models; Sect. 5 describes computing options; Sect. 6 outlines design considerations for clinical trials in which some patients may be cured; Sect. 7 proposes a competing risks cure model that accounts for cured patients who are observed to die of other causes; and Sect. 8 summarizes an analysis of the UAMS MM data by several cure models.

2 Model Options

Cure models can be classified into two groups, mixture and non-mixture. Each group will be reviewed below.

2.1 Mixture Cure Models

Mixture cure models assume that the underlying population includes both cured and uncured patients. The first cure models were motivated by cancer survival trends and assumed that survival for cured patients was different from and better than survival for uncured patients [7]. The authors assumed a simple parametric model:

$$S(t) = pS_0(t) + (1-p)S_0(t)\exp(-\lambda t), \tag{1}$$

where p denotes the proportion of cured patients, $S_0(t)$ denotes the survival of a "general" or "normal" population, and λ denotes the death rate due to cancer [7]. The authors were "surprised as well as gratified" to find that such a simple formulation with only two parameters fit observed data quite well.

Further research on mixture cure models has focused on developing more general and flexible formulations of Eq. (1). Most mixture cure models can be written as

$$S(t|X) = p(X) + (1-p(X))S_0(t|X), \tag{2}$$

where X is a set of covariates, $p(X)$ is a model for the probability that an individual is cured, and $S_0(t|X)$ is the survival function for patients who are not cured. Most mixture cure models use a logistic model for $p(X)$. Proposed models for $S_0(t|X)$ include the exponential and Weibull distributions [18], the PH model [22, 38, 41], accelerated failure time models [29], and general transformation models that can include the PH and proportional odds [6] models as special cases [32].

Recent research on mixture cure models has focused on more complicated survival data including interval censoring [31], dependent censoring [30, 36], longitudinal data [27, 37, 39, 49], current status data [20, 33], and grouped survival data [48].

2.2 Non-mixture Cure Models

Most non-mixture cure models parametrize the survival function as

$$S(t) = \exp(-\theta F(t)), \tag{3}$$

where $F(t)$ is the distribution function for a non-negative random variable. In this model, the cumulative hazard function $\theta F(t)$ is bounded and so the survival function is an improper survival function with $\lim_{t\to\infty} S(t) > 0$. In Eq. (3), the proportion of cured patients is equal to $\exp(-\theta)$. When $F(t)$ does not depend on covariates, Model (3) has a proportional hazards structure. Covariates are incorporated into this model through both θ and $F(t)$. Often θ is modeled with the relationship $\theta(X) = \exp(\beta' X)$. Common parametric forms for $F(t)$ include the Weibull, lognormal, logistic, and gamma distributions.

Parametric forms for $F(t)$ can incorporate covariates and have been considered by a number of authors [10, 40, 43]. Models with semiparametric $F(t)$ have also been proposed [44]. Some work has been done for non-mixture cure models with alternative transformations of $\theta F(t)$ [42, 50].

Non-mixture cure models are a popular framework for Bayesian cure models because mixture cure models yield improperposterior distributions for many non-informativepriors, and the PH structure of non-mixture cure models is computationally convenient [10, 21, 44]. Bayesian extensions to Eq. 3 include models for multivariate survival data [11], models for spatial data with interval censoring [1], and general transformations of $\theta F(t)$ [46, 47].

2.3 *Differences Between Mixture and Non-mixture Cure Models*

Choosing between mixture and non-mixture models is a matter of preference. Frequentist results are available for both mixture and non-mixture models, but Bayesian work has focused on non-mixture models due to computational ease. Most non-mixture models allow for a PH interpretation of covariates. Mixture models allow for separate covariate inference for cured and uncured patients.

3 Assumptions and Identifiability

All cure models (parametric and semiparametric, mixture and non-mixture) assume that a cured fraction exists. This assumption requires that there is enough data to estimate parameters related to the cure proportion. Often survival functions for populations with cured patients exhibit a plateau at the end of the curve beyond which there are no more failures and the survival curve is flat. Given this feature of cure survival curves, Kaplan–Meier plots that exhibit plateaus at the end of the curve are often interpreted to describe cured populations, and that shape of curve is often taken as evidence that a cure model may be appropriate. For mixture cure models, a test of the existence of a cure fraction based on the tail of the Kaplan–Meier curve has been proposed [34], though it is not straightforward to implement the test.

Care needs to be taken to ensure that semiparametric cure models are identifiable. Proofs of identifiability or non-identifiability exist for some general classes of semiparametric mixture and non-mixture cure models. For example, the logistic-PH model and Eq. (3) with $\log(\theta)$ linear in covariates without an intercept and $F(t)$ unspecified are both identifiable [28]. The mixture cure model Eq. (2) with survival for those not cured modeled nonparametrically and assuming a constant probability of cure ($p(x) = p$ for all x) is not identifiable [28].

Although common semiparametric mixture cure models have been proven to be identifiable, in finite samples the models can exhibit "near-nonidentifiability" in which the likelihood for cure parameters can be flat. To address this issue in mixture cure models, some authors have proposed setting the survival function for patients who are not cured [$S_0(t)$ in Eq. (2)] equal to zero after the last observed failure time [32, 38, 41]. The justification for this computational adjustment is that cure models are only appropriate when some patients are cured, and that long follow-up is required to identify the plateau of the tail of a survival curve. If there is sufficient follow-up to support the assumption of a cured proportion, authors argue that it is reasonable to set the survival function to zero after the last failure. If there is not sufficient follow-up or there is no rationale for why a cure proportion might exist, the model should not be used. Similarly, semiparametric non-mixture survival models usually assume that $F(t)$ from Eq. (3) is equal to zero at the last failure. Many Bayesian models can control the degree to which a model is semiparametric. Bayesian semiparametric non-mixture models often model $F(t)$ as having a piecewise constant hazard. The number of pieces controls the "nonparametricity" of the model and so small to moderate numbers of pieces are required to have the models behave well [11].

4 Computational Implementation

Cure models are not standard functions in most statistical packages. Below we review the limited `R` packages, SAS macros, and Stata modules available for cure analyses.

4.1 R

At this time there are three packages to fit cure models in `R`. The package `nltm` provides functions to estimate non-mixture proportional hazards and proportional odds models from [42]. The package `smcure` provides functions to estimate semiparametric PH mixture cure models and AFT mixture cure models using an EM algorithm [9]. The package `intercure` provides functions to estimate non-mixture cure models (with and without a frailty) for interval censored data. In addition, the package `NPHMC` has a function to compute power or sample size for the PH mixture cure model [8].

4.2 SAS

A SAS macro PSPMCM was published that fits some frequentist parametric and semiparametric mixture cure survival models [12].

4.3 Stata

There is a Stata module available to fit a frequentist parametric non-mixture cure model as detailed in [40]. The module can be downloaded from http://ideas.repec.org/c/boc/bocode/s446901.html. The package STGENREG has functions of parametric survival models, including parametric cure rate models [15]. Details on Stata commands to fit cure models that incorporate expected background mortality and that can estimate relative mortality have been published [23].

5 Design Considerations

Limited work has been done for power and sample size calculations assuming a proportion of patients have been cured. All of the work as focused on mixture cure survival models and most of that work has focused on power of tests of the cure proportion. Gray and Tsiatis proposed a linear rank test derived to focus power at the alternative that cure proportions are different but that survival among those not cured is the same between the two groups [19]. This test has improved power over the log-rank test when less than 50% of the population is cured. Laska and Meisner proposed a test of cure proportions based on the tails of the Kaplan–Meier curves [26]. Ewell and Ibrahim extended the results of [19] to cases in which the survival distributions for non-cured populations may differ [17]. More recently, sample size formulas for the proportional hazards cure model have published [45].

6 A Competing Risks Cure Model

Most cure models assume that cured patients will not experience an event. For some outcomes this is reasonable but for other outcomes, such as outcome overall survival, this assumption is violated. As explained in the Introduction, for a study population with finite follow-up cure models can still be useful to describe the observed and expected survival patterns for survival curves with a plateau at the tail of the curve. For some study populations, in particular studies with longer follow-up, there may be scientific rationale to expect a cured proportion, but because cured patients will eventually die of another cause, overall survival curves may not exhibit a plateau and traditional cure models may not be appropriate.

An alternative approach is to use competing risks models with cause of death data to estimate cure proportions. Such a model can be written

$$S(t|X) = p(X)S_c(t|X, \beta_{ncan}) + (1 - p(X))S_{nc}(t|X, \beta_{ncan}, \beta_{can}), \quad (4)$$

where X is a set of covariates, $p(X)$ is a model for the probability that an individual is cured, $S_c(t|X, \beta_{ncan})$ is the survival function for patients who are not cured with regression coefficient β_{ncan} corresponding to the failure due to non-cancer causes, and $S_{nc}(t|X, \beta_{ncan}, \beta_{can})$ is the survival function for patients who are not cured with regression coefficients β_{ncan} and β_{can} corresponding to failures from non-cancer and cancer causes, respectively. Patients who not cured can fail from either cancer and non-cancer causes, while patients who are cured only fail from non-cancer causes. If we assume exponential failure for both cancer and non-cancer causes, this survival function can be written

$$S(t|X) = p(X)\exp(-t\exp(\beta'_{ncan}X)) + (1 - p(X))\exp(-t[\exp(\beta'_{can}X) + \exp(\beta'_{ncan}X)]). \quad (5)$$

In contrast to previously proposed mixture models for competing risks data [25], the coefficient β_{ncan} is present in both survival function terms, not just the survival function for non-cured patients (S_{nc}). While mixture cure models for relative survival use population-based mortality data to estimate the non-cancer survival function [24, e.g., life table data], this model uses cause of death data to identify the various components of the model.

7 Analysis of Multiple Myeloma Data

In an effort to distinguish between the various cure models, we will evaluate several models on the multiple myeloma (MM) dataset mentioned in the Introduction. The University of Arkansas for Medical Sciences has developed a series of "total therapy" (TT) protocols since 1989 with the intent of curing some MM patients. The first protocol, TT1, used a tandem autotransplant approach [3, 5]. The second protocol intensified induction, added post-transplant consolidation, and randomized between the addition of thalidomide, TT2+, or no thalidomide, TT2− [4]. The more recent protocol, TT3, incorporated thalidomide and bortezomib for induction [2, 35]. Patient outcomes have improved over the protocols, so we will investigate the trends in progression-free survival (PFS) over the protocols using several cure models. PFS is defined from the date of registration to the first of death or progression, with patients last known to be alive without progression censored at the date of last contact.

First we look at the survival curves for the four groups to evaluate whether cure models are appropriate for this data. Figure 1 shows Kaplan–Meier plots of PFS stratified by TT protocol. PFS has improved over time and each PFS curve has a plateau at the tail indicating the potential that some patients may be cured.

Table 1 summarizes results for a univariate mixture cure model Eq. (2) with a constant probability of cure, $p(X) = p$, and exponential survival, $S_0(t|X) = \exp(-\lambda t)$.

The estimated cure proportions increase over the protocols, as Fig. 1 indicates. The proportion of cured patients more than doubled between TT1 and TT2+/TT3.

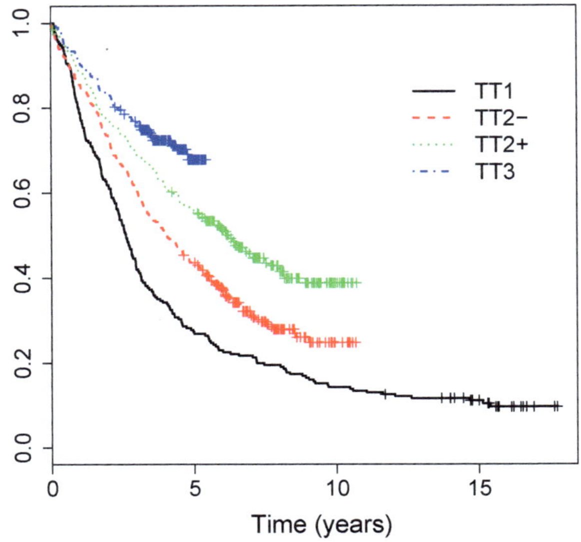

Fig. 1 Kaplan–Meier plots for PFS

Table 1 Univariate exponential cure model regression results; CI = confidence interval

	Cure proportion (%)	(95% CI)	Median PFS (years)	(95% CI)
TT1	9.4	(5.4, 13.4)	2.3	(2.0, 2.7)
TT2−	10.3	(0, 22.1)	3.5	(2.7, 4.8)
TT2+	23.2	(8.0, 38.4)	4.1	(3.0, 6.4)
TT3	52.7	(30.0, 75.1)	3.1	(1.8, 12.1)

Table 2 Logistic-proportional hazards regression results

	Cure model		PH model	
	OR	95% CI	HR	95% CI
TT1 (ref)				
TT2−	1.80	(0.99, 3.27)	0.67	(0.53, 0.86)
TT2+	3.89	(2.3, 6.98)	0.56	(0.42, 0.75)
TT3	21.60	(11.52, 40.49)	0.86	(0.61, 1.21)
Age	0.97	(0.95, 0.99)	1.01	(0.99, 1.02)
CA	0.41	(0.25, 0.66)	1.45	(1.14, 1.85)

PFS for patients who are not cured has been stable over the protocols, indicating that PFS gains over the protocols have been driven by an increase in the proportion of cured patients.

Table 2 summarizes results [odds ratios (ORs), hazard ratios (HRs), and 95% CIs)] from a semiparametric mixture cure model, the logistic-PH model, where

Table 3 Weibull non-mixture model regression results

	HR	95% CI
TT1 (ref)		
TT2−	0.64	(0.53, 0.78)
TT2+	0.45	(0.37, 0.55)
TT3	0.29	(0.22, 0.37)
Age	1.03	(1.01, 1.05)
CA	1.72	(1.47, 2.01)
Scale		
Intercept	−7.03	(−8.24, −5.83)
Age	−0.02	(−0.04, 0.01)
Shape		
Intercept	0.56	(0.18, 0.94)
Age	−0.01	(−0.01, −0.001)

Table 4 Proportional hazards model regression results

	HR	95% CI
TT1 (ref)		
TT2−	0.64	(0.53, 0.79)
TT2+	0.45	(0.36, 0.55)
TT3	0.29	(0.22, 0.37)
Age	1.01	(1.001, 1.02)
CA	1.72	(1.48, 2.01)

Table 5 Estimates of cure proportions

	Exponential mixture	PH mixture	Weibull non-mixture
TT1	9	9	6
TT2−	10	10	16
TT2+	23	22	27
TT3	53	58	43

$S(t|X) = \exp(-\exp(\beta' X)\Lambda(t))$ and $\Lambda(t)$ is an unspecified cumulative hazard function. In this model, the probability of cure increased over the protocols. Survival among those not cured in TT2− and TT2+ was significantly improved over TT1, though survival among those not cured in TT3 was not significantly improved over TT1. Increased age was associated with a decreased probability of being cured. CA were associated with a decreased probability of being cured and decreased survival for those not cured.

Table 6 Estimates from an exponential competing risks cure model

	Cure proportion (%) (95% CI)	Median survival (years) cured patients (95% CI)	Median survival (years) non-cured patients (95% CI)
TT1	28 (19, 38)	18 (14, 21)	5 (3, 7)
TT2−	21 (14, 31)	28 (24, 33)	6 (4, 8)
TT2+	32 (24, 41)	41 (35, 47)	6 (4, 8)
TT3	70 (64, 76)	31 (28, 34)	3 (2, 4)

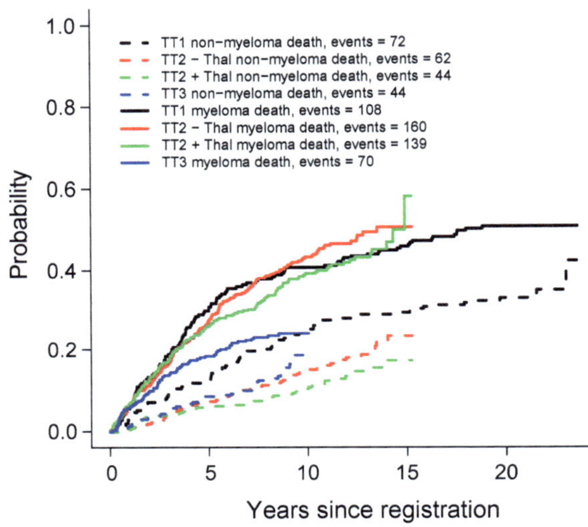

Fig. 2 Cumulative incidence curves for overall survival

An alternative semiparametric model is a non-mixture model Eq. (3). Table 3 summarizes results for $F(t)$ following the Weibull distribution and letting $\theta = \exp(\beta' X)$. The results for the non-mixture model indicate that there was continued improvement in survival for all patients, on average, from TT1 through TT3. Older age and presence of CAs are associated with decreased survival.

The standard survival model, the PH model, is summarized in Table 4. The PH model has very similar estimates as the non-mixture cure models.

Table 5 summarizes estimates of cure fractions for each of the protocols from the three cure models summarized above. Each model was fit with only covariates for the protocols. Estimates were fairly stable across the models.

Table 7 Cure competing risks model results

	Cure model		Non-myeloma survival		Myeloma survival	
	OR	95% CI	HR	95% CI	HR	95% CI
TT1 (ref)						
TT2−	0.81	(0.36, 1.83)	0.50	(0.39, 0.64)	0.80	(0.58, 1.09)
TT2+	1.32	(0.64, 2.72)	0.35	(0.27, 0.44)	0.78	(0.56, 1.08)
TT3	8.87	(4.66, 16.91)	0.41	(0.33, 0.52)	1.89	(1.21, 2.94)
Age	0.98	(0.95, 1.0)	1.04	(1.03, 1.04)	1.02	(1.01, 1.03)

One main difference between mixture and non-mixture models is parameter interpretation. Mixture models explicitly model separately the probability of being cured and the survival for those not cured, which allows for covariates to have distinct relationships for cured and uncured patients. In contrast, the interpretation of covariates within the non-mixture model is for survival averaged across patients. In this application, the mixture model picked out different trends in the cure and survival functions. The proportion of cured patients has increased continuously from TT1 to TT3, while survival in TT2± and TT3 for those not cured was fairly similar (and better than TT1).

Given the long follow-up available on these patients, if we are interested in the endpoint of overall survival (OS) a competing risks model is needed. Figure 2 summarizes the cumulative incidence of death from myeloma or non-myeloma causes for each of the protocols. Table 6 summarizes univariate results and Table 7 summarizes multivariable results.

In Table 6 the cure proportion is similar among TT1, TT2−, and TT2+ but significantly higher in TT3. Median OS for cured patients is lower among the TT1 patients, but similar in the other three cohorts. Median OS among those not cured is similar among the four cohorts, and significantly shorter than the survival of cured patients. In the multivariable analysis older age is a significant prognostic factor for poor outcomes for all components of the model. TT3 has a higher probability of cure compared to TT1, but worse myeloma-specific survival. Non-myeloma survival is improved in TT2 and TT3 compared to TT1.

8 Concluding Thoughts

Design considerations in the presence of a cured proportion have not been deeply explored as of yet. The competing risks analysis presented suggestions that further methodological development of such models would be useful. Many applications using cure models consider death an event, and the assumption that all patients who died are not cured is likely not be valid in many datasets. Competing risks models will allow more accurate estimates of cure proportions in such cases.

Acknowledgements This work was supported in part by NIH/NCI/NCTN grant CA180819.

References

1. Banerjee S, Carlin BP. Parametric spatial cure rate models for interval-censored time-to-relapse data. Biometrics. 2004;60(1):268–75.
2. Barlogie B, Anaissie E, Van Rhee F, Haessler J, Hollmig K, Pineda-Roman M, Cottler-Fox M, Mohiuddin A, Alsayed Y, Tricot G, et al. Incorporating Bortezomib into upfront treatment for multiple myeloma: early results of total therapy 3. Br J Haematol. 2007;138(2):176–85.
3. Barlogie B, Jagannath S, Vesole DH, Naucke S, Cheson B, Mattox S, Bracy D, Salmon S, Jacobson J, Crowley J, et al. Superiority of tandem autologous transplantation over standard therapy for previously untreated multiple myeloma. Blood. 1997;89(3):789.
4. Barlogie B, Tricot G, Anaissie E, Shaughnessy J, Rasmussen E, van Rhee F, Fassas A, Zangari M, Hollmig K, Pineda-Roman M, Choon L, Talamo G, Thertulien R, Kiwan E, Somashekar K, Fox M, Crowley J. Thalidomide and hematopoietic-cell transplantation for multiple myeloma. N Engl J Med. 2006;354(10):1021–30.
5. Barlogie B, Tricot GJ, Van Rhee F, Angtuaco E, Walker R, Epstein J, Shaughnessy JD, Jagannath S, Bolejack V, Gurley J, Hoering A, Vesole D, Desikan R, Seigel D, Mehta J, Singhai S, Munshi N, Dhodapkar M, Jenkins B, Attal M, Harousseau J, Crowley J. Long-term outcome results of the first tandem autotransplant trial for multiple myeloma. Br J Haematol. 2006;135(2):158–64.
6. Bennett S. Analysis of survival data by the proportional odds model. Stat Med. 1983;2 (2):273–7.
7. Berkson J, Gage R. Survival curve for cancer patients following treatment. J Am Stat Assoc. 1952;47:501–15.
8. Cai C, Wang S, Wenbin L, Zhang J. NPHMC: an R-package for estimating sample size of proportional hazards mixture cure model. Comput Methods Programs Biomed. 2014;113 (1):290–300.
9. Cai C, Zou Y, Peng Y, Zhang J. smcure: an R-package for estimating semiparametric mixture cure models. Comput Methods Programs Biomed. 2012;108(3):1255–60.
10. Chen MH, Ibrahim JG, Sinha D. A new bayesian model for survival data with a surviving fraction. J Am Stat Assoc. 1999;94(447):909–10.
11. Chen MH, Ibrahim JG, Sinha D. Bayesian inference for multivariate survival data with a cure fraction. J Multivar Anal. 2002;80(1):101–26.
12. Corbiere F, Joly P. A SAS macro for parametric and semiparametric mixture cure models. Comput Methods Programs Biomed. 2007;85(2):173–80.
13. Cox DR. Regression models and life-tables (with discussion). J R Stat Soc Ser B (Methodolgical). 1972;34:187–220.
14. Crowley J, Shaghnessy Jr J, Bolejack V, Anaissie E, van Rhee F, Barlogie B. Cure fractions modeled from event-free survival and complete response duration plots in total therapy trials for newly diagnosed multiple myeloma. under review, 2011.
15. Crowther MJ, Lambert P, et al. STGENREG: Stata module to fit general parametric survival models. Statistical Software Components, 2014.
16. Durie BGM. Role of new treatment approaches in defining treatment goals in multiple myeloma-the ultimate goal is extended survival. Cancer Treat Rev. 2010;36:S18–23.
17. Ewell M, Ibrahim JG. The large sample distribution of the weighted log rank statistic under general local alternatives. Lifetime Data Anal. 1997;3(1):5–12.
18. Farewell VT. The use of mixture models for the analysis of survival data with long-term survivors. Biometrics. 1982;38(4):1041–6.
19. Gray RJ, Tsiatis AA. A linear rank test for use when the main interest is in differences in cure rates. Biometrics. 1989;45(3):899–904.

20. Hu T, Xiang L. Efficient estimation for semiparametric cure models with interval-censored data. J Multivar Anal. 2013;121:139–51.
21. Ibrahim JG, Chen MH, Sinha D. Bayesian semiparametric models for survival data with a cure fraction. Biometrics. 2001;57(2):383–8.
22. Kuk AYC, Chen CH. A mixture model combining logistic regression with proportional hazards regression. Biometrika. 1992;79(3):531.
23. Lambert PC. Modeling of the cure fraction in survival studies. Stata J. 2007;7(3):351–75.
24. Lambert PC, Thompson JR, Weston CL, Dickman PW. Estimating and modeling the cure fraction in population-based cancer survival analysis. Biostatistics. 2007;8(3):576.
25. Larson MG, Dinse GE. A mixture model for the regression analysis of competing risks data. Appl Stat. 1985;201–11.
26. Laska EM, Meisner MJ. Nonparametric estimation and testing in a cure model. Biometrics. 1992;48(4):1223–34.
27. Law NJ, Taylor JMG, Sandler H. The joint modeling of a longitudinal disease progression marker and the failure time process in the presence of cure. Biostatistics. 2002;3(4):547.
28. Li C, Taylor J, Sy J. Identifiability of cure models. Stat Probab Lett. 2001;54:389–95.
29. Li CS, Taylor JMG. A semi-parametric accelerated failure time cure model. Stat Med. 2002;21(21):3235–47.
30. Li Y, Tiwari RC, Guha S. Mixture cure survival models with dependent censoring. J R Stat Soc Ser B (Stat Methodol). 2007;69(3):285–306.
31. Liu H, Shen Y. A semiparametric regression cure model for interval-censored data. J Am Stat Assoc. 2009;104(487):1168–78.
32. Lu W, Ying Z. On semiparametric transformation cure models. Biometrika. 2004;91:331–43.
33. Ma S. Cure model with current status data. Statistica Sinica. 2009;19:233–49.
34. Maller RA, Zhou S. Testing for sufficient follow-up and outliers in survival data. J Am Stat Assoc. 1994;89(428).
35. Nair B, van Rhee F, Shaughnessy JD Jr, Anaissie E, Szymonifka J, Hoering A, Alsayed Y, Waheed S, Crowley J, Barlogie B. Superior results of total therapy 3 (2003-33) in gene expression profiling-defined low-risk multiple myeloma confirmed in subsequent trial 2006-66 with VRD maintenance. Blood. 2010;115(21):4168.
36. Othus M, Li Y, Tiwari RC. A class of semiparametric mixture cure survival models with dependent censoring. J Am Stat Assoc. 2009;104(487):1241–50.
37. Pan J, Bao Y, Dai H, Fang H-B. Joint longitudinal and survival-cure models in tumour xenograft experiments. Stat Med. 2014;33(18):3229–40.
38. Peng Y, Dear KBG. A nonparametric mixture model for cure rate estimation. Biometrics. 2000;56(1):237–43.
39. Peng Y, Taylor JMG, Yu B. A marginal regression model for multivariate failure time data with a surviving fraction. Lifetime Data Anal. 2007;13(3):351–69.
40. Sposto R. Cure model analysis in cancer: an application to data from the Children's Cancer Group. Stat Med. 2002;21(2):293–312.
41. Sy JP, Taylor JMG. Estimation in a cox proportional hazards cure model. Biometrics. 2000;56 (1):227–36.
42. Tsodikov A. Semiparametric models: a generalized self-consistency approach. J R Stat Soc Ser B (Stat Methodol). 2003;65(3):759–74.
43. Tsodikov AD, Asselain B, Fourque A, Hoang T, Yakovlev AY. Discrete strategies of cancer post-treatment surveillance. Estimation and optimization problems. Biometrics. 1995;51 (2):437–47.
44. Tsodikov AD, Ibrahim JG, Yakovlev AY. Estimating cure rates from survival data. J Am Stat Assoc. 2003;98(464):1063–78.
45. Wang S, Zhang J, Wenbin L. Sample size calculation for the proportional hazards cure model. Stat Med. 2012;31(29):3959–71.
46. Yin G, Ibrahim JG. A general class of bayesian survival models with zero and nonzero cure fractions. Biometrics. 2005;61(2):403–12.
47. Yin G, Ibrahim JG. Cure rate models: a unified approach. Can J Stat. 2005;33(4):559–70.

48. Yu B, Tiwari RC, Cronin KA, Feuer EJ. Cure fraction estimation from the mixture cure models for grouped survival data. Stat Med. 2004;23(11):1733–47.
49. Yu M, Taylor JMG, Sandler HM. Individual prediction in prostate cancer studies using a joint longitudinal survival-cure model. J Am Stat Assoc. 2008;103(481):178–87.
50. Zeng D, Yin G, Ibrahim JG. Semiparametric transformation models for survival data with a cure fraction. J Am Stat Assoc. 2006;101(474):670–84.

Evaluation of Surrogate Endpoints Using a Meta-Analysis Approach with Individual Patient Data: Summary of a Gastric Cancer Meta-Analysis Project

Koji Oba and Xavier Paoletti

Abstract Statistical methodologies for evaluation of surrogate endpoints have been developed actively since 1989. A meta-analytic approach is frequently applied with data from several randomized controlled trials, and the surrogacy measures are evaluated at the individual level and at the trial level. This approach needs individual patient data for each trial and requires collaborative work with several professionals. In this chapter, we introduce the Global Advanced/Adjuvant Stomach Tumor Research International Collaboration (GASTRIC) project, which is an academic, worldwide project that conducts individual patient data meta-analyses of randomized controlled trials of post-operative adjuvant chemotherapy for resectable gastric cancer or chemotherapy for advanced/recurrent gastric cancer. We describe our statistical method for the evaluation of surrogate endpoints. In particular, we focus on the practical aspects of group establishment, data collection, and data analysis. Finally, future perspectives for the evaluation of surrogate endpoints are discussed.

Keywords Surrogate endpoint · Individual patient data (IPD) · Meta-analysis · Gastric cancer

K. Oba (✉)
Interfaculty Initiative in Information Studies, Graduate School of Interdisciplinary Information Studies & Department of Biostatistics, School of Public Health, Graduate School of Medicine, The University of Tokyo, 7-3-1, Hongo, Bukyo-ku, Tokyo 113-0033, Japan
e-mail: oba@epistat.m.u-tokyo.ac.jp

X. Paoletti
Department of Biostatistics and Epidemiology, Gustave Roussy Cancer Center & INSERM U1018 CESP OncoStat, 114, avenue Edouard Vaillant, 94805 Villejuif Cedex, France
e-mail: xavier.paoletti@gustaveroussy.fr

S. Matsui and J. Crowley (eds.), *Frontiers of Biostatistical Methods and Applications in Clinical Oncology*, DOI 10.1007/978-981-10-0126-0_12

1 Introduction

To determine the effectiveness of oncology drugs, improvement in the overall survival (OS) is the gold standard endpoint (sometimes called a true clinical endpoint) in randomized controlled trials (RCTs) [3]. This endpoint has various advantages, e.g., it is simple to measure, easy to interpret, clinically meaningful, and straightforward to explain. Despite its clinical relevance, this endpoint is limited for assessments of treatment effects, since the cost and length of RCTs compete with the urgency to develop, test, and market effective treatments for life-threatening diseases. In addition, treatment effects may be diluted by additional treatments after progression or relapse when OS is used as a primary endpoint. A potential strategy in these situations is to identify surrogate endpoints that can be measured more cheaply, more conveniently, more frequently, or earlier than the true endpoint of interest [16].

Surrogate endpoints frequently used in oncology trials are disease-free-survival (DFS) in the adjuvant setting (for patients whose tumor can be surgically resected with a curative intent) and progression-free survival (PFS) in the advanced disease setting (for patients whose tumor is locally advanced/metastatic or recurrent and cannot be surgically removed). DFS is defined as the time from randomization to a cancer recurrence, second cancer, or death from any cause, and PFS is defined as the time from randomization to the time of progression or death from any cause. Although DFS and PFS are common primary endpoints of phase III trials, their value as surrogate endpoints for OS has been questioned. In particular, PFS is a controversial endpoint because some new agents have a marked effect on PFS, but no statistically and clinically significant benefit on OS in some tumor types [32].

Appropriate statistical analyses are necessary to evaluate surrogate endpoints in clinical trials. In 1989, Prentice developed a framework for the validation of putative surrogate endpoints [34]. He defined a surrogate endpoint as "a response variable for which a test of the null hypothesis of no relationship to the treatment groups under comparison is also a valid test of the corresponding null hypothesis based on the true endpoint." The operational definition and well-known Prentice's criteria are often very hard to verify in single RCT, and several authors have proposed a meta-analytic approach using data collected from several RCTs [14, 18, 23]. Buyse and Molenberghs [13] introduced the concepts of individual- and trial-level surrogacy for endpoint evaluations in a single-trial setting. Two years later, these two surrogacy measures were successfully extended to the meta-analysis context meta-analysis context [14]. Individual-level surrogacy, R^2_{indiv}, measures the association between the potential surrogate endpoint and the clinical endpoint, adjusting for the effect of treatment across all trials included. Estimating R^2_{indiv} involves jointly modeling the surrogate and clinical endpoints. Trial-level surrogacy, R^2_{trial}, describes how well one can predict the treatment effect on the clinical endpoint in a future trial based on the observed association between the treatment effects on the surrogate and clinical endpoints observed in previous trials. Both R^2_{indiv} and R^2_{trial} are coefficient of determination measures, which take values between zero and one. Values of R^2_{indiv} and R^2_{trial} close to one indicate stronger surrogate endpoints than values near zero. According to some reviews, the meta-analytic approach is the most accepted statistical method to evaluate surrogate endpoints [27].

The meta-analytic approach ideally requires individual patient data (IPD) to derive R^2_{indiv} and R^2_{trial} [10]. However, IPD collection is costly, time-consuming, and requires collaboration. Therefore, it is important to establish efficient and collaborative methods for IPD collection. The GASTRIC (Global Advanced/Adjuvant Stomach Tumor Research International Collaboration) project is an academic, worldwide project that conducts IPD meta-analyses of RCTs of post-operative adjuvant chemotherapy for resectable gastric cancer or chemotherapy for advanced/recurrent gastric cancer [24, 25, 31, 33].

In this chapter, we introduce the GASTRIC project and describe our evaluation of DFS and PFS as surrogate endpoints for OS. In particular, we focus on the practical aspects of group establishment, data collection, and data analysis. Finally, future perspectives for the evaluation of surrogate endpoints are discussed.

2 The GASTRIC Project

The GASTRIC project was initiated in 2006 with the following aims: (1) to determine the usefulness of adjuvant chemotherapy in curatively resected gastric cancer and chemotherapy in advanced/recurrent gastric cancer, (2) to evaluate DFS and PFS as surrogates for OS, and (3) to evaluate the prognostic and predictive value of clinical patient characteristics. As IPD meta-analyses are often conducted retrospectively, i.e., IPD are collected after the publication of eligible RCTs, we set up a steering committee and a secretariat to manage the project. Half of the 13 steering committee members were biostatisticians and the rest were clinical researchers (medical doctors). Secretariats conducted electronic and manual searches to systematically review eligible published trials for the meta-analysis. The search strategy is summarized in the appendix of each publication [24, 25]. Secretariats also negotiated collaborations with researchers who contributed their trials to the meta-analysis after the protocols were approved. Potential collaborators were approached privately by letter or direct contact from a steering committee member to invite collaboration, explain the project, describe what participation entails, and explain how the meta-analysis will be managed and published. If a data center or study group was responsible for the management of the trial data, we contacted the group representative separately. The GASTRIC group applied terms of reference for the creation and operation of a Collaboration as follows (as of October 2016):

1. The Global Advanced/Adjuvant Stomach Tumor Research through International Collaboration is a non-profit organization.

2. The main goal of the Group is to perform meta-analyses of randomized clinical trials based on individual patient data obtained from the principal investigators of all relevant trials. A detailed protocol is written by members of the Group for each meta-analysis.
3. The principal investigators who contribute data to a meta-analysis may become members of the Group. They may request access to the data from all other trials of that meta-analysis. Such access must be approved by the principal investigators of these trials and all publication rules described below must be followed.
4. Data are sent to the Secretariat of the Group where they are kept secure. Data are not shared with anyone under any form without the written approval of the principal investigator.
5. The results of a meta-analysis are shared with the principal investigators who contributed to it, and discussed in a meeting organized by the Group Secretariat prior to presentation at scientific meetings or in publications. This meeting is restricted to the contributors to that meta-analysis. The results of that meta-analysis are not shared with anyone without approval from the principal investigators.
6. After a meta-analysis is reviewed and discussed by all principal investigators, a Writing Committee is formed. The Writing Committee ordinarily consists of the clinicians in charge of the meta-analysis, the statisticians responsible for the analyses, and the principal investigators who wish to contribute to the manuscript. A separate writing committee is formed for each sub-protocol.
7. Publication of the results of a meta-analysis is in the name of the Group. The names of all individuals in the Writing Committee are mentioned in a footnote. The contribution of other investigators is acknowledged in an appendix.
8. All other manuscripts based on data collected for a meta-analysis must be circulated to the principal investigators of all relevant trials for their approval.
9. A principal investigator who has contributed data for a meta-analysis may withdraw at any time and for any reason, and demand that the data from his or her trial be deleted from the manuscript.
10. The interpretation of the results of a meta-analysis is often complex and controversial. Should an investigator disagree with the interpretation of the Writing Committee, his or her opinion shall be mentioned as a minority opinion in the manuscript.

3 Data Collection and Management

Data collection and management were conducted separately in France (in charge of European data) and Japan (in charge of Asian and American data). Secretariats provided the data format needed for each patient with the codes list for simplicity. However, other codes were accepted and the full database for a trial could be provided if this proved to be less time consuming. The secretariat also requested trial information and the original definition of each endpoint (or other variables, if needed) from each collaborator.

After obtaining the IPD, we checked the data for accuracy (consistent with publications or information), plausibility (including checking the distributions of each variable, outliers, and missing data), appropriate randomization, and to ensure they were up-to-date. Stewart and Clarke [38] provided useful guidance, including practical advice on methods for checking and validating data. In particular, diagnostic tools for randomization quality were systematically applied to check whether baseline variables were well balanced between arms and the randomization of the accrued patients were chronologically balanced.

For the surrogate evaluation, the following data were requested for all individual patients included in all trials: center, randomization date, treatment allocated by randomization, date of last follow-up or death, survival status, cause of death (if applicable), relapse status, and type and date of relapse if any. Detailed information on the type of relapse was not always available.

4 Statistical Analysis

4.1 Statistical Methods for Evaluation of Surrogate Endpoints

Forest plots were used to display the hazard ratios (HRs) for overall and individual trials, and these HRs were used to evaluate DFS and PFS as surrogates for OS (true) and for external validation trials. HRs were estimated through the Weibull proportional hazard model, which gave acceptable goodness-of-fit in this setting.

Burzykowski et al. [8] proposed a two-stage approach for the evaluation of surrogate endpoints. First, the treatment effects on the surrogate and on the true endpoints were jointly estimated and the association at the individual level was quantified. Then, association at the trial level was obtained through the regression of the treatment effect of the surrogate endpoint on the treatment effect of the true endpoint adjusting for the treatment effects uncertainty. We used Spearman's rank correlation coefficients to assess the surrogate at the individual level and the coefficient of determination between the natural logarithm of the HRs to assess the surrogate indicators at the trial level [12, 14]. At the individual level, the association between the distribution of the true endpoint and the surrogate was evaluated using a bivariate model based on the Plackett copula combined with trial-specific Weibull models for surrogates and the true endpoint [8, 9]. The association between estimates of treatment effects obtained using the bivariate model was used to assess surrogacy at the trial level. A good surrogate was considered to provide a reliable prediction of the treatment effect on the true endpoint (e.g., the HR for OS) based on the treatment effect on the surrogate (e.g., the HR for DFS). It should be noted that HR estimates based on the bivariate model might differ from the crude estimates shown in the forest plot.

In detail, let T_{ij} and S_{ij} be random variables denoting the true and surrogate endpoints for the *j*th subject in the *i*th trial, respectively, and let Z_{ij} be the indicator variable for treatment. At the first stage, two correlated failure-time random variables were modeled using the copula function and the joint survival function of (S_{ij}; T_{ij}) was as follows:

$$F(s,t) = \Pr\left(S_{ij} \geq s, T_{ij} \geq t\right) = C_\theta\left\{F_{Sij}(s), F_{Tij}(t)\right\}$$

where F_{Sij} and F_{Tij} denote marginal survivor functions and C_θ is a copula, i.e., a distribution function on $[0; 1]^2$ with $\theta \in R^1$. Following Burzykowski et al. [9], we used Weibull proportional hazards models to determine the effect of treatment on the marginal distributions of S_{ij} and T_{ij} within the *i*th trial:

$$F_{Sij}(s) = \exp\left\{-\int_0^s \lambda_{Si}(x)\exp\left(\alpha_i Z_{ij}\right)dx\right\},$$

$$F_{Tij}(t) = \exp\left\{-\int_0^t \lambda_{Ti}(x)\exp\left(\beta_i Z_{ij}\right)dx\right\}$$

Here, $\lambda_{Si}(x)$ and $\lambda_{Ti}(x)$ are baseline hazard functions, and α_i and β_i are, respectively, the natural logarithm of the HRs of treatment Z_{ij} on the surrogate and true endpoints for trial *i*. The association parameter θ in the copula function is generally hard to interpret, but there is a link with Spearman ρ when the Plackett copula,

$$C_\theta(u,v) = \frac{1 + (u+v)(\theta-1) + \sqrt{\{1+(u+v)(\theta-1)\}^2 + 4\theta(\theta-1)uv}}{2(\theta-1)}$$

is chosen [22]:

$$\rho = 12 \iint_{I^2} C_\theta(u,v)\,du\,dv - 3$$

When the hazard functions are specified, the parameters for the joint model can be estimated using maximum likelihood. We chose to specify the marginal hazard functions for each trial parametrically using the Weibull distribution.

At the second stage, we considered a random effects model for the trial-specific treatment effects given by

$$\begin{pmatrix}\alpha_i\\ \beta_i\end{pmatrix} = \begin{pmatrix}\alpha\\ \beta\end{pmatrix} + \begin{pmatrix}a_i\\ b_i\end{pmatrix}$$

where the random effects on the right-hand side of the above equation are assumed to be normally distributed with mean zero and the following covariance matrix:

$$D = \begin{pmatrix} d_{aa} & d_{ab} \\ & d_{bb} \end{pmatrix}$$

Since α_i and β_i are estimated with estimation errors in each trial, we assume the following model for the estimated treatment effects $\hat{\alpha}_i$ and $\hat{\beta}_i$:

$$\begin{pmatrix} \hat{\alpha}_i \\ \hat{\beta}_i \end{pmatrix} = \begin{pmatrix} \alpha_i \\ \beta_i \end{pmatrix} + \begin{pmatrix} \varepsilon_{ai} \\ \varepsilon_{bi} \end{pmatrix}$$

Here, the trial-specific estimation errors ε_{ai} and ε_{bi} are assumed to be jointly normally distributed with mean zero and the following trial-specific covariance:

$$\Omega_i = \begin{pmatrix} \sigma_{aa,i} & \sigma_{ab,i} \\ & \sigma_{bb,i} \end{pmatrix}.$$

For the model parameters to be estimable, we assumed that the covariance matrices Ω_i are known and equal to their estimates obtained from the first-stage copula model. An adjusted estimate of trial-level surrogacy is given by the following:

$$\text{adjusted } R^2_{trial} = \frac{d^2_{ab}}{d^2_{aa} d^2_{bb}}$$

4.2 *Surrogate Threshold Effect*

Using a linear regression model adjusted for estimation error in the observed treatment effects, we calculated the surrogate threshold effect (STE), defined as the minimum treatment effect on a surrogate (i.e., DFS or PFS) necessary to predict a non-zero effect on the true endpoint (i.e., OS) [6] in a trial of infinite size. A future trial would require the upper limit of the confidence interval for the estimated hazard ratio for the surrogate endpoint to fall below the STE in order to predict a non-zero effect on the true endpoint.

4.3 *External Validation*

To assess the external validity of our results, we set several validation studies for the adjuvant setting and advanced setting. In the adjuvant setting, we used 4 trials for which we did not receive IPD from the principal investigators and one large-scale RCT for which only an interim analysis was available at the time of the surrogate analysis. In the advanced setting, 12 RCTs were considered validation studies. We extracted HRs for DFS or PFS and HRs for OS from the summary statistics in the published paper if we did not have IPD.

4.4 Software

All analyses were performed on an intention-to-treat basis. Two-sided 95% confidence intervals (CI) were calculated. All analyses were performed using SAS software, except for the graphical displays (double forest plots were plotted using a set of R functions developed at the International Drug Development Institute [IDDI] and other figures were prepared using STATA). Software implementations for the methods described in this paper are available at http://ibiostat.be/onlineresources/onlineresources/surrogate or in the supporting information in Buyse et al. [15].

5 Results

5.1 DFS and OS in the Adjuvant Setting

A meta-analysis of trials for patients with resected gastric cancer was used to evaluate DFS as a surrogate for OS. Data were available for 3288 patients from 14 training trials and 3281 patients from 6 validation trials with documented OS and DFS [31].

At the individual level, a Plackett copula was fitted to model the joint distribution of DFS and OS. The individual level association, quantified by the Spearman's rank correlation coefficient, was equal to 0.974 (95% CI [0.971, 0.976]), indicating a very tight correlation between DFS and OS for a given patient. At the trial level, there was also a tight association between the treatment effects on DFS and on OS (Fig. 1). Without adjustment for the estimation error in treatment effects, R^2_{trial} was 0.964 (95% CI [0.926, 1.000]). After adjusting for the estimation error, adjusted R^2_{trial} was approximately 1 (95% CI [0.999, 1.000]). It is worth noting that because the estimated R^2_{trial} value was very close to the upper limit of 1, the numerical results need to be interpreted with caution.

The linear regression model adjusted for estimation errors was $\ln(HR_{OS}) = 0.047 + 1.239 \times \ln(HR_{DFS})$. The 95% prediction limits indicate the range of effects on OS that can be expected for a given effect on DFS. The STE was 0.92; hence, in a future trial using similar treatment modalities as those in the set of trials in the meta-analysis, a HR_{DFS} of <0.92 would predict a HR_{OS} of <1. This quantifies the attenuation of the treatment effect when switching from DFS to OS.

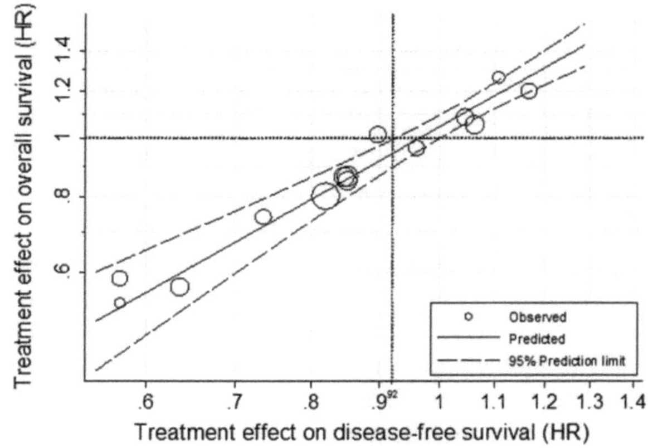

Fig. 1 Trial-level association between treatment effects on DFS and OS in resectable gastric cancer. Each trial is represented by a *bubble* whose size is proportional to the trial sample size

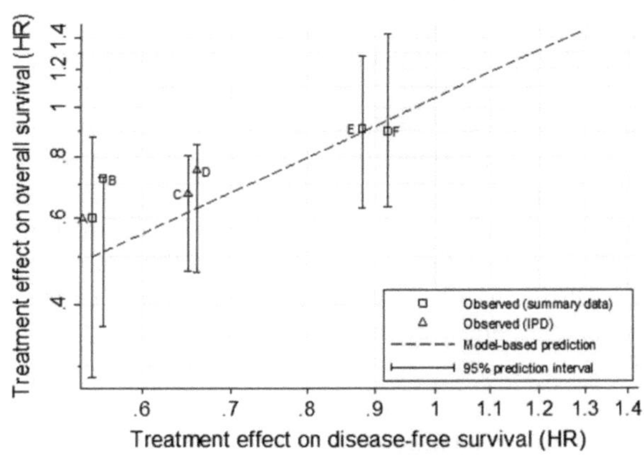

Fig. 2 Observed treatment effect on disease-free survival versus predicted treatment effect on overall survival in validation trials. The regression line, the observed treatment effects on survival (HR_{OS}) in six trials, and the treatment effects on survival predicted from the treatment effects on the surrogate (HR_{DFS}), along with their 95% prediction intervals are shown

The results of our surrogate evaluation could be externally validated using six trials not included in the meta-analysis. As shown in Fig. 2, there was excellent agreement between the observed treatment effects on survival (HR_{OS}) in these 6 trials and the treatment effects on survival predicted from the treatment effects on the surrogate (HR_{DFS}). In the three trials for which the prediction limits of HR_{OS} excluded one, the observed effects on survival actually reached statistical significance $P < 0.05$.

5.2 *PFS and OS in the Advanced Setting*

The meta-analysis of trials in advanced disease was used for the purpose of evaluating PFS as a surrogate for OS. Data were available for 4069 patients from 20 eligible randomized trials with documented OS and PFS [33]. As in the adjuvant setting, 12 RCTs were considered as validation trials.

The individual level association, quantified by Spearman's rank correlation coefficient, was 0.853 (95% CI [0.852, 0.854]), indicating a substantial correlation between PFS and OS for a given patient. At the trial level, the associations between the treatment effects on PFS and on OS were only moderate. Adjusted R^2_{trial} was 0.61 (95% CI [0.04, 1.00]). The large confidence intervals reflect the uncertainty around this estimate, due in part to the small sample sizes of some of the trials included in the meta-analysis. The linear regression model adjusted for estimation errors was $\ln(HR_{OS}) = 0.042 + 0.779 \times \ln(HR_{PFS})$ (Fig. 3).

The moderate correlation at the trial level is reflected by a STE equal to 0.56; hence, in a future trial using similar treatment modalities as those in the set of trials in the meta-analysis, a HR_{PFS} of <0.56 would predict a HR_{OS} of <1.

The results of our surrogate evaluation could be externally validated using 12 trials not included in the meta-analysis and treatment effects extracted from reports published after the conclusion of the meta-analysis. Figure 4 shows regression line, the observed treatment effects on survival HR_{OS}, and the treatment effects on survival predicted from the treatment effects on the surrogate HR_{PFS} in these trials, along with their 95% prediction intervals. As shown in Fig. 4, the prediction intervals of the regression of the observed treatment effects on survival HR_{OS} on the treatment effects on survival predicted from the treatment effects on the surrogate HR_{PFS} are wide and include one (i.e., no treatment effect on OS) in all trials, indicating that the observed effects on PFS do not enable the prediction of an effect on OS in any of these 12 trials. However, 3 of the 12 trials showed a statistically significant effect of treatment on survival [33].

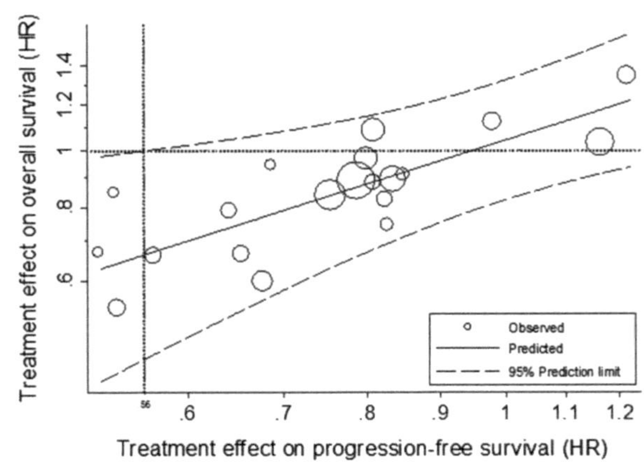

Fig. 3 Trial-level association between treatment effects on PFS and OS in advanced/recurrent gastric cancer. The regression line and the treatment effects in the 20 trials included in the analysis are shown. Each trial is represented by a bubble whose size is proportional to the trial sample size. The 95% prediction limits indicate the range of effects on OS that can be expected for a given effect on PFS

Fig. 4 Observed treatment effect on progression-free survival versus predicted treatment effect on overall survival in validation trials. The regression line, the observed treatment effects on survival HR_{OS}, and the treatment effects on survival predicted from the treatment effects on the surrogate HR_{PFS} in these trials, along with their 95% prediction intervals are shown

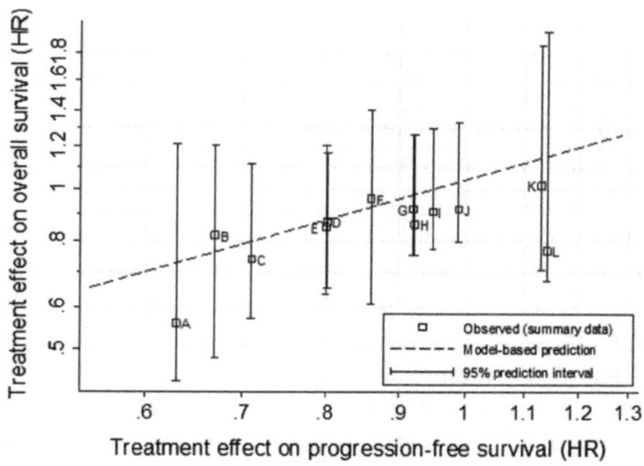

6 Discussion

The analyses summarized in Sect. 5.1 suggest that DFS is a good surrogate for OS in patients with resectable gastric cancer. These findings parallel previous results for resectable colon cancer as well as operable or locally advanced head and neck and lung cancers [28, 29, 36]. Taken together, these findings suggest that in early forms of cancer that are amenable to local treatment, DFS can be used as a reliable surrogate for OS. In contrast, the analyses described in Sect. 5.2 suggest that PFS is not a useful surrogate for OS in advanced/recurrent gastric cancer. PFS is also a poor surrogate for OS in advanced breast cancer [7, 30]. In contrast, PFS is a good surrogate in advanced ovarian cancer [9]. PFS appears to be a good surrogate for OS in advanced colorectal cancer treated with fluoropyrimidines [11], but not with more recent therapies [37]. All in all, PFS tends to be a poor surrogate for OS in advanced solid tumors.

Other validation criteria for surrogate endpoints have been proposed. Alonso and Molenberghs [2] addressed the issue that different settings lead to different measures at the individual level using an information theoretic approach. In our example, this approach yields similar conclusions to those of the copula-based meta-analysis approach [15]. Frangakis and Rubin [21] initiated a different approach for surrogate evaluation based on causal inference. They introduced so-called principal stratification to analyze data from a single trial. Drawing from the causality literature, Taylor et al. [41] suggested the use of the concepts of direct/indirect effects for surrogacy evaluation. Recently, Alonso et al. [1] revealed an interesting relationship between the causal-inference and meta-analysis approaches for the validation of surrogate endpoints. In particular, it is well known that the evaluation of survival endpoints becomes very difficult when survival post-progression is long owing to effective second-line treatments (e.g., median survival post-progression of longer than 12 months) [5]. Since the causal inference framework can be used effectively to assess the influence of second-line treatment in an RCT in comparison with the counterfactual model, these methodologies may overcome limitations of the meta-analysis approach for surrogate evaluation in the future [42] although the number of hypotheses necessary to fit causal inference models make this approach very delicate to apply in practice.

Published meta-analyses of IPD are increasing. Riley et al. [35] reported that only 57 articles were published before 2000, after which there was a considerable rise, with an average of 49 articles published per year between 2005 and 2009. We believe this growth will increase substantially in the era of data-sharing initiatives [4, 17, 20, 26, 39, 40]. IPD meta-analyses have benefited from improved data quality, increased analysis types, and advantages in achieving consensus around results and interpretation by international collaborations. However, these analyses have barriers related to resources and expertise, negotiating collaborations, data availability, and a lack of standardization with respect to variable estimation and data collection. Ideally, for prospective IPD meta-analyses, prospective collaborations with research groups establishing potentially eligible RCTs before these trials start (or before the results are disclosed) is preferable, as in the Early Breast Cancer Trialists' Collaborative Group (EBCTCG) [19].

The GASTRIC collaboration is now in its 2nd round. The aim of this project is again to investigate surrogate endpoints of PFS against OS using recent trials as well as to investigate new statistical methodologies for surrogate evaluations. We believe this kind of collaborative work between clinicians and statisticians will produce firm results and lead to breakthroughs in the medical scientific community.

References

1. Alonso A, Van der Elst W, Molenberghs G, Buyse M, Burzykowski T, et al. On the relationship between the causal-inference and meta-analytic paradigms for the validation of surrogate endpoints. Biometrics. 2015;71:15–24.
2. Alonso A, Molenberghs G. Surrogate marker evaluation from an information theory perspective. Biometrics. 2007;63:180–6.
3. Biomarkers Definitions Working Group. Biomarkers and surrogate endpoints: preferred definitions and conceptual framework. Clin Pharmacol Ther. 2001;69:89–95.
4. Bonini S, Eichler H-G, Wathion N, Rasi G. Transparency and the European Medicines Agency—sharing of clinical trial data. New Engl J Med. 2014;371:2450–2.
5. Broglio KR, Berry DA. Detecting an overall survival benefit that is derived from progression-free survival. J Natl Cancer Inst. 2009;101:1642–9.
6. Burzykowski T, Buyse M. Surrogate threshold effect: an alternative measure for meta-analytic surrogate endpoint validation. Pharm Stat. 2006;5:173–86.
7. Burzykowski T, Buyse M, Piccart-Gebhart MJ, Sledge G, Carmichael J, Lu H, et al. Evaluation of tumor response, disease control, progression-free survival, and time to progression as potential surrogate end points in metastatic breast cancer. J Clin Oncol. 2008;26:1987–92.
8. Burzykowski T, Molenberghs G, Buyse M. The evaluation of surrogate endpoints. New York: Springer; 2006.

9. Burzykowski T, Molenberghs G, Buyse M, Geys H, Renard D. Validation of surrogate end points in multiple randomized clinical trials with failure time end points. J R Stat Soc C. 2001;50:405–22.
10. Buyse M. Contributions of meta-analyses based on individual patient data to therapeutic progress in colorectal cancer. Int J Clin Oncol. 2009;14:95–101.
11. Buyse M, Burzykowski T, Carroll K, Michiels S, Sargent DJ, Miller LL, et al. Progression-free survival is a surrogate for survival in advanced colorectal cancer. J Clin Oncol. 2007;25:5218–24.
12. Buyse M, Burzykowski T, Michiels S, Carroll K. Individual- and trial-level surrogacy in colorectal cancer. Stat Methods Med Res. 2008;17:467–75.
13. Buyse M, Molenberghs G. Criteria for the validation of surrogate endpoints in randomized experiments. Biometrics. 1998;54:1014–2109.
14. Buyse M, Molenberghs G, Burzykowski T, Renard D, Geys H. The validation of surrogate endpoints in meta-analyses of randomized experiments. Biostatistics. 2000;1:49–67.
15. Buyse M, Molenberghs G, Paoletti X, Oba K, Alonso A, Van der Elst W, et al. Statistical evaluation of surrogate endpoints with examples from cancer clinical trials. Biometrical J. 2016;58:104–32.
16. Buyse M, Sargent DJ, Grothey A, Matheson A, de Gramont A. Biomarkers and surrogate end points–the challenge of statistical validation. Nat Rev Clin Oncol. 2010;7:309–17.
17. Committee on Strategies for Responsible Sharing of Clinical Trial Data. Discussion framework for clinical trial data sharing: guiding principles, elements, and activities. In: Institute of Medicine of the National Academies, editor. The Washington, DC: National Academies Press; 2014.
18. Daniels MJ, Hughes MD. Meta-analysis for the evaluation of potential surrogate markers. Stat Med. 1997;16:1965–82.
19. Darby S, Davies C, McGale P. The early breast cancer trialists' collaborative group: a brief history of results to date. In: Davison A, Dodge Y, Wermuth N, editors. Oxford: Oxford University Press; 2005.
20. Drazen JM. Sharing individual patient data from clinical trials. New Engl J Med. 2015;372:201–2.
21. Frangakis CE, Rubin DB. Principal stratification in causal inference. Biometrics. 2002;58:21–9.
22. Fredricks GA, Nelsen RB. On the relationship between Spearman's rho and Kendall's tau for pairs of continuous random variables. J Stat Plan Infer. 2007;137:2143–50.
23. Gail MH, Pfeiffer R, Van Houwelingen HC, Carroll RJ. On meta-analytic assessment of surrogate outcomes. Biostatistics. 2000;1:231–46.
24. GASTRIC (Global Advanced/Adjuvant Stomach Tumor Research International Collaboration) Group, Oba K, Paoletti X, Bang Y-J, Bleiberg H, Burzykowski T, et al. Role of chemotherapy for advanced/recurrent gastric cancer: an individual-patient-data meta-analysis. Eur J Cancer. 2013;49:1565–77.
25. GASTRIC (Global Advanced/Adjuvant Stomach Tumor Research International Collaboration) Group, Paoletti X, Oba K, Burzykowski T, Michiels S, Ohashi Y, et al. Benefit of adjuvant chemotherapy for resectable gastric cancer: a meta-analysis. JAMA. 2010;303:1729–3717.
26. Krumholz HM, Peterson ED. Editorial: open access to clinical trials data. JAMA. 2014;312:11–2.
27. Lassere MN. The Biomarker-Surrogacy Evaluation Schema: a review of the biomarker-surrogate literature and a proposal for a criterion-based, quantitative, multidimensional hierarchical levels of evidence schema for evaluating the status of biomarkers as surrogate endpoints. Stat Methods Med Res. 2008;17:303–40.
28. Mauguen A, Pignon J-P, Burdett S, Domerg C, Fisher D, Paulus R, et al. Surrogate endpoints for overall survival in chemotherapy and radiotherapy trials in operable and locally advanced lung cancer: a re-analysis of meta-analyses of individual patients' data. Lancet Oncol. 2013;14:619–26.

29. Michiels S, Le Maitre A, Buyse M, Burzykowski T, Maillard E, Bogaerts J, et al. Surrogate endpoints for overall survival in locally advanced head and neck cancer: meta-analyses of individual patient data. Lancet Oncol. 2009;10:341–50.
30. Michiels S, Pugliano L, Marguet S, Grun D, Barinoff J, et al. Progression-free survival as surrogate endpoint for overall survival in clinical trials of HER2-targeted agents in HER2-positive metastatic breast cancer. Ann Oncol. 2016;27:1029–34.
31. Oba K, Paoletti X, Alberts S, Bang Y-J, Benedetti J, Bleiberg H, et al. Disease-free survival as a surrogate for overall survival in adjuvant trials of gastric cancer: a meta-analysis. J Natl Cancer Inst. 2013;105:1600–7.
32. Ocaña A, Amir E, Vera F, Eisenhauer EA, Tannock IF. Addition of bevacizumab to chemotherapy for treatment of solid tumors: similar results but different conclusions. J Clin Oncol. 2011;29:254–6.
33. Paoletti X, Oba K, Bang Y, Bleiberg H, Boku N, Bouché O, et al. Progression-free survival as a surrogate for overall survival in advanced/recurrent gastric cancer trials: a meta-analysis. J Natl Cancer Inst. 2013; 1–4.
34. Prentice RL. Surrogate endpoints in clinical trials: definition and operational criteria. Stat Med. 1989;8:431–40.
35. Riley RD, Lambert PC, Abo-zaid G. Meta-analysis of individual participant data: rationale, conduct, and reporting. BMJ. 2010;340:c221.
36. Sargent DJ, Wieand HS, Haller DG, Gray R, Benedetti JK, Buyse M, et al. Disease-free survival versus overall survival as a primary end point for adjuvant colon cancer studies: individual patient data from 20,898 patients on 18 randomized trials. J Clin Oncol. 2005;23:8664–70.
37. Shi Q, de Gramont A, Grothey A, Zalcberg J, Chibaudel B, Schmoll H-J, et al. Individual patient data analysis of progression-free survival versus overall survival as a first-line end point for metastatic colorectal cancer in modern randomized trials: findings from the analysis and research in cancers of the digestive system databa. J Clin Oncol. 2015;33:22–8.
38. Stewart LA, Clarke MJ. Practical methodology of meta-analyses (overviews) using updated individual patient data. Cochrane Working Group. Stat Med. 1995;14:2057–79.
39. Stewart LA, Clarke M, Rovers M, Riley RD, Simmonds M, Stewart G, et al. Preferred reporting items for a systematic review and meta-analysis of individual participant data. JAMA. 2015;313:1657.
40. Taichman DB, Backus J, Baethge C, Bauchner H, de Leeuw PW, Drazen JM, et al. Sharing clinical trial data: a proposal from the International Committee of Medical Journal Editors. PLOS Med. 2016;13:e1001950.
41. Taylor JMG, Wang Y, Thiébaut R. Counterfactual links to the proportion of treatment effect explained by a surrogate marker. Biometrics. 2005;61:1102–11.
42. Vanderweele TJ, Tchetgen Tchetgen EJ. Mediation analysis with time varying exposures and mediators. J R Stat Soc B. 2016 (in press).

Machine Learning Techniques in Cancer Prognostic Modeling and Performance Assessment

Yiyi Chen and Jess A. Millar

Abstract Prognostic models for disease occurrence, tumor progression and survival are abundant for most types of cancers. Physicians and cancer patients are utilizing these models to make informed treatment decisions and corresponding arrangements. However, not all cancer prognostic models are built and validated rigorously. Some are more useful and reliable than others. In this chapter, we briefly introduce some popular machine learning methods for constructing cancer prognostic models, and discuss pros and cons of each. We also introduce the commonly used discrimination and calibration metrics for assessing predictive performance and validating the prognostic models. In the end, we outline several challenges of using prognostic models in the real world for clinical decision-making support, and propose related suggestions.

Keywords Machine learning · Prognostic model · Cancer prediction · Validation

1 Introduction

Cancer prognoses are important to facilitate early cancer diagnosis, risk assessment of future events, and clinical treatment decision-making. As a consequence, prognostic models for disease occurrence, progression and survival are abundant for nearly all type of cancers [18, 31, 42, 59, 70, 79]. An accurate prediction of risks for cancer outcomes is critical for physicians and patients to make informed decisions

Y. Chen (✉)
OHSU-PSU School of Public Health, Knight Cancer Institute,
Oregon Health & Science University, Portland, OR 97239, USA
e-mail: chenyiy@ohsu.edu

J.A. Millar
Fariborz Maseeh Department of Mathematics and Statistics,
Portland State University, Portland, OR 97006, USA
e-mail: jess.annai.millar@gmail.com

S. Matsui and J. Crowley (eds.), *Frontiers of Biostatistical Methods and Applications in Clinical Oncology*, DOI 10.1007/978-981-10-0126-0_13

on next steps. Governments and health-care departments also rely on cancer prognostic models in planning and allocating health-care resources.

A typical cancer prognostic model will predict the risk of future clinical outcomes at defined time points based on certain demographic, clinical and/or genetic factors. Only factors correlated with the clinical outcome of interest should be included in the model. These factors are called prognostic factors or risk factors, the information of which is available before the clinical endpoint of interest is observed. For example, the Prostate-Specific Antigen (PSA) and the Gleason score are known as important risk factors for prostate cancer occurrence, recurrence, and overall survival [33, 53].

Before we discuss how to construct, evaluate, and validate a cancer prognostic model, let us first clarify what the term "prognostic model" means in this chapter. Prognostic models make forecast of clinical endpoints in certain quantitative ways, and are thus often used interchangeably with the term "predictive models" by many researchers. We want to point out that prognostic models and predictive models are not the same in the medical world. While both are used for predictions, or forecasts, each has a different focus in the medical literature due to distinct definitions of prognostic biomarkers and predictive biomarkers. In oncology, prognostic biomarkers forecast the natural course and outcomes of cancer diseases, while predictive biomarkers forecast the likelihood of cancer patients responding to particular therapies [16]. As a consequence, prognostic models are often used to identify subjects most likely to experience serious clinical outcomes (e.g., shorter overall survival), while predictive models are more useful in identifying subgroups of patients most likely to benefit from certain treatments. There is no clear separation of prognostic biomarkers and predictive biomarkers. In fact, quite a few biomarkers are identified as both predictive and prognostic factors, such as the estrogen receptors and HER2/neu overexpression in breast cancer. Similarly, there is no clear separation of prognostic models and predictive models. Regardless, we want the readers to note that the prognostic models discussed in this chapter are for future outcome forecasts under *standard of care*. We omit the discussion of study design and data acquisition in this chapter because they are not as critical for prognostic models compared to predictive models.

The top-ranked endpoints of interest for cancer prognoses are cancer incidence [44, 64], recurrence [1, 40] and cancer survivability including overall survival [59], progression free survival, and chance of survival for given length of time period (e.g., 2-year survival, 5-year survival, see for example, [18, 54]). Since many factors influence clinical outcomes of cancer patients, it is challenging to build cancer prognostic models. In Sect. 2, we will introduce several popular machine learning methods used in constructing a cancer prognostic model. While different methods tackle the problem from different directions, all follow the same rule of principle: the final prognostic model should be simple enough to be generalized. A relatively parsimonious model has less chance of overfitting, is less likely to suffer from missing data problems, and is easier to be validated. For example, the breast cancer prognostic model developed by Delen et al. [18] and Lundin et al. [54], the prognostic model for stage III non-small cell lung cancer patients developed by Oberije et al. [59], the prognostic lung cancer model by Sesen et al. [70], the individualized conditional survival prognostic tool for rectal cancer by Wang et al. [79], the conditional survival prognostic model for pancreatic cancer by Katz et al. [42], and the prognostic model for metastatic cancer patients attending a palliative radiotherapy clinic by Chow et al. [14] all had a limited number of risk factors.

While plenty of prognostic models have been developed and published, they vary a lot in performances: some show more promising forecast ability than others. They also vary a lot in the targeted patient population: some are very specific while others are quite general. Not all published prognostic models are appropriately validated, and there is a lack of well accepted criteria in establishing when a prognostic model can be reliably applied to certain patient populations, and when more than one prognostic model exists, how to choose among them. Generally speaking, prognostic models developed and validated using large multi-institutional or national databases are more reliable than those built upon a single institutional database of limited size. However, if there is something unique about a single institution, and it is of specific interest to predict clinical outcomes for patients in the institution, then using single-institutional data to build and validate a prognostic model makes great sense.

Many online interactive tools are available for cancer survivability prediction for different patient populations. For example, an interactive web-based risk prediction model for prostate cancer developed by Ankerst and the team can be found in http://deb.uthscsa.edu/URORiskCalc/Pages/calcs.jsp [4]. The risk factors included in the model are: race, age, PSA level, family history, digital rectal examination and prior prostate biopsy. Once all necessary information are entered, the program will compute the risk of having a high-grade, a low-grade prostate cancer, or a negative result in next biopsy.

Another web-based nomogram about prostate cancer can be found in http://labs.fccc.edu/nomograms/main.php?nav=4&audience=1. While these online tools are informative if used cautiously, we discourage cancer patients from using publically accessible prognostic tools for survivorship estimation because patients often lack clinical and statistical knowledge to appropriately interpret the prognosis outcome.

Prognostic models can be quite helpful for clinicians if they pay close attention to the predictive quality and validity of the prognostic models before using them to support clinical decision-making. Traditionally, clinicians rely more on personal judgment in forecasting the potential clinical outcome of patients. Glare [27] showed physicians' personal judgment may not be as reliable as many people expect. They reported poor agreement between the physicians' clinical prediction of survival and the actual survival for terminally ill cancer patients based on a meta-analysis of 1563 subjects. They found that physicians tend to overestimate the duration of survival for advanced cancer patients. Clinical decisions based on poor prognostication may result in serious consequences such as overtreatment or undertreatment, unnecessary large medical expenses, and inadequate access to palliative care [15]. To obtain a more objective and reliable estimates on patients' survival, we suggest to use only validated prognostic models with good performance in both the training and validation data sets. Models with promising statistical metrics of predictive performance in the training set are not guaranteed to have good performance in the validation data set because good performance in the training set can be achieved by overfitting to the noise only.

A useful prognostic model should be developed using a database of decent sample size and a reasonable number of clinically relevant potential risk factors without serious missing information. The model should be tested on an independent sample, and should make sense to physicians. More importantly, it should be compared with other existing prognostic models in the field, and be shown to out-perform others for comparable or better prognostic accuracy.

In Sect. 2, we will introduce some useful tools to identify and combine multiple prognostic factors for forecasting the risk of future clinical outcomes in individual patients. Some of the tools are static and only utilize the available clinical and demographic information at baseline to predict the clinical outcomes, while others are dynamic and take into consideration the potential actions along the way before outcomes become available. In Sect. 3, we will discuss statistical metrics for evaluating the performance of a prognostic model before validation. Section 4 discusses several options of validating a cancer prognostic model. The chapter will conclude with a discussion of the challenges of adopting a prognostic model for clinical decision-making, and make several suggestions.

2 Machine Learning Methods for Cancer Prognostic Models

Machine learning (ML) is a branch of artificial intelligence (AI). It combines the fields of statistics, mathematics and computer science, and is used to discover hidden patterns and correlations among covariates and endpoints. While many ML methods are available for building cancer prognostic models, some are more frequently used than others. The methods we discuss in this section are those widely used in cancer prognostic modeling.

Quite a few studies are devoted to comparing multiple ML techniques for their performances using one or two selected databases. While interesting and illustrative, the findings are often technique-dependent and data-dependent. There is no ML method that consistently outperforms others. For example, Delen et al. compared decision trees (DT), artificial neural networks (ANN) and logistic regression methods in constructing a prognostic model for breast cancer survival based on over 200,000 cases from a large cancer incidence database of the Surveillance, Epidemiology, and End Results (SEER) program [18]. A similar data set was further used by Bellaachia and Guven to compare DT, Naïve Bayes (NB), and ANNs for predicting breast cancer survivability [5]. Both studies found that the DT method outperforms the other two. However, in another breast cancer study, Ahmad et al. [2] showed that the support vector machine (SVM) outperformed DT and ANN in predicting breast cancer recurrence using 1189 records from Iranian Center for Breast Cancer.

Each ML method that is used widely in practice has its own strengths and weaknesses. Although it is interesting to find out which method tends to perform better under which circumstances, this chapter does not intend to make comparisons among the methods or to make suggestions on which one to use. In most situations, the performance of a prognostic model depends more on the available database and the quality of information than on the method that is used to construct the model. With a high quality database, most ML methods will yield descent prognostic models with comparable performances.

2.1 *Logistic Regression*

Logistic regression is one of the most widely used statistical techniques for data analysis in oncology. It has also gained much popularity as a tool in the machine learning methodology. The endpoint to be predicted in the logistic regression model has to be a categorical variable (e.g., binary, ordinal or multinomial), while the prognostic factors can be of any type: binary, ordinal, multinomial or continuous. In oncology, most prognostic logistic regression models are built to predict binary endpoints.

Logistic regression is so named because it uses the logistic function to connect prognostic factors and the outcome to be predicted. The connection is sometimes also called logit link.

The standard logistic function

$$f(x) = \frac{1}{1 + e^{-x}}$$

is an S-shaped curve that is bounded by 0 and 1. Therefore, it can be used to model the probability of having an event for any particular subject. The x in the function can be viewed as a linear function of all risk factors. For example, if the prognostic model contains two risk factors: age (a continuous variable) and gender (a binary variable), then x could be $x = \beta_0 + \beta_1 * age + \beta_2 * gender$, where β_0 is the intercept term and (β_1, β_2) are the coefficients for age and gender, respectively. A major task of the logistic regression modeling is to estimate β_0, β_1, and β_2, which are learned from the training set.

While the functional form of x is linear, the logistic regression model allows more flexibility than it appears at first look. For example, instead of using age in the original scale, the model allows us to use $\ln(age)$, or $\sqrt{age}$, or age^2, if those terms fit better with the data. It also allows the same risk factor to appear multiple times in different scales. For example, the functional form of x can be $x = \beta_0 + \beta_1 * age + \beta_2 * age^2 + \beta_3 * gender$.

The logistic regression model is very transparent and easy to interpret. Unlike some other ML techniques in which the construction of the prognostic model is like a "black box", the variables selection and model building steps are very clear in logistic regression. The final functional form of the fitted logistic regression model allows researchers and physicians to evaluate the controlled influence of each covariate. In addition, the logistic function used in the model allows an easy interpretation of the effect of covariates through the odds ratio, a well-understood statistical index representing the odds of having an event for subjects with given exposures, compared with the odds of having an event for subjects without the exposures, assuming subjects are all the same for other prognostic factors.

The logistic regression model is only suitable when the endpoint of interest is a categorical variable. It cannot be used to model other popular endpoints in oncology studies: the time to a certain event (e.g., overall survival, progression free survival). For survival endpoints the most often used statistical model is the Cox regression model, also known as the proportional hazards regression model.

Although Cox regression in itself is not considered a part of the general family of ML techniques, elements of it are used to extend ML methods for survival endpoints. For this reason, we briefly go over its general use for time-to-event data here.

As with the logistic regression model, the Cox model also provides the estimated controlled effect of the prognostic factors on the endpoint. Unlike the logistic regression model, there is no link function that explicitly connects the time-to-event outcome and the prognostic factors for Cox regression. Rather, baseline hazard has to be estimated before a forecast in survival time can be made. However, if we only want to estimate the effect of risk factors on survival outcomes, computing the baseline hazard is not required, because the Cox regression model makes an important assumption of proportional hazards. The proportional hazard assumption assumes two subjects with and without exposure to certain prognostic factors should have hazard functions that are proportional over time, given all other prognostic factors are the same for the subjects. The influence of the prognostic factors on the risk of an event happening at time t for subjects with and without exposure to certain prognostic factors is expressed using the hazard ratio, which has similar interpretation as the odds ratio computed in logistic regression. To date, Cox regression is still the most often used technique in building a prognostic model for cancer studies with time-to-event endpoints.

2.2 Tree-Based Methods

The regression tree method was initially introduced in 1960s for continuous endpoints [58]. It was later extended to classification trees for categorical endpoints [41]. Tree-based methods have gained great popularity in cancer prognostic model building because simple tree-based methods are often more intuitive and easier to interpret for physicians and patients than regression models. In addition, if the outcome variable is categorical, tree-based methods provide direct prediction of classification for new subjects, while a logistic regression model only provides estimated probabilities requiring a cutoff value before classification.

Regression/Classification trees are effective tools to present complex prognostic models to laymen [17]. A complex prognostic model often has a large number of risk factors in varying scales, and two-way or three-way interaction components. While a linear regression model or a logistic regression model can provide estimated mean/probability of having an event based on a complex model, the influence of covariates and the structure of the prognostic models are not apparent. For example, for a prognostic model with multiple interaction terms, it will be difficult to tease out the influence of each covariate to the endpoint. This is because the whole covariate space is partitioned into multiple sub-spaces through the interaction terms. Such partitioning can be easily and naturally presented in a tree-based format because recursive partitioning is the exact approach taken by tree-based methods in building a prognostic model.

A simple tree-based method grows a tree from the root node, which represents the whole covariate space (Fig. 1). In the beginning, the root node is the parent node that can be split into two daughter nodes based on certain criteria (often based on a cutoff value of a continuous or ordinal prognostic factor, or a Yes/No separation of a binary prognostic factor). Each daughter node can be treated as parent node for the next level and can then be split to form its own daughter nodes. A node without daughter nodes is considered a terminal node, sometimes also referred to as a leaf of the tree. Each leaf represents a unit resulting from the partition, and subjects in the same leaf have the same predicted outcome values. The process of recursive partitioning can be repeated until all nodes became leaves. Therefore, a tree-based prognostic model centers around creating mutually exclusive and exhaustive sub-spaces from the whole covariate space for meaningful predictions. By recursively partitioning the covariate space into rectangular sets and then fitting a simple model within each partition to the response [45, 51], tree-based methods adopt a flexible nonparametric procedure in fitting a prognostic model, and thus are less restricted by the distributional assumptions of most regression models. In addition, a prognostic factor can be used multiple times in a tree, and different cutoff values of a single prognostic factor can be used at different nodes for splitting.

Different tree-based methods use different criteria to determine how to best split the parent nodes into daughter nodes. In general, the search of splitting criteria is "greedy", in that it only maximizes the split for the current step and may not be the best overall in the full model. There are also various methods to determine when to

Fig. 1 Classification tree

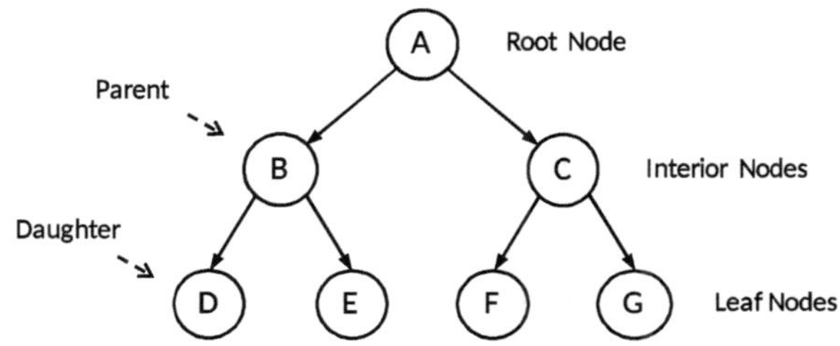

stop growing a tree, or to prune the tree once grown. This is a very important step to reduce the chance of overfitting for the prognostic model.

In this subsection, we introduce two important tree-based methods that are used in oncology: classification trees for categorical endpoints and regression trees for time-to-event endpoints. Both methods share the characteristic of binary partitions at each node; however their splitting criteria are based on different functions.

For regression trees with continuous endpoints, splits are chosen to minimize the residual sum of squares, i.e. the "deviance" between the observed and the predicted outcomes. In survival trees this was often accomplished through a log-rank statistic, which is used to compare two survival curves [10]. A popular criterion proposed by LeBlanc and Crowley uses the first step of a full likelihood estimation procedure and allows hazard functions to be unknown [47]. This criterion can be implemented using R package 'rpart'.

In classification trees there are a number of broadly used methods. Similar to residual sum of squares in regression, minimizing the misclassification rate is sometimes used as a splitting criterion. While intuitive and easy to implement, it is not sensitive to changes in node probabilities and so not often ideal for complicated trees. The most common methods use the Gini Index and Information Gain, both based on data variance within nodes. Lower variance of a node indicates its "node purity": how strongly it is dominated by a single type of observation. The Gini Index chooses a split where the resulting daughter nodes will contain the higher number of a single type of observation as possible. This creates the effects of weighted partitions, where larger and purer nodes are selected for. This option exists in many programs, with one of the more popular being the 'tree' package in R. Information Gain is slightly different in that it measures the change in homogeneity of a node due to a split compared to the parent node. This method tends to result in a large number of small, pure partitions. This is useful for new exploration of data, but trees may be overly complex. The 'party' package in R can be used for this kind of splitting. For each of these splitting criteria, smaller values indicate the variable contributes greatly to the homogeneity of the nodes.

Once a tree is grown, it is important to check whether it is too complex and overfits the training data. Instead of creating stricter splitting criteria that could potentially miss important splits if stopped too soon, a large tree is created and then pruned back into a smaller sub tree. A separate pruning criterion is required to be set, many of which involve a misclassification cost. Reduced error pruning is very simple and starts at the leaves of the tree, removing nodes and replacing them with their dominant observations. If no significant change is seen in prediction accuracy, the node is not added back. Cost-Complexity pruning is another option which has the added benefit of including a penalty parameter that controls the tradeoff between tree complexity and overall misclassification. Even with the use of pruning, single trees still have lower predictive power than many other methods discussed in this chapter. What makes the tree-based method attractive in real-world application is the improved performance in prediction once many trees are grown and "ensembled" together.

Ensemble methods in machine learning involve building a collection of classifiers (in this case, trees) and averaging them to create a new classifier. These types of classifiers are often similar in bias, but have lower variance as the number of classifiers increases. There are many algorithms that are used to accomplish this averaging, which can be characterized as either non-adaptive (bagging, random forest) or adaptive (boosting). In non-adaptive methods, each tree is built independently. One of the simpler ways of accomplishing this is through bootstrap aggregation, or bagging. In bagging, we take repeated samples from our original training data and grow trees for each of the bootstrapped sample sets. In the case of regression trees, all of the predictions are averaged to obtain an overall prediction. In classification trees, class predictions are counted and decided by a voting scheme, usually majority vote. It should be noted that none of the trees are pruned, so each has high variance, but low bias. Since averaging the trees reduces variance, the final classifier has both lower variance and bias than a single tree method.

One of the downsides of bagging that is inherited from the underlying tree building method is that the trees are still biased towards strong predictors. If one prediction variable in our set is particularly strong, most of the trees produced will use that variable for the top split, resulting in most of the trees looking very similar and will be highly correlated. To uncorrelate trees and further reduce the variance of our classifier, we can use a more general method called random forest. Random forest is very similar to bagging in that it also builds a set of decision trees from bootstrapped training sets. The main difference is that in the process of building a tree, at each split only a random subset of predictors are considered as candidates. In classification based random forests, the size of this subset is chosen to be approximately the square root of the total predictors in the dataset. For regression trees, this subset is often set to a third of the total predictors. Bagging can be viewed as a special case of random forest in which the predictor subset was set equal to the original predictors. Overfitting is of less a concern with these ensemble tree-based methods. However, we want to make sure enough bootstrapped samples are created to grow trees. Cross validations methods are sometimes used to choose an optimal number of bootstrapped trees. Using errorest in the R package ipred, testing error can be calculated and will level off after an optimal amount of trees has been reached.

Using bagging and random forest techniques, accuracy of prediction is greatly improved by lowering variance and bias. This gain is unfortunately at the expense of losing an easy interpretation of the tree structure. To aid in interpreting these models, there are several measures to gage the overall importance of our predictors. In regression trees, total reduction of residual sum of squares is measured for each predictor due to their split in a model and averaged over all trees. Those with larger residual sums of squares have greater influence over the model. For regression trees, there are two general measures used. The first is the overall mean decrease in the accuracy of our model if a variable is excluded. The other is the mean decrease in Gini Index. The Gini Index measures the variance across all our input variables. Smaller values for a node indicate its "node purity", how strongly it is dominated by a single type of observation. A larger decrease indicates the variable contributes greatly to the homogeneity of the nodes in our final model. With each of these measures, a list of predictors with relative levels of importance can be obtained, allowing for some general interpretation of the prognostic model in addition to prediction. All of these procedures can be found in the R package ‘randomForest’.

In 2008, Ishwaran introduced the idea of using random forests to model survival data [39]. This has now become one of the most common used tree-based methods in oncology prognostic modeling for survival endpoints. This random survival forest (RSF) approach was compared with both the Cox regression and the binary classification random forests, and was found to have the lowest prediction error of all three approaches. RSF was also found to be stable in the presence of noise variables, while the other methods were progressively affected as more were added to the model. Bou-Hamad et al., using a data set of 312 patients with primary biliary cirrhosis of the liver, also found RSF to have an advantage over bagging and Cox regression, which were similar to each other [10]. Yosefian et al. used the same approach on 607 acute myocardial infarction (AMI) patients. Comparing saturated survival trees, pruned survival trees, and RSF, RSF was found to be the most reliable, with the advantage of also giving the most comparable results when different datasets were used [81].

A different ensemble method mentioned before is the adaptive model averaging, the most commonly used being boosting. Instead of simply averaging many trees together, boosting involves a weighted average of successively grown trees. It is an iterative procedure, where each new tree is fit to the current model’s residuals, instead of outcome prediction, and a new tree model is created with updated residuals. Schapire and Freund created a very illustrative graph to represent the process (Fig. 2; [66]). In boosting, the data points misclassified in the previous model are given a higher weight in the next step, making it more likely to classify these points correctly. This type of model learns from the data slowly, which helps to handle the issue of overfitting that can occur from fitting single decision trees. A shrinkage parameter can be used to control how slowly the model learns from the data. The common choice of shrinkage parameter ranges from 0.1 to 0.001. The smaller the value, the more slowly the model will learn. This parameter is closely tied to the number of trees chosen to build, with smaller shrinkage parameters requiring more trees to obtain good prediction accuracy. Overfitting a boosting model is unlikely but still can occur with a large numbers of trees, as each of the boosting trees are built upon previous trees. One other parameter that needs to be specified in boosting is depth, the number of splits each tree can have. This will affect the overall complexity of the model. A depth of one involves only one variable in each tree.

Just as with random forest, boosting sacrifices a tree visual for increased accuracy. There are several alternative interpretation strategies, with one common relative importance measure found in the ‘gbm’ R package. It’s based on how often a predictor is selected for splitting and then weighted by the squared improvement to the model resulting from a split, all of which are averaged over all trees [22]. These are scaled to sum to 100, with higher values having larger relative influence. The glm package also offers the ability to graph partial dependence plots for the most

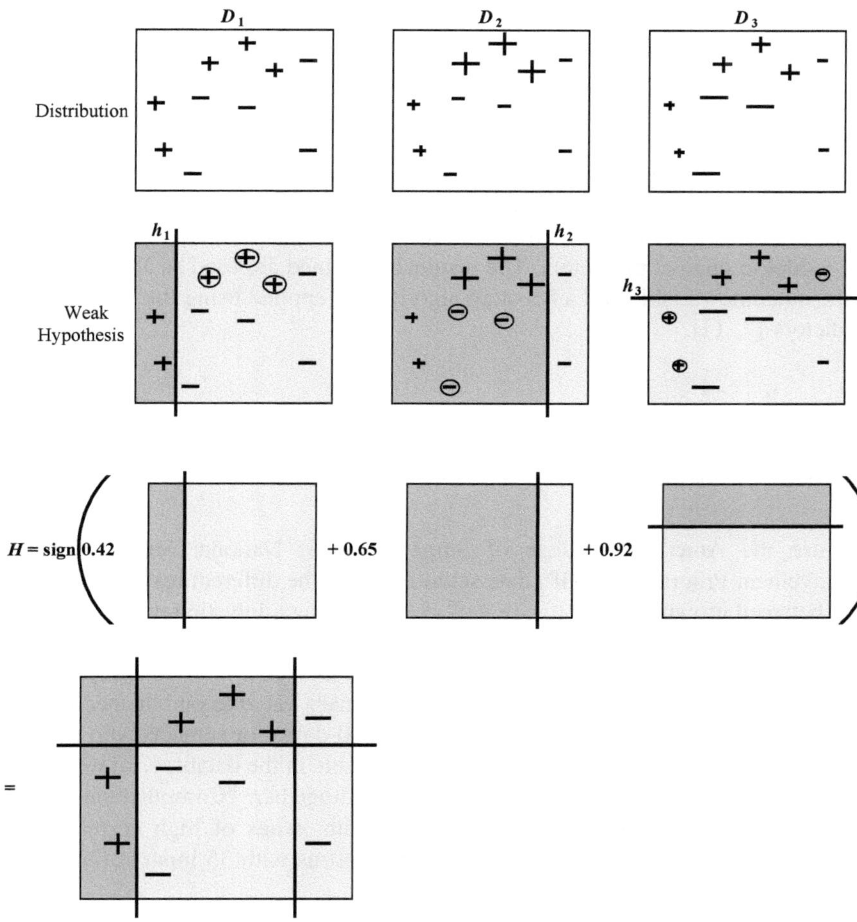

Fig. 2 Algorithm of Adaboost. In the figure, a weak hypothesis fits a decision boundary on the data set. The residuals from this model are obtained and the data points are weighted, more weight given to misclassified data points. Another decision boundary is fit on the weighted residuals of the previous model, and new residuals are calculated. Each of these are combined together to create a final decision boundary

influential variables. These show the marginal effects of a variable on the outcome after integrating out the effects of other predictors. They can be a particularly useful to aid in interpreting the underlying relationships of single predictors within the model.

Since adaptive boosting as an ensemble classifier was introduced two decades ago [21], it has been found to be useful to analyze many variables simultaneously, specifically high dimensional omics data. These include classification and survival studies on SNPS, genome wide association studies [48], gene markers [19], and cancer proteomics [26]. This approach also has been found to work well for high-dimensional, heterogeneous medical data, specifically for sample sizes less that 2500 [62]. For very large sample sizes, large predictor variable sets can have the drawback of overfitting the training set. Several papers have proposed cutting down the datasets ahead of time to correct this issue. One often used is stability selection, which involves resampling predictor variables and choosing those selected often among subsamples [37, 55]. Another proposed method of handling this involves utilizing both low dimensional clinical predictors and high dimensional omics data. Using survival based breast cancer data, Bin et al. first fit a linear cox model to clinical predictors. The residuals obtained are used as an initial offset to the outcome variable and a boosting algorithm is applied using the omics data as predictors [7, 11].

3 Illustrative Example for Logistic Regression and Classification Trees

We use the American College of Surgeon (ACS) National Surgical Quality Improvement Program (NSQIP) data set to illustrate the different results that can be seen between growing a classification model and fitting a logistic regression model. The NSQIP collects data on risk factors, operation variables, complications, and mortality outcomes of major surgical procedures. Our goal is to construct a prognostic model that will predict complications (a binary variable on whether subjects experienced a complication after surgery within 30 days) for subjects who received urology surgery. This variable is not readily available in the database, so we created it based on the following variables in Table 1. Altogether, "Complications" had a 12% occurrence rate. We removed variables with issues of high correlation or where over 5% to the data was missing, which left us with 35 input variables and 38,368 data points (Table 2).

We begin by fitting a simple classification tree to the dataset. With this particular dataset, a model with only 2 input variables was chosen (Fig. 3). Our top split is WORKRVU, which is used as a proxy for surgery complication, with values below 33.275 predicted to not have complications from the surgery. For subjects with WORKRVUs over 33.275, they are further split by what year the patient had their surgery. It is predicted that patients will have complications in 2009 and after, but not before. This is likely due to the sparsity of data collected before 2009. We can look at this closer by plotting these variables and examining the partitions assigned by the classification tree (Fig. 4). It is worth noting that general classification trees use a greedy algorithm which only maximizing at current step. For WORKRVUs over 33.275, there are far fewer data points, many of which appear to be patients with complications. There also appear to be fewer data point before 2009, which is likely why the second split was chosen here. This is a good example of how large datasets data taken over time can have an effect on the spread of the variables themselves. Our test error comes out pretty good at 12.26%, however out false

Table 1 Variables used to create "complications" outcome variable

Variable description	Variable name
Superficial Surgical Site Infection	SUPINFEC
Deep Incisional SSI	WNDINFD
Organ Space SSI	ORGSPCSSI
Wound Disrupt	DEHIS
Pneumonia	OUPNEUMO
Unplanned Intubation	REINTUB
Pulmonary Embolism	PULEMBOL
Ventilator > 48 h	FAILWEAN
Functional Health Pre-Surgery	RENAINSF
Acute Renal Failure	OPRENAFL
Urinary Tract Infection	URNINFEC
CVA/Stroke with Neurological Deficit	CNSCVA
Coma > 24 h	CNSCOMA
Peripheral Nerve Injury	NEURODEF
Cardiac Arrest Requiring CPR	CDARREST
Myocardial Infarction	CDMI
Bleeding Transfusions	OTHBLEED
Graft/Prosthesis/FF	OTHGRAFL
DVT/Thrombophlebitis	OTHDVT
Sepsis	OTHSYSEP
Septic Shock	OTHSESHOCK

negative rates comes out at 87.28%. This would in general not be a very good model to predict with.

Next, we take a look at a bagging model for the data. Compared to the single-tree method, bagging showed an improved overall prediction, with a test error rate of 10.80% and a better false negative rate of 71.13%. As other tree assembling methods, we lost tree visual using bagging. We can however look at two measures to gage the importance of our variables. The first is the overall mean decrease in the predictive accuracy if a variable is excluded (Fig. 5a). The other is the mean decrease in Gini Index (Fig. 5b). Looking at these variables, we can see that WORKRVU appears to be the most influential, with OPTIME as the second most. There are a few other variables, but their influence drops off quickly after the first five variables.

In random forests, we take the same approach as bagging, but at each split we take a random sample of the variables and are only allowed to use those as candidates. Right from the start, we can see the model is not as good as the bagging model, with a test error rate of 11.41% and a false negative rate of 79.35%. This may be due to the small number of influencing variables and their lesser ability to sway in random forest. Looking at our influential variables, OPTIME has switched with WORKRVU, but much of the rest look the same (Fig. 6).

Table 2 NSQIP prediction variables

Variable description	Variable name
Work Value Units	WORKRVU
Operation Time	OPTIME
Return to OR	RETURNOR_NUM
Days from Admin to Surgery	HTOODAY
ASA Physical Status Classification	ASACLAS_NUM
Transfusion 72 h Pre-Surgery	TRANSFUS_NUM
Admission Year	ADMYR
Age	AGE
Functional Health Pre-Surgery	FNSTATUS2_NUM
Weight	WEIGHT
Wound Classification	WNDCLAS_NUM
Weight Loss 60 Days Pre-Surgery	WTLOSS_NUM
Height	HEIGHT
Acute Renal Failure	RENAFAIL_NUM
Ventilator 48 h Pre-Surgery	VENTILAT_NUM
Transfer Status	TRANSIT_NUM
Inpatient/Outpatient	INOUT_NUM
Open Wound	WNDINF_NUM
Ascites 30 Days Pre-Surgery	ASCITES_NUM
Steroid Use for Chronic Condition	STEROID_NUM
Dyspnea	DYSPNEA_NUM
Bleeding Disorder	BLEEDDIS_NUM
History of CHF 30 Days Pre-Surgery	HXCHF_NUM
Anesthesia Technique	ANESTHES_NUM
History of Severe COPD	HXCOPD_NUM
Sepsis – SIRS	PRSEPIS_SIRS
Emergency Case	EMERGNCY_NUM
Dialysis	DIALYSIS_NUM
History of Hypertension Requiring Rx	HYPERMED_NUM
Sepsis Shock	PRSEPIS_SHOCK
Smoker	SMOKE_NUM
Admission Quarter	ADMQTR
Disseminated Cancer	DISCANCR_NUM
Sepsis	PRSEPIS_SEP
Sex	SEX_NUM

We then fit a boosting model to our data. In boosting, we need to choose shrinkage and depth parameters, which can be done through cross validation. At a smaller shrinkage value, we start to see a gradual improvement in using a depth of 3. Unlike random forests, by using too many trees we risk overfitting in boosting. We can use a shrinkage factor of 0.01 and depth of 3 (Fig. 7). For the boosting

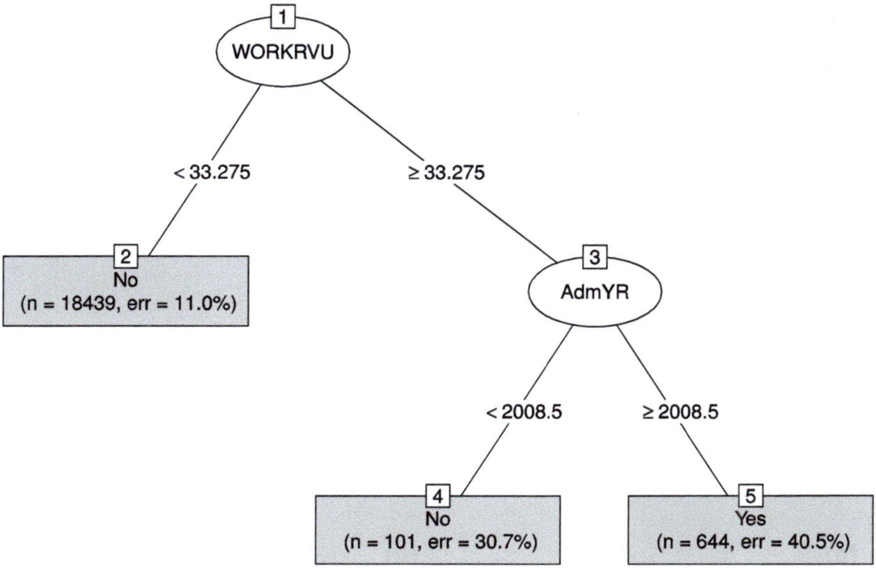

Fig. 3 Classification tree of NASQIP data set

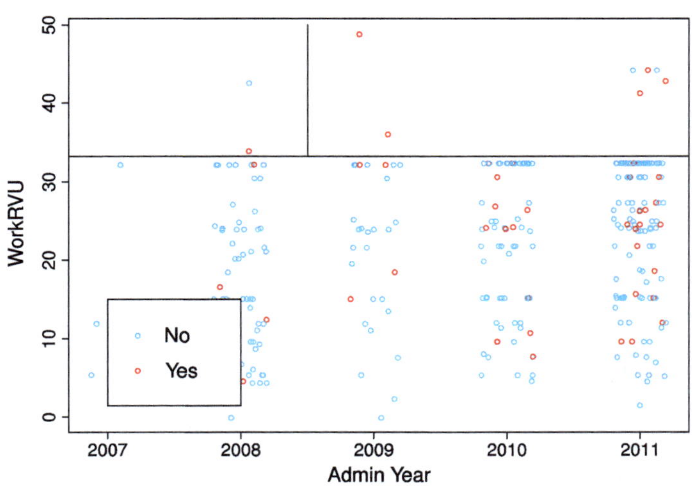

Fig. 4 Scatterplot of WORKRVU versus ADMYR data. Overlaying lies represent cutoff points chosen in classification tree

model we end up with a test error rate of 11.20% and a false negative rate of 76.29%, only slightly better than random forest. Just as before, we have lost our tree visual, but have several options to gage the importance of variables in our model. The first is a list of the relative influence of each of the variables in the model.

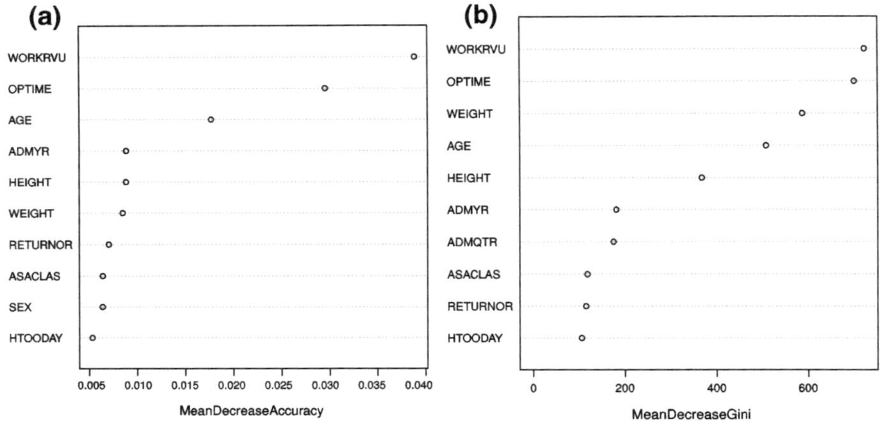

Fig. 5 Bagging influential variables based on **a** mean decreased accuracy and **b** mean decrease of Gini Index

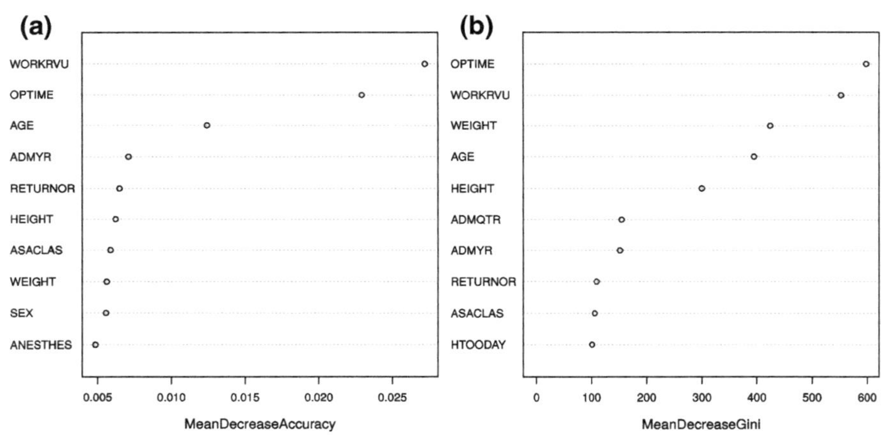

Fig. 6 Random forrest influential variables based on **a** mean decreased accuracy and **b** mean decrease of Gini Index

We can also get partial dependence plots for the most influential variables. These showcase the marginal effects of a variable on the outcome after removing the effects of other variables. In this model, WORKRVU and OPTIME are our most influential variables (Fig. 8). Both of these variables appear to have complex relationships with the complication, but in general increase at varying rates along with the probability of a complication occurring, until hitting a point of saturation.

To compare these models with a more traditional approach, we also fit a logistic regression model using Purposeful Selection (Table 3). In this model several original variables were discarded, AGE, WORKRVU, and OPTIME were transformed into splines, and seven interaction terms were included. In this model we

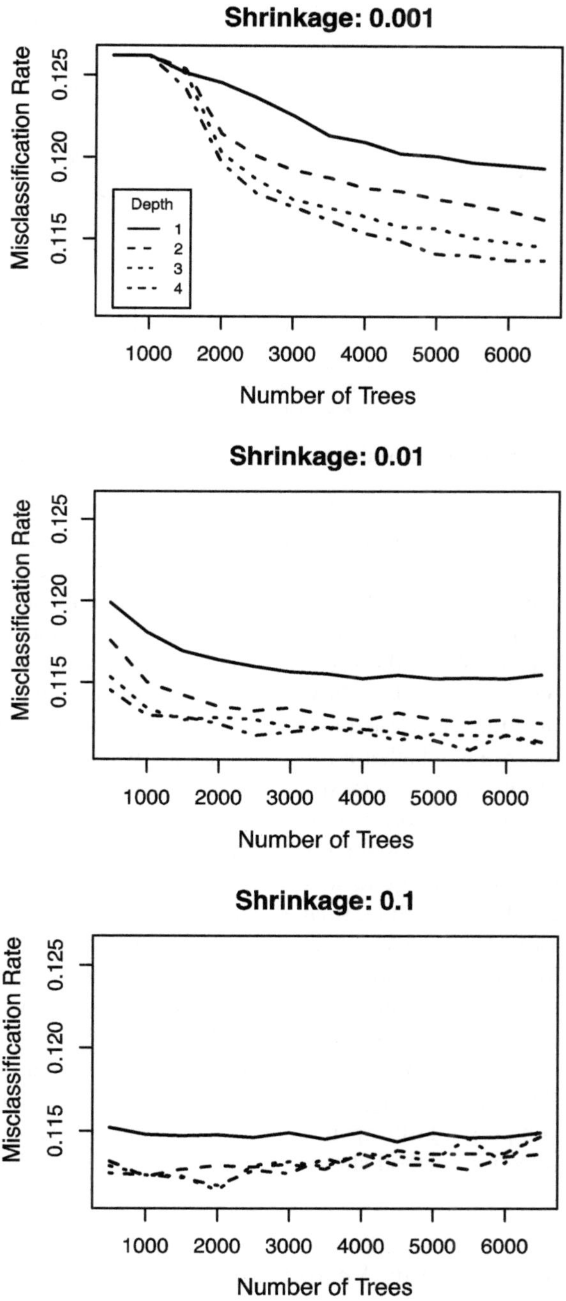

Fig. 7 Effect on test error rate over different shrinkage rates as number of trees increases

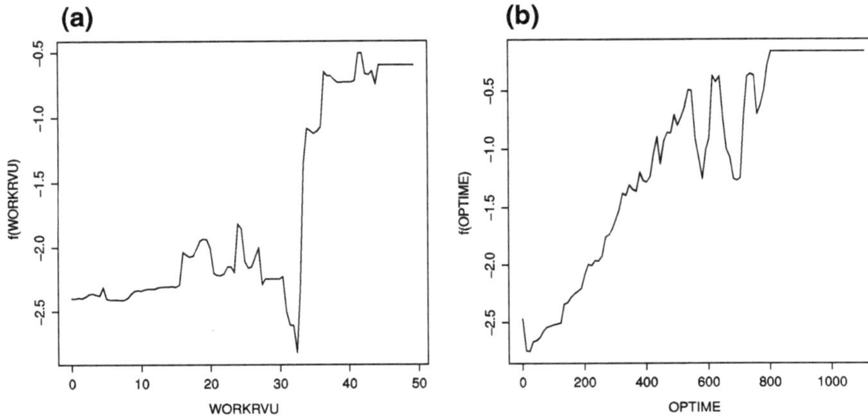

Fig. 8 Boosting partial dependence plots of **a** WORKRVU and **b** OPTIME

had a test error rate of 11.48%, false positive rate of 1.65%, and a false negative rate of 79.78%. This is not much different from our other models and highlights that the data source is the most critical factor to determine whether a good prognostic model can be achieved. It is interesting to note that the area under the ROC curve (AUC) for the logistic regression model is 0.7755, and that for the boosting model is 0.7863. We will discuss the AUC in more detail in later sections, but want to point out here that AUC above 0.7 or 0.75 is often seen as acceptable predictive power in literature. It warned us that we should not rely on one or two single parameters to determine whether a prognostic model is a good one. The high false negative rates of our models suggest the model may not be clinically useful.

One last note is that the logistic regression model is quite complex compared with the tree-based method. It contains far more risk factors compared to tree-based method with quite a few interaction terms. With comparable performance, the tree-based method, such as bagging, is more preferred as it only requires a few key variables to make predictions. The chance of overfitting is also higher for the logistic regression model due to the complexity. Then why does the logistic regression model contain so many terms? We believe it is because of the relatively large sample size of our database since the variable selected by the logistic regression model is determined by the statistical significance of the risk factors. This example suggests that we should be more cautions in getting an unnecessary complex logistic regression model when sample size is large. A different variable selection method should be implemented for databases with large sample size.

3.1 Support Vector Machines

SVM is another ML method that has gained extensive applications in cancer prognosis since its introduction in 1992 [8]. It has been used for classification,

Table 3 Logistic regression model output

Variable	Coeff.	Std. err.	χ^2	p	95% CI	
					LB	UB
ADMQTR0	0.130	0.049	6.963	0.009	0.034	0.225
ADMYRp1	269.995	21.400	159.179	<0.001	228.052	311.938
AGE						
AGE0	−2.394	0.853	7.886	0.005	−4.065	−0.723
AGE65	0.341	0.044	60.029	<0.001	0.255	0.427
ANESTHES_NUM	0.442	0.153	8.344	0.004	0.142	0.741
ASACLAS						
ASACLAS_3	0.314	0.054	33.697	<0.001	0.208	0.419
ASACLAS_4	0.716	0.107	44.845	<0.001	0.507	0.926
ASACLAS_5	2.077	1.264	2.699	0.101	−0.401	4.554
DYSPNEA_NUM	0.552	0.115	23.347	<0.001	0.328	0.776
EMERGNCY_NUM	0.427	0.146	8.605	0.004	0.142	0.712
FNSTATUS						
FNSTATUS_1	0.327	0.123	7.064	0.008	0.086	0.568
FNSTATUS_2	0.887	0.236	14.142	<0.001	0.425	1.350
HTOODAYp1	0.392	0.050	62.741	<0.001	0.295	0.489
INOUT_NUM	−1.294	0.537	5.807	0.016	−2.346	−0.242
OPTIME						
OPTIME0	1.272	0.144	78.449	<0.001	0.991	1.554
OPTIME240	0.055	0.007	74.549	<0.001	0.043	0.067
OPTIME480	0.002	0.002	1.500	0.221	−0.001	0.004
RETURNOR_NUM	−1.040	0.824	1.593	0.207	−2.654	0.575
TRANSFUS_NUM	1.280	0.191	45.268	<0.001	0.907	1.652
VENTILAT_NUM	2.293	0.850	7.284	0.007	0.628	3.958
WNDCLASS						
WNDCLAS_3	0.565	0.150	14.230	<0.001	0.272	0.858
WNDCLAS_4	0.727	0.171	18.147	<0.001	0.393	1.062
WORKRVU						
WORKRVU0	0.131	0.049	7.137	0.008	0.035	0.226
WORKRVU32p1	0.553	0.062	79.633	<0.001	0.432	0.674
WORKRVU32p2	0.416	0.030	200.832	<0.001	0.359	0.474
WORKRVU37	0.028	0.046	0.357	0.551	−0.062	0.117
WTLOSS_NUM	0.759	0.151	25.273	<0.001	0.463	1.055
AGE0xRETURNOR	3.078	1.302	5.591	0.019	0.527	5.629
AGE65xDYSPENEA_NUM	−0.2974	0.1036	8.2427	0.0041	−0.501	−0.095
ANESTHESxOPTIME0	−0.8104	0.1445	31.4647	<0.0001	−1.094	−0.528
INOUTxAGE0	2.6480	0.8848	8.9562	0.0028	0.914	4.383
WORKRVU0xRETURNOR	0.5259	0.1165	20.3843	<0.0001	0.298	0.755
WORKRVU37xOPTIME240	−0.0046	0.0022	4.4462	0.0350	−0.009	−0.001

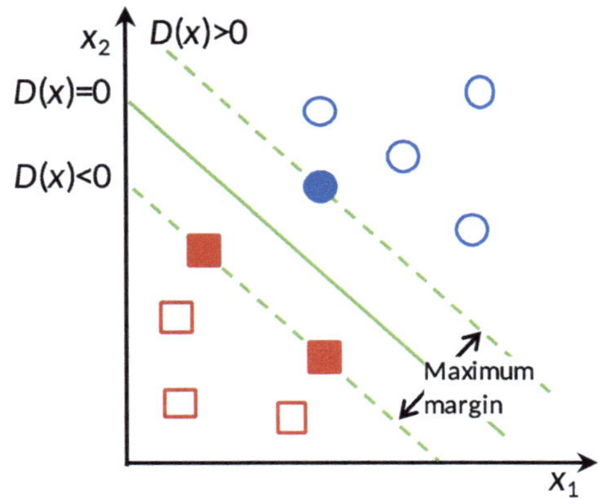

Fig. 9 Support vector machine

pattern recognition and gene separation [6, 23, 32, 50, 74]. It was first introduced as a tool of classification that maximizes the margin between the training samples and the decision boundary through a linear combination of supporting patterns. We now illustrate the idea of SVM using a simplest linear SVM with only two-dimensions (Fig. 9). In the SVM, we aim to find a decision boundary (the solid green line in the middle) which best separates the two groups, represented by the blue circles and the red squares in Fig. 9. Instead of using all samples, the SVM identifies the "support vector", which is a small subset of the training samples that are closest to the decision boundary. In Fig. 9, the support vectors are represented by the solid blue circles and the red squares.

The decision boundary is when $D(x) = 0$, which is so determined that margins are maximized on either size. $D(x)$ is the decision function:

$$D(x) = wx + b$$

where w is the weight of the support vectors and b is the bias.

Since its introduction, the SVM has been quickly extended to using a "kernel method" to allow a non-linear mapping of supporting patterns into a feature space of higher dimensionality, and then identifying the hyperplane that best separates the data into different classes. A detailed explanation on how the support vector machines work can be found in Burges [12] and Vapnik [78].

To construct an SVM, we need to determine the capacity parameter, the kernel type and its corresponding parameters. The capacity parameter, often denoted by C, is a regularization of parameters that determines the tradeoff between maximizing the margin and minimizing the classification error. Instead of minimizing the errors on the training data, the SVM uses the structural risk minimization (SRM) principle to minimize the upperbound on the expected risk. Therefore, it has more generalizability compared to ANN methods (see Sect. 3.3 below) that minimize the errors of the training data. This was partially confirmed by a study conducted by Liu et al. [50], which compared the SVM with ANN using a dataset of 683 Breast Cancer samples. The authors randomly divided the data set into two subsets: a training set of 547 samples and a test set of 136 samples. They found that ANN had smaller mean square error in the cross-validation of the training set, but the SVM preforms slightly better on the test set.

The SVM has also been applied to survival endpoints. Since survival data typically has censored observations, SVM based on observations that have actual failure (death) times will result in an underestimated survival time. Quite a few SVM methods has been developed to incorporate the censored observations in survival endpoints, see, for example, Shivaswamy et al. [71], Khan and Zubek [43] and Goldberg and Kosorok [29]. There are also SVM methods based on ranking constraints which are mainly for classifying subjects into different risk groups [75]. We are not going to discuss those further since it is not the focus of this chapter.

One disadvantage of SVMs is that they are difficult to interpret, especially when nonlinear kernel functions are used. They also do not always have great performance compared to other more traditional methods. Stiphout et al. compared proximal support vector machine with logistic regression using a dataset of 1552 cancer patients with clinical and pathological features. They concluded that proximal support vector machines do not improve the long-term rectal cancer outcome prediction as compared to logistic regression [77]. Gupta et al. also used 400 support vector machines (SVMs) with linear kernel to establish three ML models for predicting cancer survivalship at 6, 12 and 24 months. They compared AUCs of these ML models with that of clinicians' prediction using a derivation cohort of 869 patients and a validation cohort of 94 patients. The ML models only slightly outperform the clinician prediction [31]. On the other hand, Ahmad et al. showed that SVM had the best performance in terms of predictive accuracy when compared with C4.5 Decision trees and ANN [2].

3.2 Bayesian Network

Bayesian Network (BN) combines the probability theory and graph theory to a graphical model that represents dependencies and conditional independencies between variables. It uses nodes to represent input variables or features, and uses arcs to represent direct or indirect dependencies among nodes. It can be used for both supervised or unsupervised learning. The BN has been an important method in the field of artificial intelligence (AI) for a long time.

A prognostic BN is composed of two important parts. The first is the Directed Acyclic Graph (DAG), which determines the structure of the network and the relationships among the nodes. Figure 10 is an example that shows the basic relationships between three nodes: the serial connection, the divergent connection and the convergent connection. In the serial connection, nodes A, B and C are connected in serial, so that C depends on A through B. In a divergent connection, both B and C directly depend on A. The convergent connection is sometimes also called v-structure for how it looks. In this structure both A and B nodes lead to C [69]. The DAG is a graphical way of showing the connections among all nodes, so it may look like a tree or a web, but we can always identify the three basic relationships throughout the DAG.

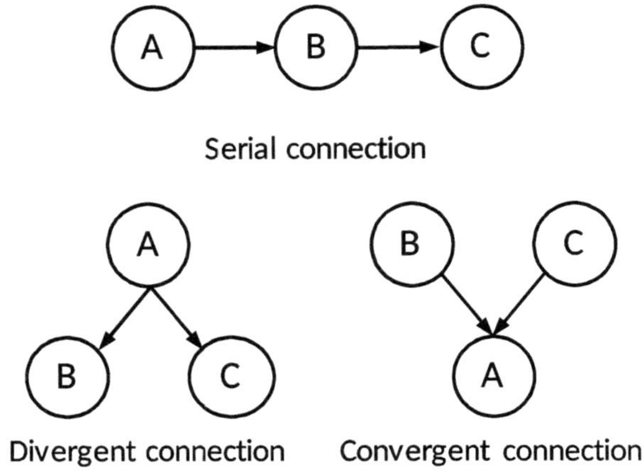

Fig. 10 Directed Acyclic Graph (DAG) types—the three basic components

Determining the DAG is a very complex task in prognostic BN, especially if the number of potential prognostic factors is quite large. When constructing DAG, it is important to include the known relationship and important prognostic factors shown in literature or other science studies. Van Gerven et al. had a nice example to follow for step by step constructions of the DAG for a carcinoid tumor model consisting 218 variables and over 74,000 parameters to estimate [76].

The second important component is the joint probability distribution of all variables represented in the nodes of DAG. The outside information such as historical studies and experts' opinions can be incorporated through specifications of prior distribution. Learning the DAG is a very complex task in prognostic BN. Conditional independence test or network scores are often used to determine which nodes should stay, and on whether two nodes are conditionally independent. The complexity of querying largely depends on the DAG. Exact inferences can be used when the DAG is relatively simple so that conditional probabilities can be computed based on a specially crafted tree constructed based on the DAG. When the DAG is large and complex, we often use approximate inference, which uses Monte Carlo simulation to randomly generate observations from the BN, and computes the query based on simulated samples.

The R package lnlearn (short for "Bayesian Network Learning") is a useful tool for constructing BNs. Aiming to unify temporal dimension with uncertainty, it started from Static Bayesian networks, and proceeded to dynamic BNs which incorporate time-dependent covariates.

3.3 *Artificial Neural Network*

ANN is a powerful tool that can handle a variety of classification and pattern recognition problems [46, 57]. It has also been applied to predict the chance of

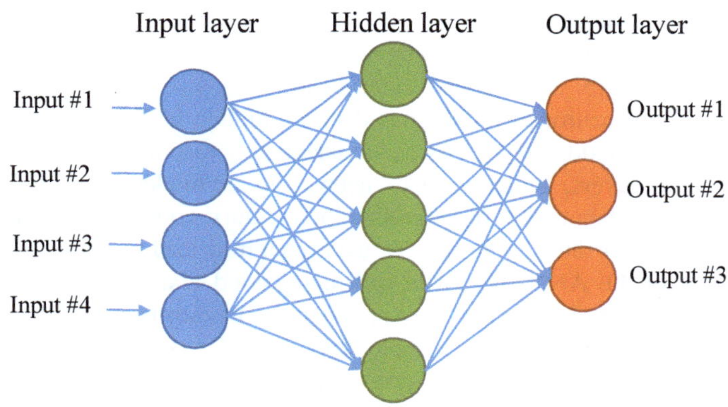

Fig. 11 Artificial neural network

survival beyond certain time points for cancer patients [13, 18]. The name of ANN was inspired by a biological neural network, as the structure of ANN looks like the network of neurons, but the algorithms used in ANN are still quite different from how the neurons work in the brain. Compared with traditional statistical methods, ANN can easily accommodate prognostic variables that change over time, and can provide a prediction based on complex multidimensional non-linear functions.

A typical ANN architecture consists of three layers: an input layer, a hidden layer and an output layer (Fig. 11). The input layer represents the input features to be used in the prognostic model, and the output layer gives the classification or the prediction of the outcomes. Multiple prognostic outcomes may be predicted from one single ANN. Figure 11 is a three-layer feed-forward fully connected ANN, the most widely used ANN structure in oncology prognostic models. This structure has a nice balance of simplicity and flexibility, and has been shown to be useful in many studies in medical fields [9]. In Fig. 11, each layer has multiple neurons, as represented by the circles. Sometimes the neurons are also called nodes in ANN literature. The network refers to the interconnection between neurons in different layers, represented by the arrowed lines. A fully connected ANN connects all input neurons with each of the neurons in the hidden layer, and each neuron in the hidden layer with each neuron in the output layer.

The number of neurons in the input layer depends on the input features in the database, and the number of neurons in the output layer is determined by the clinical outcomes to be predicted in the model. If there is only one outcome to be predicted, the ANN will have only one neuron in the output layer. While it can be challenging to determine the number of hidden layers and the associated number of neurons analytically, in most cases single hidden layer is the default choice. As Ganesan et al. [24] pointed out, the universal approximation theorem of neural networks suggested that every continuous function that maps input neurons to output neurons can be approximated arbitrarily closely by a multi-layer perception with single hidden layer. Adding multiple hidden layers will add more flexibility and complexity, but at the cost of slower training process and a higher risk of overfitting. Therefore, the dominating majority of oncology prognostic models developed using ANN used single hidden layer.

The number of neurons to be included in the hidden layer is also critical. Too few neurons in the hidden layer may fail to adequately map the association between input and output layers, while too many neurons in the hidden layer could result in overfitting. While the number of neurons to be included could be determined based on the smallest error rates in the test set, using that may lead to biased estimates on the error rate of the ANN [68]. It is well understood that a traditional statistical model requires 10 or more subjects per parameter to be estimated in the model. This means the model should be kept simple if the sample size is very limited, and a more complex model must be built upon a database with sufficient sample size and number of events. The same rule also applies to the ANN model.

In ANN, the key parameters to be estimated are the weights of each interconnection, which convert input nodes to output nodes through activation functions. The weights are estimated "adaptively" using the training data through a pre-determined learning algorithm. In oncology, the most widely used learning mechanism is the back propagation learning algorithm [9]. The estimation of the weights are adjusted over the repeated training cycles until the mean square error of the cost function that represents the difference between estimated output and real output is minimized. The number of iterations needed for the training process depends on the learning algorithm, and initial values of weights. The mechanism of iteratively training the system to learn from data and adjusting weights' computation has similarity with Bayesian estimation of posterior distributions for parameters of interest using Markov Chain Monte Carlo.

The complexity of a fully-connected ANN model thus depends on the number of weights to be trained, which is jointly determined by the number of input and output neurons, the number of hidden layers, and the number of hidden neurons. The time required to train an ANN can vary substantially depending on the complexity of the ANN models. Lisboa and Taktak have conducted a systematic review to discuss the use of ANN in decision support in cancer [49]. They have identified 27 qualified cancer clinical trials published in 1994–2003 that used ANNs modeling, including breast, prostate, cervical, bladder, head and neck, leukemia, skin, liver, lung and paediatric osteosarcoma. For example, Lundin et al. used ANN to predict 5-, 10- and 15-year survival [54].

Some studies showed a clear added benefit of using ANNs, while others suggested ANNs were comparable to traditional statistical modeling approaches. Faraggi et al. [20] showed that ANN in conjunction with regression trees can be used to find a good continuous approximation of the hazard function, which direction links to the traditional statistical modeling of time-to-event endpoints. Overall, the ANN models were shown to be a useful tool, but with limited application in routine clinical use. The reviews conducted by both Lisaboa et al. and Schwarzer et al. [68] have conveyed some major issues commonly seen in the application of ANN to oncology: (1) lack of overfitting control; (2) relatively small data sets; (3) lack of validated comparisons with other methods.

Another disadvantage of the ANN method is in its "black-box" feature, in that the final output is not a simple figure or regression function evaluating the controlled influence of each covariate. Due to the existence of the hidden layer, it can be difficult to tell what the network has learned during the process, and to figure out the rule each neuron plays in the network. It is, however, possible to extract information about the influence of variables within these networks. The weights that are connected to the neurons are similar to the weights or coefficients associated with variables in a regression problem. For each input and possible output, all possible hidden layer connecting weights can be extracted and scaled to the number of connections [25, 28]. These can then be ranked to obtain a general relative influence of the input variables with the possible outcomes, but will not be as easily interpretable as regression coefficients. While predictive accuracy is always the major concern of a prognostic model, physicians often feel more comfortable to use a method that is more understandable and trackable.

4 Evaluating the Performance of a Prognostic Model

Once a prognostic model has been developed, its performance needs to be assessed before finalizing it as the model to be validated. That is, the differences between the predicted outcomes and the observed outcomes need to be evaluated within the training dataset, at both individual and group levels. The underlying rationale is that if the predicted and observed outcomes are not close enough even for the training dataset, there is little chance the prognostic model will perform well in external datasets. Therefore, a model should be screened out if it does not have good predictive performance in the training dataset.

To evaluate the performance of a prognostic model, two types of measurements should be considered: discrimination and calibration. Discrimination is to evaluate whether the model can correctly classify subjects into one of the two categories (e.g., 1-year PFS), whereas calibration is to describe how close the predicted probabilities agree with the observed outcome. Both are important measurements that require close evaluation. We would not suggest just evaluating discrimination or calibration alone, because it is possible that a prognostic model has good discrimination but not satisfactory calibration, or vice versa.

4.1 Discrimination Measurements

One of the most popular measures of discrimination for categorical outcomes is the c-index produced in the Receiver Operating Characteristic (ROC) analysis. The *c* is a continuous measurement reflecting the area under the ROC curve (AUC), ranging from 0 to 1. To understand the c-index, let us consider a data set with a binary outcome *Y*, say, pathology complete response (pCR) Yes or No. We use P_{11} to denote the predicted probability of having pCR for a subject with pCR, and P_{12} the predicted probability of having pCR for a subject without pCR. The c-index is

$$Pr(P_{11} > P_{12}) + 0.5Pr(P_{11} = P_{12})$$

Intuitively, we can imagine the training set separated into two pools: Pool A with all subjects who had pCR and Pool B with all subjects who did not have pCR. We random sample one subject from each pool and compare the P_{11} and P_{12} for the two subjects. If $P_{11} > P_{12}$, i.e., the predicted probability of having pCR is higher for the subject who actually had pCR, we call it a prediction success. If $P_{11} < P_{12}$, it is a prediction failure. In rare situations where $P_{11} = P_{12}$, they are deemed as partial prediction successes which gain only half the credit. The procedure is repeated many times and the random draw is with replacement. The c-index is the proportion of success out of the many random draws.

The c-index is often presented together with the ROC curve, which is a plot of the sensitivity (true positive rate) against 1-specificity (false positive rate) for a continuous series of potential cutoff value (Fig. 12). If a prognostic model has both 100% sensitivity and 100% specificity at certain cutoff value, the AUC can be one, suggesting a perfect prediction. An AUC that is 50% or less suggests the prognostic model is no better than a random guess, and thus is worthless. That is why the ROC curve plots are often accompanied with a 45% degree line (which has an AUC of 50%). Any ROC curve close to or below the 45% degree line is meaningless.

Harrell et al. [34] and Pencina and D'Agostino [61] have proposed an overall c-index that can be computed for prognostic models build upon the cox regression method. When the endpoint is time-to-event, there is a time T of follow-up for each participating subject. Therefore, subjects are likely to be censored if they did not have an event before their maximum follow up time T. The overall c-index only considers the censoring due to not having the event before the end of the study period. For two randomly draw subjects, if the shorter of the two times is an event

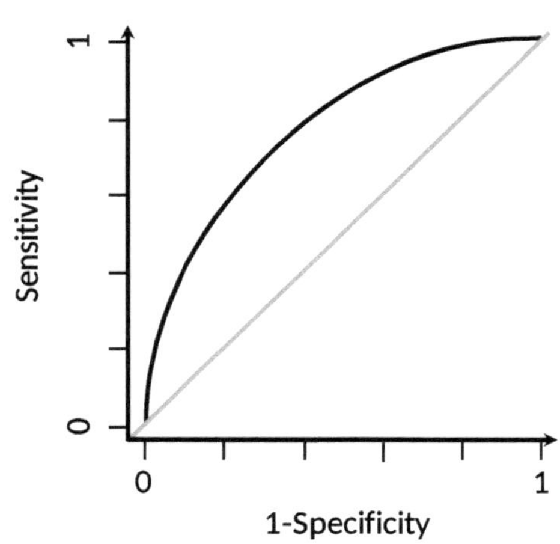

Fig. 12 Receiver Operating Characteristic (ROC) curve

(uncensored), we do the comparison. If both subjects are censored, or the shorter of the two times is censored, no comparisons will be made and the draw will be discarded as not usable, because it is unknown who had the longer time-to-event from the data. The observed and the predicted time-to-event are compared with each other within the pair. If the subjects with longer predicted time-to-event also had longer observed time-to-event, it is called a concordant pair. If the subject with longer predicted time-to-event had a shorter observed time-to-event, then the pair is a discordant pair. The overall c-index is

$$C = \frac{\pi_c}{\pi_c + \pi_d}$$

where π_c is the chance of having concordance pairs in all usable pairs.

It is suggested that the c-index be reported with a 95% confidence interval, which can easily be computed using bootstrapping.

Some other measures of discrimination focus on how much the prognostic groups are separated. For example, the discrimination slope [73] and simple index of separation [3] for categorical outcomes, and the separation parameters (SEP) [65] and D [63] for survival outcomes. These measurements are very useful in identifying whether the prognostic model effectively separates different risk groups, but not focusing on the closeness of prediction with the observed for individual subject.

4.2 Calibration Measurements

One well-known method of calibration is Hosmer-Lemeshow goodness-of-fit test [38]. The idea of the goodness-of-fit test is to first sort the data set (either the training set or the validation set) based on the predicted probabilities and then divide it into g groups. In most common cases, g is set to 10 and each group has approximately equal size. Within each group, we separate the observations into two subgroups: one with the event and the other without the event. We count the number of subjects in each subgroup and compare it with the expected counts of subjects in the group based on the computed probability. For example, if in group 1, there are 50 subjects, 5 had events and the rest 45 did not have events. Then we sum the predicted probabilities of having event for all 50 subjects as the expected counts of subjects that will have event ($\widehat{e_{1k}}$). The sum will be compared with 5 (o_{1k}). We also sum the predicted probabilities of not having events for all 50 subjects ($\widehat{e_{0k}}$, which is just 50 − $\widehat{e_{1k}}$), and compare with 45 (o_{0k}).

The Hosmer-Lemeshow goodness-of-fit test statistic, $\hat{C}$, is just the Pearson Chi-square statistic from the g group [38].

$$\hat{C} = \sum_{k=1}^{g} \left[\frac{\left(o_{1k} - \widehat{e_{1k}}\right)^2}{\widehat{e_{1k}}} + \frac{\left(o_{0k} - \widehat{e_{0k}}\right)^2}{\widehat{e_{0k}}} \right]$$

The test statistic follows a Chi-square distribution with degrees of freedom $g - 2$. The H-L goodness-of-fit statistic provides a p-value that directly helps to determine if the current model fits well. However, the H-L goodness-of-fit statistic has been criticized for lack of robustness. Depending on the different g, the H-L goodness-of-fit test may give different p-values. In addition, it is not always appropriate for certain types of prognostic models. For example, if the number of covariate patterns (J) of a prognostic model, which is simply the maximum number of covariate spaces that can be partitioned using prognostic factors included in the model, is much smaller than the sample size in the dataset, the Pearson Chi-square statistic is more appropriate for goodness-of-fit assessment [38]. This typically happens when all prognostic factors in the model are categorical.

For each covariate pattern j, as all subjects in the pattern have exact the same covariate values, they share the same predicted values, denoted by $\widehat{\pi}_j$. Let y_j denotes the number of observed events in covariate pattern j, the Pearson Chi-square statistic is computed using

$$X^2 = \sum_{j=1}^{J} \left[\frac{\left(y_j - m_j \widehat{\pi}_j\right)^2}{m_j \widehat{\pi}_j \left(1 - \widehat{\pi}_j\right)} \right]$$

The X^2 follows a Chi-square distribution with degrees of freedom equals to $J - (p + 1)$. Here p is the number of covariates included in the prognostic model. Note that it does not equal to the number of factors included in the model, unless all factors are binary (prognostic factors that are continuous without categorization suggests Pearson Chi-square statistic may not be used as the J is likely to be close to n).

Another widely used calibration measurement that directly looks at the difference in predicted and observed outcomes is the Brier score (BS). The BS computes the mean squared differences between the predicted and the observed.

$$BS = \frac{1}{N} \sum_{i=1}^{N} (predicted_i - observed_i)^2$$

where N is the sample size for either the training set or the validation set, and i represents patient i. The smaller the BS, the better the prediction. BS are often used for both continuous and categorical endpoints. Its computation can also be extended to survival outcomes using the conditional probability of being uncensored for a given time as weights [73].

5 Validating a Prognostic Model

If a prognostic model does not show promising performances in both discrimination and calibration measures in the training data set, it may be re-developed using alternative techniques, or additional prognostic factors may be added to the model.

It is not suggested to go ahead and validate a prognostic model if it does not have nice predictive ability using the same samples based on which it was developed. On the other hand, if the model performances look satisfactory, it does not mean this is a good prognostic model, as there are chances that the model overfits the sample.

Therefore, all prognostic models need to be validated because there is no guarantee that a well-constructed prognostic model will work well in practice for forcasting endpoints of interest for patients that are not used to build the model.

The variable selection and rule of prediction should be fully determined in the prognostic model before validation is conducted. For example, if the outcome variable is a binary endpoint, it is not enough to only have a predicted probability of having an event without a cutoff value that dichotomizes the predicted probabilities into two categories: having event or without event. Similarly, the hazard ratio alone is not sufficient for a prognostic model for survival outcome. A predicted time-to-event should be computable for all subjects.

The gold standard of validating a prognostic model is to evaluate the established model on a set of subjects that is not used for constructing the prognostic model, and to show that the model works well in predicting the endpoints of interest for those subjects. This is called external validation. The choice of validation sample set for external validation depends heavily on the proposed patient population that is proposed for the application of the prognostic model. For example, if the patient population is US patients who underwent surgery for a renal mass without metastatic disease, and the training set is from a single institution for qualifying subjects, the external validation set should be composed of multi-institutional data from difference places in the US. If the patient population of the model is not limited to the US patients, then external data from both US and other countries should be used for validation. It is also suggested to have a different group of researchers for external validation to ensure the generalizability.

Another well accepted approach is internal validation, where people use the same data source for build the model and validate the model. Several methods have being proposed for internal validation. Regardless of which method been used for internal validation, we cannot bypass the limitation that the validation data set is from the same source as the training data set. As a consequence, the robustness and performance of the model on samples outside the data source is still questionable. The only exception might be if the database is a huge national database that covers all patient population for the prognostic model. Otherwise, we still suggest to use external validation whenever possible.

When conducting interval validation, the data needs to be split into two sets: the training set and the validation set. The most straightforward way is to split it just once. There is no agreed upon single rule on the relative size of the two resulting datasets, but popular choices are random samples of about 2/3 for training and 1/3 for the validation data set. Before fitting the prognostic model, researchers first randomly divide the whole dataset into two parts: the training data set and the validation data set. The validation data set will not be touched until the prognostic model is fully developed and evaluated using the training data set. The performance of the prognostic model is then evaluated using the validation data set. If the good performance persists, then the model is unlikely to be overfitting.

Splitting data into definitive training and validating set is very close to the external validation, except for the data source. It is suggested when the database is large so that both the training and validation set have sufficient sample size. There are also deviations of the internal validation by using historical samples to build the model and prospectively enrolled subjects to validate the model. This is sometimes called temporal validation.

In certain situations with very limited sample size, a same database may be re-sampled multiple times so that subjects are used for both constructing the model and validating the model. This cost-efficient way of using data repeatedly for internal validation can be realized via k-fold cross-validation, jackknife or bootstrapping.

In a k-fold cross-validation, the original sample is randomly partitioned into k equal-sized subsamples. For any single process, $k - 1$ subsamples are used as the training set and the remaining single subsample is used as the validation set. The cross-validation process is then repeated k times so that each of the k subsamples are used as the validation data exactly once. The validation results are simply the average of the k-fold results produced in each single process. While researchers may choose any k as it fits the sample size, one most popular choices of k is to let $k = 10$. Another popular choice of k is $k = n$, so that in each process, only one subject was used as the validation set. The k-fold cross-validation that uses $k = n$ sometimes is also referred as the Jackknife. Draw Bootstrap samples with replacement from the original database to form multiple generated datasets which are expected to follow the sample distribution as the original database. The prognostic model can be built upon the generated dataset, and be validated in the original database, or be validated using subjects who are not used in building the prognostic models. Bootstrapping is claimed to be the most efficient interval validation method [72].

The discrimination and calibration measures can be computed in the same way for validation as we described in Sect. 3. It will be interesting to compare the measurements of discrimination and calibration computed from the validation set to those computed from the training set. While we typically expect the measurements will look more favorable for those computed in the training set, big differences in the measurements typically suggest an overfitting.

It is worth noting that statistical validation is not the same as the clinical validation. A clinically validated model should be statistically validated, and should also been shown to outperform existing models, or has comparable performance in prediction with reduced costs/requirements. A model will be practically valuable only if it is clinically validated.

6 Concluding Remarks

Cancer prognosis is an estimation on the likely course of cancer disease on a specific patient. It is very important for both physicians and patients to gain information on the cancer prognosis. In this chapter, we have introduced several machine learning techniques in building and validating cancer prognostic models. We have no doubt that more advanced tools for building and validating cancer prognostic models will be developed and adopted in the near future.

There are several existing challenges that face cancer clinicians and researchers at the moment in terms of utilizing a prognostic model to support clinical decision-making.

Challenge 1 *There are many prognostic models available for cancer studies, maybe too many.* For example, Louie et al. [52] have identified 127 unique prostate cancer models that can be used for risk prediction. Williams et al. [80] identified 15 prognostic models that are applicable to general patient population for colorectal cancer risk prediction. Meads et al. [56] identified 17 prognostic models for breast cancer. There are also many online tools that provide risk computation for cancer patients without a strong supporting publication. It is often quite difficult for clinicians to determine which one to trust and use.

Quality control of prognostic models in oncology is in urgent need. We strongly suggest (1) not to publish prognostic models that are not appropriately validated; (2) to distinguish prognostic models from other models that are developed for evaluating association between certain covariates and biomarkers with the clinical outcomes, and require authors to clearly define the purpose of the model.

We also suggest that government or a leading academic institution set up a website that includes only validated (both statistically and clinically) prognostic models, and carefully arrange them by disease categories and targeted patient population. These models should also be tested repeatedly using the new available data set to make sure they are still applicable to current patient population. No new prognostic models will be added unless they are targeting different patient population that are not covered by any of the existing models, or they show comparable or better performance compared to the models included in the website for the same patient population. With such a website available, there may not be as many overlapping efforts in building and validating prognostic models for same patient population. Instead, more efforts could be spent on validating and updating the existing prognostic models. More importantly, physicians will know a single website to look for cancer prognostic models if they need to use one for clinical reference.

Challenge 2 *The predictive accuracy of prognostic cancer models is questionable.* It is still under debate on whether any cancer prognostic models should be used to support clinical decision-making. As we discussed earlier, a good prognostic model at group or population level does not imply acceptable prediction for individual cancer patient. For example, if a prognostic model predicts that there is 69% chance for an average patient with given risk factor values to survive beyond 5 years, and if the actual observed percentage for a group of such patients is exactly 69%, the model seems to predict perfectly. However for single subject in the patient population, a probability of 69% chance to survive beyond 5 years still has a lot of uncertainty, since the actual observation can only be binary.

Henderson et al. and Schoop et al. suggested that it is unlikely to gain an accurate estimate of projected survival time for an individual cancer patient due to poor point estimates and low explained variation in survival outcomes [35, 67]. Parks has defined a "serious error" in survival prediction to be a predicted survival time that is either less than half of the actual survival time or more than twice the actual survival time, and found that the serious error rate in survival predictions is typically 50–60% for most cancer prognostic models with a survival endpoint [60]. Some researchers thus suggested to limit the use of prognostic model of survival time to group or population level [30, 36]. This is by far from ideal, as in most situations subject-specific prediction is the primary interest.

If clinicians have to predict subject-specific survival they should present it with great caution and emphasize the uncertainty in predicted outcomes. For example, they could say "My best guess is that you will live 3 months or more but there is a 60% chance I will be seriously wrong", or they may use the estimated 80% confidence interval for an individual subject and tell "My best guess is that you will live 3 months but there is an 80% chance the actual time is between 2 weeks and 2 years".

It is often more effective in communicating the survival prediction using graphics. The output of a prognostic model could be a histogram of the probabilities of surviving beyond certain month.

If there does not exist a prognostic model that is good enough for subject-specific prediction, we suggest to merely provide patients with descriptive statistics on how other patients like her/him did. Clustering or a propensity score method can be used to identify a group of patients that is similar to the patient whose outcome is to be predicted. An example is shown Fig. 13a if less than 20 subjects are in the group (Data source Oberije et al. [59]). If the number of similar patients is more than 20 subjects, Fig. 13b may be shown instead.

Challenge 3 *Most cancer prognostic models are static so that predictions cannot reflect the updated information of patients.* Most cancer prognostic models have been developed to predict the risk of having an event by given time-point from diagnosis or treatment for patients. In real world, patients may be interested in getting updated prediction based on newly available information, say, pathology complete response after the initial treatment, or no complications after surgery. Many cancer prognostic models do not contain such time dependent covariates, and thus are unable to provide predictions that take into consideration such updated information. A desirable cancer prognostic model should be dynamic at both

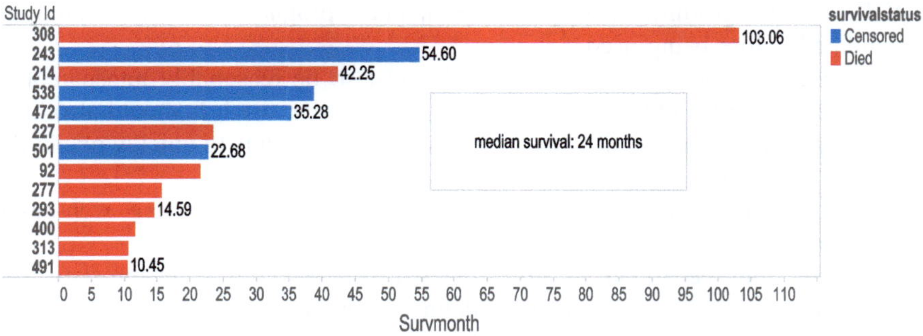

(a) Graphic Description for Similar Patients --- Smaller Group

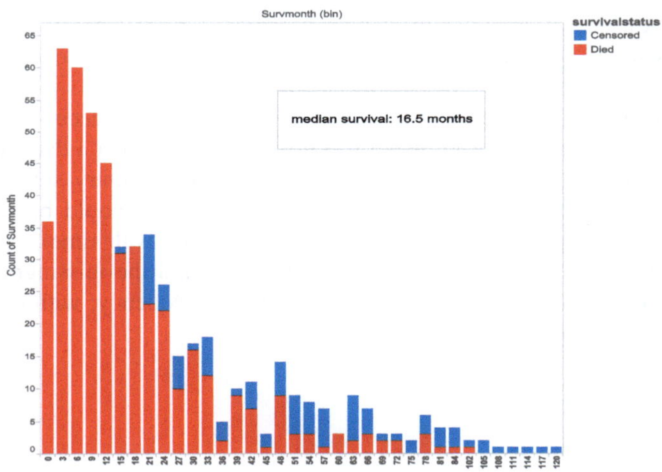

(b) Graphic Description for Similar Patients --- Larger Group

Fig. 13 Graphic description for similar patients—**a** smaller group, **b** larger group

subject-specific level and at patient population level. At the individual patient level, it would predict subject-specific survival or chance of having certain event conditioning on the current patient status. At the patient population level, it should be flexible enough to allow updates to the prognostic model based on the newly gained information about existing and new subjects. It should allow newly identified risk factors be included once sufficient information supports the new risk factor would improve the prediction, and should also gradually decrease the weights of historical patients as the database grows. Ankerst et al. have proposed using Bayesian method for updating prior knowledge with newly available data through the transformation of prior odds to posterior odds [4]. They have successfully updated an online prostate cancer prevention trial risk calculator to incorporate two new markers that became available after the tool has been developed (http://deb.uthscsa.edu/

UROR iskCalc/Pages/uroriskcalc.jsp). An updated prognostic model should be re-validated before being used.

A desirable cancer prognostic model should also be reasonably transparent in building procedures and tell which prognostic factors are used. It should also have an accompanying user-friendly tool for clinicians and patients to quickly obtain the predicted outcomes.

Currently, many cancer prognostic models are presented using web-based nomograms.

Examples can be found in https://www.mskcc.org/nomograms/prostate and http://www3.mdanderson.org/app/medcalc/index.cfm?pagename=pancreascancer.

Almost all current nomograms ask the physicians or patient to self-input necessary variables. This not only limits the number of covariates that can be included in the prognostic model, but also increases the chance of unreliable predictions due to inputting error. An ideal nomogram for cancer prognostic model should allow automatic withdrawing of necessary information from electronic health records of hospitals under privacy protection.

We should all be aware that the most critical thing to ensure the success construction and validation of a prognostic model is a great database. Such a database should be composed of multi-center, multi-region or even multi-country subjects whose information is collected using uniform standards. Patients should be followed closely for more precise endpoints (e.g., actual survival time), and time-dependent variables. The sample size should be decent and the missingness minimized. The database should be updated with reasonable frequency, with consistent close data monitoring to ensure quality.

References

1. Ahmad A. Pathways to breast cancer recurrence. ISRN Oncol. 2013;2013:290568. doi:10.1155/2013/290568.
2. Ahmad LG, Eshlaghy AT, Poorebrahimi A, et al. Using three machine learning techniques for predicting breast cancer recurrence. J Heal Med Inform. 2013;4:1000124. doi:10.4172/2157-7420.1000124.
3. Altman DG, Royston P. What do we mean by validating a prognistic model? Stat Med. 2000;19:453–73.
4. Ankerst DP, Hoefler J, Bock S, et al. Prostate cancer prevention trial risk calculator 2.0 for the prediction of low- vs high-grade prostate cancer. Urology. 2014;83:1362–7. doi:10.1016/j.urology.2014.02.035.
5. Bellaachia A, Guven E. Predicting breast cancer survivability using data mining techniques. SIAM Int Conf Data Min. 2006;6:1–4. doi:10.1109/ICSTE.2010.5608818.
6. Bharathi A, Natarajan AM. Cancer classification using support vector machines and relevance vector machine based on analysis of variance features. J Comput Sci. 2011;7:1393–9.
7. De Bin R, Sauerbrei W, Boulesteix A-L. Investigating the prediction ability of survival models based on both clinical and omics data: Two case studies. Stat Med. 2014;33:5310–29. doi:10.1002/sim.6246.

8. Boser BE, Guyon IM, Vapnik VN. A training algorithm for optimal margin classifiers. In: Proceedings of the 5th annual ACM workshop on computational learning theory. New York: ACM Press; 1992. p. 144–152.
9. Bottaci L, Drew PJ, Hartley JE, et al. Artificial neural networks applied to outcome prediction for colorectal cancer patients in separate institutions. Lancet. 1997;350:469–72. doi:10.1016/S0140-6736(96)11196-X.
10. Bou-Hamd I, Larocque D, Ben-Ameur H. A review of survival trees. Stat Surv. 2011;5:44–71. doi:10.1214/09-SS047.
11. Boulesteix A, Sauerbrei W. Added predictive value of high-throughput molecular data to clinical data and its validation. Brief Bioinform. 2011;12:215–29. doi:10.1093/bib/bbq085.
12. Burges CJC. A tutorial on support vector machines for pattern recognition. Data Min Knowl Discov. 1998;2:121–67.
13. Burke HB, Goodman PH, Rosen DB, et al. Artificial neural networks improve the accuracy of cancer survival prediction. Cancer. 1997;79:857–62.
14. Chow E, Abdolell M, Panzarella T, et al. Predictive model for survival in patients with advanced cancer. J Clin Oncol. 2008;26:5863–9. doi:10.1200/JCO.2008.17.1363.
15. Chow E, James JL, Hartsell W, et al. Validation of a predictive model for survival in patients with advanced cancer: Secondary analysis of RTOG 9714. World J Oncol. 2011;2:181–90. doi:10.4021/wjon325w.
16. Clark GM. Prognostic factors versus predictive factors: Examples from a clinical trial of erlotinib. Mol Oncol. 2008;1:406–12. doi:10.1016/j.molonc.2007.12.001.
17. Craven MW, Shavlik JW. Extracting tree-structured representations of trained networks. In: Advances in neural information processing systems. Denver: MIT Press; 1996. p. 24–30.
18. Delen D, Walker G, Kadam A. Predicting breast cancer survivability: A comparison of three data mining methods. Artif Intell Med. 2005;34:113–27. doi:10.1016/j.artmed.2004.07.002.
19. Dettling M, Bühlmann P. Boosting for tumor classification with gene expression data. Bioinformatics. 2003;19:1061–9. doi:10.1093/bioinformatics/btf867.
20. Faraggi D, LeBlanc M, Crowley J. Understanding neural networks using regression trees: an application to multiple myeloma survival data. Stat Med. 2001;20:2965–76. doi:10.1002/sim.912.
21. Freund Y, Schapire RE. A desicion-theoretic generalization of on-line learning and an application to boosting. J Comput Syst Sci. 1997;55:119–39. doi:10.1006/jcss.1997.1504.
22. Friedman JH, Meulman JJ. Multiple additive regression trees with application in epidemiology. Stat Med. 2003;22:1365–81. doi:10.1002/sim.1501.
23. Furey TS, Cristianini N, Duffy N, et al. Support vector machine classification and validation of cancer tissue samples using microarray expression data. Bioinformatics. 2000;16:906–14.
24. Ganesan N, Vankatesh K, Rama MA, Palani AM. Application of neural networks in diagnosing cancer disease using demographic data. Int J Comput Appl. 2010;1:76–85. doi:10.5120/476-783.
25. Garson DG. Interpreting neural-network connection weights. Artif Intell Expert. 1991;6:46–51.
26. Ge G, Wong GW. Classification of premalignant pancreatic cancer mass-spectrometry data using decision tree ensembles. BMC Bioinform. 2008;9:275. doi:10.1186/1471-2105-9-275.
27. Glare P. Clinical predictors of survival in advanced cancer. J Support Oncol. 2005;3:331–9.
28. Goh ATC. Back-propagation neural networks for modeling complex systems. Artif Intell Eng. 1995;9:143–51. doi:10.1016/0954-1810(94)00011-S.
29. Goldberg Y, Kosorok MR. Support vector regression for right censored data. 2012. arXiv 1202.5130v2.
30. Graf E, Schmoor C, Sauerbrei W, Schumacher M. Assessment and comparison of prognostic classification schemes for survival data. Stat Med. 1999;18:2529–45. doi:10.1002/(SICI)1097-0258(19990915/30)18:17/18<2529:AID-SIM274>3.0.CO;2-5.
31. Gupta S, Tran T, Luo W, et al. Machine-learning prediction of cancer survival: a retrospective study using electronic administrative records and a cancer registry. BMJ Open. 2014;4:e004007. doi:10.1136/bmjopen-2013-004007.

32. Guyon I, Weston J, Barnhill S, Vapnik V. Gene selection for cancer classification using support vector machines. Mach Learn. 2002;46:389–422.
33. Halabi S, Lin C-Y, Kelly WK, et al. Updated prognostic model for predicting overall survival in first-line chemotherapy for patients with metastatic castration-resistant prostate cancer. J Clin Oncol. 2014;32:671–7. doi:10.1200/JCO.2013.52.3696.
34. Harrell FE, Lee KL, Mark DB. Multivariable prognostic models: issues in developing models, evaluating assumptions and adequacy, and measuring and reducing errors. Stat Med. 1996;15:361–87.
35. Henderson R, Jones M, Stare J. Accuracy of point predictions in survival analysis. Stat Med. 2001;20:3083–96. doi:10.1002/sim.913.
36. Henderson R, Keiding N. Individual survival time prediction using statistical models. J Med Ethics. 2005;31:703–6. doi:10.1136/jme.2005.012427.
37. Hofner B, Boccuto L, Göker M. Controlling false discoveries in high-dimensional situations: boosting with stability selection. BMC Bioinform. 2015;16:144. doi:10.1186/s12859-015-0575-3.
38. Hosmer DW, Lemeshow S, Sturdivant RX. Applied logistic regression. 3rd ed. New York: Wiley Interscience; 2013.
39. Ishwaran H, Kogalur UB, Blackstone EH, Lauer MS. Random survival forests. Ann Appl Stat. 2008;2:841–60. doi:10.1214/08-AOAS169.
40. Jonsdottir T, Hvannberg ET, Sigurdsson H, Sigurdsson S. The feasibility of constructing a predictive outcome model for breast cancer using the tools of data mining. Expert Syst Appl. 2008;34:108–18. doi:10.1016/j.eswa.2006.08.029.
41. Kass GV. An exploratory technique for investigating large quantities of categorical data. Appl Stat. 1980;29:119–27. doi:10.2307/2986296.
42. Katz MHG, Hu C-Y, Fleming JB, et al. A clinical calculator of conditional survival estimates for resected and unresected pancreatic cancer survivors. Arch Surg. 2012;147:513–9. doi:10. 1001/archsurg.2011.2281.
43. Khan FM, Zubek VB. Support vector regression for censored data (SVRc): a novel tool for survival analysis. In: Eighth IEEE international conference on data mining. New York: IEEE; 2008. p. 863–868.
44. Kharya S. Using data mining techniques for diagnosis and prognosis of cancer disease. Int J Comput Sci Inf Technol. 2012;2:55–66. doi:10.5121/ijcseit.2012.2206.
45. Laber EB, Zhao YQ. Tree-based methods for individualized treatment regimes. Biometrika. 2015;102:501–14. doi:10.1093/biomet/asv028.
46. Lancashire LJ, Lemetre C, Ball GR. An introduction to artificial neural networks in bioinformatics—application to complex microarray and mass spectrometry datasets in cancer studies. Brief Bioinform. 2009;10:315–29. doi:10.1093/bib/bbp012.
47. LeBlanc M, Crowley J. Relative risk tees for censored survival data. Biometrics. 1992;48:411–25.
48. LeBlanc M, Kooperberg C. Boosting predictions of treatment success. Proc Natl Acad Sci USA. 2010;107:13559–60. doi:10.1073/pnas.1008052107.
49. Lisboa PJ, Taktak AFG. The use of artificial neural networks in decision support in cancer: a systematic review. Neural Netw. 2006;19:408–15. doi:10.1016/j.neunet.2005.10.007.
50. Liu HX, Zhang RS, Luan F, et al. Diagnosing breast cancer based on support vector machines. J Chem Inf Comput Sci. 2003;43:900–7.
51. Loh W-Y. Classification and regression trees. Wiley Interdiscip Rev Data Min Knowl Discov. 2011;1:14–23. doi:10.1002/widm.8.
52. Louie KS, Seigneurin A, Cathcart P, Sasieni P. Do prostate cancer risk models improve the predictive accuracy of PSA screening? A meta-analysis. Ann Oncol. 2015;26:848–64. doi:10. 1093/annonc/mdu525.
53. Lowrance WT, Elkin EB, Jacks LM, et al. Comparative effectiveness of surgical treatments for prostate cancer: a population-based analysis of postoperative outcomes. J Urol. 2010;183:1366–72. doi:10.1016/j.juro.2009.12.021.Comparative.

54. Lundin M, Lundin J, Burke HB, et al. Artificial neural networks applied to survival prediction in breast cancer. Oncology. 1999;57:281–6.
55. Mayr A, Hofner B, Schmid M. Boosting the discriminatory power of sparse survival models via optimization of the concordance index and stability selection. BMC Bioinform. 2016;17:288. doi:10.1186/s12859-016-1149-8.
56. Meads C, Ahmed I, Riley RD. A systematic review of breast cancer incidence risk prediction models with meta-analysis of their performance. Breast Cancer Res Treat. 2012;132:365–77. doi:10.1007/s10549-011-1818-2.
57. Menéndez LÁ, de Cos Juez FJ, Lasheras SF, Riesgo JAÁ. Artificial neural networks applied to cancer detection in a breast screening programme. Math Comput Model. 2010;52:983–91. doi:10.1016/j.mcm.2010.03.019.
58. Morgan JN, Sonquist JA. Problems in the analysis of survey data, and a proposal. J Am Stat Assoc. 1963;58:415–34. doi:10.1080/01621459.1963.10500855.
59. Oberije C, De Ruysscher D, Houben R, et al. A validated prediction model for overall survival from stage III non-small cell lung cancer: toward survival prediction for individual patients. Int J Radiat Oncol Biol Phys. 2015;92:935–44. doi:10.1016/j.ijrobp.2015.02.048.
60. Parks CM. Prognoses should be based on proved indicators not intuition. BMJ. 2000;320:473. doi:10.1136/bmj.320.7233.469.
61. Penciana MJ, D'Agostino RB. Overall C as a measure of discrimination in survival analysis: model specific population value and confidence interval estimation. Stat Med. 2004;23:2109–23. doi:10.1002/sim.1802.
62. Pölsterl S, Conjeti S, Navab N, Katouzian A. Survival analysis for high-dimensional, heterogeneous medical data: exploring feature extraction as an alternative to feature selection. Artif Intell Med. 2016;72:1–11. doi:10.1016/j.artmed.2016.07.004.
63. Royston P, Sauerbrei W. A new measure of prognostic separation in survival data. Stat Med. 2004;23:723–48. doi:10.1002/sim.1621.
64. Saritas I. Prediction of breast cancer using artificial neural networks. J Med Syst. 2012;36:2901–7. doi:10.1007/s10916-011-9768-0.
65. Sauerbrei W, Hübner K, Schmoor C, Schumacher M. Validation of existing and development of new prognostic classification schemes in node negative breast cancer. Breast Cancer Res Treat. 1997;42:149–63.
66. Schapire RE, Freund Y. Boosting—foundations and algorithms. Cambridge: MIT Press; 2012.
67. Schoop R, Graf E, Schumacher M. Quantifying the predictive performance of prognostic models for censored survival data with time-dependent covariates. Biometrics. 2008;64: 603–10. doi:10.1111/j.l541-0420.2007.00889.x.
68. Schwarzer G, Vach W, Schumacher M. On the misuses of artificial neural networks for prognostic and diagnostic classification in oncology. Stat Med. 2000;19:541–61. doi:10.1002/(SICI)1097-0258(20000229)19:4<541:AID-SIM355>3.0.CO;2-V.
69. Scutari M, Denis J-B. Bayesian networks: with examples in R. Boca Raton: CRC Press; 2014.
70. Sesen MB, Nicholson AE, Banares-Alcantara R, et al. Bayesian networks for clinical decision support in lung cancer care. PLoS ONE. 2013;8:e82349. doi:10.1371/journal.pone.0082349.
71. Shivaswamy PK, Chu W, Jansche M. A support vector approach to censored targets. In: Seventh IEEE international conference on data mining. New York: IEEE; 2007. p. 655–660.
72. Steyerberg EW, Harrell FE, Borsboom GJJM, et al. Internal validation of predictive models: efficiency of some procedures for logistic regression analysis. J Clin Epidemiol. 2001;54: 774–81. doi:10.1016/S0895-4356(01)00341-9.
73. Steyerberg EW, Vickers AJ, Cook NR, et al. Assessing the performance of prediction models: a framework for some traditional and novel measures. Epidemiology. 2010;21:128–38. doi:10.1097/EDE.0b013e3181c30fb2.Assessing.
74. Sweilam NH, Tharwat AA, Moniem NKA. Support vector machine for diagnosis cancer disease: a comparative study. Egypt Inform J. 2010;11:81–92. doi:10.1016/j.eij.2010.10.005.

75. Van Belle V, Pelckmans K, Van Huffel S, Suykens JAK. Support vector methods for survival analysis: A comparison between ranking and regression approaches. Artif Intell Med. 2011;53:107–18.
76. van Gerven MAJ, Taal BG, Lucas PJF. Dynamic Bayesian networks as prognostic models for clinical patient management. J Biomed Inform. 2008;41:515–29. doi:10.1016/j.jbi.2008.01.006.
77. van Stiphout RGPM, Postma EO, Valentini V, Lambin P. The contribution of machine learning to predicting cancer outcome. Artif Intell. 2010;350:400.
78. Vapnik VN. Statistical learning theory. New york: Wiley Interscience; 1998.
79. Wang SJ, Wissel AR, Luh JY, et al. An interactive tool for individualized estimation of conditional survival in rectal cancer. Ann Surg Oncol. 2011;18:1547–52. doi:10.1245/s10434-010-1512-3.
80. Williams TGS, Cubiella J, Griffin SJ, et al. Risk prediction models for colorectal cancer in people with symptoms: a systematic review. BMC Gastroenterol. 2016;16:63. doi:10.1186/s12876-016-0475-7.
81. Yosefian I, Mosa Farkhani E, Baneshi MR. Application of random forest survival models to increase generalizability of decision trees: a case study in acute myocardial infarction. Comput Math Methods Med. 2015;2015:576413. doi:10.1155/2015/576413.

Optimal Three-Group Splits Based on a Survival Outcome

John Crowley, Alan Mitchell, Pingping Qu, Gareth Morgan and Bart Barlogie

Abstract In clinical research it is often desirable to discretize a continuous or ordered covariate. In this paper, we investigate the use of various running ordered logrank tests for finding optimal 3-group splits based on a survival outcome and a single covariate. We first present a successful application of using the modified ordered logrank test (MOL) to find three prognostic groups on a myeloma dataset. We then evaluate through simulations the performance of the running ordered logrank tests and a hierarchical method based on recursive partitioning in different scenarios: (1) when the true underlying distribution has three-groups, (2) when there is a linear relationship between covariate and outcome, and (3) when there is no association between covariate and outcome. We conclude that the MOL is the most robust among all versions of the running ordered logrank tests if the underlying distribution truly has three-groups, although further research could help define when the MOL is the statistic of choice more generally for finding optimal 3-group splits.

Keywords Logrank test · Running ordered logrank tests · Modified ordered logrank test · Optimal three-group splits

J. Crowley · P. Qu (✉)
Cancer Research and Biostatistics, Seattle, WA, USA
e-mail: pingpingq@crab.org

J. Crowley
e-mail: johnc@crab.org

A. Mitchell
Allergan, USA Inc, Seattle, WA, USA
e-mail: alannmitchell@gmail.com

G. Morgan
Myeloma Institute, University of Arkansas for Medical Sciences, Little Rock, AR, USA
e-mail: GJMorgan@uams.edu

B. Barlogie
Mt Sinai School of Medicine, New York, NY, USA
e-mail: bart.barlogie@mssm.edu

S. Matsui and J. Crowley (eds.), *Frontiers of Biostatistical Methods and Applications in Clinical Oncology*, DOI 10.1007/978-981-10-0126-0_14

1 Introduction

The logrank test [10, 11] for comparing the survival curves $S_1(t)$ and $S_2(t)$ of two-groups is one of the most commonly used procedures in survival analysis. The running logrank plot [4] is a tool for finding an optimal split into two-groups based on all possible cutpoints of a continuous or ordered categorical covariate, where optimality is defined as the cutpoint which maximizes the logrank test for comparing the two-groups defined as having covariate values above and below the cutpoint. This tool can be used as part of a recursive partitioning scheme [6], with the first step being to look across all possible covariates and all possible cutpoints for the highest of the maximum logrank tests, and using that cutpoint on that covariate to define two-groups; the procedure then repeats within each of the groups so defined.

The extension of the logrank test for $K > 2$ groups is immediate due to Crowley [2], but this omnibus test may lack power for an ordered alternative of the form $S_1(t) < S_2(t) < \cdots < S_K(t)$. In this article we will present several versions of an ordered logrank test, and then use these to find 'optimal' splits into three-groups based on exploring all possible pairs of cutpoints of a single covariate. These new techniques for three-group splits will be applied to some data sets for patients with multiple myeloma, and then will be compared through simulations, along with a two-step recursive partitioning algorithm, and a test for trend due to Tarone [13].

2 Background on Multiple Myeloma

2.1 Clinical Setting

Multiple myeloma is a cancer involving plasma cells in the bone marrow, the cells in the B cell lineage responsible for producing immunoglobulins. Patients with myeloma typically produce large amounts of a specific clonal immunoglobulin instead of a broad spectrum, and are thus immuno-compromised. They also suffer from renal insufficiency, as their kidneys need to work overtime to clear quantities of very large molecules produced by the tumor. Fractures caused by pockets of bone destruction are also a serious issue.

At the Myeloma Institute of the University of Arkansas for Medical Sciences, newly diagnosed patients with myeloma are treated with an aggressive regimen called Total Therapy, which is based on a backbone of two cycles of high dose therapy with autologous stem cell rescue, called tandem transplants. A representative treatment schema for Total Therapy is given in Fig. 1.

Successive iterations of Total Therapy protocols, from Total Therapy 1, to Total Therapy 2 that included a randomization to thalidomide or not, to Total Therapy 3 that added the proteasome inhibitor bortezomib, have increased the 5 year progression-free survival from 27% to 65% (Fig. 2).

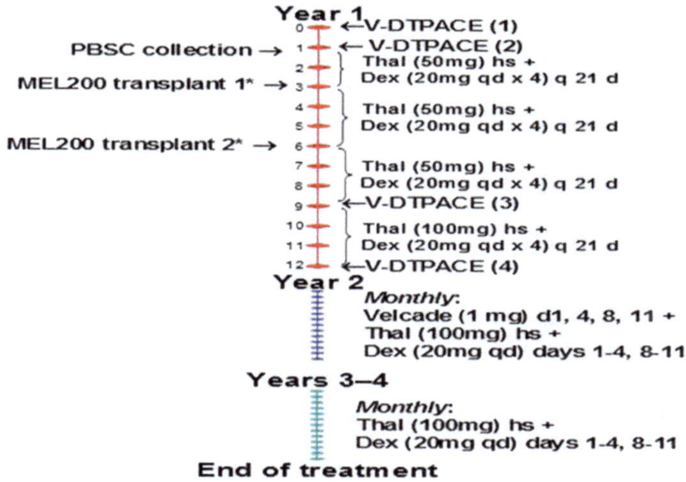

Fig. 1 Basic schema for Total Therapy at the Myeloma Institute. The backbone consists of two cycles of high dose melphalan followed by autologous stem cell rescue (tandem transplants). * Patients ≥ 70 years of age or with elevated serum creatinine (≥ 3.0 mg/dl) will receive MEL 140 mg/m^2

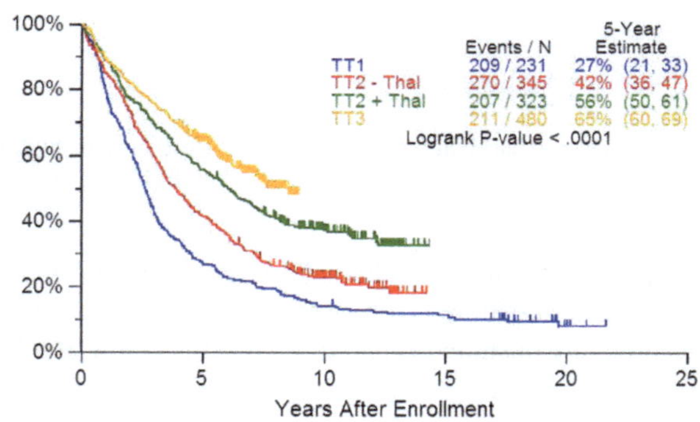

Fig. 2 Progression-free survival for successive Total Therapy protocols. TT2 ± Thal represent two arms of a randomization to thalidomide as part of the regimen or not

2.2 *Gene Expression Profiling and the GEP70 Score*

Midway through accrual to Total Therapy 2 the investigators began to take samples of the patients' tumors for gene expression profiling (GEP) using the Affymetrix platform U133Plus2. A prognostic score was developed using 70 of the 54k probesets (subunits of genes) assayed for expression levels. The distribution of this GEP70 score based on the 351 patients on Total Therapy 2 with gene expression data is shown in Fig. 3.

The apparent bimodal distribution suggests a cutpoint for GEP70 dividing the patients into two-groups. The survival experience of these two-groups on the training

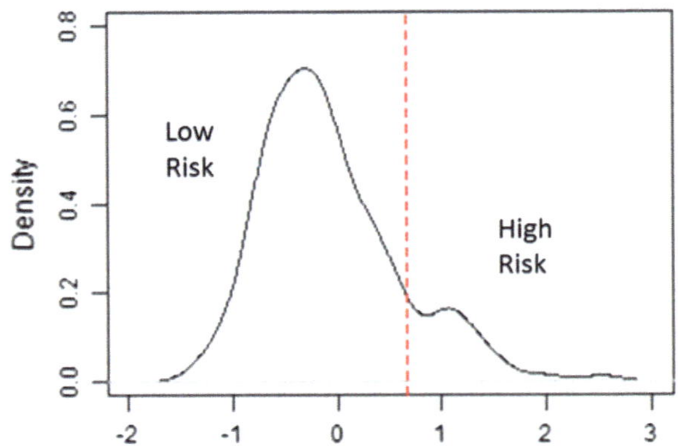

Fig. 3 Distribution of the GEP70 score in Total Therapy 2

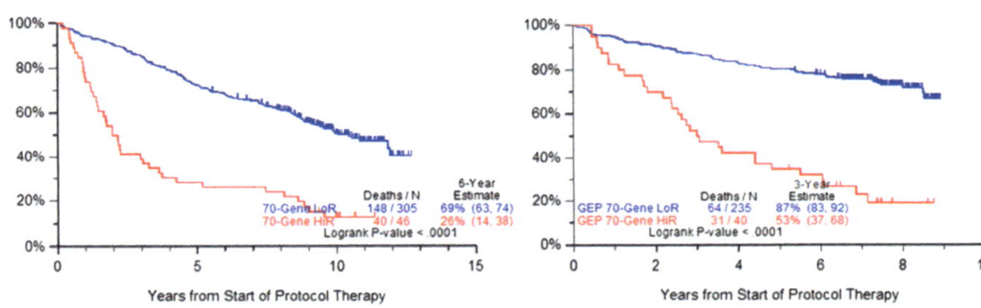

Fig. 4 Overall survival by GEP70 low risk (LoR) versus high risk (HiR) in the training set (Total Therapy 2; *left panel*) and validation set (Total Therapy 3; *right panel*)

set (Total Therapy 2) and a validation set (Total Therapy 3) is shown in Fig. 4. This prognostic signature is robust enough that the next generation of Total Therapy trials, 4 and 5, are designed separately for GEP70 low and high risk, respectively.

3 Extensions of the Logrank Test

We first introduce the two-sample logrank test, then consider some extensions. Let the ordered uncensored failure times from the combined sample be given by $t_1 < \cdots < t_n$. At time t_j, with numbers still at risk in the two samples R_{1j} and R_{2j} and numbers of deaths D_{1j} and D_{2j}, the total number at risk and dying at t_j is $R_j = R_{1j} + R_{2j}$ and $D_j = D_{1j} + D_{2j}$ (Table 1).

Define the expected number of deaths in sample i from standard contingency table arguments to be $E_{ij} = R_{ij}D_j/R_j$. Further define the variance term $V_j = R_{1j}R_{2j}D_j(R_j - D_j)/R_j^2(R_j - 1)$. Then the numerator of the logrank test for

Table 1 Contingency table at time t_j

D_{1j}	$R_{1j} - D_{1j}$	R_{1j}
D_{2j}	$R_{2j} - D_{2j}$	R_{2j}
D_j	$R_j - D_j$	R_j

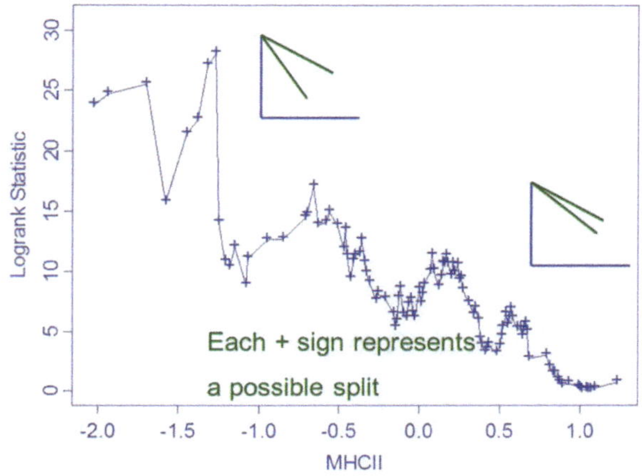

Fig. 5 An example of the running logrank test based on data from patients with non-Hodgkin lymphoma, using a covariate based on the major histocompatibility index 2 (MHCII). The y-axis is the value of the logrank test in χ^2 form for patients above and below each value of MHCII

comparing groups 1 and 2 is given by $L_{12} = \sum_{j=1}^{n} (D_{1j} - E_{1j})$, and the logrank test is $\left\{\sum_{j=1}^{n} (D_{1j} - E_{1j})\right\}^2 / \sum_{j=1}^{n} V_j$. Crowley [2] proved that the logrank test has an asymptotic χ^2 distribution with 1 degree of freedom under the null hypothesis of no association between survival and group assignment.

3.1 The Running Logrank Test

For a continuous or ordered categorical covariate X, the running logrank test is defined by performing two-sample logrank tests for all possible ways to form two-groups by those above and below a given cutpoint of X. An example plot of the resulting χ^2 statistic is given in Fig. 5, from which the optimal split can be found as the split which maximizes the logrank test.

This maximal value, and indeed the entire plot, can be judged against the permutation distribution, as illustrated in Fig. 6. A full explication is given in Crowley et al. [4]. Examples of the use of the logrank test in a recursive partitioning algorithm are given in LeBlanc and Crowley [6].

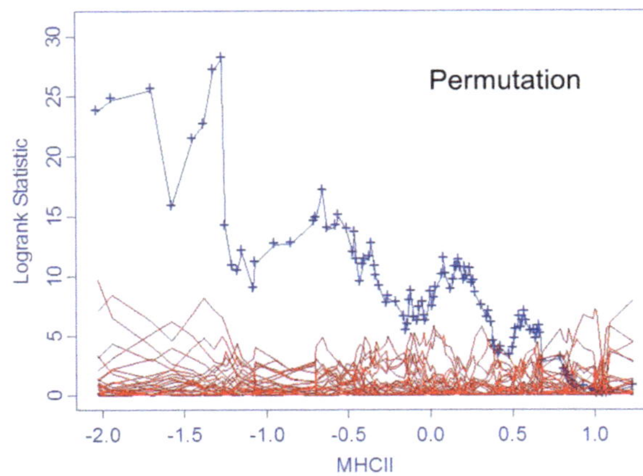

Fig. 6 Observed value of the running logrank test from Fig. 5, along with the permutation distribution. The signal clearly separates from the noise

3.2 Logrank Tests for Ordered Alternatives

Crowley [3] first proposed a modification of the logrank test sensitive to ordered alternatives of the form $S_1(t) \leq S_2(t) \leq \cdots \leq S_K(t)$, with at least one of the inequalities being strict. A Jonckheere [5] type statistic would be of the form $J = \sum_{i=1}^{K} \sum_{j=i+1}^{K} L_{ij}$, remembering that L_{ij} is the numerator of the logrank test for comparing group i to group j. It was also noted that by algebra $J = \sum_{i=1}^{K} \sum_{j=i+1}^{K} L_{ij} = \sum_{i=1}^{K-1} L^{(i)}$, where $L^{(i)}$ is the numerator of the logrank test for comparing group i to the pooled groups $i+1$ through K. This is particularly advantageous, as the $L^{(i)}$'s are uncorrelated [7]. Thus the standardized simple ordered logrank statistic is

$$SOL = \left\{ \sum_{i=1}^{K-1} L^{(i)} \right\}^2 \bigg/ \sum_{i=1}^{K-1} \operatorname{var}\left(L^{(i)}\right).$$

There are two issues with the simple ordered logrank test as defined. The first is that there is some arbitrariness in the order in which groups are compared. We can start by comparing group 1 to the combined groups 2 through K and proceed "up", as above (call this $SOL-1$), or we can start by comparing group K to the combined groups 1 through $K-1$, and proceed down ($SOL-2$). These are not the same. Secondly, as shown by Liu et al. [8], the simple ordered logrank test $SOL-1$ lacks power for alternatives of the form $S_1(t) < S_2(t) = \cdots = S_K(t)$, and symmetrically $SOL-2$ lacks power for alternatives of the form $S_1(t) = \cdots = S_{K-1}(t) < S_K(t)$. They proposed as an alternative a modified ordered logrank test. Define $L_{(i)}$ as the numerator of the logrank test for comparing the pooled groups 1 through i with the pooled groups $i+1$ through K. Then

$$MOL = \left\{ \sum_{i=1}^{K-1} L_{(i)} \right\}^2 \Big/ \left\{ \sum_{i=1}^{K-1} \mathrm{var}\left(L_{(i)}\right) + 2 \sum_{i<j} \mathrm{cov}\left(L_{(i)}, L_{(j)}\right) \right\},$$

where details of the covariance calculation are given in Liu and Tsai [9].

4 Three-Group Splits Based on a Single Covariate

We return to the example of patients with multiple myeloma treated with a Total Therapy regimen, and with gene expression profiling data as summarized in the GEP70 score. Separation into two risk groups was done by assessing the bimodal distribution of the score, resulting in a cutpoint of 0.66 (the optimal split based on the running logrank test is quite close to this value). The question arose—how best to define 3 risk groups?

Qu et al. [12] addressed this issue by defining a latent class model, which assumes that there ARE two-groups, but that there is an area of uncertainty in the score, in which it is unclear to which group the patient belongs (a grey zone). Their model assumed a Weibull distribution for progression-free survival within each risk group, and a logistic model for the probability of being in a risk group given the GEP70 score. The grey zone was defined by having a score such that the 95% confidence limits for the logistic probability included the value 0.5. This resulted in cutoffs of 0.49 and 1.07 for the score in the Total Therapy 2 training set. The resulting 3 progression-free survival curves are shown in Fig. 7, along with the results of applying these cutoffs to a test set of patients on Total Therapy 3.

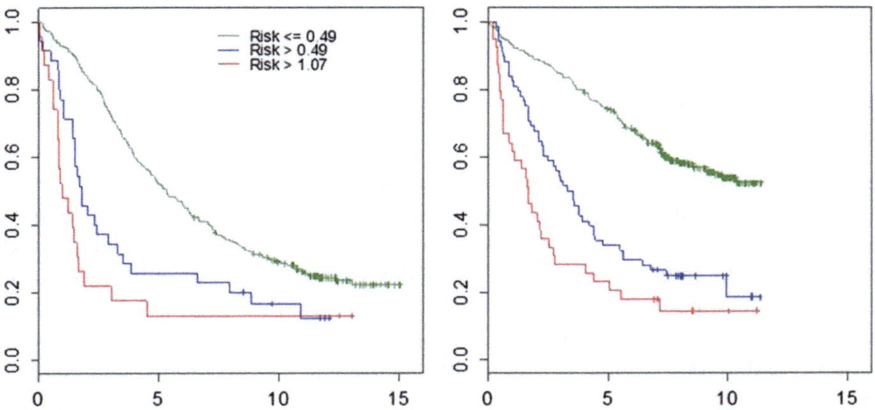

Fig. 7 Progression-free survival for groups defined by the grey zone model, the middle group being those who by the model are not clearly in either the high or low GEP70 risk groups. In the legend Risk > 0.49 is the middle group, for whom the risk score is between 0.49 and 1.07. The *left panel* is the training set Total Therapy 2, and the *right panel* applies the same cutpoints to the validation set Total Therapy 3

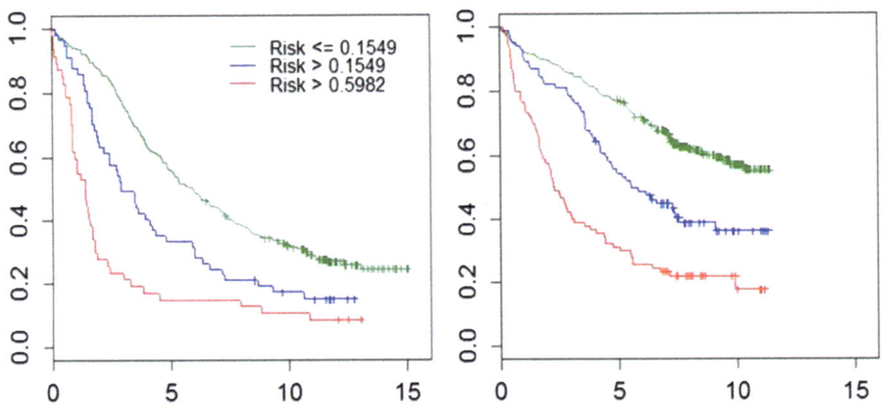

Fig. 8 Progression-free survival for groups determined by the MOL procedure in the training set (Total Therapy 2; *left panel*) and the validation set (Total Therapy 3; *right panel*). Note that in the legend Risk > 0.1549 is the intermediate group, with risk score between 0.1549 and 0.5982

The grey zone methods validates well, but note that the three resulting groups do not have comparable separations, the two higher risk groups being fairly similar. This motivated us to try the modified running ordered logrank test *MOL* to these same data. Thus instead of searching for all possible cutpoints of a single covariate, we search for all possible *pairs* of cutpoints, and choose the pair that maximizes the *MOL*. Applying this procedure to the Total Therapy 2 progression-free survival data gives cutpoints of 0.1549 and 0.5982. The resulting 3 curves are shown in Fig. 8, along with curves for the Total Therapy 3 validation set using the same cutpoints. Note that there is comparable separation among the 3-groups, which we consider a desirable outcome.

5 Simulations

In an effort to see whether the proposed method for finding optimal three-group splits based on a single covariate can uncover underlying structure, we performed a simulation study based on an exponential model and a uniformly distributed covariate on the interval [0,2]. The first model specified the exponential parameter as a step function, $\lambda = 3 - I(x \geq 0.67) - I(x \geq 1.33)$, that is, 3 risk groups with hazards 3, 2 and 1, with cutpoints 0.67 and 1.33, and equal sample sizes for each group. We did 500 simulations, each with sample size 300, and found cutpoints for each simulation. For comparison we did a hierarchical running logrank split into 3-groups using two steps of a recursive partitioning algorithm, applying the running logrank test at each step (the first step chooses an optimal cutpoint, the next step fixes that cutpoint and chooses the next best split on the covariate, in either of the original groups). We also included in the simulations Tarone's trend test [13],

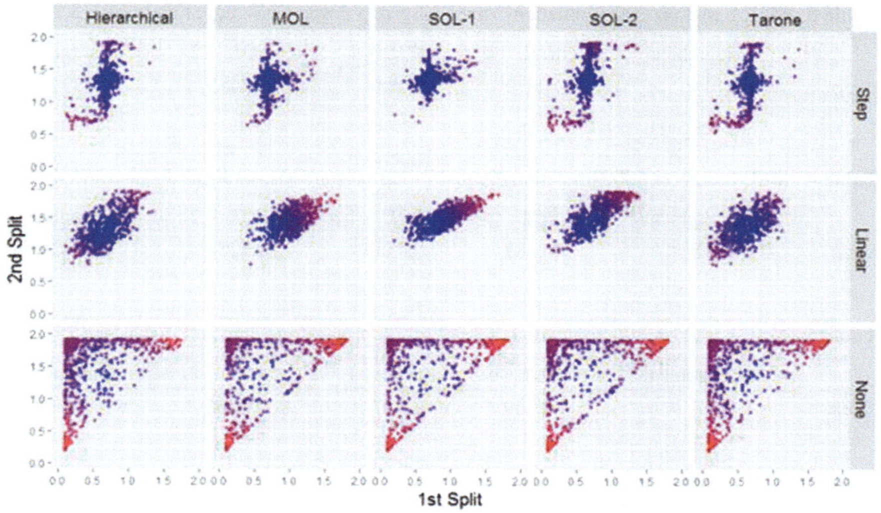

Fig. 9 Results of 500 simulations for a step function covariate (*top row*), a linear covariate (*middle row*) and a null model (*bottom row*). *Blue dots* are closer to the "true" cutpoints, *red dots* are farther away

Table 2 MSE based on 500 simulations (equal group proportions, equal distances (3,2,1))

	Hierarchical	*MOL*	*SOL* − 1	*SOL* − 2	Tarone
Step	0.0950	0.0653	0.0414	0.1327	0.1090
Linear	0.1177	0.2058	0.1916	0.1834	0.1122

which is a Cox regression [1] with covariate (3,2,1) for the 3-groups, respectively. We chose for simplicity not to include censoring in the simulations. The results are plotted in Fig. 9 (top row), from which it is apparent that the two ordered logrank procedures *MOL* and *SOL* − 1 produce somewhat tighter clustering around the true cutpoints of 0.67 and 1.33 than the 3 other methods. From the pattern in Fig. 9 it seems that *SOL* − 2, Tarone's trend test and the hierarchical procedure tend to be less sensitive to the choice of the second cutpoint. The middle row of Fig. 9 shows the results of a model which is linear in the covariate, which should favor the trend test, and the bottom row is from a null model, showing no apparent clustering.

We also calculated the mean squared error (MSE), the Euclidean distance between the estimated and true cutpoints averaged across the 500 simulations, for both the step function and linear models. (For the linear model we took the "true" cutpoints to be at 0.67 and 1.33, giving equal sample sizes to the 3-groups.) The results are given in Table 2, from which it can be seen that for the step function model *SOL* − 1 is the best of the 5 procedures, followed closely by *MOL*. For the linear model Tarone performs best as expected, with the hierarchical procedure nearly the same, while the 3 ordered logrank procedures perform relatively poorly.

Table 3 MSE based on 500 simulations (unequal group proportions, equal distances (3,2,1))

	Hierarchical	MOL	$SOL-1$	$SOL-2$	Tarone
Step	0.1144	0.0679	0.0858	0.2455	0.0999

Table 4 MSE based on 500 simulations (equal group proportions, unequal distances (5,4,1))

	Hierarchical	MOL	$SOL-1$	$SOL-2$	Tarone
Step	0.1798	0.2187	0.0359	0.3284	0.3133

Table 5 MSE based on 500 simulations (equal group proportions, unequal distances (5,2,1))

	Hierarchical	MOL	$SOL-1$	$SOL-2$	Tarone
Step	0.0165	0.2359	0.3107	0.0666	0.0211

We varied the cutpoints and proportions in each group and found that sometimes MOL is the best of the 5 procedures, followed closely by $SOL-1$, and otherwise there are no substantive differences in the rankings of the procedures. For example, a step function model with cutpoints 0.5 and 1.0, and sample fractions 1/4, 1/4, and 1/2 yields results for MSE as in Table 3.

Varying the distance between the groups made a larger difference in the simulation results. With the step function model with cutpoints 0.67 and 1.33 and equal group sizes, but hazards 5,4,1, the results are in Table 4, and with hazards 5,2,1, Table 5.

From these and other simulations, some observations emerge. When there are 3-groups, the comparison between $SOL-1$ and $SOL-2$ depends on whether groups 1 and 2 are close together, or groups 2 and 3, because of the way groups are combined in the test statistic. The modified ordered logrank test MOL represents a more robust alternative test. Tarone's test often performs similarly to the hierarchical running logrank procudeure, and is the best when the linear model holds.

6 Computational Considerations

The computational burden in finding optimal 3-group splits via the ordered logrank tests is heavy, with calculations being on the order of n^2 rather than order n as with 2-group splits (and thus the hierarchical procedure). This is of course especially important for simulation studies and for permutation assessment of the null distribution. An important shortcut for the ordered logrank and hierarchical recursive partitioning procedures is an updating algorithm for the running logrank test due to LeBlanc and Crowley [6] which increases the computational speed by eliminating the need for a recalculation of all the risk sets from scratch. It is possible that a

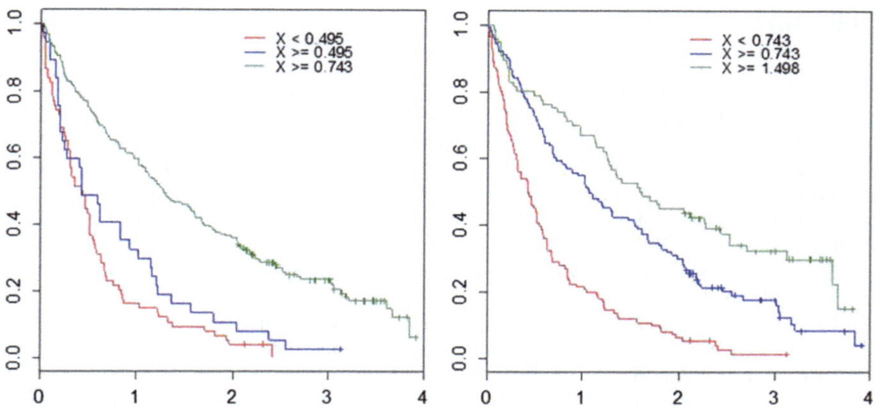

Fig. 10 Simulated survival based on cutpoints determined by the MOL procedure (*left panel*) and the hierarchical procedure (*right panel*) in a case where the MOL does poorly while the hierarchical does well

one-step version (first step of the Newton–Raphson algorithm) of Tarone's test might entail similar improvements in computational speed, but perhaps at the price of an increase in MSE.

7 Concluding Remarks

We have attempted to motivate the use of some version of a running ordered logrank test as an algorithm for creating 3 risk groups based on a single covariate. The idea appears promising based on its application to data on myeloma patients from the Myeloma Institute of the University of Arkansas for Medical Sciences. The modified ordered logrank procedure *MOL* appears to be the best among the 3 ordered logrank tests for a step function model for the covariate, though in certain situations the hierarchical procedure is better. In an effort to understand the differing results with the modified ordered logrank test *MOL* compared to the hierarchical recursive partitioning algorithm, we chose one simulation where the hierarchical procedure did well and *MOL* did not. The results are given in Fig. 10, from which it is apparent that the procedure using *MOL* might preferentially choose cutpoints where the survival of 2 of the 3-groups is relatively close.

Tarone's trend test and the hierarchical procedure perform best under a linear model ideally suited for Tarone's test, but the hierarchical procedure is to be preferred, being comparable in terms of MSE and much better in terms of speed. Further simulations could help define when the *MOL* is the statistic of choice for optimal 3-group splits.

References

1. Cox DR. Regression models and life tables. J R Stat Soc Ser B. 1972;34:187–202.
2. Crowley J. Non-parametric analysis of censored survival data, with distribution for the *k*-sample generalized savage statistic. Ph.D. dissertation, University of Washington; 1973.
3. Crowley J. Some extensions of the logrank test. In: Lindberg DAB, Reicherts PL, editors. Medical informatics, Lecture Notes, vol. 4; 1979, p. 213–23.
4. Crowley J, LeBlanc M, Gentleman R, Salmon S. Exploratory methods in survival analysis. In: IMS Lecturer notes, vol. 27; 1995, p. 55–77.
5. Jonckheere AR. A distribution-free *k*-sample test against ordered alternatives. Biometrika. 1954;41:133–45.
6. LeBlanc M, Crowley J. Survival trees by goodness of split. J Am Stat Assoc. 1993;88:457–67.
7. Liu PY, Greeen S, Wolf M, Crowley J. Testing against ordered alternatives for censored survival data. J Am Stat Assoc. 1993;88:153–60.
8. Liu PY, Tsai WY, Wolf M. Design and analysis for survival data under order restrictions with a modified logrank test. Stat Med. 1998;17:1469–79.
9. Liu PY, Tsai WY. A modified logrank test for censored survival data under order restrictions. Stat Probab Lett. 1999;41:57–63.
10. Mantel N. Evaluation of survival data and two new rank order statistics arising in its evaluation. Cancer Chemother Rep. 1966;50:163–70.
11. Peto R, Peto J. Asymptotically efficient rank invariant test procedures. J R Stat Soc Ser A. 1972;135:185–98.
12. Qu P, Barlogie B, Crowley J. Using a latent class model to refine risk stratification in multiple myeloma. Stat Med. 2015;34:2971–80.
13. Tarone RE. Tests for trend in life table analysis. Biometrika. 1975;62:679–82.

A Smooth Basis for Clinical Subgroup Analysis

Michael LeBlanc

Abstract Data partitioning methods, including regression trees, have been widely used to describe subgroups of cancer patients with differing prognosis. We describe an alternative technique based on a modeling that characterizes subgroups through a smooth basis function representation of subgroups. The strategy allows the user to control the expected number of patients in the subgroup as well as the anticipated survival in the targeted group. An example based on data from a clinical trial for patients with Myeloma is used to illustrate the new method.

Keywords Regression · Tree-based Regression · Prognostic Groups

1 Introduction

There is a continuing need to expand the current set of analytic tools to better understand the complex heterogeneity of patient outcomes in cancer clinical trials. Our focus will be on extending statistical modeling tools that are helpful in facilitating the development of new clinical trials. We will discuss methods that give well defined and interpretable prognostic groups and are potentially less variable than the results obtained from tree-based algorithms. In addition, it is often useful to control the mass of the prognostic groups (or size of the subgroups), and as such the new method allows for that control.

In this chapter we propose a simple procedure based on combining existing algorithmic components that yields model components that can lead to decision rules. We first provide more motivation for constructing subgroups first in the univariate setting, but then with multiple variables. We then describe a transformation of regression variables using a basis function representation, and show how the new method fits into a general regression model formulation. We end with a clinical trial data set example.

M. LeBlanc (✉)
SWOG Statistical Center, Fred Hutchinson Cancer Research Center,
Seattle, WA, USA
e-mail: mleblanc@fredhutch.org

S. Matsui and J. Crowley (eds.), *Frontiers of Biostatistical Methods and Applications in Clinical Oncology*, DOI 10.1007/978-981-10-0126-0_15

2 Background

Providing simple descriptions of individuals with extreme risk, differing prognosis or even greater treatment effect has long been an interest in oncology. Many methods have been proposed that lead to simple logical or Boolean descriptions of subgroups of patients. The most widely utilized is the decision rule (or cut-point) developed on a single ordered biomarker related to patient outcome. This optimization has even been extended to simultaneously look for multiple sub-groups ([4], this monograph). For cases of more than one marker or predictor, many techniques have been developed that yield simple decision rules. These methods include tree-based models [3, 5, 10, 11, 18, 7, 15], rule induction methods sometimes called bump hunting or peeling [6, 12], extreme regression [13] and methods that construct Boolean combinations of binary predictors using a method called Logic Regression [14]. While these methods have been useful, alternative rule based methods that yield less variable results that can be used for decision making and trial design are worthy of investigation.

As general motivation, below we consider a single gene expression variable for a group of patients with Diffuse B-Cell Lymphoma (DBCL). The gene called DR-Alpha (a member of MHC-Class II) genes is shown in Fig. 1. The smooth line is a non-parametric estimate of the logarithm of the hazard ratio as a function of values of the marker based on B-spline basis in Cox regression (e.g. [16]. One can see here the hazard estimate decreases with increases in the marker. In other words, survival is worse for patients with low values of the marker. In addition to this relationship, it could be important to describe that rule for the region or the subgroup R = {log DR-Alpha < −1}, the fraction of the patients that would fall into that group, v(R), and the outcomes associated with that group.

While the strategy to select a single subgroup is relatively straightforward in the univariate setting, obtaining decision rules in more than one dimension is more complex. The best known class of algorithms is called tree-based or recursive partitioning. In Fig. 2 we provide an example, this time with patients that have been

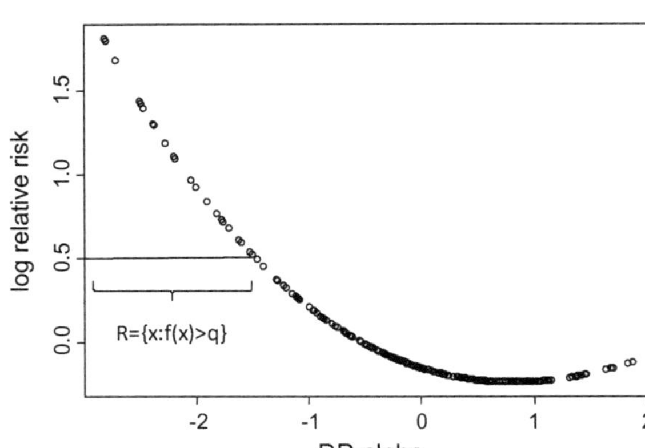

Fig. 1 Smooth estimate of relative risk as a function of gene expression DR-alpha for diffuse large B-Cell Lymphoma patients. The region or subgroup of patients corresponding to those with poor survival or high hazard is indicated by region R

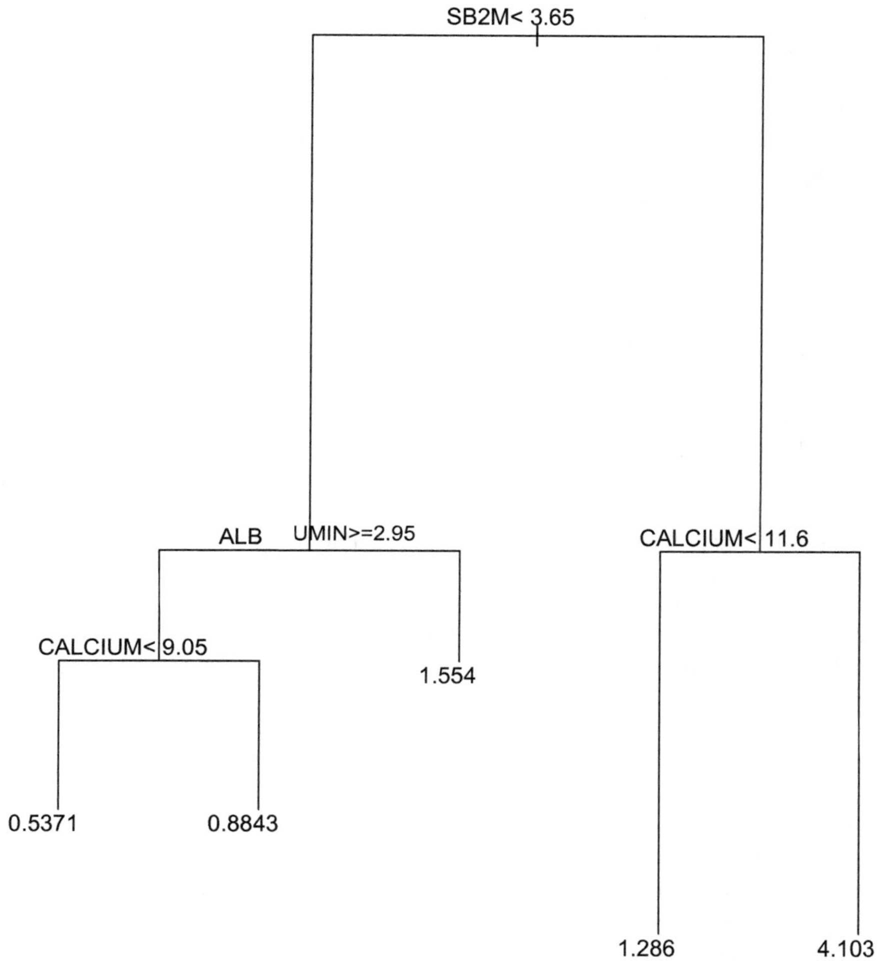

Fig. 2 Survival tree for patients with multiple myeloma. The terminal nodes in the tree give hazard ratios relative to the root node

treated for multiple myeloma. Without going into the details of how the model is built, the rule appears as in Fig. 2. Successive univariate rules are estimated from the data. Individuals associated with a terminal node (the end of any branch) are those where the covariate rules apply for all the univariate rules down the path. Thus the right-most node of the tree, corresponding to patients with high SB2M (Serum beta2 microglobulin) and high CALCIUM (Serum Calcium) have the worst survival, corresponding to a hazard ratio of 4.1 relative to the root node or overall group hazard. For individuals in each group one could describe the prognosis or survival for patients falling into that group.

While it has been recognized that trees yield useful descriptions, their extreme discreteness can lead to relatively poor prediction and in some settings where calibrating the size of the prognostic group is important, they are also too discrete to achieve that goal. To address these issues, ensembles of trees and other machine learning methods [2, 8] have been proposed, but the trade-off is that one can lose the simple or parsimonious decision rule interpretation. This proposal works by first viewing the prognostic subgroup modeling problem in terms of a regression function representation.

2.1 Examples of Basis Function Regression

First we review some useful regression methods that are comprised of combinations of simple univariate functions. While applications typically considered in oncology use time-to-event (survival) data, or response binary data, we present background and develop the ideas in terms of a general regression model set up. For instance, with survival data there would be an observed time under observations T and an indicator of whether the subject was observed to fail at the time denoted as $\delta = \{0, 1\}$. The underlying survival model is assumed to be modulated by patient characteristics $\mathbf{x}$ through an index regression function $\eta(\mathbf{x})$. We start with the simple linear model and reference some extensions. The linear model

$$\eta(\mathbf{x}) = \sum_{i=1}^{p} \beta_i \mathbf{x}_i$$

can also be used as the starting point for non-linear, non-additive, multivariate regression methods. In the survival data setting the linear model could represent the linear regression component in a proportional hazards model. Assume that the regression function $\eta(\mathbf{x})$ is in some and let $B_1(\mathbf{x}), \ldots, B_p(\mathbf{x})$ be a basis for linear functions useful to model the outcome distributions. Then we can write a generalized regression function as follows:

$$\eta(\mathbf{x}) = \sum_{i=1}^{p} \beta_i B_i(\mathbf{x}). \tag{1}$$

The linear model most widely used model in prognostic settings, is frequently based on the Cox's proportional hazards model.

Several nonparametric multivariate regression methodologies use a basis function approach, but rather than fixing the initial set of basis functions, these approaches select the space at the same time the coefficients of the basis functions are estimated. Some extensions are highlighted below:

- Multivariate Adaptive Regression Splines (MARS) and related spline methods (e.g. [9]): The basis functions that are used for MARS and related methods are piecewise polynomials (splines) and their tensor products.
- Regression tree methods, such as Classification and Regression Trees (CART, [3]): The basis functions that are used for tree methods are indicator functions corresponding to rectangular regions of the predictor space.
- Logic Regression [14] is discussed below. The basis functions that are used for Logic Regression are Boolean combinations of binary predictors.
- Rule Induction or Peeling [6, 12]: For this method there is a sequence of basis function $B_i(\mathbf{x})$ representing nested boxes in the covariate space, but only one is chosen for a given model.

Smooth regression methods using splines likely better capture the underlying association but do not lead to simple descriptive subset rules. Regression tree or Logic Regression methods are similar with respect to defining subsets or subgroups of subjects based on Boolean or logical rules.

2.2 *Trees via Basis Functions*

Tree-based models have been described in many publications. However, a key aspect of these models that needs to be emphasized is the concept of recursive data splitting. Each split is induced by a rule of the form "$x \in S$" where $S \subset X$. For ordered variables the rule is of the form

$$S = \{x : x_j \leq c\},$$

or S is a subset rule

$$S \subset B = \{v_1, v_2, \ldots, v_r\}$$

of the r values of x_j for categorical variables. The tree model is grown in a forward stepwise fashion. For the remaining data set and predictor space, each variable and potential split point is evaluated. The algorithm can be represented as generating a sequence of indicator basis functions. Any split at a node h yields two nodes that can also be represented with a pair of basis functions. Here, focusing only on the ordered variable setting, the new basis function would be

$$b^{+}_{h(j)}(\mathbf{x}) = I\{x_{h(j)} > c_{h(j)}\} \text{ and } b^{-}_{h(j)}(\mathbf{x}) = I\{x_{h(j)} \leq c_{h(j)}\}.$$

Each step in the growing tree replaces a current node h with a left and right daughter nodes $l(h)$ and $r(h)$, or in other words, the current basis function $B_h(x)$ for node h with the basis functions $B_{l(h)}(\mathbf{x})$ and $B_{r(h)}(\mathbf{x})$

$$B_{l(h)}(\mathbf{x}) = B_h(\mathbf{x})b^{+}_{h(j)}(\mathbf{x}) \text{ and } B_{r(h)}(\mathbf{x}) = B_h(\mathbf{x})b^{-}_{h(j)}(\mathbf{x}).$$

This split is equivalent to just creating a new basis function in the regression model (1). For example, a typical regression function representing a node in a tree would be

$$L(\mathbf{x}) = I\{x_1 > c_1\} \text{ and } I\{x_2 \leq c_2\} \text{ and } I\{x_3 > c_3\}.$$

2.3 Logic Regression and Basis

While Logic Regression models are constructed differently than trees, they can still can be viewed as having a similar regression function representation:

$$f = \beta_0 + \sum \beta_j L_j(X).$$

The Logic Regression method used combinations of variables through basis functions of binary data of

$$L_{ij} = \{X_{ij} = 1\} \text{ OR } \overline{L}_{ij} = \{X_{ij} = 0\}$$

for covariate j and observation i. For instance, a three term logic expression is

$$L_{i1} \text{ AND } L_{i2} \text{ OR } \overline{L}_{i3}.$$

This is a natural method for binary or discrete variables but "AND" or "OR" is not a natural combination function for ordered variables. The primary reason we are re-introducing Logic regression as part of this work is to motivate a modification to regression modeling that would be appropriate for ordered variables and combinations.

2.4 A New Smooth Basis Function and Combinations of Variables

We propose to evaluate a new function approximation method that characterizes individual ordered or continuous factors in terms of quantiles of their distribution function, which can be used to describe regions or subgroups, R, described above. In prior work, we used extreme functions (maximum and minimum) to construct extreme regression functions, but that work used linear sub-functions and was applicable only to continuous predictors [13]. However, optimization of the individual component functions is quite complex for that method. Here we focus on a simpler model building method analogous to tree-based regression or step-wise regression.

First we replace the step function transformation used in regression trees (with ordered variables) with something smoother. For instance, we propose that

$$I\{x_1 > c_1\} \text{ or } 1 - I\{x_1 > c_1\}$$

could be just replaced with the rank transformation of the covariate, in terms of the empirical distribution or survival distribution of the ordered covariate,

$$F_n(X) \text{ or } 1 - F_n(X).$$

The empirical distribution function of the ordered feature is a natural extension of the binary feature variable $\{0, 1\}$ used in trees or Logic Regression. One could also consider parameterized transformations of the distribution function

$$g_a(F_n(X)) : [0, 1] \rightarrow 0, 1]$$

to control for the impact of the variable X relative to other variables in the model. An example of simple transformation would be

$$g_a(F_n(X)) = F_n(X)^a$$

which is the power basis. Alternatively one could use a truncated spline a

$$\begin{aligned} F_n(X)^{(c+)} &= aF_n(X) \text{ if } aF_n(X) < c \\ &= 1 \text{ if } aF_n(X) > c. \end{aligned}$$

Limiting our discussion to the power basis one could use the complement function,

$$\overline{g}_a(F_n(X)) = 1 - g_a(F_n(X)),$$

or use these empirically transformed variables

$$b^+_{h(j)}(\mathbf{x}) = g_a(F_n(X_{h(j)})) \text{ and } b^-_{h(j)}(\mathbf{x}) = 1 - g_a(F_n(X_{h(j)})).$$

An obvious choice is to consider products of the basis functions for each node in the tree,

$$L_j(X) = g_a(F_n(X_1))g_a(F_n(X_2))(1 - g_a(F_n(X_3))).$$

However, this definition is not directly useful in deriving regression rules. However, a special surface is obtained by replacing the product term with the minimum function. For instance, the term

$$L_j(X) = \min(g_a(F_n(X_1)), g_a(F_n(X_2)), 1 - g_a(F_n(X_3))$$

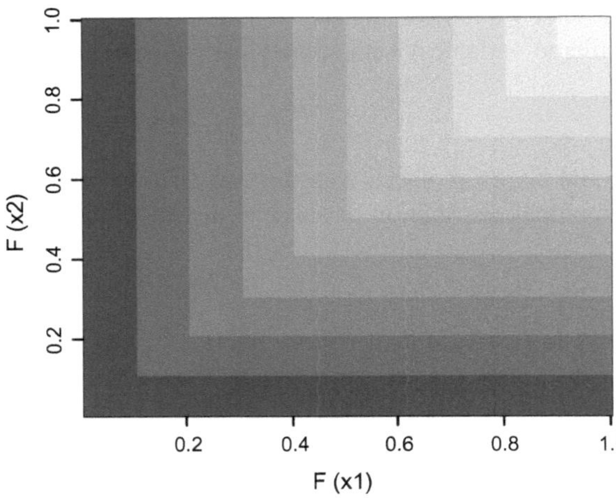

Fig. 3 Example of the combination of two basis functions $\min(F_n(X_1), F_n(X_2))$. The surface is locally univariate and the threshold rule would be in the form of the simple binary decision rule

results in a simple inverse function for the component term, $L_j(X)$. That is, for each component term lead, any level $\beta_j L_j(X) > q$ describes a Boolean decision rule. In this case, the level sets or contours of the function move along coordinate axes, and the subset of patients defined by any $L_j(X) < q$ is a Boolean combination of individual thresholds $F_n(X_j) < q_j$ or $F_n(X_j) \geq q_j$. That is, each basis function for a given level output $L_j(X) > q$ results q-level set $\Omega = \{x : L_j(x) \geq q\}$. There are strong connections to our prior work, Extreme Regression, but here we just construct simple rank based transformations to construct regression models, rather than trying to jointly specify a complex regression function of a combination of minima and maxima of component terms used as part of extreme regression.

In Fig. 3, we give an example of a component term using the new method. Note that the surface for the minimum-based basis function is locally univariate; so any decision rule is an AND function. There is considerable flexibility with respect to shapes depending on the power parameters. Some examples are given in Fig. 4.

3 Algorithm: Expand and Select

We propose to use standard regression function methods to combine the component functions

$$f = \beta_0 + \beta Z + \sum \beta_j L_j(\boldsymbol{X}).$$

We propose a simple model building strategy. For each variable X_j, consider a range of transformation parameters $a_1, \ldots, a_k$. This creates a set of potential basis functions:

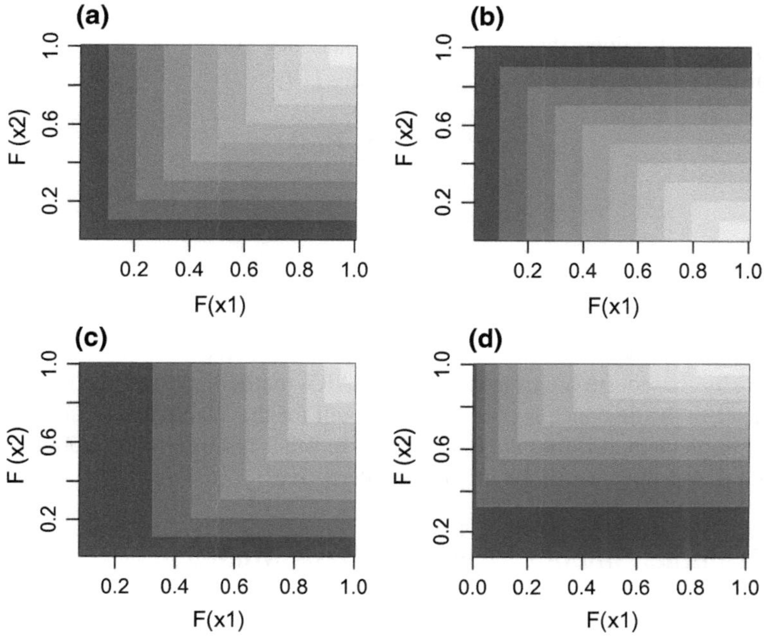

Fig. 4 Four examples of the combination of two basis functions **a** $\min(F_n(X_1), F_n(X_2))$, **b** $\min(F_n(X_1), 1 - F_n(X_2))$, **c** $\min(F_n(X_1)^{.5}, F_n(X_2))$, **d** $\min(F_n(X_1)^2, F_n(X_2)^{.5})$

$$\{g_{a_1}(F_n(X_1)), \ldots g_{a_k}(F_n(X_1)), \ldots g_{a_1}(F_n(X_p)), \ldots g_{a_k}(F_n(X_p))\}.$$

Once that set of basis functions is constructed, consider that set for inclusion in the model. In addition, allow for more complex basis functions to be considered by combining them with one of the existing sets of basis functions

$$\{B_{m+1}(X) = \min(B_m(X), g_{a_j}(F_n(X_r))\}.$$

Here, the combination uses the minimum function, unlike most adaptive regression function settings where the combinations used to construct interactions are products. This stepwise process is continued, adding terms to grow a model to a full size of K terms.

Now we use Lasso [17] regression (or elastic net) to choose which terms to retain in the model and to estimate the component terms,

$$-l(\beta, \lambda) = -\sum_{i=1}^{n_k} l_i(\beta) + \lambda P(\beta),$$

where $P(\beta)$ represents a penalty term, λ is a positive penalty parameter, and $\beta = (\beta_1, \ldots \beta_p)$. Given that simplicity and variance control are both critical, it is natural to consider an elastic net type penalty [19],

$$P_\alpha(\beta) = \sum_j P_\alpha(\beta_j)$$

where

$$P_\alpha(\beta_j) = [(1 - \alpha)\beta_j^2 + \alpha|\beta_j|].$$

Although in many settings the elastic net will give better predictions, because we want simple models the Lasso method is preferred. We choose to select model complexity based on a variation of the AIC method, where the usual 2 per parameter in the deviance is doubled to account for the adaptive selection. We have not yet implemented k-fold cross-validation or other resampling techniques for this algorithm, but they would be a feasible alternative.

4 Example: Smooth Prognostic Basis Modeling

We will demonstrate the modeling method on data generated from patients treated for multiple myeloma on a clinical trial conducted by SWOG. The study was a randomized Phase III study considering Standard Dose Versus Myeloablative Therapy for Previously Untreated Symptomatic Multiple Myeloma [1]. Data considered in this example used five prognostic factors [Calcium, WBC, Serum beta 2 microglobulin, Albumin and Lactate Dehydroginase (LDH)], and survival times as outcomes. For this example we chose to only use cases with complete data elements. In addition, because this was only to be intended as an exploration of the new method, we chose to simulate the data via empirical bootstrap to achieve 600 cases from the existing data set of 432 cases. Thus this can be viewed as an empirically motivated simulated data set.

We used the stepwise version of the method described above. We chose to select the model complexity number of terms based on the AIC type penalty rather than cross-validation to simplify computation. However, to acknowledge the additional selection bias due to basis set selection, we used an AIC penalty of 4 rather than the standard value of 2.

Ultimately the model selected had 3 terms with two terms involving a single variable and the final term involving 3 variables:

$$f(\text{serum b2}) + f(\text{calcium}) + f(\text{serum b2, calcium, wbc}).$$

Importantly, since the goal is to be able to describe decision rules, we also present the inverse of the component functions. It allows us to describe the rule that corresponds to the worst (or best) grouping of patients based on that component function. Figure 5 shows each of the inverse component functions, which happened to correspond to the 1st, 2nd and 4th terms in the model before it was simplified, and are denoted as eta 1, eta 2 and eta 4. For example, if one wanted the group of patients where the hazard ratio estimator for the term *f*(serum b2, calcium, wbc) > .15, then that would approximately correspond to patients described by

$$\{\text{calcium} > 9.2\}\text{AND}\{\text{serum b2} > 3.5\}\text{AND}\{wbc < 7\}.$$

To explore the marginal impact of each component term, Fig. 6 presents survival curves for all patients as divided by the 25th, 50th and 75th percentiles of the data.

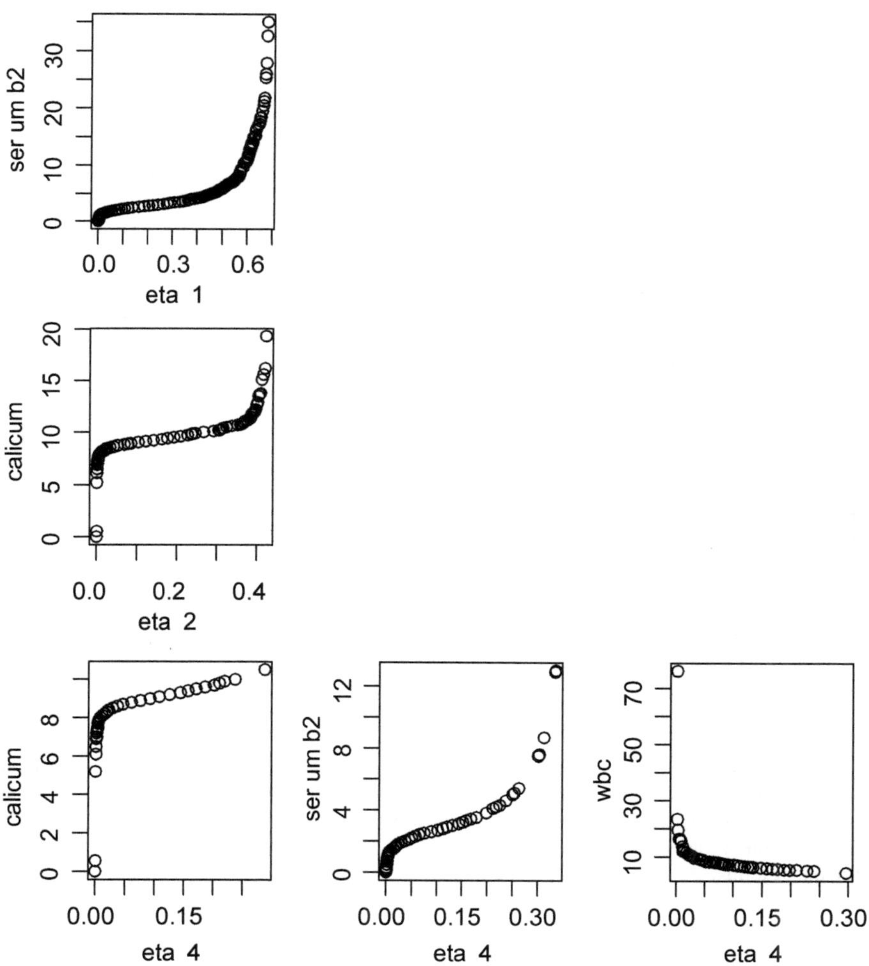

Fig. 5 Inverse function representation of each of the component functions of the new method. The y-axis of each plot give the prognostic variable in the original scale. The x-axis for each plot is the regression component function value $\widehat{\beta}_j g_j(X)$.

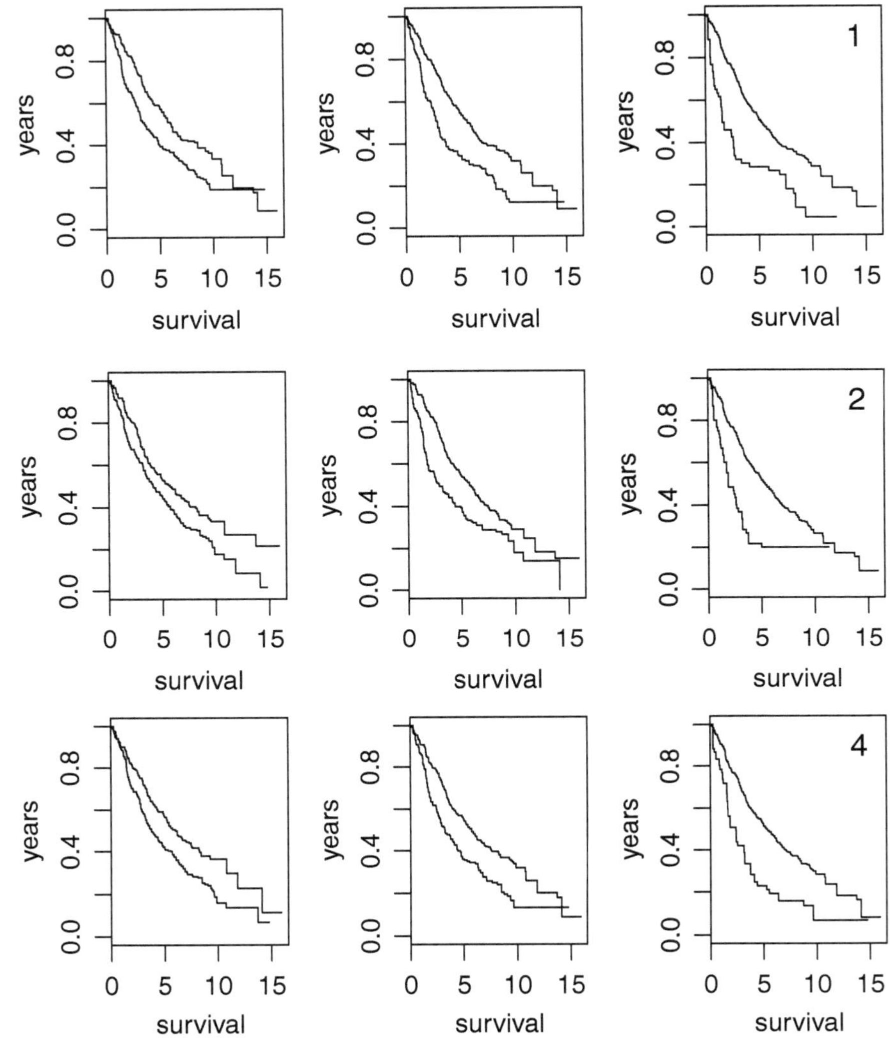

Fig. 6 A panel showing the impact of splitting patients into two groups based on 25th, 50th and 75th percentile of each of the component functions(terms) in the final model. The model terms are (1) serum beta 2, (2) serum calcium, (3) combination of serum beta 2, serum calcium and wbc. Therefore, these plots represent the "marginal" association with survival for each of these component terms

5 Discussion

We presented a simple experimental extension to standard regression models. It consists of two parts: first, each covariate is rank transformed (or transformed to its empirical distribution or survival function) and then different power transformations are evaluated. Second, a model building method is used where interactions are built up with minimum functions rather than products. These two small changes result in a procedure that is covariate transformation invariant. In addition, any value of the component of the regression function can be represented by a simple rule consisting of an AND function, which leads to cut-point or decision rules for individual model terms.

References

1. Barlogie B, Kyle RA, Anderson KC, Greipp PR, Lazarus HM, Hurd DD, McCoy J, Moore DF Jr, Dakhil SR, Lanier KS, Chapman RA, Cromer JN, Salmon SE, Durie B, Crowley JC. Standard chemotherapy compared with high-dose chemoradiotherapy for multiple myeloma: final results of phase III US Intergroup Trial S9321. J Clin Oncol. 2006;24 (6):929–36.
2. Breiman L. Random forests. Mach Learn. 2001;45:5–32.
3. Breiman L, Friedman J, Olshen R, Stone C. Classification and regression trees. Pacific Grove: Wadsworth; 1984.
4. Crowley J. Optimal three group splits for survival data based on a running ordered logrank test, Frontiers of Biostatistical Methods. Berlin: Springer; 2016.
5. Davis R, Anderson J. Exponential survival trees. Stat Med. 1989;8:947–62.
6. Friedman J, Fisher N. Bump hunting in high dimensional data(with discussion). Stat Comput. 1999;9:123–62.
7. Gordon L, Olshen R. Tree-structured survival analysis. Cancer Treat Rep. 1985;69:1062–9.
8. Ishwaran H, Kogalur UB, Blackstone EH, Lauer MS. Random survival forests. Ann Appl Stat. 2008;2:841–60.
9. Kooperberg C, Stone C, Truong Y. Hazard regression. J Am Stat Assoc. 1995;90:78–94.
10. LeBlanc M, Crowley J. Relative risk regression trees for censored survival data. Biometrics. 1992;48:411–27.
11. LeBlanc M, Crowley J. Survival trees by goodness of split. J Am Stat Assoc. 1993;88:457–67.
12. LeBlanc M, Moon J, Crowley J. Adaptive risk group refinement. Biometrics. 2005;61:370–8.
13. LeBlanc M, Moon J, Kooperberg C. Extreme regression. Biostatistics. 2006;13(106–122):2006.
14. Ruczinski I, Kooperberg C, LeBlanc M. Logic regression. J Graph Comput Stat. 2003;12:475–511.
15. Segal MR. Regression trees for censored data. Biometrics. 1988;44:35–47.
16. Sleeper LA, Harrington DP. Regression splines in teh cox model with application to covariate effects in liver disease. J Am Stat Assoc. 1990;85:941–9.

17. Tibshirani R. Regression shrinkage and selection via the lasso. J R Stat Soc B. 1996;58:267–88.
18. Zhang H, Singer B. Recursive partitioning in the health sciences. New York: Springer; 1999.
19. Zou H, Hastie T. Regularization and variable selection via the elastic net. J R Stat Soc B. 2005;67:301–20.

Meta-Analysis of Prognostic Studies Evaluating Time-Dependent Diagnostic and Predictive Capacities of Biomarkers

Satoshi Hattori and Xiao-Hua Zhou

Abstract Prognostic biomarker studies, which examine the association between biomarkers and patients' prognoses, have played important roles in clinical decision making. Since prognostic studies are often conducted with small sample sizes in a limited number of centers, meta-analysis is expected to be a powerful tool to obtain sound evidence on prognostic biomarkers. However, the application of meta-analysis of prognostic studies has been limited partly due to the lack of sound statistical methods. In this chapter, we introduce some recently developed methods useful for the evaluation of diagnostic or predictive capacities of biomarkers for binary or time-to-event outcomes. In addition, we newly present a novel method to estimate the time-dependent positive and negative predictive value curves based on meta-analysis.

Keywords Cutoff value · Diagnostic studies · Prognostic studies · Meta-analysis · Time-dependent predictive value curve · Time-dependent receiver operating characteristics

1 Introduction

Prognostic studies have been widely conducted to determine whether specific biomarkers or other demographic factors such as age are associated with patients' prognoses. Such studies are very useful to understand disease progression and to

---

S. Hattori (✉)
Department of Integrated Medicine, Biomedical Statistics, Osaka University, 2-2, Yamada-Oka, Suita, Osaka 565-0871, Japan
e-mail: hattoris@biostat.med.osaka-u.ac.jp

X.-H. Zhou
HSR&D Center of Excellence, VA Puget Sound Health Care System, Seattle, USA

X.-H. Zhou
Department of Biostatistics, University of Washington, Seattle, WA 98195, USA

S. Matsui and J. Crowley (eds.), *Frontiers of Biostatistical Methods and Applications in Clinical Oncology*, DOI 10.1007/978-981-10-0126-0_16

identify subgroups of patients with poor/good prognoses. Therefore, they have played important roles in clinical decision making, healthcare policy, and patient management [18]. However, as noted by several authors [1, 19, 23, 31, 32], prognostic studies are often conducted with small sample size data from a single or a few centers. Therefore, the findings in a prognostic study should be further assessed, and meta-analysis is expected to be useful for this purpose [32]. In the context of evaluating treatment efficacy in clinical trials, meta-analysis based on multiple independent studies has been widely applied as a powerful tool to derive more reliable evidence. Findings by well-conducted meta-analyses are regarded as highly reliable evidence [2].

However, the application of meta-analyses to prognostic studies has been very limited. Among meta-analyses of prognostic studies recently reported, Becattini et al. [3] conducted a meta-analysis to examine the association between troponins and short-term death (binary outcomes) in patients with an acute pulmonary embolism. They reported the combined odds ratio of the high-expression group of troponin relative to the low-expression group for short-term death. Meta-analyses of prognostic studies with time-to-event outcomes include de Azambujya et al. [11] for the antigen Ki-67 in early-stage breast cancer, Callagy et al. [5] for the protein BCL-2 in breast cancer, and Pak et al. [27] and Na et al. [26] for FDG-PET in head and neck cancer and lung cancer, respectively. They reported the combined hazard ratio of the high-expression group of a biomarker relative to the low-expression group across studies. The definition of high- and low-expression depends on a cut-off value for the biomarker, which is often study-specific. All the above-mentioned meta-analyses of prognostic studies simply applied standard meta-analysis techniques (such as fixed-effects or random-effects modelling), ignoring the presence of heterogeneous cut-off values and making it difficult or impossible to accurately interpret the combined odds or hazard ratio. This has been one of the pressing issues in the meta-analyses of prognostic studies [19, 31, 42].

The issue of using different marker cut-off values across studies also arises in meta-analyses of diagnostic studies. For meta-analysis of diagnostic studies, the summary receiver operating characteristics (sROC) curve based on a pair of the true positive rate (TPR) and the false positive rate (FPR) provides a way to make an inference freely from the specification of cut-off values [22, 25, 30]. Here the TPR and FPR are defined as conditional probabilities that a subject has an observation of the biomarker more than a cut-off value, given that he/she does have an event and does not, respectively. Recently, Hattori and Zhou [15] re-analyzed the acute pulmonary embolism data by Becattini et al. [3] by using the sROC curve and found that troponin T had a better diagnostic capacity than troponin I, which could not be clearly concluded by the combined odds ratios by Becattini et al. [3].

Another methodological perspective in the meta-analysis of prognostic studies is the application of other diagnostic measures, the positive predictive value (PPV) and the negative predictive value (NPV), rather than the sROC curve based on the TPR and FPR. Here the PPV is defined as the conditional probability that a subject will experience an event given that his/her biomarker is equal to or higher than the cut-off value, while the NPV is defined as the conditional probability that a subject will experience no event given that his/her biomarker value is less than the cut-off value. The PPV and NPV provide useful information to medical doctors and patients about the likely outcome for a given biomarker value [47]. Chu et al. [8] and Leeflang et al. [21] proposed to make a summary of pairs of the PPV and NPV with the summary operating point by applying the mixed-effect model. Riley et al. [34] proposed to show a predictive region of the pair, PPV and NPV, of future populations in presenting results of meta-analyses of diagnostic studies. However, the summary indices proposed by these authors were dependent on the cut-off values in the studies enrolled in the meta-analysis, so that it can be very hard to compare predictive capacities of two or more biomarkers based on the results by these methods. Hattori and Zhou [15] proposed a meta-analysis method for estimating the positive/negative predictive value curves, that was earlier introduced by Moskowitz and Pepe [24] in the presence of individual-level data (not in the setting of meta-analysis).

Another new direction in methodological research on meta-analysis of prognostic studies is to extend the sROC curve to time-to-event outcomes. Combescure et al. [9] proposed a method to estimate a time-dependent ROC curve [17, 41, 46] among others) in a meta-analysis of prognostic studies. Using the Kaplan–Meier estimate of the survival function from each study at several time points as data, Combescure et al. [9] proposed to apply a mixed-effect-based joint model with a piecewise constant hazards function for time-to-event and a parametric distribution of the biomarker. Hattori and Zhou [16] proposed two alternative methods, one an extension of the bivariate normal model by Reitsma et al. [30] and the other an extension of the bivariate binomial model by Macaskill [22].

In this chapter, we introduce the existing and some recently developed statistical methods for meta-analysis of prognostic studies. In Sect. 2, we briefly introduce some methods for meta-analysis of diagnostic studies with binary outcomes. In Sect. 2.1, we briefly review how to estimate the sROC curve. Although the use of a bivariate normal model by Reitsma et al. [30] provides a simple method to estimate the sROC curve, we focus on the method based on a bivariate binomial model by Macaskill [22], since it outperformed that based on the bivariate normal model when the number of studies is small [12]. In Sect. 2.2, we introduce a method to estimate the predictive value curves based on meta-analysis [15]. In Sect. 3, following Hattori and Zhou [16], we introduce a method to estimate the time-dependent summary ROC curve based on the bivariate binomial model. The key idea in this method is to impute the number of subject with the event before the time point of interest both in the high- and low-expression groups from the censored observations, and then to apply the bivariate binomial model. In Sect. 4, we introduce a new statistical methods to estimate the time-dependent positive/negative predictive curves [44, 45, 48] based on meta-analysis through applying the imputation idea to the method in Sect. 2.2. In Sect. 5, we illustrate the methods given in Sects. 3 and 4 using the data of BCL2 in breast cancer [5]. Lastly, we conclude this chapter with some discussion in Sect. 6.

2 Statistical Methods for the Meta-Analysis of Diagnostic Studies (Binary Outcome)

2.1 Data

Suppose we are interested in conducting a meta-analysis of S diagnostic studies (or prognostic studies with a binary outcome). Let D be a binary outcome (disease/non-disease) and X be a continuous biomarker of a subject. We assume the range of X is $[0, \infty)$. We consider to make an inference based on information from published papers. In this case, individual-level data of D and X are not observed. Suppose we have the following study-level data. Let $n^{(s)}$ be the number of subjects in the sth study and $n = \sum_{s=1}^{S} n^{(s)}$. Each study has a study-specific cut-off value for X, which is observable and denoted by $v^{(s)}$. For notational convenience, denote $v_0^{(s)} = 0, v_1^{(s)} = v^{(s)}$ and $v_2^{(s)} = \infty$. If a subject has X such as $X < v^{(s)}$, the subject is classified as the low-expression group, and otherwise as the high-expression group. Let $Z = I(X \geq v^{(s)})$ and $N_{zd}^{(s)}$ be a random variable, which denotes the number of subjects with $Z = z$ and $D = d$ in the sth study. Denote $N_{z+}^{(s)} = N_{z0}^{(s)} + N_{z1}^{(s)}$ and $N_{+d}^{(s)} = N_{0d}^{(s)} + N_{1d}^{(s)}$. Notation is summarized in Table 1. A realization of $N_{zd}^{(s)}$ is denoted by $n_{zd}^{(s)}$. Similarly, a realization of $N_{z+}^{(s)}$ and $N_{+d}^{(s)}$ is denoted by $n_{z+}^{(s)}$ and $n_{+d}^{(s)}$, respectively. Our observations are $\{n_{zd}^{(s)} : z = 0, 1, d = 0, 1\}$ and $v^{(s)}$ for $s = 1, 2, \ldots, S$.

2.2 Summary Receiver Operating Characteristics

Rutter and Gastoni [36] proposed a hierarchical model for a pair of binomial variables, the number of subjects in a high-expression and that in a low-expression group. They proposed a Baysian inference procedure to estimate unknown parameters. Later, Macaskill [22] proposed to apply the maximum likelihood method. The maximum likelihood estimator can be obtained with a software package covering the non-linear mixed-effect model such as the NLMIXED PROCEDURE of SAS (SAS Institute, Cary, NC).

Table 1 Notations for cell frequencies of 2 × 2 table for the sth study

	$D = 0$	$D = 1$	
$Z = 0 : X < v^{(s)}$	$N_{00}^{(s)}$	$N_{01}^{(s)}$	$N_{0+}^{(s)}$
$Z = 1 : X \geq v^{(s)}$	$N_{10}^{(s)}$	$N_{11}^{(s)}$	$N_{1+}^{(s)}$
	$N_{+0}^{(s)}$	$N_{+1}^{(s)}$	$n^{(s)}$

Define $\pi_d^{(s)} = P(X \geq v^{(s)}|D = d)$. Suppose that, conditional on $N_{+d}^{(s)} = n_{+d}^{(s)}, N_{1d}^{(s)} \sim Bin(n_{+d}^{(s)}, \pi_d^{(s)})$ for $d = 0, 1$. Consider the model,

$$logit(\pi_d^{(s)}) = \{\delta + \delta^{(s)} + (a + a^{(s)})Z_d^{(s)}\} \times \exp(-bZ_d^{(s)}), \tag{1}$$

where $logit(x) = \log\{x/(1-x)\}, Z_1^{(s)} = 0.5$ and $Z_0^{(s)} = -0.5$. The quantities δ, a and b are fixed-effects, and $\delta^{(s)}$ and $a^{(s)}$ are random effects following a zero-mean normal distribution independently. We call this model the bivariate binomial model. The random effects $\delta^{(s)}$ and $a^{(s)}$ are shared by $\pi_0^{(s)}$ and $\pi_1^{(s)}$, which account for the effects of a study-specific cut-off value.

Setting the random effects $\delta^{(s)}$ and $a^{(s)}$ at zero and eliminating δ in (1), the summary receiver operating characteristics (sROC) curve is defined by

$$sROC(x; a, b) = \left[1 + \exp\left\{-\alpha e^{-\frac{\beta}{2}} - logit(x)e^{-\beta}\right\}\right]^{-1}.$$

We employ the maximum likelihood method for parameter estimation. The sROC curve can be estimated by $sROC(x; \hat{a}, \hat{b})$, where $\hat{a}$ and $\hat{b}$ are maximum likelihood estimators for a and b, respectively. The area under the sROC curve (sAUC) is estimated by

$$s\hat{AUC} = sAUC(\hat{a}, \hat{b}) = \int_0^1 sROC(x; \hat{a}, \hat{b})dx. \tag{2}$$

The variance of $\hat{s}AUC(\hat{a}, \hat{b})$ is estimated by using the delta-method and the standard likelihood theory for the bivariate binomial model (1).

2.3 Summary Predictive Value Curves

The sROC curve is very useful to evaluate the diagnostic capacity of a biomarker in the presence of heterogeneous cutoff values. In this subsection, following Hattori and Zhou [15], we introduce a method to estimate the predictive value curves, which is an alternative to the ROC curve.

We assume that the distribution of the biomarker X has a parametric probability density function $f(x : \theta)$, where θ is a column vector of unknown parameters in a parameter space. The cumulative distribution function of X is denoted by $F(x : \theta)$. Further, we assume a parametric model for relationship between the biomarker and the response. For this purpose, we adopt the logistic regression,

$$P(D=1|X)=\frac{\exp(\alpha+\beta X)}{1+\exp(\alpha+\beta X)}, \tag{3}$$

where α and β are unknown parameters. Denote $\eta^T=(\theta^T,\alpha,\beta)$, and their true values are denoted by $\eta_0^T=(\theta_0^T,\alpha_0,\beta_0)$. The cumulative distribution function of X is denoted by $F(x)$. The likelihood function for the multinomial sample $\{n_{zd}^{(s)}\}$ is given by

$$\prod_{s=1}^{S}\prod_{z=0,1}\prod_{d=0,1}P\left(N_{zd}^{(s)}=n_{zd}^{(s)}\right)=\prod_{s=1}^{S}\prod_{z=0,1}\prod_{d=0,1}\left\{P(D=d,v_z^{(s)}<X\leq v_{z+1}^{(s)})\right\}^{n_{zd}^{(s)}}$$

$$=\prod_{s=1}^{S}\prod_{z=0,1}\prod_{d=0,1}\left[\int_{v_z^{(s)}}^{v_{z+1}^{(s)}}\left\{\frac{\exp(\alpha+\beta x)}{1+\exp(\alpha+\beta x)}\right\}^d\left\{\frac{1}{1+\exp(\alpha+\beta x)}\right\}^{1-d}f(x:\theta)dx\right]^{n_{zd}^{(s)}}.$$

Then, one can estimate the unknown parameter $\eta^T=(\theta^T,\alpha,\beta)$ with the maximum likelihood estimator $\hat{\eta}^T=(\hat{\theta}^T,\hat{\alpha},\hat{\beta})$.

Following Moskowitz and Pepe [24], the positive predictive value curve is defined as $PPV(u)=P\{D=1|F(X)\geq u\}$, which is the positive predictive value with subjects with the biomarker value X at or above the v th percentile regarded as the positive test result. In a similar fashion, the negative predictive value curve is defined as $NPV(u)=P\{D=0|F(X)<u\}$. Following Huang et al. [20], we call $F(X)$ the percentile value of the biomarker X, which is the standardized measurement of X and enables us to compare the predictive values of several biomarkers of their own scale.

Since $PPV(u)=(1-u)^{-1}P\{D=1,X\geq F^{-1}(u)\}$, if the parametric model $\{f(x:\theta)\}$ correctly specifies the true distribution and the model (3) for the relationship between the biomarker and the outcome is correctly specified, one can estimate $PPV(u)$ by $PPV(u:\hat{\eta})$, where

$$PPV(u:\eta)=\frac{1}{1-u}\int_{F^{-1}(u:\theta)}^{\infty}Q(x:\alpha,\beta)f(x:\theta)dx,$$

and $Q(x:\alpha,\beta)=\exp(\alpha+\beta x)/\{1+\exp(\alpha+\beta x)\}$. We call $PPV(u:\hat{\eta})$ the summary predictive value (sPPV) curve. As shown in Appendix A of Hattori and Zhou [15], $PPV(u:\hat{\eta})$ follows a normal distribution approximately and thus, a $100(1-\gamma)\%$ pointwise confidence interval is constructed by $PPV(u:\hat{\eta})\pm z_{\gamma/2}\hat{\sigma}_{PPV}(u)/\sqrt{n}$, where $z_{\gamma/2}$ is the $100(1-\gamma/2)\%$ percentile of the standard normal distribution and $\hat{\sigma}_{PPV}^2(u)$ is a consistent variance estimator obtained following the standard likelihood theory, whose definition is presented in Hattori and Zhou [15].

Similarly, $NPV(u) = u^{-1}P\{D = 0, X < F^{-1}(u)\}$ can be estimated by $NPV(u : \hat{\eta})$, where

$$NPV(u : \eta) = \frac{1}{u} \int_{0}^{F^{-1}(u:\theta)} \{1 - Q(x : \alpha, \beta)\} f(x : \theta) dx.$$

We call $NPV(u : \hat{\eta})$ the summary negative predictive value (sNPV) curve. A $100(1-\gamma)\%$ pointwise confidence interval is constructed by $NPV(u : \hat{\eta}) \pm z_{\gamma/2}\hat{\sigma}_{NPV}(u)/\sqrt{n}$. The definition of $\hat{\sigma}_{NPV}(u)$ is given in Hattori and Zhou [15]. Some further inferential tools, including simultaneous confidence bands for the PPV and NPV curves, are presented in Hattori and Zhou [15].

3 Time-Dependent Summary Receiver Operating Characteristics

3.1 Data

Suppose we enroll S prognostic studies of a right-censored time-to-event outcome into a meta-analysis. Let T and C be the time-to-event and the potential censoring time of a subject, respectively, and X is a measurement at baseline of a biomarker of interest. We assume that each study is subject to right-censoring by C. Let the cut-off value for the s th study be denoted by $v^{(s)}$, and $S_0^{(s)}(t) = P(T > t | X \le v^{(s)})$ and $S_1^{(s)}(t) = P(T > t | X > v^{(s)})$ be the survival functions of the low- and the high-expression groups, respectively. We assume that T is a continuous random variable, and T and C are independent conditional on X. The distribution function of C is assumed to be common across studies and C is independent of X. These facts lead to independence between T and C.

We suppose that the individual-level data T, C and X are not observed and the following study-level data are available. The number of subjects in the low-expression group and that in the high-expression group are denoted by $n_{0+}^{(s)}$ and $n_{1+}^{(s)}$, respectively, and denote $n^{(s)} = n_{0+}^{(s)} + n_{1+}^{(s)}$. Let $\hat{S}_0^{(s)}(t)$ and $\hat{S}_1^{(s)}(t)$ be Kaplan–Meier estimates of the low- and the high-expression groups, respectively. At $t = t_1 < t_2, \ldots < t_K$, $\hat{S}_0^{(s)}(t)$ and $\hat{S}_1^{(s)}(t)$ are extracted from the graphical plots of Kaplan–Meier estimates. Graph scan software packages such as the *digitize* package [29] can be used for this purpose. We assume that $n_{0+}^{(s)}$, $n_{1+}^{(s)}$ and the Kaplan–Meier estimates are available in each study. We further assume that the cut-off value of each study is observed. Let the follow-up time be defined as $Y = min(T, C)$. The median follow-up time is defined as the sample median of Ys, where the median is taken over the entire sample (not separately by the high- or the low- expression group) of each study, which is often reported in prognostic studies. We assume that in some studies enrolled in the meta-analysis, the median follow-up time is reported to estimate the common censoring distribution.

3.2 Multiple-Imputation and Bivariate Binomial Model

Suppose we are interested in estimating the time-dependent ROC curve at $t = t_K$. Denote $D = D(t_K) = I(T \le t_K)$ and $Z = Z(t_K) = I(X \ge v^{(s)})$. We use the same notation presented in Table 1. That is, let $N_{zd}^{(s)}$ denote the number of subjects with $D = d$ and $Z = z$. Denote $N_{+d}^{(s)} = N_{0d}^{(s)} + N_{1d}^{(s)}$. Note that $N_{zd}^{(s)}$ is not observed in the presence of censoring. Our proposal is to impute $\{N_{zd}^{(s)}\}$ and then apply methods for the meta-analyses of diagnostic studies, which have binary outcomes. To make a valid inference accounting for variation in the imputation, we employ the multiple imputation technique [14, 35]. The multiple imputation accounting for uncertainty of the parameter estimation in the imputation model is called proper. To conduct a proper multiple imputation, we need to draw samples from the conditional distribution of missing observations given observed data. Let $\hat{p}_z^{(s)}(t_K) = N_{z0}^{(s)}/n_{z+}^{(s)}$. To impute $N_{z0}^{(s)}$, which is missing in all the studies, we generate $\hat{p}_z^{(s)}(t_K)$ from its conditional distribution given observed data $\hat{S}_z^{(s)}(t_K)$,

$$f(\hat{p}_z^{(s)}(t_K)|\hat{S}_z^{(s)}(t_K)) = \int_0^1 f(\hat{p}_z^{(s)}(t_K)|\hat{S}_z^{(s)}(t_K), S_z^{(s)}(t_K)) f(S_z^{(s)}(t_K)|\hat{S}_z^{(s)}(t_K)) dS_z^{(s)}(t_K), \tag{4}$$

where, $f(\hat{p}_z^{(s)}(t_K)|\hat{S}_z^{(s)}(t_K), S_z^{(s)}(t_K))$ is the probability density function of $\hat{p}_z^{(s)}(t_K)$ given observed data $\hat{S}_z^{(s)}(t_K)$ and the true survival function $\hat{S}_z^{(s)}(t_K)$, $f(S_z^{(s)}(t_K)|\hat{S}_z^{(s)}(t_K))$ is a posterior distribution of $S_z^{(s)}(t_K)$ given observed data $\hat{S}_z^{(s)}(t_K)$ and $dS_z^{(s)}(t_K)$ is the Lebesgue measure on (0, 1). Let $g(x)$ be a smooth and monotone function from $(0, 1)$ to $(0, \infty)$. The function g is introduced to make samples for $\hat{p}_z^{(s)}(t_K)$ of between 0 and 1, and a choice is the logit function $g(x) = \log x - \log(1 - x)$. As shown by Hattori and Zhou [16], it holds that

$$\sqrt{n_{z+}^{(s)}} \begin{pmatrix} g(\hat{p}_z^{(s)}(t_K)) - g(S_z^{(s)}(t_K)) \\ \hat{S}_z^{(s)}(t_K) - S_z^{(s)}(t_K) \end{pmatrix} \xrightarrow{d} N\left(\begin{pmatrix} 0 \\ 0 \end{pmatrix}, \sum\nolimits_z^{(s)} \right), \tag{5}$$

where $\xrightarrow{d}$ implies a convergence in distribution,

$$\sum\nolimits_z^{(s)} = \begin{pmatrix} g_{11}, g_{12} \\ g_{12}, g_{22} \end{pmatrix} = \begin{pmatrix} \dot{g}^2(S_z^{(s)}(t_K))u_z^{(s)}(t_K), \dot{g}(S_z^{(s)}(t_K))u_z^{(s)}(t_K) \\ \dot{g}(S_z^{(s)}(t_K))u_z^{(s)}(t_K), \{\sigma_z^{(s)}(t_K)\}^2 \end{pmatrix},$$

$u_z^{(s)}(t_K) = S_z^{(s)}(t_K)\{1 - S_z^{(s)}(t_K)\}$, which is the variance of the binomial distribution, and $\{\sigma_z^{(s)}(t_K)\}^2$ is the Greenwood variance for the Kaplan–Meier estimator [16]. Then, the conditional distribution of $\sqrt{n_{z+}^{(s)}}\{g(\hat{p}_z^{(s)}(t_K)) - g(S_z^{(s)}(t_K))\}$ given $\hat{S}_z^{(s)}(t_K) - S_z^{(s)}(t_K)$ is given by

$$N\left(\frac{g_{12}}{g_{22}}\sqrt{n_{z+}^{(s)}}\left\{\hat{S}_z^{(s)}(t_K) - S_z^{(s)}(t_K)\right\}, g_{11}\left(1 - \frac{g_{12}}{\sqrt{g_{11}g_{22}}}\right)\right).$$

Thus, conditional on $\hat{S}_z^{(s)}(t_K)$ and $S_z^{(s)}(t_K)$,

$$g(\hat{p}_z^{(s)}(t_K)) \sim N\left(g(S_z^{(s)}(t_K)) + \frac{g_{12}}{g_{22}}\left\{\hat{S}_z^{(s)}(t_K) - S_z^{(s)}(t_K)\right\}, \frac{1}{\sqrt{n_{z+}^{(s)}}}g_{11}\left(1 - \frac{g_{12}}{\sqrt{g_{11}g_{22}}}\right)\right), \tag{6}$$

which holds approximately.

Let $h(x)$ be a smooth and monotone function from $(0, 1)$ to $(0, \infty)$. From an asymptotic property of the Kaplan–Meier estimator with the delta method,

$$h\{\hat{S}_z^{(s)}(t_K)\}|S_z^{(s)}(t_K) \sim N(h\{S_z^{(s)}(t_K)\}, \sigma_{h,z}^2(t_K))$$

holds approximately, where $\sigma_{h,z}^2(t_K) = \dot{h}^2\{S_z^{(s)}(t_K)\}\{\sigma_z^{(s)}(t_K)\}^2/n_{z+}^{(s)}$ and $\dot{h}$ is the derivative of h. With a vague prior distribution $h\{S_z^{(s)}(t_K)\} \sim N(h_*, \infty)$, the posterior distribution of $h\{S_z^{(s)}(t_K)\}$ is given by

$$h\{S_z^{(s)}(t_K)\}|\hat{S}_z^{(s)}(t_K) \sim N\left(h\{\hat{S}_z^{(s)}(t_K)\}, \sigma_{h,z}^2(t_K)\right). \tag{7}$$

If the Greenwood variance $\{\sigma_z^{(s)}(t_K)\}^2$ is known, one can generate $\hat{p}_z^{(s)}(t_K)$ from the conditional distribution (4) given observed data $\hat{S}_Z^{(s)}(t_K)$ by sampling from (7) and (6). Thus a proper multiple imputation can be conducted. However, in practice, $\{\sigma_z^{(s)}(t_K)\}^2$ is unknown. Hattori and Zhou [16] proposed a consistent estimator of $\{\sigma_z^{(s)}(t_K)\}^2$ by utilizing observations of the median follow-up time. To be precise, we propose to generate samples according to the following steps:

Step 1: Generate $U \sim N(h\{\hat{S}_z^{(s)}(t_K)\}, \hat{\sigma}_{h,z}^2)$, where $\hat{\sigma}_{h,z}^2(t_K) = \dot{h}\{\hat{S}_z^{(s)}(t_K)\}$ $\{\hat{\sigma}_z^{(s)}(t_K)\}^2/n_{z+}^{(s)}$, and set $S_z^{(s)}(t_K) = h^{-1}(U)$.

Step 2: Generate

$$V \sim N\left(g(S_z^{(s)}(t_K)) + \frac{g_{12}}{\hat{g}_{22}}\left\{\hat{S}_z^{(s)}(t_K) - S_z^{(s)}(t_K)\right\}, \frac{1}{n_{z+}^{(s)}} g_{11}\left(1 - \frac{g_{12}}{\sqrt{g_{11}\hat{g}_{22}}}\right)\right),$$

where $\hat{g}_{22} = \{\hat{\sigma}_z^{(s)}(t_K)\}^2$ and set $\hat{p}_z^{(s)}(t_K) = g^{-1}(V)$.

Step 3: Set $N_{z0}^{(s)}$ as the nearest integer of $n_{z+}^{(s)}\hat{p}_z^{(s)}(t_K)$ and $N_{z1}^{(s)} = n_{z+}^{(s)} - N_{z0}^{(s)}$.

For $s = 1, 2, \ldots, S$, L imputed 2×2 tables at time t_K are generated. We can apply any meta-analysis methods for a binary response. Here, we apply the bivariate binomial model [22].

By applying the bivariate binomial model (1) to the L sets of cell frequencies $\{N_{zd}^{(s)}\}$, we have L sets of the sROC curves and their sAUCs. Then, an inference can be made according to the standard multiple-imputation methodology [14, 35]. The simulation study by Hattori and Zhou [16] demonstrated that this multiple-imputation-based method worked very well in practical situations.

4 Time-Dependent Summary Predictive Value Curves

The time-dependent PPV and NPV curves for the biomarker X are defined as $PPV(u;t) = P\{D(t) = 1|F(X) \geq u\}$ and $NPV(u;t) = P\{D(t) = 0|F(X) < u\}$, respectively, where $D(t) = I(T \leq t)$. Suppose we are interested in estimating the PPV and NPV curves at t_K. Using individual participant data (i.e., in a non-meta-analysis setting), Zheng et al. [44, 45] and Zhou et al. [48] proposed inference procedures for the time-dependent PPV and NPV curves. In this section, we propose a method to estimate them based on meta-analysis of prognostic studies, that have the data defined in Sect. 3.1.

Our idea is to apply the multiple imputation explained in Sect. 3.2, which was developed for the time-dependent sROC curve, to the method presented in Sect. 2.3. We assume that X has a parametric probability density function $f(x;\theta)$, which has the range of $[0, \infty)$, and T follows the Cox proportional hazard model [10],

$$\log\{-\log\{S(t|X)\}\} = \log\{-\log\{S_0(t)\}\} + \beta X, \tag{8}$$

where $S_0(t)$ is a baseline survival function. Alternatively, one may employ the proportional odds model [4], which is defined as

$$\log\left\{\frac{1 - S(t|X)}{S(t|X)}\right\} = \log\left\{\frac{1 - S_0(t)}{S_0(t)}\right\} + \beta X. \tag{9}$$

More generally, these models can be regarded as special cases of the linear transformation model [6, 7],

$$g_*\{S(t|X)\} = g_*\{S_0(t)\} + \beta X, \tag{10}$$

where $g_*(.)$ is a known function. If $g_*(x) = \log\{-\log(x)\}$ and $g_*(x) = \log(1-x)/x$, the linear transformation model (10) lead to the proportional hazards model (8) and the proportional odds model (9), respectively. Since $P\{D(t_K) = 1|X\} = 1 - S(t_K|X)$, setting $\alpha = g\{S_0(t_K)\}$, (10) leads to

$$P\{D(t_K) = 1|X\} = 1 - g_*^{-1}(\alpha + \beta X). \tag{11}$$

By applying the imputation method in Sect. 3.2, one can generate L sets of imputed cell frequencies $\{n_{zd}^{(s)}\}$, which is regarded as a realization of $\{N_{zd}^{(s)}\}$. Then, one can estimate unknown parameters $\eta = (\theta^T, \alpha, \beta)$ by maximizing the multinomial likelihood

$$\prod_{s=1}^{S}\prod_{z=0,1}\prod_{d=0,1} P\left(N_{zd}^{(s)} = n_{zd}^{(s)}\right) = \prod_{s=1}^{S}\prod_{z=0,1}\prod_{d=0,1}\left\{P(D(t_K) = d, v_z^{(s)} < X \le v_{z+1}^{(s)})\right\}^{n_{zd}^{(s)}}$$

$$= \prod_{s=1}^{S}\prod_{z=0,1}\prod_{d=0,1}\left[\int_{v_z^{(s)}}^{v_{z+1}^{(s)}} \{Q_g(x:\alpha,\beta)\}^d\{1 - Q_g(x:\alpha,\beta)\}^{1-d} f(x:\theta)dx\right]^{n_{zd}^{(s)}},$$

where $Q_g(x:\alpha,\beta) = 1 - g^{-1}(\alpha + \beta x)$. The maximum likelihood estimator for η based on the lth imputed cell frequencies is denoted by $\hat{\eta}^{[l]}$. Following the inference procedure presented in Sect. 2.3, one can estimate the PPV and NPV curves and their standard errors for the lth imputed cell frequencies. Then, following Rubin's multiple-imputation methodology, the PPV curve is estimated by $P\bar{P}V(u) = L^{-1}\sum_{l=1}^{L} PPV(u:\hat{\eta}^{[l]})$, which is called the time-dependent sPPV curve, and its variance can be estimated by $V\{P\bar{P}V(u)\} = A(t_K) + (1 + L^{-1})B(t_K)$, where $A(t_K) = L^{-1}\sum_{l=1}^{L}\{\hat{\sigma}_{PPV}^{[l]}(u)\}^2$, $B(t_K) = (L-1)^{-1}\sum_{l=1}^{L}\{PPV(u:\hat{\eta}^{[l]}) - \bar{P}PV(u)\}^2$, and $\{\hat{\sigma}_{PPV}^{[l]}(u)\}^2$ is the variance estimate for the lth imputed cell frequencies. The construction of pointwise confidence intervals can be done with a t-distribution of the degree of freedom $v(t_K)$, where $v(t_K) = (L-1)\{1 + \rho^{-1}(t_K)A(t_K)\}^2$ and $\rho(t_K) = (1 + L^{-1})B(t_K)$. Inference for the time-dependent sNPV curve can be made in a similar way.

5 Application to BCL-2 Data

Callegy et al. [5] reported the results of a meta-analysis of 18 prognostic studies for BCL-2, which is an anti-apoptosis protein in breast cancer patients. We illustrate our proposed methods by re-analyzing this data. Among the 18 studies, 9 studies provided a graphical plot of the Kaplan–Meier estimate of the survival functions of the overall survival for the high-expression and low-expression groups. The cut-off values of the 9 studies ranged from 0.1 to 0.33. We extracted the Kaplan–Meier estimate every six months. Among the 9 studies, 5 studies reported their median follow-up times, which were required to estimate the Greenwood variance. We applied the bivariate binomial model for estimation of the sROC curve at $t = 4$ (year) with the proposed multiple-imputation. The exponential distribution was assumed for censoring and 30 imputed samples were generated. In Fig. 1, the estimated sROC curve at $t = 4$(year) is presented with the observed pairs of the sensitivity and the specificity of the 9 studies plotted. The estimated sROC curves appeared to fit well to the observed data. The sAUC was estimated as 0.65 (95% CI: 0.59, 0.71). The lower limit of the 95% CI was higher than 0.5, indicating that BCL-2 was significantly associated with the overall survival.

In addition, we estimated the time-dependent sPPV and sNPV curves. We assumed that the overall survival followed the proportional hazards model (8) or the proportional odds model (9). For simplicity of illustration, we considered only the log-normal distribution for BCL-2. Using these models, we applied our method with 10,000 random numbers for Monte-Carlo integration in the likelihood function. The average of the log-likelihood over the 30 imputed samples was −2611 with the proportional hazards model and was −2561 with the proportional odds model. We therefore employed the proportional odds model. In Fig. 2, the

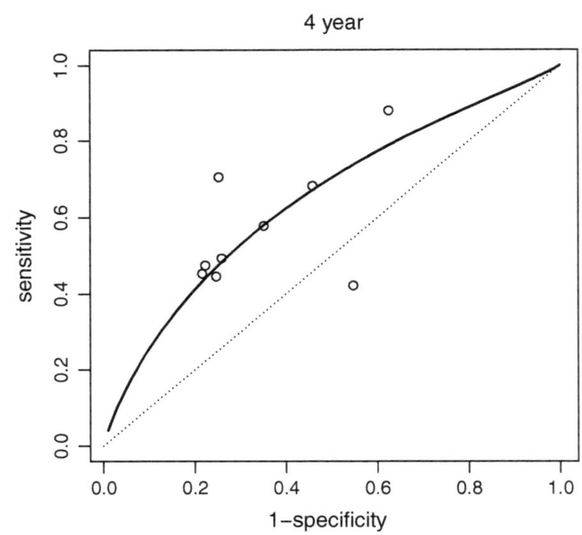

Fig. 1 Summary ROC curve for BCL-2 at $t = 4$ (year) estimated by bivariate binomial model with pairs of observed sensitivity and specificity

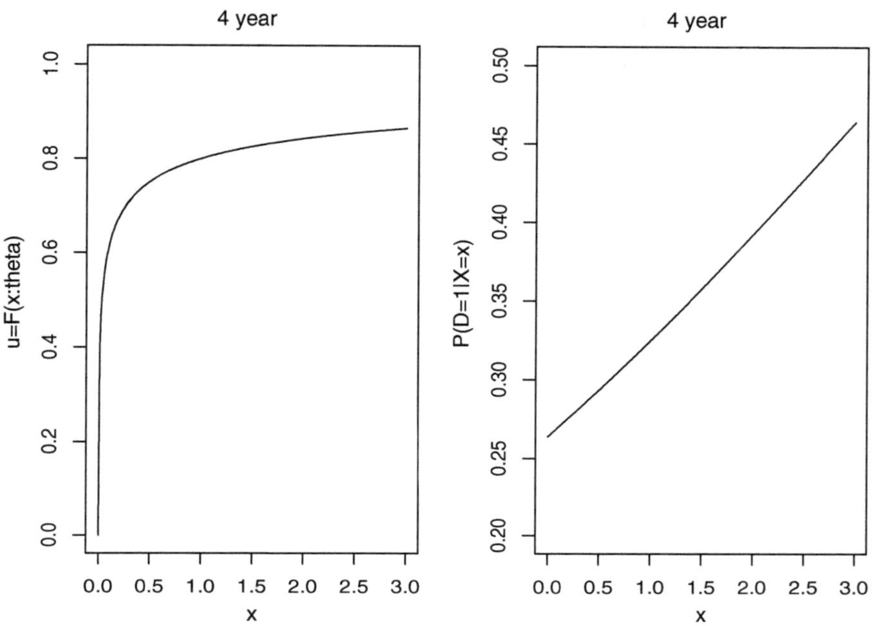

Fig. 2 Estimated cumulative distribution function $F(x : \hat{\theta})$ (*left panel*) and $P(D = 1|X)$ (*right panel*) curves

estimated cumulative distribution function $u = F(x : \hat{\theta})$ and $P\{D(t_K) = 1|X\}$ are presented. In Fig. 3, the estimated time-dependent sPPV and sNPV curves at t = 4 are presented with 95% pointwise confidence intervals. The right panel of Fig. 3 suggests that the sNPV curve was almost invariant up to u = 0.8. On the other hand, the sPPV curve increased from about u = 0.7. The corresponding x was calculated as $0.67 = F^{-1}(0.7; \hat{\theta})$, indicating that the subjects with BCL-2 measurement of more than 0.67 comprised the upper 30% of subjects of the population enrolled in the meta-analysis, and this subpopulation had a much higher risk of dying before t = 4.

6 Discussion

Although meta-analysis is expected to be useful for prognostic biomarker studies, methodological development and application remained very limited. In this chapter, we introduced some recently or newly developed statistical methods for the meta-analysis of prognostic biomarker studies: the time-dependent summary ROC curve [9, 16] and the time-dependent summary predictive value curves. Alternative to these methods related to diagnostic medicine, Riley et al. [33] and Sadashima

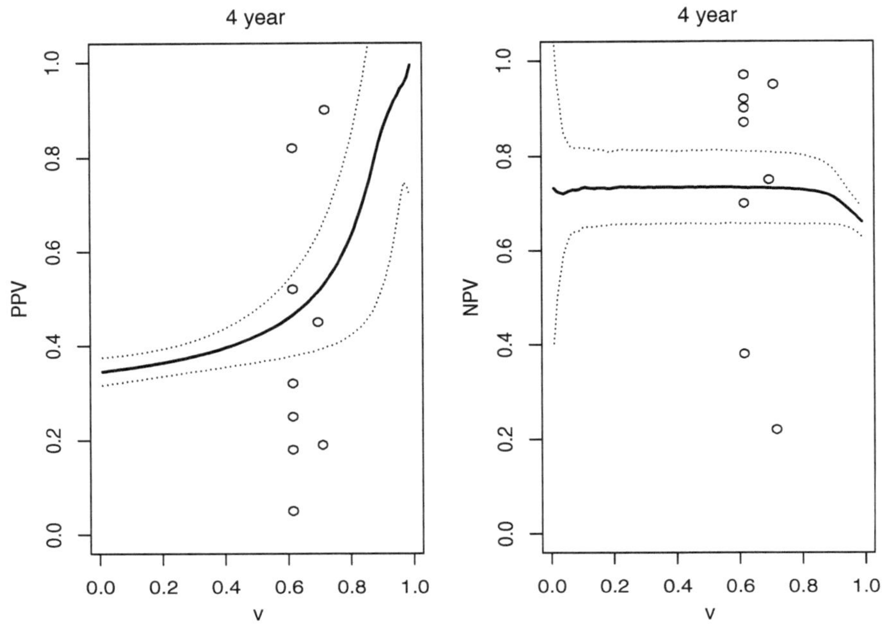

Fig. 3 Estimated PPV (*left panel*) and NPV (*right panel*) curves (*solid* and *bold line*) with 95% pointwise confidence intervals (*broken line*) based on the proportional odds model and the log-normal distribution for BCL-2: $u = F^{-1}(x)$ is the percentile value of BCL-2, and *open circles* are observed PPV and NPV of each study with the estimated percentile value of the cut-off value

et al. [37] proposed to perform a summary based on a combined hazard ratio. Riley et al. [33] proposed to apply a multivariate meta-regression model, in which the study-specific cut-off value was incorporated as a study-level covariate. Their focus was on examining the association between hazard ratios and cut-off values. Sadashima et al. [37] proposed to make a summary of reported hazard ratios with a study-specific cut-off value by estimating the individual-level biomarker-hazard relationship by applying the meta-analysis techniques for the dose-response [39, 43]. To the best of our knowledge, these references constitute all the main proposals for the meta-analysis of prognostic studies. In other words, this research area has only just opened.

As presented in Sects. 3 and 4, inference of the time-dependent summary ROC or predictive value curves requires the Kaplan–Meier estimates as input data. On the other hand, the methods of Riley et al. [33] and Sadashima et al. [37] utilized the hazard ratios and their standard errors. Accordingly, the hazard-based approaches by Riley et al. [33] and Sadashima et al. [37] can incorporate more studies, since one can extract a hazard ratio estimate from a Kaplan–Meier estimate [28]. Moreover, it is our impression that researchers will be more likely to display Kaplan–Meier estimates to highlight their findings. Therefore, the time-dependent summary ROC or predictive value curves may suffer from more severe publication bias issues. Future research should address how to detect and adjust for publication bias for these methods.

Finally, although we have overviewed how to make an inference for the time-dependent summary predictive value curves, many issues should be addressed in future research. As can be seen in Fig. 3, there was large heterogeneity in the observed PPVs and NPVs among studies. To capture the heterogeneity, one can consider extensions of the model (11) such as $P\{D(t_K) = 1|X\} = 1 - g^{-1}(\alpha + \gamma W^{(s)} + e^{(s)} + \beta X)$, where $W^{(s)}$ is a study-level covariate and $e^{(s)}$ is a zero-mean random-effect. This model allows study-specific prevalences and thus would be useful to predict the PPV and NPV with a given cut-off value and a prevalence of the population of interest.

In our analysis of the BCL data in Sect. 5, we selected the model with larger average log-likelihood values over imputed samples in an intuitive matter. The development of model-selection procedures for multiple imputation is a highly important goal [38, 40] in the analysis of missing data. It is therefore imperative that model-selection procedures also be developed for our method relying on multiply-imputed samples.

References

1. Altman DG. Systematic reviews of evaluations of prognostic variables. BMJ. 2001;323:224–8.
2. American Society of Clinical Oncology. Clinical practice guidelines for the treatment of unresectable non-small-cell lung cancer. J Clin Oncol. 1997;15:2996–3018.
3. Becattini C, Vedovati MC, Agnelli G. Prognostic value of troponin in acute pulmonary embolism. Circulation. 2007;116:427–33.
4. Bennett S. Analysis of survival data by the proportional odds model. Stat Med. 1982;2:273–7.
5. Callagy GM, Webber MJ, Pharoa PDP, Carldas C. Meta-analysis confirms BCL2 is an independent prognostic marker in breast cancer. BMC Cancer. 2008;8:153–62.
6. Cheng SC, Wei LJ, Ying Z. Analysis of transformation models with censored data. Biometrika. 1995;82:835–45.
7. Chen K, Jin Z, Ying Z. Semiparametric analysis of transformation models with censored data. Biometrika. 2002;89:659–68.
8. Chu H, Nie L, Cole ST, Poole C. Meta-analysis of diagnostic accuracy studies accounting for disease prevalence: alternative parametrizations and model selection. Stat Med. 2009;28:2384–99.
9. Combescure C, Daures JP, Foucher Y. A literature-based approach to evaluate the predictive capacity of a marker using time-dependent summary receiver operating characteristics. Stat Methods Med Res. 2016;25:674–85.
10. Cox DR. Regression models and life tables. J R Stat Soc B. 1972;34:187–220.
11. de Azambujya E, Cardoso F, de Castro Jr G, Colozza M, Mano MS, Durbecq V, Sotiriou C, Larsimont D, Piccart-Gebhart MJ, Paesmans M. Ki-67 as prognostic marker in early breast cancer: a meta-analysis of published studies involving 12155 patients. Br J Cancer. 2007;96:1504–13.
12. Hamza TH, van Houwelingen HC, Stijnen T. The binomial distribution of meta-analysis was preferred to model within-study variability. J Clin Epidemiol. 2008;61:41–51.

13. Harbord RM, Deeks JJ, Egger M. A unification of models for meta-analysis of diagnostic accuracy studies. Biostatistics. 2007;8:239–51.
14. Harel O, Zhou XH. Multiple imputation: review of theory, implementation and software. Stat Med. 2007;26:3057–77.
15. Hattori S, Zhou XH. Evaluation of predictive capacities of biomarkers based on research synthesis. Stat Med. 2016;35:4559–72.
16. Hattori S, Zhou XH. Time-dependent summary receiver operating characteristics for meta-analysis of prognostic studies. Stat Med. 2016;35:4746–63.
17. Heagerty PJ, Lumley T, Pepe MS. Time-dependent ROC curves for censored survival data and a diagnostic marker. Biometrics. 2000;56:337–44.
18. Hemingway H, Croft P, Perel P, Hayden JA, Abrams K, Timmis A, Lindsay AB, Udumyan R, Moons KGM, Steyerberg EW, Robert I, Schroter S, Altman DG, Riley RD, for the PROGRESS Group. Prognosis research strategy (PROGRESS) 1: A framework for researching clinical outcomes. Br Med J. 2013; 346:e5595.
19. Hemingway H, Riley RD, Altman DG. Ten steps towards improving prognosis research. BMJ. 2010;340:410–4.
20. Huang Y, Pepe MS. Biomarker evaluation using the controls as a reference population. UW biostatistics working paper series. Working paper 306;2007.
21. Leeflang MMG, Deeks JJ, Rutjes AWS, Reitsma JB, Bossuyt PMM. Bivariate meta-analysis of predictive values of diagnostic tests can be an alternative to bivariate meta-analysis of sensitivity and specificity. J Clin Epidemiol. 2012;65:1088–97.
22. Macaskill P. Empirical Bayes estimates generated in a hierarchical summary ROC analysis agreed closely with those of a full Bayesian analysis. J Clin Epidemiol. 2004;57:925–32.
23. McShane LM, Altman DG, Sauerbrei W, Taube SE, Gion M, Clark GM. Reporting recommendations for tumor marker prognostic studies (REMARK). J Natl Cancer Inst. 2005;97:1180–4.
24. Moskowitz CS, Pepe MS. Quantifying and comparing the predictive accuracy of continuous prognostic factors for binary outcome. Biostatistics. 2004;5:113–27.
25. Moses LE, Shapiro D, Litterberg B. Combining independent studies of a diagnostic test into a summary ROC curve: data-analytic approaches and some additional considerations. Stat Med. 1993;12:1293–316.
26. Na F, Wang J, Li C, Deng L, Xue J, Lu Y. Primary tumor standardized uptake value measured on F18-fluorodeoxyplucose positron emission tomography is of prediction value for survival and local control in non-small-cell lung cancer receiving radiotherapy: meta-analysis. J Thorac Oncol. 2014;9:834–42.
27. Pak K, Cheon GJ, Nam HY, Kim SJ, Kang KW, Chung JK, Kim EE, Lee DS. Prognostic value of metabolic tumor volume and total lesion glycolysis in head and neck cancer: a systematic review and meta-analysis. J Nucl Med. 2014;55:884–90.
28. Parmar M, Torri V, Stewart L. Extracting summary statistics to perform meta-analyses of the published literature for survival endpoints. Stat Med. 1998;17:2815–34.
29. Poisot T. The digitize package: extracting numerical data from scatterplots. R J. 2011;3:25–6.
30. Reitsma JB, Glas AS, Rutjes AW, Scholten RJPM, Bossuyt PM, Zwinderman AH. Bivariate analysis of sensitivity and specificity produces informative summary measures in diagnostic reviews. J Clin Epidemiol. 2005;58:982–90.
31. Riley RD, Abrams KR, Sutton AJ, Lambert PC, Jones DR. Reporting of prognostic markers: current problems and development of guidelines for evidence-based practice in the future. Br J Cancer. 2003;88:1191–8.
32. Riley RD, Hayden JA, Steyerberg EW, Moons KGM, Abrams KR, Kyzas PA, Malats N, Briggs A, Schroter S, Altman DG, Hemingway H, The PROGRESS Group. Prognosis research strategy (PROGRESS) 2: prognostic factor research. PLOS Med. 2013;10(2): e1001380.
33. Riley RD, Elia EG, Malin G, Hemming K, Price MP. Multivariate meta-analysis of prognostic factor studies with multiple cut-points and/or methods of measurement. Stat Med. 2015;34:2481–96.

34. Riley RD, Ikhlaaq A, Debray TP, Willis BH, Noordzij JP, Higgins JPT, Deeks J. Summarising and validating test accuracy results across multiple studies for use in clinical practice. Stat Med. 2015;34:2081–103.
35. Rubin DB. Multiple imputation for non-response in surveys. New York: Wiley; 1987.
36. Rutter CM, Gatsonis CA. A hierarchical regression approach to meta-analysis of diagnostic test accuracy evaluations. Stat Med. 2001;20:2865–84.
37. Sadashima E, Hattori S, Takahashi K. Meta-analysis of prognostic studies for a biomarker with a study-specific cut-off value. Res Synth Methods. 2016;7:402–419.
38. Shen CW, Chen YH. Model selection of generalized estimating equations with multiply imputed longitudinal data. Biometrical J. 2013;55:899–911.
39. Shi QJ, Copas JB. Meta-analysis for trend estimation. Stat Med. 2004;23:3–19.
40. Schomakera M, Heumannb C. Model selection and model averaging after multiple imputation. Comput Stat Data Anal. 2014;71:758–70.
41. Song XJ, Zhou X-H, Ma S. Nonparametric receiver operating characteristic-based evaluation for survival outcomes. Stat Med. 2012;31:2660–75.
42. Sutton AJ, Higgins JPT. Recent developments in meta-analysis. Stat Med. 2008;27:625–50.
43. Takahashi K, Tango T. Assignment of grouped exposure levels for trend estimation in a regression analysis of summarized data. Stat Med. 2010;29:2605–16.
44. Zheng Y, Cai T, Pepe MS, Levy WC. Time-dependent predictive values of prognostic biomarkers with failure time outcome. J Am Stat Assoc. 2008;103:362–8.
45. Zheng Y, Cai T, Stanford JL, Feng Z. Semiparametric models of time-dependent predictive values of prognostic biomarkers. Biometrics. 2010;66:50–60.
46. Zheng Y, Katsaros D, Shan JCS, Longrais IR, Porpiglia M, Scorilas A, Kim NW, Wolfert RL, Simon I, Li L, Feng Z, Diamandis PD. A multiparameteric panel for ovarian cancer diagnosis, prognosis, and response to chemotherapy. Clin Cancer Res. 2007;13:6984–92.
47. Zhou XH, Obuchowski NA, McClish DK. Statistical methods in diagnostic medicine. New York: Wiley; 2011.
48. Zhou XH, Ma Y, Gary Chan KC. Covariate-specific and covariate-adjusted predictive values of prognostic biomarkers with survival outcome. In: Fang JQ, Lu Y, Tian L, Jin H, editors. Advanced medical statistics. 2nd ed. Singapore: World Science Publishing Co; 2015.

Statistical Methodology and Engineering for Next Generation Clinical Risk Calculators

Donna Pauler Ankerst, Andreas Strobl and Sonja Grill

Abstract In today's practice of medicine, a variety of online clinical risk calculators are available to assist doctors and patients in informed decision-making. These tools may have unparalleled accuracy when founded on large cohorts or clinical trial populations; they may have passed the litmus test of multiple validations. However, evolving clinical practice, technology and population characteristics, as well as the discovery of new markers, can quickly outdate an existing risk tool, making it non-optimal for the contemporary patient. The traditional path of waiting for the next clinical trial or grant collective to end in order to amass fresh data and build a brand new model is too slow for today's rapid science society, suggesting novel re-calibration methods applied to compartmentalized models that can be incrementally updated in real time. While Electronic Health Records promise an inexpensive, uninhibited and institution-tailored data flow, the percent usable data can be crippled by selection bias, non-ignorable missing data mechanisms and entanglement in indeterminate text fields, requiring novel big-data and record-linkage approaches to unravel. In this chapter we outline statistical methods and engineering approaches that can be used to tackle these challenges, and thereby keep risk calculators up to date in a continually evolving clinical care landscape. To illustrate we outline our experience adapting the Prostate Cancer Prevention Trial Risk Calculator during the past decade to meet the evolving challenges to risk prediction, and new research needed for the next generation of clinical risk prediction tools.

D.P. Ankerst · A. Strobl · S. Grill
Department of Mathematics, Technical University Munich, Munich, Germany
e-mail: a.strobl@tum.de

S. Grill
e-mail: sonja.grill@tum.de

D.P. Ankerst (✉)
Departments of Urology and Epidemiology/Biostatistics,
University of Texas Health Science Center at San Antonio,
San Antonio, TX, USA
e-mail: ankerst@tum.de

S. Matsui and J. Crowley (eds.), *Frontiers of Biostatistical Methods and Applications in Clinical Oncology*, DOI 10.1007/978-981-10-0126-0_17

Keywords Dynamic prediction · Likelihood ratio · Prediction model · Discrimination · Calibration

1 Introduction

As clinical research has become more translational and patient-focused, so too have individualized online risk calculators flourished as a means for fast-tracking academic results into patient practice and population validation. It is now commonly the case for these tools to serve as tangible products of clinical trials or large cohorts where substantial resources have been invested to prospectively and completely collect the relevant data elements. For example, based on a three-generation cardiovascular study initiated with 5000 members of Framingham, Massachusetts, the Framingham Risk Calculator asks 7 simple questions in order to calculate one's 10-year risk of having a heart attack [1]. The commonly used Breast Cancer Risk Assessment Tool (BCRAT) first produced in 1989 based on data from 6000 participants in the Breast Cancer Detection Demonstration Project, asks five simple questions on medical and reproductive history in order to estimate a woman's risk of developing breast cancer during the next five years [2]. And more recently, the Prostate Cancer Prevention Trial Risk Calculator (PCPTRC) established in 2006 calculates the risk of finding prostate cancer on biopsy based on 6 clinical and demographic questions, including the commonly used screening biomarker, prostate-specific antigen (PSA) [3].

The posting online of these risk tools has spurred external validation, pushing the boundaries of generalizability to other populations differing in substance from those on whom the risk tool was developed, for example to Asian or minority populations. The absolute risk prediction webpage on the National Cancer Institute's website conveniently lists all available prediction models according to cancer type, with links to published validation studies and papers citing the tools. For some of the risk calculators the actual data set used to build the model has been posted, which serves as a valuable education tool for young researchers new to the field. Users can submit their own model to be posted, though this is not required as the website periodically queries the internet for new published risk tools.

What is common to most of the major clinical risk calculators is that they only contain a small handful of the established predictors, making them well-powered, unlikely prone to overfitting, and easy to use by patients and doctors. However, their smallness derives from necessity rather than these considerations. For all cancers, risk factors currently in use are not perfect, and most models have operating characteristics far from optimal. Expansive research groups, such as the Early Detection Research Network (EDRN) and the genome-wide association study (GWAS) consortia, continually invest an immense amount of effort at all junctures of the biomarker discovery and validation pipeline in the search for better markers to improve cancer prediction. In the meantime, developed risk tools serve the clinical world by providing state-of-the-art estimates of risk to improve patient-doctor communication and decision-making, and the biomarker research community by providing a benchmark against which to assess the independent predictive value of new markers.

Posed as a state-of-the-art estimate, the challenge to current cohort-based risk models is that the conditions under which the models were developed, including diagnostic technology, clinical practice patterns and population characteristics, undergo constant evolution. This raises the possibility that any risk tool can become outdated at any time. As a reminder, nearly all major risk calculators were founded on large populations extracted from well-conducted trials or observational studies that took decades to perform. For example, the PCPTRC was based on an 18,882-participant prevention trial with annual screening of healthy men over a period of 7 years, with the exclusive requirement that all men were requested to undergo prostate biopsy at the end of the study regardless of their risk [3, 4]. It is not optimal to toss out older models built on the large well-organized studies in favor of finding more recent cohorts to build new models, as the typical observational cohort that is lying around is smaller, likely to have data errors, and be prone to bias because its data collection was not subject to a protocol or quality check. What is needed is a change from the traditional philosophy towards building risk calculators, to move away from static single cohort-based models towards dynamic multiple cohort-based ones.

In this chapter, we show the statistical methods that can be used to enact this new philosophy towards building contemporary risk tools. For concreteness, we use as a running example throughout our ongoing experience in adapting the PCPTRC to keep it current. The original PCPTRC predicted the binary outcome of cancer or not on biopsy using logistic regression, so we will restrict the scope of the chapter to this model. However, PCPTRC 2.0 implemented multinomial logistic regression for the prediction of the tri-variate outcome of no cancer, low-grade, and high-grade cancer, so we state briefly how our proposed techniques straightforwardly scale to this case. Extensions to survival models to predict the chance of developing a cancer over an extended period of years, as used in the Framingham and Gail risk tools, have been recently addressed in the literature using variations on what we propose here, and are not covered.

Specifically, the remainder of this Chapter proceeds as follows. In Sect. 2, we outline the Bayesian prior to posterior approach to updating an existing risk tool for new markers, in Sect. 3 we provide methods for dynamically updating existing risk prediction tools using annually collected data on the same risk factors, and in Sect. 4 we provide concluding remarks.

2 Incorporating New Biomarkers into Existing Risk Tools

Novel genetic and biological markers are continually being discovered in the laboratory and pushed through the validation pipeline, bringing with them the potential to improve cancer prediction. It becomes imperative then to incorporate them into clinical decision-making, by merging the information they provide with that of the established risk factors into a coherent forecast. As an example, the PCPTRC was built in 2006 using the primary screening marker PSA in addition to the digital rectal examination (DRE) and a few other demographic and clinical variables. But already as it was being constructed, new markers were coming into clinical practice, including percent free PSA and the urine marker PCA3. These markers could not be retrospectively measured on stored specimens from the original PCPT participants, making it seemingly impossible to include them in the PCPTRC. It appeared necessary to find a new cohort that measured the new markers in addition to the established risk factors in order to build a clean-slate model. While this might be the only option under a single-cohort philosophy to risk model building, it is not under an alternative multi-cohort compartmentalized approach, which will be outlined here.

We demonstrate the approach in the context of the PCPTRC, and thereby denote the vector of risk factors used in the PCPTRC, including PSA, DRE, race, age, prior biopsy history and first-degree family history of prostate cancer, by X [5]. We denote new markers not contained in X by Y. The PCPTRC provided a prior risk model for cancer based on factors X, $P(Cancer \mid X)$, but what was needed was an updated posterior risk based on the new information Y: $P(Cancer \mid X, Y)$. By the definition of conditional probabilities, this could be written as $P(Cancer, Y \mid X)/P(Y \mid X)$, and following factorization of the numerator, as $P(Y \mid Cancer, X)P(Cancer \mid X)/P(Y \mid X)$. The expression for $P\ (No\ Cancer \mid X, Y)$ follows the same formula, with *No Cancer* replacing *Cancer*. Taking ratios yields the following relationship:

$$\frac{P(Cancer|X,Y)}{P(No\,Cancer|X,Y)} = \frac{P(Y|X,Cancer)}{P(Y|X,No\,Cancer)} \times \frac{P(Cancer|X)}{P(No\,Cancer|X)}, \qquad (1)$$

which in layman's terms can be stated as *Posterior odds = Likelihood ratio × Prior odds.*

To evaluate (1) a patient enters their X and Y values, which are evaluated in the two terms on the right-hand side. The function for the prior odds comes from the existing risk tool. If logistic regression was used to construct the prior model, as was the case for the PCPTRC, then the prior odds assume the simple expression exp $(\beta'X)$, where β is the vector of parameters that have been estimated in the PCPTRC logistic regression. Parameters of the likelihood ratio (LR) have been estimated from a separate study to the PCPTRC, one that measured Y and ideally as many components as X as are predictive of the distributions of Y in cancer cases and non-cancer cases. The distributions appearing in the LR depend on the variable type of Y, for example, whether Y is continuous or discrete. A separate model selection and fitting procedure has been performed in the external study to optimize the densities appearing in the numerator and denominator of the LR.

The resulting LR is now a ratio of two densities to be evaluated as a function of a new input Y, thus comparing how likely it would have been to observe Y under the cancer case compared to non-cancer case distribution in the external study. If the LR equals 1 then the likelihood of observing Y would have been the same under both distributions, if it exceeds 1, Y was more likely to be observed among cancer cases, and if it is less than 1, then Y was more likely to be observed among non-cancer cases. The LR shifts the prior odds either in favor of a high risk of cancer, or of non-cancer, or adds no information to the prior odds, depending on the value of Y. Once the LR is multiplied by the prior odds to achieve the posterior odds, the posterior risk is obtained as *Posterior Odds*/[1 + *Posterior Odds*], and remains a monotonic function of the LR.

It can be helpful to plot the LR and the posterior risk as a function of Y for fixed values of X to see how the new marker moves the existing model risk. If the distributions of the new marker Y are largely overlapping between cases and controls in the external study, then Y has little discriminatory power and the LR will be nearly constant at 1 over most of the Y range. The variance of the posterior risk estimate can be obtained using the delta rule, which convolves the variance resulting from the external study used to form the LR with that resulting from the prior risk. Typically the former is much larger than the latter and contributes most of the variability. Ninety-five percent confidence intervals can be calculated on the log-scale, where the function behaves more nearly as a Normal distribution, and then transformed to the risk scale.

2.1 Example: Updating with Continuous Markers

Suppose that Y is a single continuous marker that can be assumed to follow a Normal distribution with mean depending on the risk factors X and estimated via separate linear regressions in cancer cases and controls. These were the assumptions used to build the LR when the urine marker PCA3 was added to the PCPTRC [6]. The LR becomes:

$$\begin{aligned} LR &= \frac{1/\sqrt{2\pi}\sigma_c \exp\left\{-(Y-\gamma_c' X)^2/(2\sigma_c^2)\right\}}{1/\sqrt{2\pi}\sigma_n \exp\left\{-(Y-\gamma_n' X)^2/(2\sigma_n^2)\right\}} \\ &= \frac{\sigma_n}{\sigma_c}\exp\left\{\left(Y-\gamma_n' X\right)^2\Big/\left(2\sigma_n^2\right) - \left(Y-\gamma_c' X\right)^2\Big/\left(2\sigma_c^2\right)\right\}, \end{aligned} \tag{2}$$

where the subscripts c and n refer to cancer cases and non-cancer cases, respectively, the γ's refer to regression slope parameters and the σ's to standard deviations. When different standard deviations for Y are assumed for cancer cases and non-cancer cases ($\sigma_c \neq \sigma_n$), the logarithm of the LR is quadratic in Y, implying that the logarithm of the posterior odds is also quadratic in Y. This case is equivalent to quadratic discrimination analysis used in classification theory. However, under the assumption of equal standard deviations ($\sigma_c = \sigma_n$), the square term for Y cancels out of the LR, making it linear and thus monotonic in Y, corresponding to linear discriminant analysis. Our prior simulation studies and real data experiments have shown that constraining the variance to be equal among the cancer cases and non-cancer cases increases stability and reduces bias, resulting in more accurate confidence interval coverage [7, 8].

For Y a vector of continuous multivariate markers that can be assumed to follow multivariate Normal distributions, the densities in the numerator and denominator can be replaced accordingly. Our experience with incorporating the markers proPSA and percent free PSA into the PCPTRC using bivariate Normal distributions indicated that constraining the variance matrices to be equal among cancer cases and non-cancer cases became even more critical to avoid large non-monotonic fluctuations in the posterior risk as a function of the two markers [9]. The problem became exacerbated when we considered more flexible distributions in the numerator and denominator to accommodate skewness and outliers [unpublished report].

2.2 Example: Updating with Categorical Marker

Many markers are by nature categorical, and these may also be accommodated by substituting the multinomial distribution into the numerator and denominator of the LR. As an example, the PCPTRC includes as a risk factor the question of whether or not a participant has a first-degree relative that has been diagnosed with prostate cancer, coded as a binary yes/no variable. It has been established that more refined measures of the extent of family history can improve risk estimates. Researchers maintaining the Swedish Family-Cancer Database (SFCD), a comprehensive registry covering the entire population of Sweden, provided LR estimates corresponding to more detailed family history patterns, including the number of first-degree and second-degree male relatives diagnosed with prostate cancer, whether these relatives were diagnosed under the age of 60, as well as the number of female first-degree relatives ever diagnosed with breast cancer.

To incorporate a single detailed family history question, if we denote by Y the presence of a particular detailed family history pattern, the LR becomes

$$LR = \frac{\pi_{cancer}^{I(Y=1)}(1-\pi_{cancer})^{I(Y=0)}}{\pi_{no\ cancer}^{I(Y=1)}(1-\pi_{no\ cancer})^{I(Y=0)}}, \tag{3}$$

where $I(A)$ denotes the indicator function equal to 1 if A is true and 0 otherwise. The π's were estimated as empirical proportions from the SFCD, by counting among men diagnosed with prostate cancer the proportion with the family history pattern for the numerator, and similarly for men not diagnosed with prostate cancer in the SFCD for the denominator. To accommodate multiple detailed family history questions, we established 23 disjoint categories of family history and used multinomial distributions in the numerator and denominator; details can be found in [10].

LRs for detailed family history were not conditioned on the PCPTRC risk factors X, in part due to necessity and in part by choice. Clinical risk factors, such as PSA, DRE and prior biopsy, which are immediate risk factors measured close to diagnosis, would not be surmised to be associated with detailed family history. Because detailed family history patterns are so rare, the SFCD population was restricted to

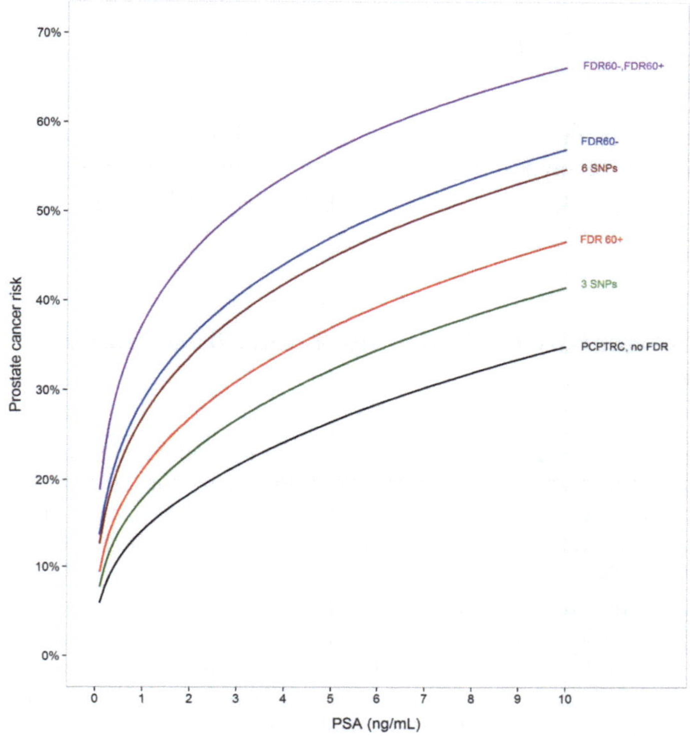

Fig. 1 Comparison of the PCPTRC with and without updates for specific family history patterns and single nucleotide polymorphisms (SNPs) as a function of PSA, adopted from [11]; FDR: first-degree relative diagnosed with prostate cancer, 60+: relative was diagnosed over 60 years of age, and 60−, under 60 years of age

men over 55 years and was predominantly Caucasian, dependence on race and age was not modeled. First-degree relative prostate cancer history is in the PCPTRC but was turned off in the prior odds model so as not to double measure it through the LRs. Because of the SFCD confidentiality rules, the data could not be exported outside of the source, which posed no inconvenience for the LR approach since the LRs could be calculated on site and exported. Resulting posterior risk curves for updated PCPTRC estimates incorporating family history patterns compared to the PCPTRC itself are shown in Fig. 1.

Multinomial distributions were also used to update the PCPTRC for single nucleotide polymorphisms (SNPs) associated with prostate cancer [12]. SNPs are characterized by two alleles, such as A and G, with one denoted as the risk allele due to past associations with prostate cancer. There are three outcomes to a SNP corresponding to how many copies of the risk allele occur, 0, 1 or 2, and these comprise the categorical SNP variable *Y*. Assuming no dependence of Y on the PCPTRC risk factors, the LR becomes

$$LR = \frac{\pi_{0,cancer}^{I(Y=0)}\pi_{1,cancer}^{I(Y=1)}\pi_{2,cancer}^{I(Y=2)}}{\pi_{0,no\,cancer}^{I(Y=0)}\pi_{1,no\,cancer}^{I(Y=1)}\pi_{2,no\,cancer}^{I(Y=2)}}, \quad (4)$$

where the π's in the numerator sum to 1 and similarly for the denominator. Frequencies of genotypes (π's) in cases and controls are usually reported in GWAS's, and hence can be directly imported to analytically update the risk calculator.

2.3 Meta-analysis for Importing Results from Multiple Studies

The compartmentalized LR approach allows one to input results straightforwardly from an external study to update the PCPTRC using the efficient case control design, the method of choice for biomarker studies. GWAS reported SNPs are frequently validated across all the major gene consortia, with resulting odds ratios reported in the form of a meta-analysis.

When multiple studies report information that can be used to construct an LR, the LR may also be subjected to a meta-analysis, with the average meta-analysis estimate used for the LR, thus reducing the component of variability due to the LR in the estimate of posterior risk. The meta-analysis proceeds as follows. First S independent studies are identified that provide estimates of the parameters comprising the LR, these are denoted by $\Theta_1, \ldots, \Theta_S$ and may be vectors. For example, in (4) Θ would be a vector of the four independent π*'s* comprising the proportions of cases and controls obtaining the 3 genotypes (two of π*'s* are determined since the vector of probabilities need to sum to one for cases and controls). The studies should also provide the required estimates to construct variances of the Θ*'s*, using the delta rule if necessary, denoted by $V_1, \ldots, V_S$. Although estimated, study variances are treated as fixed and known in the analysis, they will be non-diagonal matrices whose forms depend on the distribution of the component elements of Θ. Continuing the SNP example, the variance matrix will be block diagonal, with dependence among the π*'s* within sets of cases and controls and independence between them. It is assumed that studies are independent with sufficiently large sample sizes so that

$$\theta_i \sim N(\mu_i, V_i) \text{ independently for } i = 1, \ldots, S. \quad (5)$$

Transformations, such as the log for parameters restricted to positive values, can be used for this purpose. Assuming that the independent studies arise from a common population, the heterogeneity among the study estimates is captured by specifying

$$\mu_i \sim N(\mu, D) \text{ independently and identically for } i = 1, \ldots, S. \tag{6}$$

Equations (5) and (6) imply that, marginally, $\Theta_i \sim N(\mu, V_i + D)$ independently for $i = 1,\ldots,S$. The parameters μ and D can be estimated using a meta-analysis function available in many statistical software packages. Estimates of μ and its standard error from the meta-analysis are then used to form the LR and to compute its variance.

We performed a meta-analysis to incorporate 30 multiply-validated SNPs for prostate cancer into the PCPTRC in [11]. GWAS studies tend to report and validate SNPs not in linkage disequilibrium (LD). Under the assumption of independence of SNPs, the joint effect of multiple SNPs on the LR can still be estimated by separate meta-analyses for each SNP due to the factorization:

$$LR = \frac{P(Y_1, \ldots, Y_r|X, Cancer)}{P(Y_1, \ldots, Y_r|X, No\ Cancer)} = \frac{\prod_{i=1}^{r} P(Y_i|X, Cancer)}{\prod_{i=1}^{r} P(Y_i|X, NoCancer)} = \prod\nolimits_{i=1}^{r} LR_i \tag{7}$$

for markers $Y_1,\ldots, Y_r$ independently distributed given X and cancer status. In (7) LR_i is the likelihood ratio for each Y_i that can be estimated from separate meta-analyses. Due to independence, the update to the PCPTRC for incorporation of the 30 SNPs allows any combination to be used, examples of some updates are shown in Fig. 1.

Groups of SNPs reported across different publications may be in LD, which should be accounted for when analyzing them jointly in a meta-analysis for simultaneous incorporation into the LR. Several genomic databases are available that report estimates of LD based on haplotype studies, which can be incorporated into the within-study variance V_i by back-solving haplotype probabilities [12]. Our experience implementing this approach for the 30 prostate cancer SNPs showed negligible differences to the independent analyses, likely due to the observed low LD. However, simulation studies with artificially increased LD revealed only minor increases in the width of confidence intervals [11].

2.4 Issues and Open Research

The simplicity of the LR approach to updating risk models with new information is not without its limitations. The first is that typically the detailed collection of risk factors X that makes the prior risk tool so powerful is not performed in the external studies used to update the LR, forcing an assumption of independence to be made. The large SFCD that contributed the detailed family history information based on the entire population of Sweden certainly did not have current PSA or DRE available at the individual level; out of necessity the assumption of independence of detailed family history to these clinical factors was assumed. Similarly, the large genomic consortia that collect millions of individuals in order to capture rare variants could not be expected to rigorously collect established risk factors.

Different studies specialize in the collection of alternative types of information, which do not necessarily overlap. The strategy is to use relevant information from all sources to the extent possible, making assumptions or approximations when necessary. The naive Bayes classifier, commonly used in machine learning, ignores dependence among multiple features, but in many practical scenarios and simulation studies has shown accuracy approaching that of more complicated methods that model the dependence [13]. The LR assuming independence is a function of the naive Bayes classifier.

Grill et al. examined the impact of assuming independence between X and Y in the LR, finding considerable bias when data were generated under various dependence settings [7]. The bias was less pronounced for situations where the prior risk of disease was not small, the so-called non-rare-disease setting, which while the case for prostate cancer, is not for most diseases. Considering dependence between X and Y in the LR but assuming equal standard deviations among the cancer cases and controls was unbiased in all considered settings and showed accurate predictive performance. Not constraining variances to be equal resulted in poor calibration for higher risks in some of the settings.

How to link the dependence between Y and X when the new study measuring Y does not measure X remains an open issue. If a separate study could be found and used as a surrogate for estimating the correlation then some sort of imputation could be performed, the accuracy of which would depend on the sample size of the separate study.

Another issue that confronts the LR method is the potential difference in patient attributes between cohorts supplying estimates for the LR and prior risk tool. Mitigating these differences is the motivation behind conditioning the LR on the prior risk factors X. However, even when X has been measured in both cohorts there may be un-measured cohort differences beyond these factors that present contradictory information to the dual parts of the model. For our prostate cancer studies we typically restricted patients used in the LR to be 55 years or older, the minimal age of men who were used to build the PCPTRC population. For the GWAS reported SNPs this was not possible since individual patient age was unavailable. The GWAS and SFCD markers were only available for Caucasian men, so the updated PCPTRC for these markers was restricted to Caucasian men. However, there are many lifestyle differences between European and US men, the populations comprising the SFCD/GWAS and PCPTRC cohorts, respectively. For incorporating the new sera and urine markers, the case control studies that supplied them were collected as part of Early Detection Research Network (EDRN) grants mandating measurement of X. However, these were symptomatic patients presenting to a tertiary care clinic, and not the healthy men who had been pre-screened to have low PSA and normal DRE values to enter the seven year PCPT. Simulation studies are needed to understand the extent of bias that can occur as the dissimilarity between cohorts in terms of X and unmeasured factors increases.

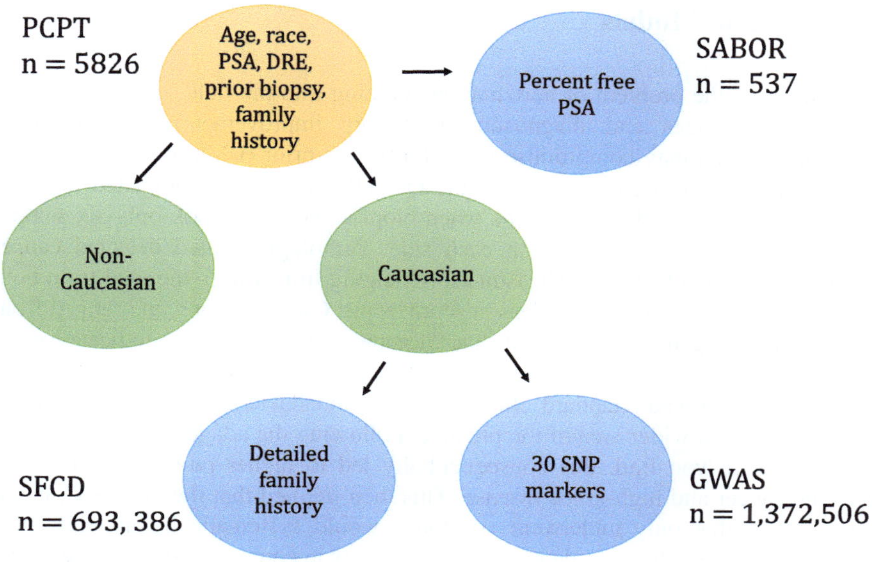

Fig. 2 Current options for incorporating markers into the PCPTRC, population sources, and sample sizes (*n*) on which they were built: PCPT: Prostate Cancer Prevention Trial [8], SABOR: San Antonio Biomarkers Of Risk of prostate cancer [8], SFCD: Swedish Family-cancer database [10], GWAS: multiple published genome-wide association studies [12]

2.5 Away from Single Cohort-Based to Multiple Cohort Compartmentalized Models that can be Updated One Component at a Time

New markers with promise to improve prediction and the lives of patients continually traverse the pipeline from discovery to validation to clinical practice. This dynamic necessitates a forward-looking view of risk models that may start with an exclusive cohort, but builds in modular fashion, taking advantage of all the information that specialized population-based studies have to offer as soon as the data are available. This process of merging information from multiple data sources, termed data transfer in the informatics literature, has the potential to result in increased power due to larger sample sizes. It capitalizes on the use of "found data", a recent term for data that has been carefully constructed for other purposes, but that becomes available for new objectives. Figure 2 shows the current new marker options to the PCPTRC that are all available online to facilitate validation in new populations.

3 Dynamic Models

In addition to the problem of new markers coming into the field, clinical practice, population changes and diagnostic technology improvements are constantly occurring, which may compromise the validity of a prior risk tool itself. Precisely such changes were occurring even as the PCPTRC was being completed in 2006. The PCPT started in the late 1990's when biopsies normally took only six sample cores from the prostate, three on each side. Pathologists rated detected cancer lesions on either side using a Gleason score ranging from 1 to 5, the total from both sides was denoted as the total Gleason score or just Gleason score, and ranged from 2 to 10. It was generally accepted that Gleason score 7 or higher indicated more aggressive disease, which was termed high-grade cancer. In the early 2000s, as technology improved, standard clinical practice mandated 12 biopsy cores rather than 6 to cover a wider area of the prostate. Following the adage that the more you look the more you find, this consequentially led to higher rates of detection of prostate cancer and high-grade disease. This then implied that the PCPTRC, based on a cohort that only underwent six cores, would systematically underestimate prostate cancer and high-grade prostate cancer rates in contemporary practice where the biopsy took twelve cores.

Additionally, with the turn of the century, the extent of over-diagnosis of prostate cancers became an issue, and the clinical field recognized different treatment options for low grade or non-significant cancers. Watchful waiting or active surveillance of patients with low grade cancers was endorsed, with periodic biopsies and no action taken until indication of an upgrading of the cancer. This change in treatment recommendation was accompanied by an upgrading shift in the field of pathology, whereby cancers that were normally graded under 7 by the Gleason score were more liberally graded as 7 or above, perhaps unconsciously in response to anxiety about a missed serious cancer. This upward shift in labeling over time threatened the risk of high-grade disease produced as one of the PCPTRC outputs, implying that the PCPTRC might underestimate the current risk of high-grade disease.

When fundamental changes such as these occur, one is faced with similar options as for incorporating new markers: either rebuild the model from scratch using a new cohort, with the same drawback of inefficiency, or patch up the existing risk tool. We again suggest the second approach using the statistical method of re-calibration of a risk model. As for incorporating the new markers, this approach also requires additional data, but in this case the additional data is easier to obtain as it just requires outcomes along with the established risk factors.

3.1 Updating a Statistical Model

Updating refers to any method of altering a risk model built on one population to optimize its performance on a new population. The last decade has witnessed a sharp increase in methods applied to dynamically updating models in intensive stations and critical care wards, where patient measurements flow in continuously. Our interest focused on simple intuitive methods for updating a risk tool built from logistic regression for application to a new or expanding population, where the update could happen in real time, as soon as more data became available. Specifically, we were interested in updating the PCPTRC to reflect patients seen under current clinical practice conditions, including with elevated PSA for those who were referred to a clinical practice versus normal PSA values for those undergoing regular screening, and for patients receiving the more commonly used 10- or 12-core biopsy procedure. Noting that the established risk factors are routinely collected in the clinic and can be automatically de-identified, we were motivated to see how serial updates applied to data from different institutions would diverge. The following case study shows how we arrived at our recommendation for dynamically updating logistic regression models.

3.2 Case Study: The Prostate Biopsy Collaborative Group

The Prostate Biopsy Collaborative Group (PBCG) was initially founded by the epidemiologist Andrew Vickers in response to the observation that a vast number of risk calculators were being produced in the urologic oncology field that gave widely varying predictions of whether cancer would be indicated if biopsy were to be performed. Concurrently he observed that multiple validation studies of a single risk tool often produced conflicting conclusions as to the generalizability of the tool, adding further confusion to the field. Collecting retrospective risk factor and outcome data from ten international institutions, Vickers and colleagues noticed that cancer risk, as a function of PSA, varied substantially from center to center, and that the differences between centers could not be accounted for by adjustment for measured risk factors, ushering in a conclusion that one-size-fits-all risk tools would not be optimal [14]. To illustrate we performed a multiple validation of the PCPTRC on the ten cohorts, and investigated the area-underneath-the-receiver-operating-curve (AUC), a measure of the discrimination power of a risk tool that ranges from 50% (no better than flipping a coin) to 100% (perfect ability to discriminate a cancer case from control). We obtained AUCs ranging from 56.2 to 72.0%, which to put in context, produced larger changes than those due to any improvement in a risk tool ever seen [15].

For a more detailed look at the institutional and temporal variation, we examined the yearly number of biopsies performed and positive biopsy rate at five of the PBCG cohorts in Table 1 and Fig. 3. The two urological referral centers, the Durham VA and Cleveland Clinic, which also happen to be in areas with high African American representation (a risk factor for prostate cancer), had cancer rates much higher than the remaining primarily screening cohorts. The Tyrol cohort was part of an Austrian screening study, where personal communication revealed that the principal investigator led an aggressive screening program, referring men to biopsy even with very minimal risk factors. The Durham VA clinic experienced large fluctuations in the positive biopsy rate in some years, which we later learned coincided with changes in personnel. Examination of the temporal cancer rate profiles revealed that specific local tendencies or changes incurred long-term and/or fleeting impacts on risk.

As seen in Table 1, the number of biopsies performed annually in large centers is quite high, meaning that these centers accrue enough patients to build their own calculator in only a handful of years. Since the required variables to build a risk tool are mandated by current clinical practice, we reasoned from Fig. 3 that procedures could in principle be developed allowing local data trustees to build their own institution-specific risk tools, which would be dynamically updated at intervals of convenience, yearly, monthly or even daily. The PCPTRC could be used as an initializing risk calculator for the institutions until enough data were available to overrule it as a prior risk. Smaller institutions or those without the need to invest in data cleaning and quality checks could use the default global PCPTRC, which had accumulated its patients from across the US and Canada. The choice between using a regional versus global calculator could be made akin to deciding whether to read the local versus global news.

Once procedures were in place to accumulate data at regular temporal intervals, a temporal validation procedure could be effortlessly established. The risk calculator could be built on all data up to a current year, say Year 1, and then validated on the next year, Year 2. Only when validation was acceptable on Year 2, could the Year 1 or Year 1 + Year 2 updated calculator be implemented for Year 3, and so forth.

With these data collection mechanisms in place, the next question becomes how to actually construct a dynamically changing risk calculator. Considering commonly-used modeling techniques, we arrived at the six methods in Table 2. It was prudent to compare all dynamic methods to just using the static PCPTRC, which would require no work to implement, as well as to the other extreme of building a clean-slate model using the institution's specific data and ignoring the PCPTRC altogether. Recalibration and revision are ad hoc frequentist methods that are straightforward to implement, using the linear predictor of a prior risk model as a single covariate in a new model; see [16, pp. 363–370] for an overview of these methods. The Bayesian approach fits a new logistic regression model to the data, but uses the PCPTRC parameter and variance estimates as a prior for the parameters comprising the log odds ratios. The specific details of these methods can be found in [17]. Proceeding year by year, the six approaches were fit using as a training set all data up to the current year and for validation, data from the next year.

There are currently many metrics available for evaluating risk predictions [16, pp. 255–280]. We chose two aimed at complementary aspects, one for discrimination and one for calibration. Since we were to perform many external validations, essentially the number of years of data from each cohort, we restricted ourselves to single summary measures. For discrimination we chose the AUC, which can be calculated as the Wilcoxon statistic for non-parametric two sample testing, available in standard statistical packages.

For calibration we chose the Hosmer-Lemeshow goodness-of-fit statistic, whose algorithm for calculation is shown in Fig. 4. Large values of the Hosmer-Lemeshow statistic indicate that predicted risks from the training data do not match observed

Table 1 Number of biopsies performed by year for five cohorts of the PBCG

	1994	1995	1996	1997	1998	1999	2000	2001	2002	2003	2004	2005	2006	2007	2008	Total
SABOR									138	96	147	202	126	84	105	898
Cleveland clinic							256	294	261	296	314	359	632	705	140	3257
Protect									629	872	1049	1272	1259	1261	918	7260
Tyrol		365	418	577	430	335	409	410	455	395	323	295	337			4749
Durham VA	77	99	119	129	80	83	104	145	198	220	212	228	185	173	133	2185

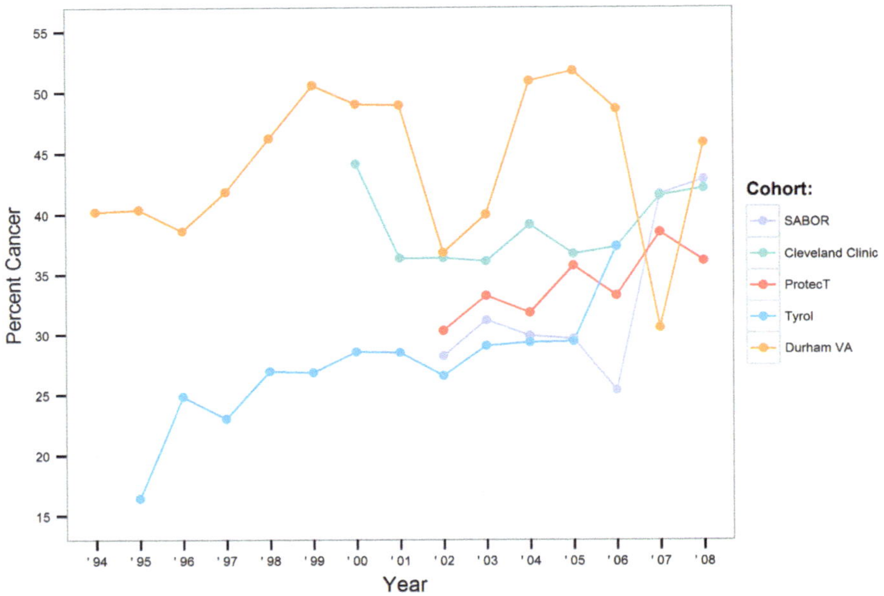

Fig. 3 Percent biopsies positive for cancer according to year performed for five cohorts of the PBCG; reproduced with permission from [17]

Table 2 Six alternative approaches for a prostate cancer risk calculator, five that change yearly by incorporating institutional information compared to a baseline approach of just using the static PCPTRC

PCPTRC: Use no institution-level data at all, just the online PCPTRC
Recalibration: Fit a new logistic regression with the PCPTRC linear predictor ($\beta'X$) as the only covariate in the model
Revision: Use the PCPTRC linear predictor ($\beta'X$) as one potential covariate among the other risk factors in logistic regression
Bayesian: Use prior to posterior updating on parameters in a logistic regression
Clean-slate: Build a new model each year using logistic regression
Random forests: An ensemble learning method that fits a series of random classification and regression trees

risks in the test data at least somewhere across the range from low to high risks. The smaller the statistic value the better the fit, and with the null hypothesis indicating goodness-of-fit, the less likely to reject the null hypothesis. We did not interpret p-values of the statistic since a property of hypothesis testing is that with large sample sizes the null hypothesis has a greater chance of being rejected. Our experience showed that indeed good calibration was only achieved for small test sets. We therefore restricted attention to the size of the test statistic itself. Although the statistic is restricted to evaluation over deciles, there is a slight dependence on

ALGORITHM:

1.) Compute the predicted risk for each individual in the test set.

2.) Calculate the deciles (10% lowest value, 20% lowest value,...) of the predicted risks : $\pi_{(.1)}, \pi_{(.2)}, \ldots, \pi_{(.9)}$.

3.) Make 10 intervals according to decile of risk : $[0, \pi_{(.1)}), [\pi_{(.1)}, \pi_{(.2)}), \ldots, [\pi_{(.9)}, 1.0]$.

4.) Calculate the observed number of people with predicted risk in each of the intervals, $n_1, \ldots, n_{10}$, the average predicted risk in each group, $\bar{\pi}_1, \bar{\pi}_2, \ldots, \bar{\pi}_{10}$, and the observed number of events (cancer cases) in each group, $O_1, O_2, \ldots, O_{10}$.

5.) To test H_0 : Goodness - of - fit of predicted risks versus H_A : not, use

$$X^2 = \sum_{i=1}^{10} \frac{(O_i - n_i \bar{\pi}_i)^2}{n_i \bar{\pi}_i (1 - \bar{\pi}_i)} \sim \chi^2_8 \text{ (chi - square distribution with 8 degrees of freedom).}$$

Fig. 4 Algorithm for computing the Hosmer-Lemeshow Goodness-of-fit test

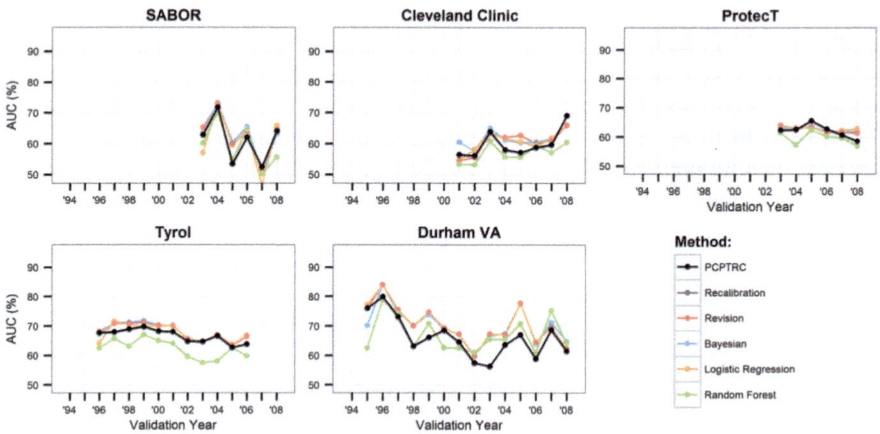

Fig. 5 Annual AUC values for the six methods evaluated on the five cohorts of the PBCG; higher AUC values indicate better discrimination of cancer cases from non-cancer cases; reproduced with permission from [17]

sample size, but since sample sizes did not vary dramatically over the years within a cohort, the statistic values were comparable. We performed extra analyses overlaying confidence intervals over the best methods, which revealed when changes were statistically significant. These matched years of extreme fluctuations, but because they made for busy graphs they are not shown.

Figure 5 shows how the AUCs of the different methods evolved annually over the sequential test sets across the five cohorts. As a reminder, higher AUCs indicate a greater probability for a model to assign higher risk to the cancer case among a randomly chosen cancer case-control pair in the test set. The first observation from Fig. 5 was that across all cohorts the AUCs did not improve with time, which was unexpected since the training set cumulatively aggregated more past data with each additional year. In Durham the AUC actually decreased during the initial years. Durham had the oldest series, beginning in 1994 and at a time when PSA-based screening was first becoming commonplace. Throughout the rest of the decade clinical practice patterns surrounding the emphasis on PSA were likely undergoing changes. The second observation was the lack of difference among the methods, except for random forests, which always seemed to perform more poorly than all others no matter how much its internal cross-validation parameters were tuned. As a rank-based measure, the AUC is notoriously robust to minor changes in model-based predictions, which could explain its lack of sensitivity for differentiating among the methods. It is invariant to monotonic transformations, hence the PCPTRC and recalibration yielded identical AUCs. The conclusion from Fig. 5 was that if discrimination was the sole objective, the static PCPTRC, requiring no local work, was good enough.

On the other hand, Fig. 6 revealed that calibration was where institution-specific data mattered. For interpretation, high values of the Hosmer-Lemeshow test statistic indicated poor rather than good fit as for the AUC. The PCPTRC performed markedly worse than all the other adaptive methods, except for random forests, whose values were so bad they fell off the graph, despite all the tweaking of tuning parameters to optimize their performance. Still apparent was that calibration did not improve with time, as one might have expected with the accumulation of more training data. In the SABOR screening cohort all methods showed high fluctuation, which could have resulted from changes over time in the screening protocol, such as a retreat from annual PSA testing in the later years (personal communication).

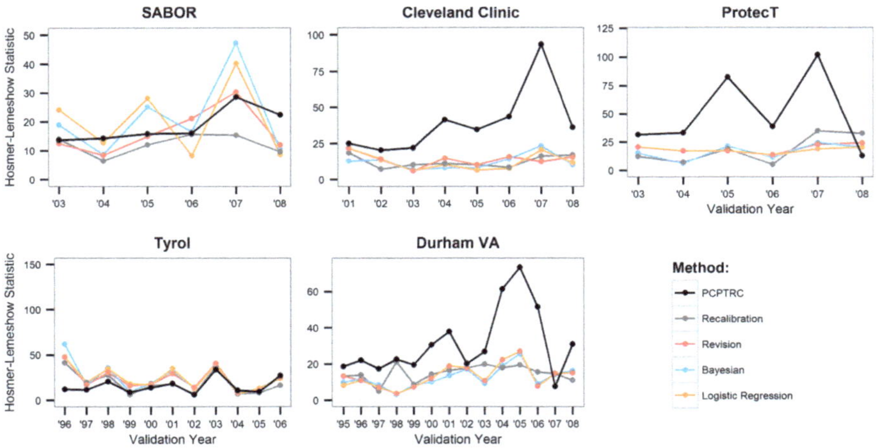

Fig. 6 Annual Hosmer-Lemeshow test statistic values for the six methods evaluated on the five cohorts of the PBCG; higher values indicate worse agreement between predicted and observed risks; reproduced with permission from [17]

All adaptive methods besides the random forests appeared to work equally well in terms of calibration.

Based on this empirical study of five real study cohorts, our recommendation was that if feasible, recalibration of a model to tailor it to a local data situation was always preferable to use of a global risk tool. Five alternative updating methods were investigated, all yielding equal performance except for random forests, which appeared to over-fit. We therefore recommended the simplest, recalibration, which only involves fitting a logistic regression with the single covariate, the logit of the PCPTRC risk estimate. Discrimination based on the rank-based AUC measure is a crude evaluation only of whether a risk tool provides higher values for cancer cases compared to non-cases. Doubling all risk predictions or halving them yields the same AUC since ranks are invariant to monotonic transformations. In this study, recalibration tended to primarily act on the intercepts of the risk models, to capture the large heterogeneity among cancer prevalence among the cohorts as witnessed in Fig. 3. Therefore, recalibration essentially served as a monotonic transformation of PCPTRC risks, thus not impacting the AUCs.

4 Discussion

In this chapter we have presented some of the contemporary issues facing risk prediction tools and argued the case for updating with external data in order to keep such tools relevant. The proposed methods were simple to implement, yet shown to be as adequate as more complicated alternatives. Challenges to their widespread use remain however, with future practical solutions and research needed.

4.1 Data Cleaning and Missing Values: Garbage in, Garbage out

One of the major persistent hurdles for risk prediction tool construction is messy data, which continues to plague most retrospective data archives despite all the improvements in data storage technology. We hid the dirty details in our analysis of the PBCG, but these ten international data sets, which took on average two years to assimilate locally, were no exception. Some of the cohorts did not collect certain PCPTRC risk factors at all, in particular family history, prior biopsy history and race. With 100% missing data on these fields within a cohort, imputation was not an option. To circumvent this issue, we derived alternative versions of the PCPTRC that allowed missing fields, by fitting the reduced models to the PCPT population. Other fields, such as DRE, were only collected sporadically by some of the cohorts, and contained up to 75% missing values. We deleted these records for the comparison of the methods, but have for other analyses used within-cohort multiple imputation. Imputation methods assume data are missing at random; techniques to handle non-random missing data require advanced statistical models with untestable specifications.

Post hoc imputation for missing values is not as optimal as correct prospective design to collect the right risk factors and prevent missing-ness altogether. Indeed this is why most risk calculators are founded on large well-planned study populations rather than retrospectively collected databases. Motivated by the poor and uneven quality of the retrospective PBCG data, we wrote a grant to prospectively standardize collection of the established risk factors for prostate biopsy across the ten centers. As the work has started it has become apparent that even some intuitive data entry requirements require education, such as recording the date of risk factors in relation to the date the outcome was assessed in order to ensure the risk factor was not measured after the outcome or too early in advance of the predictive window. Our grant has had to fund local administrative assistants to implement the data entry, which is an expensive and time-consuming process.

4.2 The Promise and Pitfalls of Electronic Health Records (EHR)

As an automated daily supply of hospital risk factors and procedure outcomes, the EHR would appear to offer a simple alternative to manual preparation of data for risk model construction. In principle, data quality control checks and risk model building could be built directly into the EHR, sidestepping all the ethical hurdles surrounding the collection and de-identification of data. With so much data available, models could be dispensed altogether in favor of non-parametric techniques such as nearest-neighbor clustering that would just search for similar patients in terms of their risk factors, returning the proportion of these that experienced the outcome as the estimated risk.

However, the current state of most EHR systems offers little above that witnessed by manual extraction, with data irregularly coded and often masked indecipherably in text fields. Work needs to be done to design doctor charts prospectively to enable automated data entry. Such systems have been implemented in the Kaiser Permanente HealthCare system, where all infant beds have a computer entry system attached, and all information has to be entered through drop-down selection menus, with only certain notes typed and no hand-writing allowed [18].

The necessary resources are out there for keeping our valuable risk tools up to state-of-the-art in order to benefit patients optimally. We have to keep working on both levels, data and methods, to accelerate the progress.

References

1. Mahmood SS, Levy D, Vasan RS, Wang TJ. The framingham heart study and the epidemiology of cardiovascular disease: a historical perspective. Lancet. 2014;383 (9921):999–1008.
2. Gail MH. Twenty-five years of breast cancer risk models and their applications. J Natl Cancer Inst. 107(5):djv042. doi:10.1093/jnci/djv042.
3. Thompson IM, Goodman PJ, Tangen CM, et al. The influence of finasteride on the development of prostate cancer. N Engl J Med. 2003;349(3):215–24.
4. Thompson IM, Pauler DK, Goodman PJ, et al. Prevalence of prostate cancer among men with a prostate-specific antigen level $\leq$ or = 4.0 ng per milliliter. N Engl J Med. 2004;350(22):2239–46.
5. Thompson IM, Ankerst DP, Chi C, Goodman PJ, Tangen CM, Lucia MS, Feng Z, Parnes HL, Coltman CA Jr. Assessing prostate cancer risk: results from the Prostate Cancer Prevention trial. J Natl Cancer Inst. 2006;98(8):529–34.
6. Ankerst DP, Groskopf J, Day JR, Blase A, Rittenhouse H, Pollock BH, Tangen C, Parekh D, Leach RJ, Thompson I. Predicting prostate cancer risk through incorporation of prostate cancer gene 3. J Urol. 2008;180(4):1303–8.
7. Grill S, Ankerst DP, Gail MH, et al. Comparison of approaches for incorporating new information into existing risk prediction models Stat Med. 2017;36(7):1134–56.
8. Ankerst DP, Hoefler J, Bock S, Goodman PJ, Vickers A, Hernandez J, Sokoll LJ, Sanda MG, Wei JT, Leach RJ, Thompson IM. The prostate cancer prevention trial risk calculator 2.0 for the prediction of low—versus high-grade prostate cancer. Urology. 2014;83(6):1362–7, Reply in 83(6):1368, 2014.
9. Ankerst DP, Koniarski T, Liang Y, Leach RJ, Feng Z, Sanda MG, Partin AW, Chan DW, Kagan J, Sokoll L, Wei JT, Thompson IM. Updating risk prediction tools: a case study in prostate cancer. Biometrical J. 2012;54(1):127–42.
10. Grill S, Fallah M, Leach RJ, Thompson IM, Freedland S, Hemminki K, Ankerst DP. Incorporation of detailed family history from the Swedish-family cancer database into the prostate cancer prevention trial risk calculator. J Urol. 2015;193(2):460–5.
11. Grill S. Incorporation of external methods into clinical prediction models. Ph.D. thesis, Technical University Munich. 2016.
12. Grill S, Fallah M, Leach RJ, Thompson IM, Hemminki K, Ankerst DP. A simple-to-use method incorporating genomic markers into prostate cancer risk prediction tools facilitated future validation. J Clin Epidemiol. 2015;68(5):563–73.
13. Hand DJ, Yu K. Idiot's Bayes: not so stupid after all? Int Stat Rev. 2001;69(3):385–98.
14. Vickers AJ, Cronin AM, Roobol MJ, Hugosson J, Jones JS, Kattan MW, Klein E, Hamdy F, Neal D, Donovan J, Parekh DJ, Ankerst D, Bartsch G, Klocker H, Horninger W, Benchikh A, Salama G, Villers A, Freedland SJ, Moreira DM, Schroeder FH, Lilja H. The relationship between prostate-specific antigen and prostate cancer risk: the Prostate Biopsy Collaborative Group. Clin Cancer Res. 2010;16(17):4374–81.
15. Ankerst DP, Boeck A, Freedland SJ, Thompson IM, Cronin AM, Roobol MJ, Hugosson J, Jones JS, Kattan MW, Klein EA, Hamdy F, Neal D, Donovan J, Parekh DJ, Klocker H, Horninger W, Benchikh A, Salama G, Villers A, Moreira DM, Schroeder FH, Lilja H, Vickers AJ. Evaluating the PCPT risk calculator in ten international biopsy cohorts: results from the prostate biopsy collaborative group. World J Urol. 2012;30(2):181–7.
16. Steyerberg DW. Clinical prediction models. New York: Springer; 2010.
17. Strobl AN, Vickers AJ, van Calster B, Steyerberg E, Leach RJ, Thompson IM, Ankerst DP. Improving patient prostate cancer risk assessment: moving from static, globally-applied to dynamic, practice-specific cancer risk calculators. J Biomed Inform. 2015;56:87–93.
18. Escobar GJ, LaGuardia JC, Turk BJ, Ragins A, Kipnis P, Draper D. Early detection of impending physiologic deterioration among patients who are not in intensive care: development of predictive models using data from an automated electronic medical record. J Hosp Med. 2012;7(5):388–95.

Evaluation of Cancer Risk in Epidemiologic Studies with Genetic and Molecular Data

Aya Kuchiba

Abstract Epidemiology has made significant contribution to better understanding cancer etiology and improving public health. Recently, with increasingly available genetic and molecular data, methodology in cancer epidemiology has been greatly progressing through incorporation of those data. This chapter focuses on some topics in Genome-Wide Association Studies and also provides some discussion of investigating etiologic heterogeneity among molecular subtypes of cancer.

Keywords Genome-wide association studies · Multiple testing · Meta-analysis · Prediction · Cancer heterogeneity

1 Introduction

In the past decade, a number of disease-associated genetic variants have been identified by Genome-Wide Association Studies (GWAS) [1]. GWAS have become larger-scaled, for example, recent GWAS for breast cancer included nearly 100,000 participants from several studies in the consortium, and evaluated more than hundreds of thousands of SNPs [2]. In addition to advances in knowledge of the human genome [3–7] and in technology for measuring genetic variants, considerable effort in developing strategies for association analysis contributes to successful GWAS [8].

On the other hand, somatic genome or other molecular features of the cancers have been investigated to understand the underlying pathogenesis mechanisms. In parallel catalogs for variants in the human genome, The Cancer Genome Atlas (TCGA) project (https://cancergenome.nih.gov/) and the International Cancer Genome Consortium (ICGC) project (icgc.org) have discovered major cancer-causing genomic alterations for more than 30 tumor types. Epidemiologic research has increasingly examined the associations of risk factors with a cancer,

A. Kuchiba (✉)
Biostatistics Division, Center for Research Administration and Support,
National Cancer Center, Tokyo, Japan
e-mail: akuchiba@ncc.go.jp

S. Matsui and J. Crowley (eds.), *Frontiers of Biostatistical Methods and Applications in Clinical Oncology*, DOI 10.1007/978-981-10-0126-0_18

taking into account the inherent molecular heterogeneity of a cancer, which might reflect distinct processes of tumor development.

This chapter will provide an overview of some topics in GWAS, including gene discovery and prediction model development. We also discuss studies of etiologic heterogeneity among molecular subtypes of cancer.

2 Genome-Wide Association Studies

GWAS is an approach to scan associations of genetic variants with disease across the whole genome by genotyping hundreds of thousands of SNPs simultaneously. Typically, GWAS is carried out in a population-based case-control study. While a genome-wide approach was proposed in 1996 as a most powerful method for discovering genes associated with common complex diseases [9], recent advances in the understanding of the human genome structure and in genotyping technology have made an efficient genome-wide approach feasible.

The Human Genome Project [3, 4] and the HapMap Project [5–7] have revealed human genome structures, including the positions of single nucleotide polymorphisms (SNPs) and the linkage disequilibrium (LD) patterns in the population by ancestry groups. A SNP is a single base change in DNA, which is the most common type of genetic variant in the human genome. LD is a phenomenon, where alleles at flanking loci on the same chromosomes tend to occur together in the population, and consequently SNPs in the region of strong LD tend to be correlated. This is generated as a result of sharing ancestry of a population of chromosomes at some regions. This knowledge enables us to use a SNP set with about 1 million SNPs in order to obtain sufficient information on roughly 10 million SNPs over the human genome.

SNPs are used as markers indicating the location in the genome. SNPs themselves may be causative variants or the flanking markers that are highly correlated with the causative variants through LD (Fig. 1). The more SNPs are measured, the more likely one of the SNPs is located near the causative variants. The coverage of the genome is one of the components for successful GWAS. Imputation has become a routine approach to search the genome, in which unmeasured variants are predicted using existing catalogs and observed genotype data [10]. Imputation accuracy will depend on SNP density as well as the similarity of LD patterns between the data used and the HapMap populations. Imputation is also potentially useful for combining GWAS data sets in meta-analysis (discussed later) because the studies often use different SNP panels and have partially overlapped genotyped data.

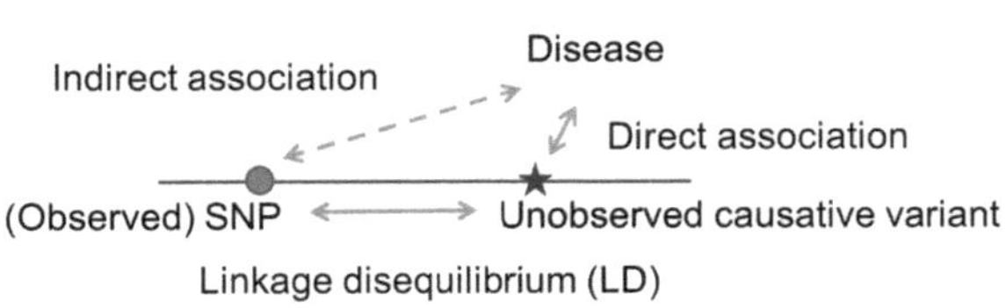

Fig. 1 Direct and indirect associations

GWAS evaluates the SNP-disease associations without distinction of direct or indirect association, and involves narrowing down the regions that would include the causative variants. The following sections will discuss some of the specific topics in GWAS.

2.1 Summarizing GWAS Results Visually

Hypothesis testing of each SNP sequentially for comparing allele or genotype frequencies between the cases and the controls is the common approach for GWAS analysis; the *P*-value is usually used as a primary summary measure of association. Logistic regression is often used for controlling potential confounders. Consequently, we will have a million of *P*-values in a single GWAS. The whole set of results with the huge number of *P*-values is visually summarized with quantile-quantile (Q-Q) plots and Manhattan plots.

The Q-Q plot is a plot of the quantiles of the negative logarithm of the observed *P*-values (i.e., $-\log_{10}(P)$) on the y-axis against the same quantiles of the expected values assuming a uniform distribution on the x-axis (e.g., Supplemental Fig. 1 in [11]). That is, if all SNPs are under the null hypothesis of no association, the Q-Q plots will approximately lie on the y = x line. This plot is useful in the quality control process on genotype data. Since most of SNPs will have no association, some SNPs with extremely small *P*-values will deviate from the y = x line. If the Q-Q plot departs from the y = x line overall, this may suggest that the genotype data still contain a substantial amount of typing errors. It may be solved, at least partially, by applying more strict criteria for the quality control checking of genotype data (such as minor allele frequency, missing genotype frequency for a SNP and for an individual, and violation of the Hardy-Weinberg equilibrium). The difference in accuracy of genotyping between cases and controls will result in biased estimates; in consequence, false positives can arise.

The Q-Q plot is also used to evaluate potential population stratification. Population stratification is the differences in allele frequencies between cases and controls due to systematic differences in ancestry, rather than association of genes with disease. Allele frequencies vary among populations of different genetic ancestry. Similarly, disease risk often varies among the populations for some reasons, such as lifestyle differences. Evaluating whether population stratification exists in the GWAS population is an important part of the quality control process on genotype data. The genomic inflation factor [12] (usually denoted by λ), which is defined as the ratio of the median of the observed distribution of a test statistic to the expected median, is often used to quantify the deviation with the Q-Q plot.

Also, hidden population structure can be estimated by principal component analysis, which infers continuous axes of genetic variation using genotype data [13]. The principal components can be included in the logistic regression model to adjust for population stratification, as for the other potential confounders.

The Manhattan plot represents the whole set of *P*-values from a different point of view. In this plot, $-\log_{10}(P)$ for each SNP is displayed on the y-axis, along with the positions on chromosomes on the x-axis (e.g., Fig. 1 in [11]). Because a majority of SNPs will be under the null hypothesis, the *P*-values look to be uniformly distributed, except for the smallest *P*-values deviating from such a trend. This plot gives us a rough sense of the associations.

2.2 P-Value Adjustment

Given the hundreds of thousands of hypothesis tests, the multiplicity of comparisons should be accounted for to make a decision on whether the marker is "significant" or not. Table 1 shows the results when testing *m* SNPs. In early GWASs, a threshold of $P \leq 10^{-7}$ or $P \leq 5 \times 10^{-7}$ was typically used to control family-wise error rate (FWER), which is defined as $\Pr(V \geq 1)$. However, in current practice more SNPs are genotyped or imputed with higher quality, a more strict threshold, $P \leq 5 \times 10^{-8}$, is commonly accepted as a genome-wide significant level, which is roughly corresponding to a Bonferroni correction to maintain FWER of 5% for 1 million independent comparisons for SNPs [14].

False discovery rate (FDR) is the other definition of error in the context of multiple comparisons. FDR is defined to be the expectation of *V*/*R*, that is, the expected proportion of the truly non-associated SNPs among the SNPs for which the null hypotheses are rejected. FDR is represented as the function of the proportion of truly associated SNPs (defined as a prior), and the power and alpha level of each test.

FDR was originally proposed in the frequentist framework by Benjamini and Hochberg [15], and further formulated in the Bayesian framework [16, 17]. The threshold of *P*-value can be obtained to maintain the FDR at a pre-specified level (e.g., 0.05), or the FDR can be estimated for the decision based on hypothesis testing. The *q* value, which is the minimum FDR that can be attained when declaring a significant association, is proposed as an FDR-based measure of significance for a particular SNP [18]. FDR is popular and successfully used in omics studies, e.g., gene expression studies with microarrays, where the proportion of non-null associations is generally not small. In contrast, the proportion of non-null associations may be very close to 0 in many GWASs. In this case, the FDR approach may not give much advantage over the FWER approach. That may be the reason that the standard Bonferroni correction remains the most commonly used adjustment for GWAS.

Table 1 Results when testing *m* hypotheses

	Accept null	Reject null	Total
Null true	U	V	m_0
Non-null true	T	S	m_1
Total	$m - R$	R	m

It would be worthwhile to mention that empirical evaluation suggested that a substantial portion of associations with borderline *P*-values (i.e., $P \leq 10^{-7}$ and $P > 5 \times 10^{-8}$) may be genuine associations [19]. This suggests that making a prioritized list of SNPs to be studied in other secondary analyses or further studies, not only identifying statistically significant SNPs, would be an important purpose for GWAS analysis. Although the *P*-value is commonly used as a summary measure of association to prioritize (rank) the SNPs, there has been debate about summary measures of associations in GWAS. As for combining the Bayesian idea and classical statistical significance, false positive report probability (FPRP) has been proposed, which is the joint probabilities from the hypothesis testing and the probability of truth of the alternative hypothesis [20]. FPRP is defined as $FPRP = p(1 - \pi)/\{p(1 - \pi) + (1 - \beta)\pi\}$, where p is the level of statistical significance for a single test of association, $1 - \beta$ is the power of the test, and π is the prior probability that the alternative hypothesis is true. Bayes factor may be another option. The Bayes factor is defined as the ratio of the probability of the observed data under the null hypothesis to the probability of the observed data under the alternative hypothesis, requiring assumptions for effect sizes of SNP-disease associations. Wellcome Trust Case Control Consortium has used Bayes factor to prioritize the SNP as a complement to *P* value [21, 22].

2.3 Meta-analysis

GWAS findings should be followed in further independent studies to confirm whether the significant associations are replicated, regardless of which decision rules or summary measures are used. Meta-analyses are usually used to evaluate evidence from the replication studies. Furthermore, GWAS focuses on selection of potential disease-associated SNPs, and usually the effect size estimation is a secondary purpose. Indeed, the effect estimates (e.g., odds ratio) of the top hit SNPs from discovery studies tend to be upward biased, which is known as "winner's curse" [23, 24]. Meta-analysis of replication studies has role of obtaining unbiased effect size estimates.

In addition to confirmation, meta-analysis has become popular approach to discovery new disease-associated variants. Basically, meta-analysis for this purpose is to combine the effect estimates of each SNP across the studies, for all of SNPs genotyped in GWASs. Statistical power will be increased and the true associated SNPs are expected to rise to the top of the list. Also, the false positives caused by random errors are expected to be reduced over those from a single study.

Suppose that genotype data from the same M SNPs are available for S case-control studies. Let β_{ij} and v_{ij} denote the effect size and its variance of the ith SNP ($i = 1, \ldots, M$) in the jth study ($j = 1, \ldots, S$). β_{ij} is typically logarithm of odds ratio for the ith SNP in the jth study. The SNP specific combined estimate can be expressed:

$$\hat{\beta}_i = \frac{\sum_{j=1}^{s} \hat{\beta}_{ij}\hat{w}_{ij}}{\sum_{j=1}^{s} \hat{w}_{ij}},$$

where $\hat{w}_{ij}$ is the jth study-specific weight for the ith SNP. In the standard fixed-effects model, $\hat{w}_{ij}$ can be the inverse of the variance estimate of $\hat{\beta}_{ij}$, and the asymptotic variance of the combined estimate can be obtained as:

$$\hat{V}_i = \frac{1}{\sum_{j=1}^{s} \hat{w}_{ij}}.$$

The fixed-effects meta-analysis approach assumes that the true effect of each SNP is the same across the studies. The random-effects meta-analysis approach allows the true effects to vary across studies, rather than assuming one true effect. The combined estimate from a random-effects model represents the mean of all potential populations. w_{ij} includes two sources of the variance, within studies and between studies.

There would be no standard rule for choosing between a fixed or random effects model for discover. In either case, quality control in each study, which includes accuracy of imputed genotypes, is essential to avoid unnecessary between-study heterogeneity. Also, all of the analyses must be planned to be as similar as possible across the studies. In the sense of prioritizing SNPs, a random-effects meta-analysis approach can be considered to penalize the SNPs showing heterogeneity between studies and appears to be reasonable to discover new disease-associated SNPs. The disadvantage of a random-effects meta-analysis approach will be to unnecessarily penalize the SNPs that show heterogeneity by chance, leading those SNPs to be moved downward in the priority list. The strengths and weaknesses of random effects meta-analysis have been discussed in [25], although not in the context of GWAS. Indeed, a fixed-effects approach is generally more powerful in terms of raising the true positives to the top of the list [26]. In practice, both models can be applied. If there are SNPs which show differences in rankings or effects by models, the investigators should see the results in each study and explore the reasons for the differences to judge whether the further studies for those SNPs are warranted.

The question may be raised as to resource allocation, i.e., how many studies should be used for discovery studies and how many for replication studies. Meta-analytic GWAS may give some reason to skip independent replication studies, because the approach includes investigation of heterogeneity in effect estimates of SNPs between studies.

2.4 Beyond a Single Locus Analysis

Single-SNP analyses are predominant in GWAS practice. This single-SNP approach is sometimes referred to as "unbiased" since it requires no prior knowledge of location or function of genetic variants, but also it can be viewed as a preliminary step in the gene identification process. Increasingly available knowledge of human genome can extend GWAS analysis. Pathway-analysis is one of the approaches (e.g., [27, 28]). These methods combine the effects from multiple SNPs within given genes or biological pathways and examine the association of the joint effect of a set of SNPs with an outcome. It could have a potential role as a complement to single-SNP analysis, and provide an additional insight to identify the disease-associated genes, especially where each SNP within a given pathway or gene has relatively small effects on the disease.

Also, all SNPs may not be equally likely to have influence on disease, depending on the location or function of the variants. It has been demonstrated that SNPs identified in GWASs are enriched in protein-coding exons, in promoters, and in untranslated regions (UTRs) [29]. A Bayesian framework can incorporate this prior knowledge into the gene discovery process from the beginning. In particular, a Bayesian hierarchical modelling approach would have promise for further analysis using GWAS data [30, 31], although it is still less used in practice.

The importance of the potential interplay of environmental and genetic factors has been discussed extensively [32, 33]. Studying the interaction is expected to improve the power to discover underlying susceptibility loci and identify susceptible subpopulations. Understanding gene-environmental interactions involved in complex disease may also improve performance and utility of risk prediction models for disease prevention and treatment. Gene-environment interaction has been commonly explored with a test for the interaction term based on a logistic regression model. However, most such studies have shown disappointing results, suggesting that multiplicative interactions, even if present, are likely to have relatively small impact for complex diseases and may not be easily detected in GWAS approaches [34, 35]. The effective way to assess interactions in the context of GWAS remains unclear. Statistical methods to detect the interaction have been discussed in the several papers, which include a joint test of marginal association and gene-environment interaction, case-only analysis, and shrinkage estimators (e.g., [36–39]).

3 Prediction Model

In hereditary cancer, which is caused primarily by mutations in the cancer-susceptibility genes, the high-penetrance genes such as *BRCA1* and *BRCA2* genes for breast and ovarian cancers are important for clinical management of individuals. For example, a recent study suggests that the risk of developing breast cancer by age 70 years is around 55% for *BRCA1* mutation carries and 47% for *BRCA2* mutation carries [40]. The presence of mutations in the cancer-susceptibility genes is clinically used in genetic testing and counseling of individuals in high-risk families.

For common complex diseases, stratifying the population based on distinct disease risks could greatly contribute to the development of public health strategies for disease prevention in the general population. For this purpose, the absolute risk, which is the probability that an individual will develop the disease over a certain time interval, is critical. Studying prediction models for estimating absolute risk has been carried out with non-genetic risk factors for common cancers. For example, the Gail model is one of the popular models for breast cancer risk prediction, which provides the probability that a woman with given age and risk factors will develop breast cancer over an age interval $[a, a + s]$. This probability, R, can be defined from [41] with a vector of risk factors, $\boldsymbol{x}$, as following:

$$R = \int_{a}^{a+s} \lambda(t|\boldsymbol{x}) \exp(-\int_{a}^{t} [\lambda(u|\boldsymbol{x}) + h(u)]du)dt,$$

where $\lambda(t|\boldsymbol{x})$ is the age-specific incidence rate, $h(u)$ is the age-specific mortality from other causes than breast cancer. In this model, the absolute risk of developing the disease over a specific age interval is defined as the sum of the probability that a woman will develop the disease at a given age, t, given that the woman is disease-free and alive until that age. In a prospective cohort study, $\lambda(t|\boldsymbol{x})$ can be commonly modeled using the Cox proportional hazards model: $\lambda(t|x) = \lambda_0(t) \exp(\boldsymbol{\beta}'\boldsymbol{x})$, where $\lambda_0(t)$ is a baseline hazard for the disease and $\boldsymbol{\beta}$ is a vector of regression coefficients for $\boldsymbol{x}$. The risk factors originally used in Gail model were age at menarche, age at first live birth, number of previous biopsies, and number of first-degree relatives with breast cancer [41]. The Gail model was actually used for patient selection criteria in the tamoxiphen chemopreventive intervention trial [42].

Wacholder et al. [43] investigated the model including adding 10 SNPs to the original Gail risk factors, then compared the prediction performance of models by the concordance index (known as C-index or C-statistics). Although the inclusion of an additional 10 SNPs showed no substantial impact on prediction performance, interestingly, their data suggested that a SNP-only model had almost the same prediction performance (C-index: 58.0% for original Gail model; 59.7% for SNP-only model). Early development of prediction models with GWAS findings may be disappointing, since including the associated SNPs did not dramatically improve prediction performance as expected.

In a recent prediction model development, the Polygenic Risk Score (PRS) (or Genetic Risk Score (GRS)) has been used as genetic susceptibility for individuals, instead of including each of the disease-associated SNPs into the model. PRS is defined as a weighted combination of any type of variants that cause disease susceptibility, and considered to be summary measure of genetic susceptibility to the disease for an individual. PRS may not be interpretable in itself, but the variation of PRS in the population can be related to the heritability, which is the proportion of phenotypic variation attributed to genetic variation among individuals in a population. The detailed explanation of the relationship of PRS and heritability has been described in [44].

Several studies have shown that a substantial proportion of heritability in most common cancers can be explained by GWAS SNPs [45, 46]. From the GWAS findings, the PRS for each individual may be estimated as:

$$PRS_j = \sum_{i=1}^{m} \hat{\beta}_i x_{ij},$$

where $\hat{\beta}_i$ is an estimate of the per-minor allele log odds ratio for the *i*th SNP, x_{ij} is the number of minor alleles for the *i*th SNP (0, 1, or 2), and m is the total number of SNPs. Note that the *PRS* summarizes the effects of the susceptible SNPs and, here, ignores the interaction effects between SNPs.

A number of SNPs with modest or small effects can be involved defining genetic susceptibility for common complex diseases. Recently, Mavaddat et al. investigated the absolute risk estimate for breast cancer based on PRS using 77 SNPs with genome-wide significant levels [47]. This study showed that the estimated risk of developing breast cancer by age 80 years for women in the lowest and highest 1% of the PRS was 3.5 and 29.0%, respectively, although discrimination ability was still modest with C-index = 0.622 [47].

Constructing an optimal PRS may be challenging. Estimating PRS essentially requires two parts: selecting SNPs for constructing PRS and estimating the weights, usually the estimates of regression coefficients on disease, for each SNP. Generally, SNPs with genome-wide significant level are used for PRS calculation, suggesting that sufficient large sample size is required to detect true SNPs with small effects. Incorporating additional SNPs showing evidence for association, but not reaching genome-wide statistical significance, may have potential to improve the prediction performance. As more risk factors are identified for a disease and incorporated in a model, estimated risks will be more variable between individuals. As a result, a larger proportion of people could be identified as belonging more extreme risk categories [44]. A potential challenge would be to include non-associated noisy SNP. So far, empirical investigations for breast cancer and prostate cancer showed that including non-significant SNPs into PRS have no impact on the prediction performance [48]. The other concern may be that the effect size estimate (i.e., the weight for each SNP) from a discovery data set can be upward biased and should be obtained from independent samples. Consequently, the process for constructing optimal PRS requires a large number of samples. Furthermore, regardless of using PRS or not, evaluating predictive performance of the developed prediction model will generally require an independent data set to avoid the over-fitting problem. It can be easily expected that an enormous sample size is required to complete the process of developing a prediction model. The optimum strategy for developing prediction model would be an important future issue.

The utility of a prediction model depends on the prediction performance and also on available actions based on the predicted risks. The evaluation of a prediction model should be suited to the available strategies for disease prevention. Risk-prediction models first need careful calibration to ensure they provide unbiased estimates of risk for individuals given their risk factor profiles. In addition to calibration ability, good discrimination ability will be required in the high-risk intervention, such as chemoprevention [49]. However, good discrimination ability may be difficult in the PRS prediction model, because the risk factors must have very large relative risks to achieve high discriminatory accuracy [50].

Genetic variants can be considered as a basis of individual susceptibility for the diseases. There is potential for a stronger impact in modifying non-genetic factors in higher risk group from PRS model. The distribution of modifiable risk factors in the risk categories based on underlying genetic risk might provide useful information to develop cost-effective intervention programs for prevention and health management in the population.

4 Cancer Heterogeneity

The previous sections have focused on the germline genome and discussed studies for understanding genetic contribution to cancer etiology. On the other hand, the cancer of interest can often be classified into molecularly distinct subtypes. There has been tremendous progress in using such cancer classification for the study of prognosis in cancer patients and differences in treatment response. In this section, we discuss cancer heterogeneity from the etiological perspective, in which molecular data are used to define outcomes. For example, fatty acid synthase (FASN) plays an important role in energy metabolism of fatty acids and is overexpressed in subset of colorectal cancers. Although obesity is one of the established

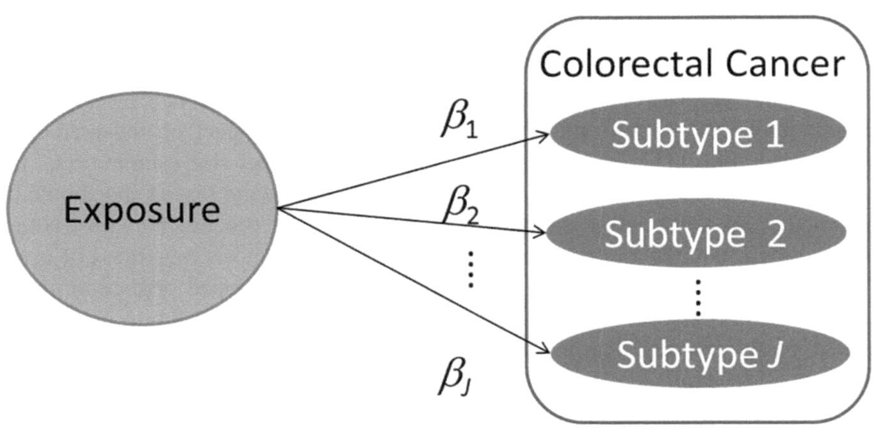

Fig. 2 Subtype-specific effect and heterogeneity parameter Heterogeneity parameter between *i*th subtype and *j*th subtype, $\alpha_{ij}=\beta_j-\beta_i$

risk factors of colorectal cancer, a recent study has suggested that obesity may be associated with increased risk of FASN-negative (no or weak expression) colorectal cancer but not associated with increased risk of FASN-positive (moderate to strong expression) colorectal cancer [51]. Colorectal cancer subtypes by FASN may have distinct etiology, in terms of obesity.

Basically, the study can evaluate the associations of a risk factor with each subtype, separately, then compare the associations among subtypes (Fig. 2). In a cohort study, a competing risks framework can be applied to model the hazards for each subtype. Suppose that there are J molecular subtypes of interest for evaluating etiologic heterogeneity. Let T_i denote time to the first occurrence of the cancer of interest or the censoring. Y_i denote an event indicator with $Y_i = j\ (1, \ldots, J)$ if the jth subtype occurs during follow-up, otherwise $Y_i = 0$ (the censoring). Let $\boldsymbol{X_i}$ denote a vector of the exposures of interest of the ith participant. For simplicity, $\boldsymbol{X_i}$ is assumed to be time independent. The cause-specific proportional hazards model [52] can be used to model a subtype-specific hazard at time t, $\lambda_j(t)$, as following:

$$\lambda_i(t|\boldsymbol{X}_i) = \lambda_{0j}(t)\exp(\boldsymbol{\beta}_j'\boldsymbol{X}_i), \tag{1}$$

where $\lambda_{0j}(t)$ is a baseline hazard at time t for the jth subtype and $\boldsymbol{\beta}_j$ is a vector of the jth subtype-specific regression coefficient for $\boldsymbol{X}_i$. In the above case of the association between obesity and colorectal cancer subtypes, $J = 2$, and suppose that $j = 1$ for FASN-negative colorectal cancer and $j = 2$ for FASN-positive colorectal cancer. $\boldsymbol{X}$ is BMI (kg/m^2), which is one of the measurements of obesity, at baseline. $\exp(\boldsymbol{\beta}_2)$ and $\exp(\boldsymbol{\beta}_2)$ are the hazard ratios of BMI for FASN-negative colorectal cancer and FASN-positive colorectal cancer, respectively.

To estimate subtype-specific effects, $\boldsymbol{\beta}_j$, the standard Cox regression analysis can be performed for each subtype separately, where the occurrence of the other subtypes is treated as a censoring. Heterogeneity parameter between the kth subtype and jth subtype can be defined as $\boldsymbol{\alpha}_{jk} = \boldsymbol{\beta}_k - \boldsymbol{\beta}_j$, which is equivalent to the ratio of the hazard ratio for the kth subtype to the hazard ratio for the jth subtype. The data duplication method [53] provides the joint estimation of subtype-specific parameters and heterogeneity parameters. Each record for a participant is augmented for each subtype and new exposure variable $\boldsymbol{X}_{ji}$ is created as $\boldsymbol{X}_{ji} = \boldsymbol{X}_i$ for the jth subtype and $\boldsymbol{X}_{li} = 0$ for the lth subtype ($l \neq j$) in the augmented data set. Table 2 illustrates

Table 2 Example of an augmented data set with $J = 2$

ID = 1 in the original data set

ID	Y	T	X
1	1	20	23.6

ID = 1 in the augmented data set

ID	Y	T	X	X_1	X_2	CENSOR	TYPE
1	1	20	23.6	23.6	0	1	1
1	1	20	23.6	0	23.6	0	2

Table 3 3 × 2 table with 2 subtypes and controls

	Exposed	Non-exposed
Subtype 1	*a*	*b*
Subtype 2	*c*	*d*
Control	*e*	*f*

augmented data, when $J = 2$, for a participant with $ID = 1$ who developed the 1st subtype ($Y = 1$) at 20 months from the start of study ($T = 20$) and had body mass index (BMI) of 23.6 kg/m^2 at baseline ($X = 23.6$). X_1 and X_2 are the augmented exposure variables. Two new variables will be also created: $TYPE = 1$ if the record is for the 1st subtype and $TYPE = 2$ if the record is for the 2nd subtype; and $CENSOR = 1$ if a participant developed the subtype indicated by *TYPE*, otherwise $CENSOR = 0$. Model (1) can be rewritten on the augmented data set as follows:

$$\begin{aligned}\lambda_j(t|\boldsymbol{X}_i) &= \lambda_{0j}(t)\exp(\boldsymbol{\beta}_1'\boldsymbol{X}_{1i} + \boldsymbol{\beta}_2'\boldsymbol{X}_{2i} + \cdots + \boldsymbol{\beta}_J'\boldsymbol{X}_{Ji}) \\ &= \lambda_{0j}(t)\exp(\boldsymbol{\beta}_1'\boldsymbol{X}_i + \boldsymbol{\alpha}_{12}'\boldsymbol{X}_{2i} + \cdots + \boldsymbol{\alpha}_{1J}'\boldsymbol{X}_{Ji}).\end{aligned}$$

In the association between obesity and colorectal cancer subtypes, the hazard ratios for BMI $\geq$ 30.0 (obese) compared to BMI of 18.5–22.9 (normal) were estimated to be 2.25 (95% CI 1.49–3.40) for FASN-negative colorectal cancer and 1.27 (95% CI 0.88–1.83) for FASN-positive colorectal cancer; and the likelihood test for $\boldsymbol{\alpha}_{12} = \boldsymbol{\beta}_2 - \boldsymbol{\beta}_1 = 0$ indicated statistical significance ($P = 0.03$) [51].

Note that the heterogeneity parameter can be estimated in case-only studies [54, 55]. This can be illustrated in the simple 3 × 2 table shown in Table 3. Here, the subtype-specific effect is represented by odds ratio. The ratio of the odds ratio for subtype 2 to the odds ratio for subtype 1 can be written as $\frac{cf/de}{af/be} = \frac{bc}{ad}$, which is the same as the odds ratio for subtype 1 versus subtype 2.

When the subtypes are characterized by multiple markers, the question of interest might be which markers reflect the influence of the risk factors. For example, microsatellite instability (MSI), CpG island methylator phenotype (CIMP), and *BRAF* mutation status are known to be important molecular markers in colorectal cancer. These markers are associated with each other, where CIMP-high is associated with MSI-high and *BRAF* mutated in colorectal cancers [56, 57]. Previous studies have suggested that smoking may be associated with increased risk of MSI-high colorectal cancer, but not with increased risk of MSI-low [58–61]. Similarly, smoking has been suggested to have an association with increased risk of CIMP-high colorectal cancer, but not with that of CIMP-low colorectal cancer; and to have association with increased risk of *BRAF* mutated colorectal cancer, but not with that of *BRAF* wild-type colorectal cancer [59, 60, 62]. So far, it remains unclear whether smoking is directly associated with increased risk of each of colorectal cancer subtypes; or smoking may be directly associated with one of three subtypes and the association with the subtypes classified by the other two markers may be observed indirectly through the direct association of smoking with the one subtype.

The model for a subtype-specific hazard described above has been extended to address this question [63–66]. For simplicity, we will illustrate the approach with focusing on a single and scalar exposure variable, for example smoking status. Essentially, the *j*th subtype-specific effect of the exposure variable, β_j, is further modeled with the marker variables. Suppose that there are K markers ($k = 1, \ldots, K$) which comprise the molecular subtypes. Let m_{kj} denote the level of the *k*th marker variable corresponding to the *j*th subtype. Potential model for β_j may be $\beta_j = \gamma_0 + \sum_{k=1}^{K} \gamma_k m_{kj}$, where γ_k is a measure of the degree of etiologic heterogeneity among subtypes classified by the *k*th marker, under the other markers' levels to be the same. This model reduces the number of parameters, ignoring higher-order interaction between molecular markers. Considering the three binary markers ($k = 1, 2, 3$): CIMP (high/non-high), MSI (high/non-high) and *BRAF* (mutant/wild-type), $2^3 = 8$ subtype-specific effects will be modeled with 4 parameters. $\exp(\gamma_1)$ is the ratio of the hazard ratio of smoking for CIMP-high colorectal cancer to that for CIMP-non-high colorectal cancer, adjusted for the other markers' influence. Similarly, $\exp(\gamma_2)$ and $\exp(\gamma_3)$ are the ratios of the hazard ratios between the subtypes by MSI and between the subtypes by *BRAF*, respectively. These ratios of the hazard ratios for CIMP, MSI and *BRAF* have been estimated to be 1.23, 1.34, and 0.78, respectively [63].

In the GWAS context, restricting the analysis on each subtype may improve the power to discover subtype specific associations and new loci. Focusing on subtypes would lead to decreased sample size and loss of statistical power for common genetic factors across the subtypes. On the other hand, some SNPs may have subtype-specific effects. In this case, focusing on those subtypes may increase the power to detect such effects even if sample size decreases. Etiologically homogeneous subtypes would be unknown, but similar molecular features in cancers are likely to share common etiology. Previous study showed a relatively modest degree of etiologic heterogeneity is necessary for the subtyping strategies to have improved statistical power [67]. In addition, subset-based approach has been proposed for heterogeneous traits [68].

Under similar rationale for investigating etiologic heterogeneity, common etiology for related diseases or phenotypes can be investigated. Conceptually, subtype can be defined by overall etiological differences [69]. Etiologically distinct subtypes may provide a new classification method, as a complement for anatomic sites or molecular subtypes.

Revealing etiologic heterogeneity has potential to contribute to risk-based prevention strategy, through improving absolute risk prediction. Some intervention may be effective in reducing some specific cancer subtypes. If the preventable subtypes can be linked to specific risk factor profiles, identifying this subtype more specifically would provide an advance with a potential prevention strategy.

5 Remarks

In this chapter, we discussed some topics in cancer epidemiology, focusing on genetic risk factors and genomic features in tumor tissues. Biomarker data from both genomes (germline and somatic) have been increasingly and rapidly available in epidemiologic researches, providing valuable opportunities and challenges to refine genetic and biological cancer etiology. It would also require analysis methods that are statistically powerful and unbiased, as well as sufficiently large study samples from populations that effectively provide information regarding the research question.

Next generation sequencing (NGS) technology opens new opportunities. In terms of genetic risk factors, NGS will make it possible to evaluate the impact of rare variants on developing cancer, which cannot be captured by typical GWAS with SNP genotyping, although there have been debates about the "common disease common variant" versus the "common disease rare variant" [70]. Statistical power in a standard single variant analysis would be low due to a low frequency, and novel statistical analysis methods will be required to overcome this problem. Finer cancer subtyping may facilitate a deeper insight into the mechanisms between exposure and disease, while improving public health with that information may require developing a conceptual framework along with actual available actions.

This growing and promising area requires further development of statistical framework and methodology for utilizing the full potential of such data and making a positive impact on public health.

References

1. Hindorff LA, MacArthur J (European Bioinformatics Institute), Morales J (European Bioinformatics Institute), et al. A catalog of published genome-wide association studies. www.genome.gov/gwastudies (2015).
2. Michailidou K, Hall P, Gonzalez-Neira A, et al. Large-scale genotyping identifies 41 new loci associated with breast cancer risk. Nat Genet. 2013;45(4):353–61, 361e351–352.
3. Venter JC, Adams MD, Myers EW, et al. The sequence of the human genome. Science. 2001;291(5507):1304–51.
4. Lander ES, Linton LM, Birren B, et al. Initial sequencing and analysis of the human genome. Nature. 2001;409(6822):860–921.
5. International HapMap, C. The international HapMap project. Nature. 2003;426(6968): 789–96.
6. International HapMap, C. A haplotype map of the human genome. Nature. 2005;437 (7063):1299–320.
7. International HapMap, C, Frazer KA, Ballinger DG, et al. A second generation human haplotype map of over 3.1 million SNPs. Nature. 2007;449(7164):851–61.
8. Balding DJ. A tutorial on statistical methods for population association studies. Nat Rev Genet. 2006;7(10):781–91.
9. Risch N, Merikangas K. The future of genetic studies of complex human diseases. Science. 1996;273(5281):1516–7.

10. Marchini J, Howie B, Myers S, McVean G, Donnelly P. A new multipoint method for genome-wide association studies by imputation of genotypes. Nat Genet. 2007;39(7):906–13.
11. Amundadottir L, Kraft P, Stolzenberg-Solomon RZ, et al. Genome-wide association study identifies variants in the ABO locus associated with susceptibility to pancreatic cancer. Nat Genet. 2009;41(9):986–90.
12. Devlin B, Roeder K. Genomic control for association studies. Biometrics. 1999;55(4): 997–1004.
13. Price AL, Patterson NJ, Plenge RM, Weinblatt ME, Shadick NA, Reich D. Principal components analysis corrects for stratification in genome-wide association studies. Nat Genet. 2006;38(8):904–9.
14. Pe'er I, Yelensky R, Altshuler D, Daly MJ. Estimation of the multiple testing burden for genomewide association studies of nearly all common variants. Genet Epidemiol. 2008;32 (4):381–5.
15. Benjamini Y, Hochberg Y. Controlling the false discovery rate: a practical and powerful approach to multiple testing. J R Stat Soc Ser B Methodol. 1995; 289–300.
16. Efron B, Tibshirani R. Empirical Bayes methods and false discovery rates for microarrays. Genet Epidemiol. 2002;23(1):70–86.
17. Storey JD, Tibshirani R. Statistical significance for genomewide studies. Proc Natl Acad Sci USA. 2003;100(16):9440–5.
18. Storey JD. A direct approach to false discovery rates. J R Stat Soc Ser B Stat Methodol. 2002;64(3):479–98.
19. Panagiotou OA, Ioannidis JPA. What should the genome-wide significance threshold be? Empirical replication of borderline genetic associations. Int J Epidemiol. 2012;41(1):273–86.
20. Wacholder S, Chanock S, Garcia-Closas M, El Ghormli L, Rothman N. Assessing the probability that a positive report is false: an approach for molecular epidemiology studies. J Natl Cancer Inst. 2004;96(6):434–42.
21. Consortium, W.T.C.C. Genome-wide association study of 14,000 cases of seven common diseases and 3,000 shared controls. Nature. 2007;447(7145):661–78.
22. Wakefield J. Bayes factors for genome-wide association studies: comparison with P-values. Genet Epidemiol. 2009;33(1):79–86.
23. Garner C. Upward bias in odds ratio estimates from genome-wide association studies. Genet Epidemiol. 2007;31(4):288–95.
24. Zollner S, Pritchard JK. Overcoming the winner's curse: estimating penetrance parameters from case-control data. Am J Hum Genet. 2007;80(4):605–15.
25. Higgins JP, Thompson SG, Spiegelhalter DJ. A re-evaluation of random-effects meta-analysis. J R Stat Soc Ser A. 2009;172(1):137–59.
26. Pfeiffer RM, Gail MH, Pee D. On combining data from genome-wide association studies to discover disease-associated SNPs. Stat Sci. 2009;24(4):547–60.
27. He Q, Cai T, Liu Y, et al. Prioritizing individual genetic variants after kernel machine testing using variable selection. Genet Epidemiol. 2016;40(8):722–31.
28. Yu K, Li Q, Bergen AW, et al. Pathway analysis by adaptive combination of P-values. Genet Epidemiol. 2009;33(8):700–9.
29. Schork AJ, Thompson WK, Pham P, et al. All SNPs are not created equal: genome-wide association studies reveal a consistent pattern of enrichment among functionally annotated SNPs. PLoS Genet. 2013;9(4):e1003449.
30. Lewinger JP, Conti DV, Baurley JW, Triche TJ, Thomas DC. Hierarchical Bayes prioritization of marker associations from a genome-wide association scan for further investigation. Genet Epidemiol. 2007;31(8):871–82.
31. Pickrell JK. Joint analysis of functional genomic data and genome-wide association studies of 18 human traits. Am J Hum Genet. 2014;94(4):559–73.
32. Mechanic LE, Chen HS, Amos CI, et al. Next generation analytic tools for large scale genetic epidemiology studies of complex diseases. Genet Epidemiol. 2012;36(1):22–35.

33. Khoury MJ, Wacholder S. Invited commentary: from genome-wide association studies to gene-environment-wide interaction studies–challenges and opportunities. Am J Epidemiol. 2009;169(2):227–30 discussion 234–225.
34. Aschard H, Chen J, Cornelis MC, Chibnik LB, Karlson EW, Kraft P. Inclusion of gene-gene and gene-environment interactions unlikely to dramatically improve risk prediction for complex diseases. Am J Hum Genet. 2012;90(6):962–72.
35. Hein R, Flesch-Janys D, Dahmen N, et al. A genome-wide association study to identify genetic susceptibility loci that modify ductal and lobular postmenopausal breast cancer risk associated with menopausal hormone therapy use: a two-stage design with replication. Breast Cancer Res Treat. 2013;138(2):529–42.
36. Kraft P, Yen YC, Stram DO, Morrison J, Gauderman WJ. Exploiting gene-environment interaction to detect genetic associations. Hum Hered. 2007;63(2):111–9.
37. Cornelis MC, Tchetgen EJ, Liang L, et al. Gene-environment interactions in genome-wide association studies: a comparative study of tests applied to empirical studies of type 2 diabetes. Am J Epidemiol. 2012;175(3):191–202.
38. Aschard H, Lutz S, Maus B, et al. Challenges and opportunities in genome-wide environmental interaction (GWEI) studies. Hum Genet. 2012;131(10):1591–613.
39. Aschard H. A perspective on interaction effects in genetic association studies. Genet Epidemiol. 2016;40(8):678–88.
40. Chen S, Parmigiani G. Meta-analysis of BRCA1 and BRCA2 penetrance. J Clin Oncol (Off J Am Soc Clin Oncol). 2007;25(11):1329–33.
41. Gail MH, Brinton LA, Byar DP, et al. Projecting individualized probabilities of developing breast cancer for white females who are being examined annually. J Natl Cancer Inst. 1989;81 (24):1879–86.
42. Fisher B, Costantino JP, Wickerham DL, et al. Tamoxifen for prevention of breast cancer: report of the National Surgical Adjuvant Breast and Bowel Project P-1 Study. J Natl Cancer Inst. 1998;90(18):1371–88.
43. Wacholder S, Hartge P, Prentice R, et al. Performance of common genetic variants in breast-cancer risk models. N Engl J Med. 2010;362(11):986–93.
44. Chatterjee N, Shi J, Garcia-Closas M. Developing and evaluating polygenic risk prediction models for stratified disease prevention. Nat Rev Genet. 2016;17(7):392–406.
45. Sampson JN, Wheeler WA, Yeager M, et al. Analysis of heritability and shared heritability based on genome-wide association studies for thirteen cancer types. J Natl Cancer Inst. 2015;107(12):djv279.
46. Lee SH, Wray NR, Goddard ME, Visscher PM. Estimating missing heritability for disease from genome-wide association studies. Am J Hum Genet. 2011;88(3):294–305.
47. Mavaddat N, Pharoah PD, Michailidou K, et al. Prediction of breast cancer risk based on profiling with common genetic variants. J Natl Cancer Inst. 2015;107(5).
48. Machiela MJ, Chen CY, Chen C, Chanock SJ, Hunter DJ, Kraft P. Evaluation of polygenic risk scores for predicting breast and prostate cancer risk. Genet Epidemiol. 2011;35(6): 506–14.
49. Gail MH. Personalized estimates of breast cancer risk in clinical practice and public health. Stat Med. 2011;30(10):1090–104.
50. Pepe MS, Janes H, Longton G, Leisenring W, Newcomb P. Limitations of the odds ratio in gauging the performance of a diagnostic, prognostic, or screening marker. Am J Epidemiol. 2004;159(9):882–90.
51. Kuchiba A, Morikawa T, Yamauchi M, et al. Body mass index and risk of colorectal cancer according to fatty acid synthase expression in the nurses' health study. J Natl Cancer Inst. 2012;104(5):415–20.
52. Kalbfleisch JD, Prentice RL. The statistical analysis of failure time data, vol. 360. New York: Wiley; 2011.
53. Lunn M, McNeil D. Applying Cox regression to competing risks. Biometrics. 1995;51(2): 524–32.

54. Begg CB, Zhang ZF: Statistical analysis of molecular epidemiology studies employing case-series. Cancer Epidemiol Biomark Prev: A Publication of the American Association for Cancer Research, Cosponsored by the American Society of Preventive Oncology. 1994;3(2): 173–5.
55. Wang M, Spiegelman D, Kuchiba A, et al. Statistical methods for studying disease subtype heterogeneity. Stat Med. 2016;35(5):782–800.
56. Hughes LA, Khalid-de Bakker CA, Smits KM, et al. The CpG island methylator phenotype in colorectal cancer: progress and problems. Biochim Biophys Acta. 2012;1825(1):77–85.
57. Tanaka N, Huttenhower C, Nosho K, et al. Novel application of structural equation modeling to correlation structure analysis of CpG island methylation in colorectal cancer. Am J Pathol. 2010;177(6):2731–40.
58. Chia VM, Newcomb PA, Bigler J, Morimoto LM, Thibodeau SN, Potter JD. Risk of microsatellite-unstable colorectal cancer is associated jointly with smoking and nonsteroidal anti-inflammatory drug use. Cancer Res. 2006;66(13):6877–83.
59. Limsui D, Vierkant RA, Tillmans LS, et al. Cigarette smoking and colorectal cancer risk by molecularly defined subtypes. J Natl Cancer Inst. 2010;102(14):1012–22.
60. Samowitz WS, Albertsen H, Sweeney C, et al. Association of smoking, CpG island methylator phenotype, and V600E BRAF mutations in colon cancer. J Natl Cancer Inst. 2006;98(23):1731–8.
61. Poynter JN, Haile RW, Siegmund KD, et al. Associations between smoking, alcohol consumption, and colorectal cancer, overall and by tumor microsatellite instability status. Cancer Epidemiol Biomark Prev: A Publication of the American Association for Cancer Research, Cosponsored by the American Society of Preventive Oncology. 2009;18(10): 2745–50.
62. Rozek LS, Herron CM, Greenson JK, et al. Smoking, gender, and ethnicity predict somatic BRAF mutations in colorectal cancer. Cancer Epidemiol Biomark Prev: A Publication of the American Association for Cancer Research, Cosponsored by the American Society of Preventive Oncology. 2010;19(3):838–43.
63. Wang M, Kuchiba A, Ogino S. A meta-regression method for studying etiological heterogeneity across disease subtypes classified by multiple biomarkers. Am J Epidemiol. 2015;182(3):263–70.
64. Chatterjee N, Sinha S, Diver WR, Feigelson HS. Analysis of cohort studies with multivariate and partially observed disease classification data. Biometrika. 2010;97(3):683–98.
65. Chatterjee N. A two-stage regression model for epidemiological studies with multivariate disease classification data. J Am Stat Assoc. 2004;99(465):127–38.
66. Rosner B, Glynn RJ, Tamimi RM, et al. Breast cancer risk prediction with heterogeneous risk profiles according to breast cancer tumor markers. Am J Epidemiol. 2013;178(2):296–308.
67. Begg CB, Zabor EC. Detecting and exploiting etiologic heterogeneity in epidemiologic studies. Am J Epidemiol. 2012;176(6):512–8.
68. Bhattacharjee S, Rajaraman P, Jacobs KB, et al. A subset-based approach improves power and interpretation for the combined analysis of genetic association studies of heterogeneous traits. Am J Hum Genet. 2012;90(5):821–35.
69. Begg CB, Zabor EC, Bernstein JL, Bernstein L, Press MF, Seshan VE. A conceptual and methodological framework for investigating etiologic heterogeneity. Stat Med. 2013;32(29): 5039–52.
70. Schork NJ, Murray SS, Frazer KA, Topol EJ. Common versus rare allele hypotheses for complex diseases. Curr Opin Genet Dev. 2009;19(3):212–9.

Effect of *Helicobacter pylori* Eradication on Gastric Cancer Prevention in Korea: A Randomized Controlled Clinical Trial

Jin Young Park, Byung-Ho Nam, Rolando Herrero and Il Ju Choi

Abstract Despite the decreasing trend shown worldwide, considering the remaining high seroprevalence of *H. pylori* in the middle-aged population in the Republic of Korea (Korea) and the notable increase in gastric cancer (GC) incidence in specific age groups in the US, searching for and eradicating *H. pylori* may offer a great opportunity to reduce GC incidence dramatically. However, mass use of antibiotics that are necessary to eradicate the bacteria is likely to result in substantial overtreatment and may not be feasible. There are still some doubts about the effectiveness of *H. pylori* eradication in preventing GC and uncertainty about the eradication programs to maximize effectiveness and minimize possible adverse effects. A population-based double-blinded, randomized controlled clinical trial has therefore been proposed and being conducted in Korea to investigate the effectiveness of *H. pylori* eradication on GC prevention, addressing remaining unresolved issues. A total of 11,000 people between 40 and 65 years of age who are invited to the National Cancer Screening Program (NCSP) in Korea will be included in this study, among which about 60% of them are expected to be

J.Y. Park (✉) · R. Herrero
Prevention and Implementation Group, International Agency for Research on Cancer, Lyon, France
e-mail: parkjy@iarc.fr

R. Herrero
e-mail: herreror@iarc.fr

B.-H. Nam
Department of Cancer Control and Policy, Graduate School of Cancer Science and Policy, National Cancer Center, Goyang, Korea
e-mail: byunghonam@heringsglobal.com

Present Address:
B.-H. Nam
HERINGS, The Institute of Advanced Clinical and Biomedical Research, Seoul, Korea

I.J. Choi
Center for Gastric Cancer, National Cancer Center, Goyang, Korea
e-mail: cij1224@ncc.re.kr

S. Matsui and J. Crowley (eds.), *Frontiers of Biostatistical Methods and Applications in Clinical Oncology*, DOI 10.1007/978-981-10-0126-0_19

H. pylori positive. Eligible participants who agree to participate and sign informed consent undergo medical history and physical examination, and are administered a detailed lifestyle questionnaire. Blood (15 ml) is also collected in selected centers for ancillary studies. All participants undergo upper endoscopy and standard collection of gastric biopsies is made for histology and *H. pylori* diagnosis. Individuals who have already undergone their endoscopies as part of the NCSP or outside the NCSP scheme but could not be enrolled in the study prior to their gastroscopy are contacted for study participation and *H. pylori* status is determined with a breath test. *H. pylori* positive subjects are randomly assigned to either the treatment or placebo group in double-blind fashion. For those assigned to the treatment group, *H. pylori* eradication treatment with a 10-day course of bismuth-based quadruple therapy is provided while the others receive a placebo. Participants with no evidence of *H. pylori* infection or baseline chronic atrophic gastritis constitute the unexposed group to investigate natural history of the infection and GC precursors. All trial participants are followed up within the NCSP at least for 10 years to collect systematic information on medical conditions, in particular gastric cancer and causes of death. The primary endpoint of this trial is the incidence of histologically confirmed gastric adenocarcinoma. This study will be the first large clinical trial with endoscopic follow-up to provide comprehensive clinicopathological information about the *H. pylori* eradication effect on the GC incidence. Based on the results from this study, effective guideline for GC prevention could be established.

Keywords *Helicobacter pylori* · Gastric cancer · Prevention · Randomised controlled trial

1 Background

Gastric cancer is the fifth most commonly diagnosed cancer in the world with an estimated 952,000 new cases in 2012 [1]. It is also the third leading cause of cancer death in both men and women (723,000 deaths, 8.8% of the total) [1]. There is a considerable geographical variation in the incidence of GC with some of the lowest rates seen in North America and Western Europe and the highest rates in Central and South America, Eastern Europe and East Asia [2]. Generally, age-standardized incidence rates (ASRs) are about twice as high in men as in women, ranging from 4.3 in Northern Africa to 35.4 in Eastern Asia for men, and from 2.7 in Northern Africa to 13.8/100,000 in Eastern Asia for women [1]. Almost half of the world total is estimated to occur in China, Japan and Korea and several Latin America countries including Costa Rica and Ecuador [1].

Over the past decades, the overall incidence of GC has markedly declined in most countries irrespective of whether the background risk of GC is high or low [3]. However, a recent study demonstrated unexpectedly increasing GC (non-cardia) incidence rates among whites aged 25–39 years over the last 30 years in the US

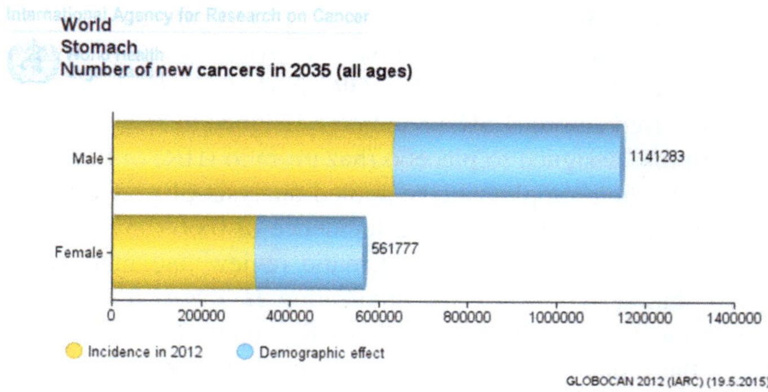

Fig. 1 Estimated number of new gastric cancer cases in 2035. Figure drawn using GLOBOCAN 2012 database; population forecasts were extracted from the United Nations, World Population prospects, the 2012 revision; numbers are computed using age-specific rates and corresponding populations for 10 age-groups

(estimated annual percentage change, EAPC +2.7% among whites) [4], emphasizing importance of age-specific trends rather than summary rates. Nonetheless, one should note that even with the overall declining incidence trends, the absolute burden is likely to remain static in coming years due to demographic effect, i.e. growth in world population combined with increased longevity [2] as illustrated in Fig. 1 [1].

Gastric cancer has been the most commonly diagnosed cancer in Korea in men since 1999 when the Korea Central Cancer Registry (KCCR) first reported nationwide cancer incidence [5]. According to the most recent national statistics in 2013, it remains the most common cancer in men (ASR 55.3) while it is the fourth most common cancer in women (ASR 22.4) [5]. Gastric cancer incidence significantly increases with age; age-specific incidence rates were: 2.3 and 3.4 for 15–34 years old; 88.3 and 38.8 for 35–64 years old; and 396.3 and 149.3/100,000 for 65 years old or over in men and women, respectively. Gastric cancer is the third most fatal cancer both in men (ASR 16.4) and in women (ASR, 6.1), having shown a continuous decreasing trend since mid-1990s [5].

2 *Helicobacter pylori* Eradication and Gastric Cancer Risk

2.1 *Previous Studies on Helicobacter pylori Eradication and Gastric Cancer Risk*

A meta-analysis of seven randomized trials that compared eradication treatment with no treatment in *H. pylori*-positive patients in relation to GC risk showed a pooled relative risk (RR) of 0.65 (95% confidence interval (CI), 0.43–0.98) in the treatment group [6]. However, the data included in this meta-analysis were questioned due to inclusion of redundant data [7]. In 2012, Ma and colleagues published their 15-year follow-up results of a randomized trial in China showing that GC was diagnosed in 3.0% of subjects who received *H. pylori* treatment and in 4.6% of those who received placebo (odds ratio (OR) 0.61, 95% CI 0.38–0.96). Gastric cancer deaths occurred among 1.5% of subjects assigned to *H. pylori* treatment and among 2.1% of those assigned to placebo (hazard ratio (HR) of death = 0.67, 95% CI 0.36–1.28) [8]. Their supplementary pooled analysis of previous four randomized trials resulted in relative risk of GC incidence of 0.66 (95% CI 0.46–0.95) in the treatment group. A most recent systematic review and meta-analysis of six RCTs suggests that searching for and eradicating *H. pylori* infection reduces the subsequent GC incidence by 34% (a pooled RR = 0.66, 95% CI 0.46–0.95), with the caveat that these data cannot be extrapolated to other populations because the majority of the included studies were conducted in East Asia [9].

2.2 *Helicobacter pylori* Seroprevalence in Korea

In Korea, according to the most recent estimate, the seropositivity rate of *H. pylori* was 54.4% among subjects aged >16 years who had no history of *H. pylori* eradication nor current gastrointestinal symptoms [10]. The seroprevalence increased with age and was the highest in people in their 60s (62%). This study showed a statistically significant decrease in seroprevalence compared with the figures estimated from the earlier surveys conducted in 1998 [11] and 2005 [12].

2.3 *Helicobacter pylori* Treatment in Korea

Considering high seroprevalence of *H. pylori* and substantial burden of GC in the country, searching for and eradicating *H. pylori* may be considered as an effective strategy for GC prevention. However, the revised guidelines for diagnosis and treatment of *H. pylori* infection in Korea do not indicate *H. pylori* eradication for the general population while definite indications for identifying and treating the infection include (1) early GC, (2) previous indications of peptic ulcer including scar, (3) Marginal zone B cell lymphoma (MALT type) and (4) idiopathic thrombocytopenic purpura [13]. Currently in Korea, standard triple therapy with a proton pump inhibitor (PPI), amoxicillin, and clarithromycin is recommended as a primary regimen for *H. pylori* treatment [14].

2.4 Antimicrobial Resistance

There is an increasing trend of *H. pylori* treatment failure with traditional triple therapy in many parts of the world [15]. Studies have shown that unsuccessful treatments significantly increase resistance [16, 17]. It is therefore important to choose the most effective first-line treatment regime in order to avoid treatment failure and subsequent secondary resistances. In Korea, prevalence of primary antibiotic resistance among *H. pylori* isolates was estimated to be 18.5% for Amoxicillin, 13.8% for Clarithromycin, and 66.2% for Metronidazole in 2003 [17]. The study also compared *H. pylori* strains isolated from Korean patients in 1987, 1994 and 2003 and showed that the distribution of minimal inhibitory concentrations (MIC) for amoxicillin, clarithromycin, metronidazole, tetracycline, azithromycin, and fluoroquinolone (ciprofloxacin, levofloxacin, and moxifloxacin) have shifted to higher concentrations [17].

3 Cancer Screening and Registry in Korea

3.1 National Cancer Screening Program in Korea

The NCSP in Korea was first introduced in 1999 to reduce the high burden and mortality from cancer, as part of a national 10-year plan for cancer control [18]. The NCSP provides GC screening every 2 years for those aged 40 or over using direct or indirect upper gastrointestinal series (UGIS) or endoscopy [19]. The proportion of participants who chose UGIS as a GC screening modality has steadily decreased, and approximately 73% of participants were estimated to choose endoscopy as a preferred modality in 2011 [20].

The impact of GC screening on GC mortality has been observed since early 2000 and the difference in mortality between people with and without screening effect has steadily increased (National Cancer Center, Korea (NCC) internal data). It has been projected that GC mortality during the periods of 2015–2019 will be at least 30% less among those who undergo GC screening compared with who do not (NCC internal data).

3.2 Korea Central Cancer Registry

The KCCR was initiated by the Korean Ministry of Health and Welfare as a hospital-based cancer registry in 1980 [21]. In 1999, the KCCR expanded cancer registration to cover the entire population under the Population-Based Regional Cancer Registry program. The completeness of incidence data for 2013 was estimated to be 97.8% [5].

4 HELPER—Effect of *Helicobacter pylori* Eradication on Gastric Cancer Prevention in Korea: A Randomized Controlled Clinical Trial

4.1 Motivation for the Study

Despite the decreasing trend shown worldwide, considering the remaining high seroprevalence of *H. pylori* in Korea and the notable increase in GC incidence in specific age groups in the US, *H. pylori* screening and eradication may have a great impact in reducing GC incidence dramatically. However, as pointed out in previous studies, mass use of antibiotics is likely to result in substantial overtreatment and may not be feasible [22]. Today, no country has yet implemented a population-based *H. pylori* eradication program for GC prevention. This may reflect some doubts about the effectiveness of *H. pylori* eradication in preventing gastric cancer and about the generalizability of previous study results from China and Japan to other populations. In addition, there exists uncertainty about how best to apply eradication programs to maximize effectiveness and minimize possible adverse effects including weight gain, gastroesophageal reflux disease and antibiotic resistance. Specifically, there is only limited information on the program feasibility, appropriate target groups for intervention in different regions, and potential harms of population-based *H. pylori* screening and treatment programs [23].

To address these issues and implement effective population-based GC prevention strategies, a prevention trial has been developed [24]. It is a multi-center, double-blind, randomized controlled clinical trial in Korea to evaluate the effect of *H. pylori* eradication to prevent GC incidence in middle aged adults. The effect of *H. pylori* eradication on the incidence of gastric dysplasia and other conditions that may be associated with *H. pylori* infection or its eradication will also be investigated. This study will be able to address possible adverse events caused by antibiotic treatment as well as the role of environmental and host genetic factors in development of GC and its precursors and as modifiers of the treatment. All participants will be followed up for at least 10 years to assess the GC incidence. This study will greatly benefit from already existing cancer control activities in the country, such as the NCSP and the KCCR.

4.2 Study Hypothesis

H. pylori infection is an important cause of GC development. Therefore, the risk of GC can be reduced by antibiotic eradication of *H. pylori* infection in individuals in Korea.

4.3 Objectives of the Study

Main Objective
The primary objective of the study is to determine if *H. pylori* eradication reduces GC incidence in Korean population among 40–65 years old subjects.

Secondary Objectives

1. To determine if *H. pylori* eradication reduces incidence of gastric dysplasia
2. To assess adverse events caused by antibiotic treatment for *H. pylori* eradication
3. To evaluate the impact of *H. pylori* eradication on the occurrence of selected medical conditions potentially associated with the infection or its eradication (e.g. obesity, diabetes, cerebrovascular disease, coronary artery disease, asthma, esophageal diseases, other cancers, cognitive functions)
4. To evaluate the role of demographic, lifestyle, nutritional, environmental and host genetic factors, compliance with treatment, and *H. pylori* strains in development of gastric cancer and its precursors and as modifiers of the treatment
5. To assess whether the *H. pylori* treatment would result in similar gastric cancer incidence compared to the Unexposed Group without *H. pylori* infection
6. To assess whether gastric cancer incidence in the group with successful eradication is different from those refusing/failing eradication within the treated *H. pylori* positive (treatment) group
7. To examine the difference in all-cause mortality between the treated *H. pylori* positive group (treatment group) and untreated *H. pylori* positive group (placebo group)
8. To assess the difference in gastric cancer incidence between the untreated *H. pylori* positive group (placebo) and the *H. pylori* negative group (Unexposed Group)
9. To investigate the role of cofactors for gastric cancer development among untreated *H. pylori* positive subjects (e.g. demographic, dietary, lifestyle, host genetic, factors and inflammatory markers)
10. To assess the impact of *H. pylori* eradication on precancerous lesions (atrophy score)

4.4 Overview of Study Design

The study design has been described previously [24]. Briefly summarizing the study design with an additional recruitment method that has been newly adopted, men and women between 40 and 65 years of age at entry who are invited to NCSP in Korea are asked to participate in this trial until a total number of 11,000 are recruited at local centers where the NCSP takes place. Eligible participants who agree to participate and sign informed consent undergo medical history, physical examination and blood collection, and are administered a detailed lifestyle questionnaire. Participants who visit study sites to undergo endoscopy outside the NCSP scheme are also contacted for study participation. The participants are excluded if they meet any of the following criteria: (1) personal history of GC; (2) family history of GC in a first-degree relative; (3) history of other organ cancers within 5 years; (4) clinical indication of *H. pylori* eradication; (5) other serious medical illnesses or conditions that preclude adequate participation.

All participants undergo upper endoscopy and gastric biopsies are collected according to the Updated Sydney System for histology [25] and *H. pylori* diagnosis. *H. pylori* status is determined either by the rapid urease test (RUT) on an endoscopic biopsy specimen or pathology reading. Individuals who have already undergone their endoscopies as part of the NCSP or outside the NCSP but could not be enrolled in the study prior to their endoscopy receive Urea Breath Test (UBT) for determination of *H. pylori* infection. Study participants undergo medical history, physical examination and blood collection, and are administered a detailed lifestyle questionnaire. Subjects who are *H. pylori* positive are randomly assigned to either the treatment group (50%) or the control group (50%) (Fig. 2). Randomization is performed using random permutation block size design stratified by sex and participating center, generating an allocation sequence in which the number of assignments to intervention groups satisfies a specified allocation ratio after every "block" of specified size, by nQuery Advisor® (version 7.0, Cork, Ireland). This will ensure the continued equivalence of group size. Both participants and investigators are blinded to the identity of the interventions.

For those assigned to the treatment group, eradication treatment with a 10-day course of a bismuth based quadruple therapy (metronidazole 500 mg, 3 times a day, tetracycline 500 mg, 4 times a day and, bismuth 300 mg, 4 times a day, and a PPI (Lansoprazole) 30 mg, twice a day for 10 days) are provided. Participants assigned to the control group receive a placebo with lookalike medications. Participants with no evidence of *H. pylori* infection or baseline chronic atrophic gastritis will constitute the unexposed group to investigate natural history of *H. pylori* infection and GC precursors (Fig. 2).

All the trial participants will be followed up at least for 10 years to collect systematic information on medical conditions, in particular GC incidence and cause of death. Subjects who are identified outside the NCSP and agree to participate in the study will be included in NCSP for regular follow-up within the program as other participants. We anticipate approximately 80% of all participants will undergo upper endoscopy every two years as part of the NCSP, assuming an active follow-up. Extra efforts will be made to encourage participants to attend the follow-up endoscopic examination. Gastric cancer cases will be identified during a biennial endoscopic follow-up for those who participate in the NCSP. For those lost to endoscopic follow-up, GC cases will be identified through a record linkage with the KCCR. At the first follow-up visit in routine screening another biopsy collection will be made for blinded assessment of the presence of *H. pylori* with the RUT method. At the end of the follow-up all the examinations done at the baseline will be repeated for all participants.

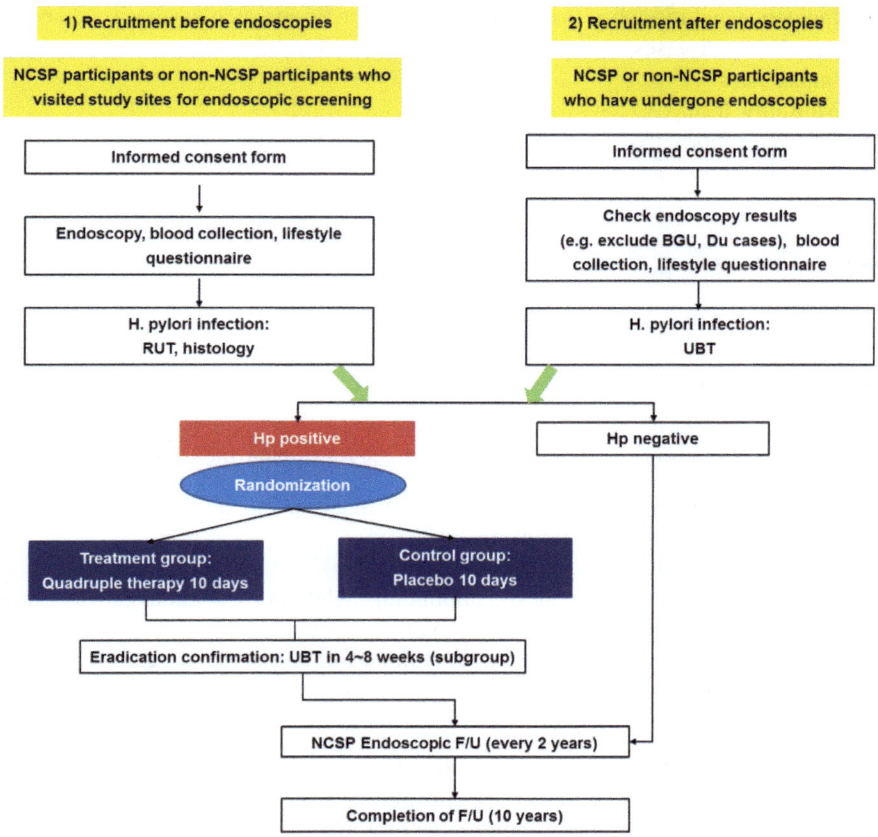

Fig. 2 Overview of the study design with two different ways to recruit participants into the study

4.5 *Trial Endpoints*

Primary Endpoint

The primary endpoint of the trial is the incidence of histologically confirmed gastric adenocarcinoma. The incidence of GC will be compared between the treatment and placebo groups at 10 years or when enough cases accumulate to satisfy the power analysis outlined below.

Secondary Endpoints

In addition to the incidence of GC as the primary endpoint of the study, endpoints to achieve the secondary objectives are the following:

- Incidence of gastric dysplasia
- Occurrence of adverse events caused by antibiotic treatment

- Incidence and mortality from other medical conditions such as obesity, diabetes, circulatory diseases, oesophageal diseases as well as other cancers and cognitive impairment
- Mortality from GC
- All-cause mortality
- Modification of atrophy score

4.6 Unblinding Criteria

The following events may require unblinding of the study:

- Compelling medical need as determined by the treating physician, such as:
  - Occurrence of a serious adverse event where the knowledge of the participant's assignment would directly influence or affect his immediate care.
- Ingestion of the study drugs in excessive quantity by the participant or by a person other than the participant.
- Ingestion of study drugs by a child.
- Participant adamantly requests unblinding. Unblindings endanger the trial; therefore, participants should be strongly discouraged from finding out their treatment assignments before the completion of the study drugs. However, a participant who is adamant in requesting his treatment assignment may refuse to cooperate with follow-up efforts if he is not given this information.

Unblinding of individual participants, at the request of the Data and Safety Monitoring Board (DSMB) and the Institutional Review Boards will also be allowed. This individual unblinding will be performed in a manner that assures that the overall study blinding is maintained, that staff involved in the conduct, analysis, or reporting of the study remain blinded, and that any unblinding is appropriately documented.

4.7 Stopping Criteria

Although the final evaluation between the treatment and placebo groups according to GC incidence is planned to be conducted at 10 years from the last inclusion, the evaluation in respect to the main end-point may be conducted as soon as the specified total number of planned cases is reached. The DSMB will be responsible for evaluating unblinded data on case accrual, efficacy and safety of the intervention to recommend on continuation or interruption of the study. If major differences in the management recommendations are put in place in Korea, the strategy of the study will be revised in consultation with the DSMB to introduce the necessary adjustments. Under the circumstances if a definite risk would be revealed for the control group, the planned follow-up strategy may be stopped for the individuals at risk or the entire group. At the same time longer follow-up period (up to life-time follow-up) may be justified to reach secondary end-points and conduct ancillary studies after the primary end-point is reached. At any time points when the study reveals clear benefits of *H. pylori* treatment for GC prevention, all the participants including those who belong to the placebo group will be given the treatment.

4.8 Questionnaires and Data Management

Questionnaires are administered by trained staff following administration instructions and manuals. The staff involved in this process have to comply with the requirements in the manual as well as with the potential further amendments to it. Data are entered into the internet-enabled eVelos system operated by NCC which serves the research team through a centralized platform (Fig. 3). This system creates participant clinical profiles to include diagnosis, lab results, and family histories helping with managing participants online during the research process, including recruitment, registration, scheduling, visit tracking, data entry, notifications and monitoring and data cleaning. The data in this database are kept strictly confidential as required by law and available only to investigators and institutions who have received approval from the Clinical Research Coordination Center at NCC after certifying their adherence to patient data protection policies for the project.

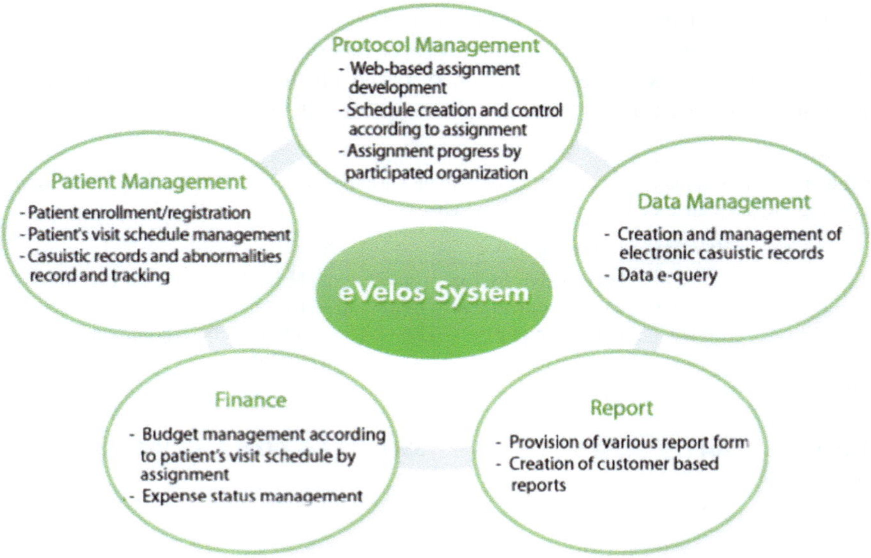

Fig. 3 Velos system structure

4.9 Data Linkage

Information on participants' GC screening examination, diagnosis of cancer or other diseases including obesity, diabetes, cerebrovascular disease, coronary artery disease, asthma, esophageal diseases, cognitive functions, or survival data will be obtained from the KCCR, National Health Insurance Corporation of Korea, NCSP, Health Insurance Review & Assessment Service, Statistics Korea, or other national data through a record linkage using participants resident registration numbers during or at the end of the study. All the participants' data collected will be treated strictly confidential under the law.

4.10 Sample Size Calculation

The expected number of GC cases was estimated based on the assumptions of a risk reduction in the GC incidence due to the intervention at least by 47%. Our assumption for the effect size was based on the available literature [8, 26] as well as the more recent Japanese study of early GC patients that reported a HR of 0.497 (95% CI 0.297–0.831) in the eradicated group for the incidence of metachronous GC after endoscopic resection after maximum 10 years of follow-up [27]. When we applied a significance level of 5% and a statistical power of 90%, we would need 104 GC cases (Table 1, in bold). Overall GC incidence (men and women combined) in *H. pylori* positive population in Korea was calculated as 165 cases/100,000/year, using 5 year follow-up data from the NCSP in Korea (NCC, internal communication). *H. pylori* prevalence was estimated to be 60% in Korean adults aged 40–65 years old [12] and a relative risk of GC for *H. pylori* positives to *H. pylori* negatives was assumed to be 6, based on the available evidence in the literature [28]. Assuming a 10% of follow-up loss, it was estimated that the total

Table 1 Study sample sizes required to determine various effect sizes of *H. pylori* eradication in reducing GC incidence at 10 years of follow-up

	10 years of follow-up				
	GC outcome needed	Hp positive (N for each treatment and placebo group)	+10% follow-up loss	N for both treatment and placebo groups	Total (treatment group, placebo group and unexposed group)
HR 0.50 power 90%	87	2400	2667	5334	8890
HR 0.53 power 90%	**104**	**2917**	**3241**	**6482**	**10,804**
HR 0.55 power 90%	118	3332	3702	7404	12,340
HR 0.60 power 90%	161	4710	5234	10,468	17,446

sample size of 11,000 (6600 *H. pylori* positive participants in both treatment and placebo groups plus 4400 participants in the *H. pylori* negative group) with all participants to be followed up for 10 years, would meet the requirement of the study design to investigate a 47% reduction of GC risk (HR 0.53) in the treatment group compared to the placebo group. nQuery (Statistical Solutions Ltd. Boston, USA) Version 2.0 was used to calculate the sample size based on the log-rank test assuming proportionality of hazard for the time to event analysis.

4.11 Statistical Analysis

This study is a randomized, phase III superiority trial. The primary objective of the study is to compare treatment (*H. pylori* eradication) group against placebo group to determine if *H. pylori* eradication reduces GC incidence in Korean population among 40–65 years old subjects.

The primary endpoint of this study is the event free survival (EFS), which is defined as the time from randomization to the incidence of histologically confirmed gastric adenocarcinoma. The primary analysis will be performed based on intention to treat (ITT) including all subjects who are randomized. Unstratified and stratified log-rank test will be used to compare the two survival curves between the two groups at the interim and/or final analyses. The event time associated with each group will be summarized using the Kaplan-Meier method and displayed graphically where appropriate. Confidence intervals for the 25th, 50th and 75th percentiles will be reported. The proportionality of the HR will be examined and if this is satisfied, the Cox proportional hazard model will be used to estimate the HR and the corresponding 95% CI. Both stratified and unstratified Cox regression models will be used. The secondary endpoints include gastric dysplasia, GC mortality and all-cause mortality. Similar survival analysis methods will be used for these secondary endpoints.

The χ^2 test and logistic regression model will be employed for analyzing categorical variables including adverse events. T-test or appropriate non-parametric methods such as Wilcoxon's rank-sum test will be used to compare some baseline characteristics with continuous measures between the two groups.

Information on interruptions, changes or discontinuation of treatments will be documented in order to perform additional analyses restricted to subjects who completed their treatments. We will also perform a per-protocol analysis with data obtained from subjects who complete this trial. In the per-protocol analysis, subjects who are included in interruptions or exclusion criteria will be excluded. Interruptions will be considered for subjects who are categorized as one of the following:

- Violation of inclusion or exclusion criteria
- Subjects in the control group who decided to receive *H. pylori* eradication
- Subjects taking treatment regimen for less than 7 days (<70%)

The main analysis planned for this trial will be conducted by the NCC and the International Agency for Research on Cancer (IARC) investigators and will focus on the primary outcome, histologically confirmed gastric adenocarcinoma as defined in the trial endpoints section. All statistical calculations will be performed using SAS, version 9.1 (SAS institute, Cary, NC) and a 2-tailed $p < 0.05$ will be considered statistically significant.

4.12 Interim Analysis

Independent statisticians will prepare the interim unblinded reports for the independent DSMB, which oversee participant's safety and the quality of trial conduct. One formal interim analysis will be conducted using a two-sided significance test with the O'Brien–Fleming spending function and a type I error rate of 5%. The criteria for deciding on the timing of this analysis will be made by the members of the DSMB after initiation of the study (without regard to any information on treatment efficacy observed in the trial). The DSMB may recommend termination of the study, on the basis of their assessment that the excess risk of adverse events in the treatment group cannot be offset by a reduction in GC events or whenever an interim analysis reveals a remarkably significant difference between the two groups, whichever comes first.

5 Concluding Remarks

This prevention trial will generate evidence to demonstrate to what extent *H. pylori* eradication can reduce the risk of GC. Furthermore, it will be able to identify not only the target groups where the eradication would be most beneficial, but also its potential deleterious effects, in addition to important environmental, genetic and bacterial factors associated with GC and its preneoplastic lesions. The study would have major public health implications by providing leads for prevention activities in populations with elevated rates of GC, not only in Asia, but also other regions including Latin American countries.

References

1. Ferlay J, Soerjomataram I, Ervik M, Dikshit R, Eser S, Mathers C, Rebelo M, Parkin D, Forman D, Bray F. GLOBOCAN 2012 v1.0, Cancer Incidence and Mortality Worldwide: IARC CancerBase No. 11 [Internet]. http://globocan.iarc.fr. Accessed 28 Feb 2017. Lyon, France: International Agency for Research on Cancer; 2013.
2. Forman D, Sierra M. The current and projected global burden of gastric cancer. http://www.iarc.fr/en/publications/pdfs-online/wrk/wrk8/index.php. In: IARC *Helicobacter pylori* Working Group *Helicobacter pylori* Eradication as a Strategy for Preventing Gastric Cancer IARC Working Group Reports, No 8. Lyon, France: International Agency for Research on Cancer; 2014. p. 5–15.

3. Ferlay J, Bray F, Steliarova-Foucher E, Forman D. Cancer incidence in five continents, CI5plus. IARC CancerBase No. 9. http://ci5.iarc.fr. Accessed 28 Mar 2017. Lyon: International Agency for Research on Cancer; 2014.
4. Anderson WF, Camargo MC, Fraumeni JF Jr, Correa P, Rosenberg PS, Rabkin CS. Age-specific trends in incidence of noncardia gastric cancer in US adults. JAMA. 2010;303(17):1723–8.
5. Oh C-M, Won Y-J, Jung K-W, Kong H-J, Cho H, Lee J-K, Lee DH, Lee KH. Cancer Statistics in Korea: incidence, mortality, survival, and prevalence in 2013. Cancer Res Treat. 2016;48(2):436–50.
6. Fuccio L, Zagari RM, Eusebi LH, Laterza L, Cennamo V, Ceroni L, Grilli D, Bazzoli F. Meta-analysis: can *Helicobacter pylori* eradication treatment reduce the risk for gastric cancer? Ann Intern Med. 2009;151(2):121–8.
7. Ford AC, Moayyedi P. Redundant data in the meta-analysis on *Helicobacter pylori* eradication. Ann Intern Med. 2009;151(7):513 author reply 513–514.
8. Ma JL, Zhang L, Brown LM, Li JY, Shen L, Pan KF, Liu WD, Hu Y, Han ZX, Crystal-Mansour S, et al. Fifteen-year effects of *Helicobacter pylori*, garlic, and vitamin treatments on gastric cancer incidence and mortality. J Natl Cancer Inst. 2012;104(6):488–92.
9. Ford AC, Forman D, Hunt RH, Yuan Y, Moayyedi P. *Helicobacter pylori* eradication therapy to prevent gastric cancer in healthy asymptomatic infected individuals: systematic review and meta-analysis of randomised controlled trials. BMJ Br Med J. 2014;348.
10. Lim SH, Kwon J-W, Kim N, Kim GH, Kang JM, Park MJ, Yim JY, Kim HU, Baik GH, Seo GS, et al. Prevalence and risk factors of *Helicobacter pylori* infection in Korea: nationwide multicenter study over 13 years. BMC Gastroenterol. 2013;13(1):104.
11. Kim JH, Kim HY, Kim NY, Kim SW, Kim JG, Kim JJ, Roe IH, Seo JK, Sim JG, Ahn H, et al. Seroepidemiological study of *Helicobacter pylori* infection in asymptomatic people in South Korea. J Gastroenterol Hepatol. 2001;16(9):969–75.
12. Yim JY, Kim N, Choi SH, Kim YS, Cho KR, Kim SS, Seo GS, Kim HU, Baik GH, Sin CS, et al. Seroprevalence of *Helicobacter pylori* in South Korea. Helicobacter. 2007;12(4):333–40.
13. Kim SG, Jung HK, Lee HL, Jang JY, Lee H, Kim CG, Shin WG, Shin ES, Lee YC, Korean College of H, et al. Guidelines for the diagnosis and treatment of *Helicobacter pylori* infection in Korea, 2013 revised edition. Korean J Gastroenterol. 2013;62(1):3–26.
14. Kim SG, Jung HK, Lee HL, Jang JY, Lee H, Kim CG, Shin WG, Shin ES, Lee YC. Guidelines for the diagnosis and treatment of *Helicobacter pylori* infection in Korea, 2013 revised edition. J Gastroenterol Hepatol. 2014;29(7):1371–86.
15. Graham DY, Shiotani A. New concepts of resistance in the treatment of *Helicobacter pylori* infections. Nat Clin Pract Gastroenterol Hepatol. 2008;5(6):321–31.
16. Romano M, Iovene MR, Russo MI, Rocco A, Salerno R, Cozzolino D, Pilloni AP, Tufano MA, Vaira D, Nardone G. Failure of first-line eradication treatment significantly increases prevalence of antimicrobial-resistant *Helicobacter pylori* clinical isolates. J Clin Pathol. 2008;61(10):1112–5.
17. Kim JM. Antibiotic resistance of *Helicobacter pylori* isolated from Korean patients. Korean J Gastroenterol (Taehan Sohwagi Hakhoe chi). 2006;47(5):337–49.
18. Lee KS, Oh DK, Han MA, Lee HY, Jun JK, Choi KS, Park EC. Gastric cancer screening in Korea: report on the national cancer screening program in 2008. Cancer Res Treat. 2011;43(2):83–8.
19. Yoo KY. Cancer control activities in the Republic of Korea. Jpn J Clin Oncol. 2008;38(5):327–33.
20. Lee S, Jun JK, Suh M, Park B, Noh DK, Jung K-W, Choi KS. Gastric cancer screening uptake trends in Korea: results for the national cancer screening program from 2002 to 2011: a prospective cross-sectional study. Medicine. 2015;94(8):e533.
21. Jung KW, Park S, Kong HJ, Won YJ, Lee JY, Seo HG, Lee JS. Cancer statistics in Korea: incidence, mortality, survival, and prevalence in 2009. Cancer Res Treat. 2012;44(1):11–24.
22. Forman D, Pisani P. Gastric cancer in Japan—honing treatment, seeking causes. N Engl J Med. 2008;359(5):448–51.

23. Park JY, Forman D, Greenberg ER, Herrero R. *Helicobacter pylori* eradication in the prevention of gastric cancer: are more trials needed? Curr Oncol Rep. 2013;15(6):517–25.
24. Choi IJ, Park JY, Herrero R. Effect of *Helicobacter pylori* eradication on gastric cancer prevention in the Republic of Korea: a randomized controlled clinical trial. http://www.iarc.fr/en/publications/pdfs-online/wrk/wrk8/index.php. In: IARC *Helicobacter pylori* Working Group *Helicobacter pylori* Eradication as a Strategy for Preventing Gastric Cancer IARC Working Group Reports, No 8. Lyon, France: International Agency for Research on Cancer; 2014. p. 154–60.
25. Dixon MF, Genta RM, Yardley JH, Correa P. Classification and grading of gastritis. The updated Sydney system. International workshop on the histopathology of gastritis, Houston 1994. Am J Surg Pathol. 1996;20(10):1161–81.
26. Fukase K, Kato M, Kikuchi S, Inoue K, Uemura N, Okamoto S, Terao S, Amagai K, Hayashi S, Asaka M. Effect of eradication of *Helicobacter pylori* on incidence of metachronous gastric carcinoma after endoscopic resection of early gastric cancer: an open-label, randomised controlled trial. Lancet. 2008;372(9636):392–7.
27. Kato M, Asaka M, Kikuch S. 9 Long-term follow-up study about preventive effect of *H. pylori* eradication for the incidence of metachronous gastric cancer after endoscopic resection of primary early gastric cancer. Gastroenterology. 2012;142(5):S-3.
28. Helicobacter, Cancer Collaborative G. Gastric cancer and *Helicobacter pylori*: a combined analysis of 12 case control studies nested within prospective cohorts. Gut. 2001;49 (3):347–53.

Contemporary Evaluation of Breast Cancer Screening

William E. Barlow

Abstract Mammography screening has been shown in randomized trials to reduce breast cancer mortality by at least 20%, though it has risks as well due to radiation exposure and overtreatment of benign conditions. However, mammography technology and breast cancer treatment have improved since these trials were conducted and it is unlikely that large scale trials will ever be conducted again. Therefore, prospective observational data need to be used to continuously assess improvements in the screening process. We consider the successive steps for a woman undergoing screening and attempt to measure and improve each step in that process to maximize benefits while monitoring harms of screening. A large population-based study entitled PROSPR is assessing longitudinal performance of screening mammography and showing areas where improvements in follow-up of positive mammograms need to be made. In this assessment we consider sources of bias in evaluation of observational data when assessing efficacy of screening. We also propose a chained statistical model to look at steps in the overall process from screening participation to mortality.

Keywords Cancer screening · Observational data bias · Test performance · Risk modeling · Sequential processes

1 Introduction

Randomized trials of mammographic screening to detect early breast cancer have demonstrated a breast cancer mortality reduction benefit in women aged 50 years or greater. Three separate meta-analyses of existing randomized trials of mammography screening have shown very similar results: (1) RR = 0.80 with 95% confidence interval (CI) 0.73–0.89; (2) RR = 0.82 (95% CI 0.74–0.94); (3) RR = 0.81 (95% CI 0.74–0.87) despite differences in the computational methods [1]. Thus, regardless of analytic approach there seems to be strong evidence showing a reduction in breast cancer

W.E. Barlow (✉)
Cancer Research and Biostatistics, 1730 Minor Ave, Suite 1900,
Seattle, WA 98101, USA
e-mail: williamb@crab.org

S. Matsui and J. Crowley (eds.), *Frontiers of Biostatistical Methods and Applications in Clinical Oncology*, DOI 10.1007/978-981-10-0126-0_20

mortality due to screening for women aged 50 years or above. However, there is conflicting evidence of a benefit for screening women 40–49 [2, 3], and there is not strong evidence for a particular interval between screens [1]. Furthermore, there are downsides to screening due to costs, radiation exposure, an increase of false positive biopsies, and over-diagnosis, i.e. the detection of cancers that would not have been lethal or perhaps ever clinically detected had they not been found by screening. Therefore, there is a need to balance screening risks and benefits. For the most part, guidelines for recommendations for screening of average risk women are typically dependent solely on age, but may be modified by breast cancer risk factors and co-morbidity [4].

Having already shown that screening mammography is beneficial for some women, it is now unlikely that any new trials of mammography screening comparing screening to no screening will ever be conducted. The intent-to-treat analyses in the randomized trials compared offering screening to women versus not offering screening. Many women assigned to the screening group refused to be screened and thus the hazard ratio may not represent the true efficacy of mammography screening. Adjusting the meta-analysis for adherence to screening showed an estimated ITT risk decrease of 22% (95% CI 15–28%) in breast cancer mortality that became stronger after adjustment for adherence (30% with 95% CI 18–42%) [5]. However, it also showed that the over-diagnosis rate increased from 19% (95% CI 15–23%) in the ITT analysis to 30% (95% CI 18–42%) after adjustment. Thus, in an observational setting one might expect the benefit and harms of screening to be comparable to these adjusted results if one was able to rule out bias in screening uptake, i.e. participation in screening.

The percentage uptake of screening in a randomized trial can be seen to be a large factor in determining the likelihood of finding a statistically significant result. However, even if compliance is high, other factors would affect likely success. These include the ability of the screening mammogram to detect the cancer at an earlier stage than would be possible clinically. Secondly, suspicious lesions detected on a screening mammogram must be confirmed with additional imaging, and ultimately a biopsy would be performed if indicated. If a cancer is indeed detected, then there must be effective treatment available that would decrease the likelihood of recurrence or metastasis compared to a cancer detected clinically at a later time. Finally, early detection must reduce actual mortality from breast cancer. In short, there are many steps that must go well in order for a screening trial to show a significant benefit. Below we try to decompose the steps in the screening process in order to improve how well screening works in actual practice.

2 Various Aspects, Issues, and Challenges in Assessing Mammography Screening Using Observational Data

2.1 Biases in Evaluation of Screening from Observational Studies

When it became clear that new trials of mammography screening were unlikely to be conducted, many attempted to use existing observational data to show a benefit to screening. This has led to some biased evaluations of screening. The most pernicious analysis is a comparison of screen-detected versus clinically-detected women with regard to survival or clinical presentation of the cancer. For example, if one compares survival from the time of diagnosis between screen-detected women versus clinically-detected women, then survival might appear to confer a survival benefit [6]. However, this observation is subject to many biases including lead-time bias [6]. Suppose that regardless of diagnosis method, the cancer begins in a pre-detectable state, as it becomes larger it becomes detectable by screening, and finally it becomes large enough to be detectable clinically. However, suppose treatment is completely ineffective, and the patient ultimately succumbs to the disease. It may be that screening has not actually led to a better clinical outcome, but has merely shifted the diagnosis date earlier, but not changed the ultimate outcome. Thus survival appears to be longer even though there has been no benefit from screening. Similarly, comparisons of screen-detected cancers to clinically-detected cancers with regard to tumor size, proliferation rates, and poor prognostic characteristics may be misleading since faster growing cancers are less likely to be detected by periodic screening and more likely to be clinically detected (length-biased sampling) [7]. Therefore, it is still necessary to demonstrate in observational data that screening improves outcomes while avoiding bias.

2.2 *Use of a Surrogate Outcome for Breast Cancer Mortality*

One method that has been suggested to address this bias is to focus on an earlier surrogate for mortality, late stage disease incidence, which should theoretically be prevented by screening. If one can show a reduction in late stage disease in a screened group, it would suggest a downstream effect on death due to breast cancer. In an attempt to determine whether late-stage disease may be a surrogate for future breast cancer mortality, we evaluated the association of screening with this outcome in a population-based study [8]. We characterized screening as a time-dependent covariate in an analysis of time to late stage diagnosis followed by the effect on mortality. We were unable to conclude that late stage disease was an appropriate surrogate for breast cancer mortality. We also evaluated what were the potential precursors for failing to diagnose late stage disease at an earlier screen [9]. We determined that it was primarily a failure to conduct a screen at all, but also there was a failure to diagnose even among women screened, and failure to appropriately treat women who were diagnosed. Since failures can occur at each step in the screening process, it is necessary to study each part of the screening process and the factors that each part depend on.

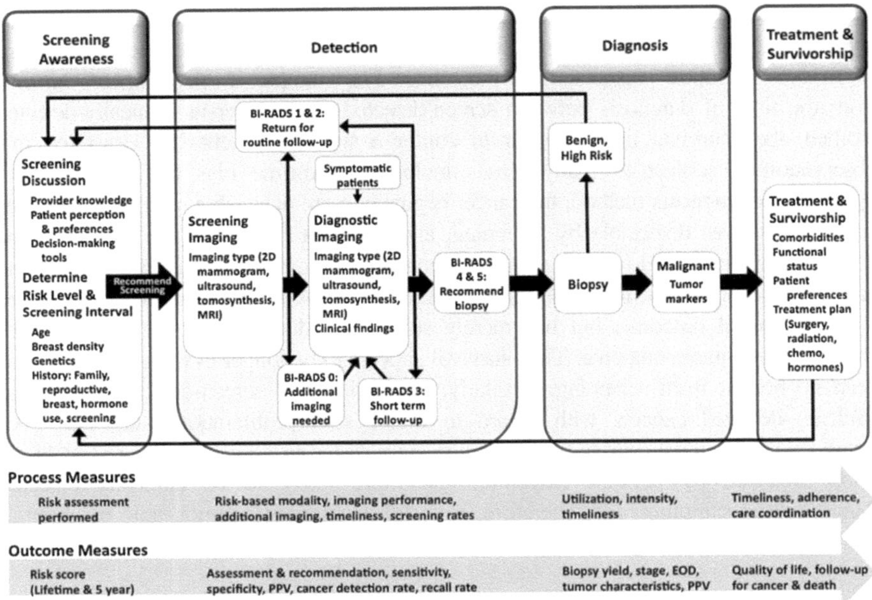

Fig. 1 The PROSPR ("Population-based Research Optimizing Screening through Personalized Regimens") conceptual model of breast cancer screening that represents risk-based and preference-based care within diverse multilevel systems. *BI-RADS* indicates Breast Imaging-Reporting and Data System, *2D* 2-dimensional, *MRI* magnetic resonance imaging; chemo, chemotherapy, *PPV* positive predictive value, *EOD* extent of disease

3 Decomposition of the Screening Process

3.1 Conceptual Model of Breast Cancer Screening

We have created a conceptual model of the screening process for breast cancer shown in Fig. 1 [10; figure reproduced with permission].

So a randomized trial of screening requires that each step in this process work well in order to achieve a mortality reduction. Even if randomized trials of screening could be done, the overall timeline to find a mortality reduction would be 10–15 years from start of the trial. Therefore, it is necessary to decompose these steps and deal with each separately. Each part of the process can be tested in a randomized trial or more likely evaluated with observational data adjusting for perceived major confounding.

3.2 Population Undergoing Screening

The very first part of the process is to identify those most at risk for breast cancer and prioritize screening for that population. The first and most common risk model for breast cancer was developed by Gail [11]. This model includes age, family history, age at menopause, number of live births, and previous diagnosis of atypical hyperplasia, a benign breast condition. However, other than older age, risk factors with high prevalence are few. Family history is a well-known risk factor but is not common and not as predictive as most would believe. The specific mutations of BRCA1 and BRCA2 are highly related to future breast cancer, but most women are not tested for these mutations routinely unless there is a family history of early onset of breast cancer or other compelling evidence for such testing.

Using data from 2.4 million screening mammograms from the Breast Cancer Surveillance Consortium (BCSC [12]) we predicted a diagnosis of breast cancer within one year [13]. Because the risk factors differ dramatically by menopausal status, separate models were fit to premenopausal and postmenopausal women. For premenopausal women only four risk factors were identified: (1) age; (2) breast density; (3) prior breast procedure (e.g. biopsy); and (4) first-degree family history. Breast density is the percentage of breast volume comprised of dense versus fatty tissue. It is judged subjectively from the screening mammogram by the radiologist and classified into four categories determined by BI-RADS [14]. Category 1 is the least dense and category 4 the most dense. Higher density has higher risk for breast cancer as well as making it more difficult to detect the breast cancer in a mammogram [13, 15]. Using these four risk factors yielded a prediction AUC of 0.63. For post-menopausal women many additional risk factors were identified including: race, Hispanic ethnicity; age at first birth; current use of exogenous hormones; surgically induced menopause; body mass index (BMI); and having had a previous false positive mammogram. Nonetheless, even with many highly significant predictors of breast cancer risk the ability to discriminate high risk from low risk remains poor (AUC of 0.62). Thus, it would be difficult at the current time to recommend to women above age 50 that they not be screened due to low risk. However, one could tailor the screening interval to risk level. That strategy is being tested in a randomized trial funded by Patient-Centered Outcomes Research Institute (PCORI) led by Dr. Laura Esserman [16]. They will randomize 10,000 women aged 40–74 years to annual screening or a personalized schedule based on risk factors.

Until that trial is conducted, one may need to rely on information from observational studies about participation in screening for breast cancer and how it depends on measured risk factors. For that reason the National Cancer Institute initiated an observational cohort study "Population-based Research Optimizing Screening through Personalized Regimens (PROSPR)" [17]. This initiative studies the actual application of screening for breast, cervical, and colorectal cancer in the population. For example, one can identify each person in the population and whether they have undergone screening and the outcome of that screening. Therefore, using population-based data one can infer screening benefit (or harm) to the entire population and not just individuals who are screened. The latter has been a limitation of other research efforts that start follow-up at the point of the screen. Furthermore, we can cluster individuals in their primary care practice and determine the association of each primary care physician with likelihood of screening. PROSPR has surveyed primary care physicians in order to understand how their beliefs about the effectiveness and optimal timing of screening actually are associated with screening by their patients [18]. Furthermore, we are looking at initiation of screening when one becomes an appropriate age to be screened. Beaber and colleagues have shown that even though screening is recommended at age 40 for many women, it still takes one to two years to reach 50% screened after their 40th birthday [19].

3.3 Mammography Interpretation and Cancer Detection

There has been extensive work on actual screening performance and how it depends on patient and radiologist factors as well as technology [20]. The initial screening mammogram is assigned a BI-RADS measure of suspicion of cancer that ranges from 1 (least likely) to 5 (most likely) [14]. Scores of 1 and 2 are considered "normal" and the patient is advised to return for screening in 1–2 years depending on age or risk factors [21]. Scores of 3 are rarely used as it indicates an ambiguous finding and the patient may be given a shorter screening interval (typically 6 months) until it is resolved. Scores of 4 or 5 may lead to consult with a surgeon or a breast biopsy though few patients receive a 4 or 5 directly from the initial screening mammogram. In cases where additional information is needed such as more imaging or access to past mammograms, a 0 may be assigned as a placeholder until the screening episode is resolved. Women assigned a 0 typically undergo additional imaging such as a more focused diagnostic mammogram, ultrasound, or a MRI image. After completion of this imaging, a final BI-RADS score may be assigned with the woman either referred back to a return to screening in the future or to an immediate surgical consult or biopsy. When forced to classify the initial mammogram we typically call 0, 4, and 5 as a "positive" mammogram although the underlying probability of cancer differs across those scores. The total positivity rate of the initial screening exam will range from about 8 to 20% depending on age, breast density, and whether this is the first screening examination for that woman. Often this is characterized as the recall rate even though there may be no actual recall and the woman is referred to biopsy.

4 Common Measures of Mammography Performance

4.1 Retrospective Measures Sensitivity and Specificity

To determine sensitivity and specificity, it is typical to determine the "actual" cancer state, preferably at the time of the screening examination. However, to do so would require invasive procedures such as a breast biopsy for each patient, and that would not be feasible or ethical in the absence of evidence of any breast cancer. Instead, it is common to adopt a follow-up period of one year to determine if cancer is diagnosed in that interval [19]. So sensitivity and specificity become conditional on the observed disease state one year after the screening mammogram. This has certain problems as well. First a rapidly growing cancer may not have been present at time of the negative screening mammogram, but the screen is still classified as a false negative examination in order to compute sensitivity. Secondly, the decision to perform a biopsy is often conditional on the screening result, leading to ascertainment bias of the true disease state. We have developed a doubly robust estimator that considers the probability of ascertainment in order to address this bias [22].

Sensitivity and specificity require a dichotomization of the BI-RADS scale into positive and negative that can lose valuable information. One can use a ROC approach that uses each value to generate either an empirical or modelled ROC curve. For the empirical AUC the area the comparison of every cancer case to every non cancer case with respect to which had the larger ordinal BI-RADS value. The modeling uses an ordinal probit model with BI-RADS assessment as an ordinal response (1, 2, 3, 0, 4, 5) reflecting increasing likelihood of a cancer diagnosis [20]. Disease status is the primary covariate that determines the AUC which can be computed from the parameter estimates. The curve itself represents choice of cutoffs determining true positive rate (sensitivity) and false positive rate (1-specificity) while the area under the curve (AUC) is characterized as the overall discriminatory ability of screening mammography. The modeled curve allows for adjustment for covariates as main effects (moving along the ROC curve) or as interactions with disease status (different ROC curves). Nonetheless, some difficulty in interpretation remains, particularly for unrealistic values of sensitivity or specificity. Consequently, use of direct modeling of sensitivity and specificity may be more common.

4.2 Prospective Measures of Positive and Negative Predictive Value

Sensitivity and specificity are "retrospective" as they condition on disease status and then look backwards to determine screening assessment. This also allows sampling of controls which are often more numerous than cases. However, one may prefer probabilistic statements about the likelihood of cancer given a positive or negative screening mammogram. Therefore, positive and negative predictive value may be valuable as prospective measures to guide patients. However, they are highly dependent on the overall level of disease in the population of interest. Since incident breast cancer is still rare in a population undergoing screening, negative predictive value is often 99% or greater. Positive predictive value may be 5–20% depending on the constellation of risk factors [23]. Thus, there may be considerable anxiety associated with an initial positive screening mammogram until it is resolved though further testing. Typically, additional imaging would be performed using diagnostic (focused) mammography, ultrasound, or magnetic resonance imaging (MRI). A new BI-RADs score may be assigned after this imaging. If the imaging is negative, a woman may be returned to the usual screening interval. If positive, she would likely be scheduled for a definitive biopsy.

There are actually three positive predictive values in common use named PPV_1, PPV_2, and PPV_3 [21]. PPV_1 is the more usual definition of PPV which uses as a denominator all positive screens and a numerator of all breast cancers diagnosed within a year of the screen. PPV_2 conditions on a recommendation of a biopsy either from the initial screen or more likely from subsequent diagnostic imaging as the denominator. PPV_3 conditions on actual receipt of a biopsy that was initially prompted by screening or follow-up imaging.

While we largely see PPV as being a "test" characteristic it is highly dependent on risk factors and individual risk for cancer so may vary widely with age, breast density, and other factors. It also includes BI-RADS categories 0, 4, and 5 which have very different likelihood for cancer [20]. Since 4 and 5 are rare as the initial screening result, this consolidation may have little impact.

4.3 *Survival and Mortality Outcomes*

Survival from point of initial diagnosis is often used as an outcome measure, but as previously discussed this can be biased if comparing screened women to unscreened women. Similarly, showing that screening is associated with smaller earlier stage breast cancer is a necessary condition, but not a sufficient condition, for demonstration of screening benefit. One actually has to show that there has been a change in the outcome trajectory due to screening. This is best done in individualized or group randomized trials of screening programs. In the absence of randomization, mortality rates may be instructive provided one can adjust for numerous sources of bias. Mortality in a population is measured from an arbitrary point in time (e.g. beginning of a calendar year) and modeled in survival time models with screening as a time-dependent covariate. Screening may be modeled as "ever-screened" which would confer a life-time benefit or may be modeled as time-limited such as "screened within the last 3 years prior to the current time point". Again such analyses are highly subject to the indication for screening requiring collection and modeling of potential confounders.

While the objective of screening is to reduce mortality due to breast cancer, this can be a difficult outcome to study requiring lengthy follow-up. Our previous attempts to use a surrogate outcome such as advanced disease were not successful [8]. Screening may also reduce morbidity even if not reducing mortality. That is, the intensity of treatment may be reduced in order to achieve the same outcome. Since treatments have improved dramatically one may no longer observe a mortality difference, but quality of life during treatment is higher and healthcare costs lower.

5 Current Research

5.1 New Technology in Imaging

Screening trials have used mostly film based mammography from two screening views. Digital mammography has largely replaced film and appears to offer better resolution. Mammography screening appears to improve each year [24]. Recently, tomosynthesis (3-dimensional) mammography has started to replace 2-dimensional digital mammography. It appears to have better performance than digital mammography [25]. Thus, studies of mammography become outdated quickly and modeling of benefit must adjust for these improvements.

5.2 Overtreatment Prevention

Breast cancer screening is a balance between reducing morbidity and mortality by detecting early stage breast cancer earlier, but at the same time not identifying lesions which would not be life-threatening. This is particularly true with an early form called Ductal Carcinoma in Situ (DCIS) which may be a precursor to invasive breast cancer in some, but not all, cases. It is almost universally detected by mammography screening. One current goal of screening is to identify DCIS with malignant potential usually requiring biomarker analysis of the DCIS specimen. Current models are not sufficiently accurate to deter treatment resulting in possible overtreatment. The tradeoff between overtreatment and early detection is largely responsible for differing recommendations for screening initiation and interval. Therefore, efforts are underway to use molecular tools (e.g. Oncotype DX DCIS Recurrence Score) to determine the level of treatment needed when DCIS is detected.

5.3 Population-Based Research of Screening Mammography

The Breast Cancer Surveillance Consortium (BCSC) was originally funded by the National Cancer Institute to quantify and describe mammography screening metrics

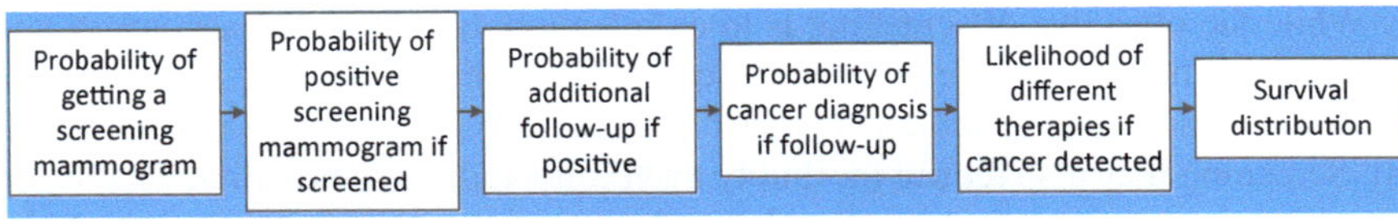

Fig. 2 Statistical model of the process of undergoing and evaluating screening

[12]. They have been very productive with extensive publications describing factors affecting mammography performance. The limitation was primarily that it captured mostly a screening population and therefore little was known about those not undergoing screening. Accordingly, the NCI began PROSPR to study population-based screening in breast, cervical, and colorectal cancer. The intent is to track large populations and ascertain level of screening and subsequent outcomes. The initiative has started to be productive computing screening metrics for all three cancers. It also allows an opportunity to develop statistical methodology that will cover the entire screening process from screening participation, to diagnosis, and subsequent morbidity and mortality. This prospective statistical model can be simplified as conditional steps in the process (Fig. 2).

The first step is to characterize the potential screening population requiring a full enumeration of all eligible for screening and whether they have been recently screened. This probability depends on personal characteristics such as age and other breast cancer risk factors as well as her primary care provider, health plan guidelines, and higher level system variables. This numerator then becomes the denominator in assessing the likelihood of the screen being deemed positive. This is also affected by personal risk characteristics and demographics, screening history, imaging equipment, and radiologist characteristics. Women who have positive initial screens undergo subsequent exams with some probability based on their level of concern or fear and the level of communication between the radiology facility, primary care provider, and the woman. If the woman does receive appropriate follow-up, the likelihood of cancer detection depends on both imaging and pathologic assessments. Given a breast cancer diagnosis, treatment options depend on the staging and type of breast cancer as well as individual preferences of the woman and her oncologist. Finally, among women treated for breast cancer there is great variability in survival even with similar characteristics. In practice it is quite common for each step to be estimated separately. However, it would be possible to characterize the complete process either by microsimulation or statistical modeling.

6 Conclusions

Overall, breast cancer screening has been successful, though it can continue to be refined. Most recommendations are age-based and may need to depend more on other risk factors such as breast density. Technology is improving which increases the benefit and decreases the likelihood of overtreatment. It is clear that the entire process needs to be continuously scrutinized and a prospective statistical model needs to be developed that can comprehensively assess the importance of person-level, provider-level, and system-level factors. This model can then be generalized to other cancer screening arenas and to other health conditions.

References

1. Myers ER, Moorman P, Gierisch JM, Havrilesky LJ, Grimm LJ, Ghate S, Davidson B, Mongtomery RC, Crowley MJ, McCrory DC, Kendrick A, Sanders GD. Benefits and harms of breast cancer screening: a systematic review. JAMA. 2015;314(15):1615–34.
2. Magnus MC, Ping M, Shen MM, Bourgeois J, Magnus JH. Effectiveness of mammography screening in reducing breast cancer mortality in women aged 39–49 years: a meta-analysis. J Womens Health. 2011;20(6):845–52.
3. Miller AB, Wall C, Baines CJ, Sun P, To T, Narod SA. Twenty five year follow-up for breast cancer incidence and mortality of the Canadian National Breast Screening Study: randomised screening trial. BMJ. 2014;348:g366.
4. US Preventive Services Task Force. Screening for breast cancer: U.S. preventive services task force recommendation statement. Ann Intern Med. 2009;151(10):716–26.
5. Jacklyn G, Glasziou P, Macaskill P, Barratt A. Meta-analysis of breast cancer mortality benefit and overdiagnosis adjusted for adherence: improving information on the effects of attending screening mammography. Br J Cancer. 2016;114(11):1269–76.
6. Morrison AS. The effects of early treatment, lead time and length bias on the mortality experienced by cases detected by screening. Int J Epidemiol. 1982;11(3):261–7.
7. Kramer BS, Croswell JM. Cancer screening: the clash of science and intuition. Ann Rev Med. 2009;60:125–37.
8. Thompson RS, Barlow WE, Taplin SH, Grothaus L, Immanuel V, Salazar A, Wagner EH. A population-based case-cohort evaluation of the efficacy of mammographic screening for breast cancer. Am J Epidemiol. 1994;140(10):889–901.
9. Taplin SH, Ichikawa L, Yood MU, Manos MM, Geiger AM, Weinmann S, Gilbert J, Mouchawar J, Leyden WA, Altaras R, Beverly RK, Casso D, Westbrook EO, Bischoff K, Zapka JG, Barlow WE. Reason for late-stage breast cancer: absence of screening or detection, or breakdown in follow-up? J Natl Cancer Inst. 2004;96(20):1518–27.
10. Onega T, Beaber EF, Sprague BL, Barlow WE, Haas JS, Tosteson AND, Schnall M, Armstrong K, Schapira MM, Geller B, Weaver DL, Conant EF. Breast cancer screening in an era of personalized regimens: a conceptual model and National Cancer Institute initiative for risk-based and preference-based approaches at a population level. Cancer. 2014;120 (19):2955–64.
11. Gail MH, Brinton LA, Byar DP, Corle DK, Green SB, Schairer C, Mulvihill JJ. Projecting individualized probabilities of developing breast cancer for white females who are being examined annually. J Natl Cancer Inst. 1989;81(24):1879–86.
12. Ballard-Barbash R, Taplin SH, Yankaskas BC, Ernster VL, Rosenberg RD, Carney PA, Barlow WE, Geller BM, Kerlikowske K, Edwards BK, Lynch CF, Urban N, Chrvala CA, Key CR, Poplack SP, Worden JK, Kessler LG. Breast cancer surveillance consortium: a national mammography screening and outcomes database. AJR Am J Roentgenol. 1997;169 (4):1001–8.
13. Barlow WE, White E, Ballard-Barbash R, Vacek PM, Titus-Ernstoff L, Carney PA, Tice JA, Buist DS, Geller BM, Rosenberg R, Yankaskas BC, Kerlikowske K. Prospective breast cancer risk prediction model for women undergoing screening mammography. J Natl Cancer Inst. 2006;98(17):1204–14.

14. American College of Radiology. Illustrated breast imaging reporting and data system (BI-RADS™). 4th ed. Reston: American College of Radiology; 2003.
15. Kolb TM, Lichy J, Newhouse JH. Comparison of the performance of screening mammography, physical examination, and breast US and evaluation of factors that influence them: an analysis of 27,825 patient evaluations. Radiology. 2002;225(1):165–75.
16. http://www.pcori.org/research-results/2015/enabling-paradigm-shift-preference-tolerant-rct-personalized-vs-annual. Accessed 24 Aug 2016.
17. National Cancer Institute. Population-based Research Optimizing Screening through Personalized Regimens (PROSPR). National Cancer Institute. http://healthcaredelivery.cancer.gov/prospr/. Accessed 24 Aug 2016.
18. Haas JS, Barlow WE, Schapira MM, MacLean CD, Klabunde CN, Sprague BL, Beaber EF, Chen JS, Bitton A, Onega T, Harris K, Tosteson ANA. On behalf of the PROSPR consortium. Primary care providers' beliefs and recommendations and use of screening mammography by their patients. J Gen Intern Med. 2016 (in press).
19. Beaber EF, Tosteson AN, Haas JS, Onega T, Sprague BL, Weaver DL, McCarthy AM, Doubeni CA, Quinn VP, Skinner CS, Zauber AG, Barlow WE. Breast cancer screening initiation after turning 40 years of age within the PROSPR consortium. Breast Cancer Res Treat. 2016;160:323–31.
20. Barlow WE, Chi C, Carney PA, Taplin SH, D'Orsi C, Cutter G, Hendrick RE, Elmore JG. Accuracy of screening mammography interpretation by characteristics of radiologists. J Natl Cancer Inst. 2004;96:1840–50.
21. http://www.acr.org/~/media/ACR/Documents/PDF/QualitySafety/Resources/BIRADS/MammoGlossary.pdf. Accessed 24 Aug 2016.
22. Zheng Y, Barlow WE, Cutter G. Assessing accuracy of mammography in the presence of verification bias and intrareader correlation. Biometrics. 2005;61(1):259–68.
23. Domingo L, Hofvind S, Hubbard RA, Román M, Benkeser D, Sala M, Castells X. Cross-national comparison of screening mammography accuracy measures in U.S., Norway, and Spain. Eur Radiol. 2016;26(8):2520–8.
24. Ichikawa LE, Barlow WE, Anderson ML, Taplin SH, Geller BM, Brenner RJ. National Cancer Institute-sponsored breast cancer surveillance consortium. Time trends in radiologists' interpretive performance at screening mammography from the community-based Breast Cancer Surveillance Consortium, 1996–2004. Radiology. 2010;256(1):74–82.
25. Conant EF, Beaber EF, Sprague BL, Herschorn SD, Weaver DL, Onega T, Tosteson AN, McCarthy AM, Poplack SP, Haas JS, Armstrong K, Schnall MD, Barlow WE. Breast cancer screening using tomosynthesis in combination with digital mammography compared to digital mammography alone: a cohort study within the PROSPR consortium. Breast Cancer Res Treat. 2016;156(1):109–16.

Mediation Analysis for Multiple Causal Mechanisms

Masataka Taguri

Abstract In many health studies, researchers are interested in estimating the treatment effects on the outcome around and through an intermediate variable. Such causal mediation analyses aim to understand the mechanisms that explain the treatment effect. Although multiple mediators are often involved in real studies, most of the literature considers mediation analyses with one mediator at a time. In this article, we review some recent advances in mediation analyses when there are multiple causal pathways. We discuss the cases that (1) there is a mediator-outcome confounder that is affected by the treatment when we are interested in one mediator and (2) there are causally non-ordered multiple mediators.

Keywords Causal inference · Mediation analysis · Multiple mediators · Natural direct effect · Natural indirect effect

1 Introduction

In many health studies, researchers are interested in estimating the treatment effects on the outcome around and through an intermediate variable (called a mediator), where the corresponding effects are called direct and indirect effects respectively, and their sum is the total effect of the treatment on the outcome of interest. Such mediation analyses aim to understand the mechanisms that explain the treatment effect. Robins and Greenland [1] originally put forward a formal study of causal mediation analysis using the potential outcome framework. Following their work, Pearl [2] showed that a total effect can always be broken down into natural direct and indirect effects. There is a growing literature on evaluating natural direct and indirect effects [3–11]. Although a treatment often affects the outcome through multiple mediators in real studies, most of the literature considers a mediation analysis with a single mediator only.

M. Taguri (✉)
Department of Biostatistics, Yokohama City University
School of Medicine, Yokohama, Japan
e-mail: taguri@yokohama-cu.ac.jp

S. Matsui and J. Crowley (eds.), *Frontiers of Biostatistical Methods and Applications in Clinical Oncology*, DOI 10.1007/978-981-10-0126-0_21

The goal of this chapter is to review some recent advances in mediation analysis in the presence of multiple causal pathways. Figure 1 presents two causal diagrams with multiple causal pathways from the treatment or exposure variable A to the outcome Y. For example, A is a cavity prevention intervention, M_1 and M_2 are oral bacteria level and fluoride level at 12 months of follow-up, and Y is the number of tooth decay at 24 months. Another example in cancer epidemiology is that A is obesity, M_1 and M_2 are insulin resistance and increasing low-grade chronic inflammatory state, and Y is the incidence of colorectal cancer. In addition, we may use Fig. 1 for the surrogate endpoints evaluation. For example, A is a cancer treatment (e.g. presence or absence of a new chemotherapy), M_1 and M_2 are tumor response and standardized uptake value on PET/CT imaging after introduction of the study treatment, and Y is the overall survival.

The critical difference between Fig. 1a, b is that in the former a mediator M_1 may possibly affect the other mediator M_2, whereas in the latter M_1 and M_2 are assumed to have no causal relationship with one another. In this chapter, we discuss the cases that (1) there is a mediator-outcome confounder that is affected by the treatment when we are interested in one mediator but not the other (Fig. 1a; see also Fig. 2a) and (2) there are causally non-ordered multiple mediators (Fig. 1b). See Daniel et al. [12] and the references therein for mediation analysis when there are causally ordered multiple mediators and all are of interest.

The remainder of this chapter is organized as follows. In Sect. 2, we briefly review the direct and indirect effects in the single mediator setting and present identification assumptions when there is a mediator-outcome confounder that is affected by the treatment. In Sect. 3, we discuss mediation analysis when there are causally non-ordered multiple mediators. We conclude with a discussion in Sect. 4.

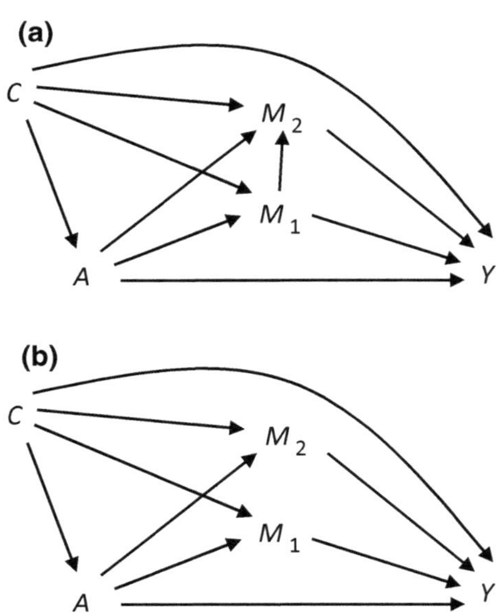

Fig. 1 A causal diagram with treatment A, mediators M_1 and M_2, outcome Y, and confounding factors C under **a** M_1 causally affects M_2, and **b** M_1 does not causally affect M_2

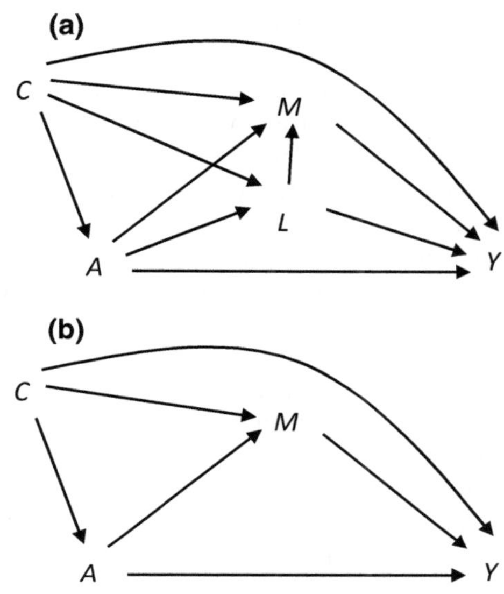

Fig. 2 A causal diagram in a single mediator setting with treatment A, mediator M, outcome Y, and confounding factors C under **a** there exists a treatment-induced mediator-outcome confounder L, and **b** L does not exist

2 Mediation Analysis with a Single Mediator

We first briefly review the causal mediation analysis with a single mediator. Let Y denote an observed outcome for an individual, A denote a binary treatment or exposure (1: treatment or exposure, 0: control or non-exposed), C denote a set of confounding variables that may affect the treatment, mediator and/or outcome, and M denote a single potential mediator that may be on the pathway from the exposure to the outcome (Fig. 2). There may be other mediators as well but when focusing on only one mediator, the effect through other mediators would be included in the direct path from A to Y and not through M, as long as such mediators are not causally related with M (Fig. 2b). When there exists a confounder L that is affected by the treatment and itself affects the mediator and outcome (Fig. 2a), it is in fact also a second mediator. That is, L lies on the pathway from the treatment to the outcome and we are in a setting with multiple mediators even when we were only interested in one mediator.

2.1 *Notation and Assumptions for Identification When There Is No Mediator-Outcome Confounder That Is Affected by the Treatment*

To conduct a causal mediation analysis, we use the potential outcome framework [13, 14]. Let $Y(a)$ and $M(a)$ respectively denote the potential outcome and potential mediator that would be observed if, possibly contrary to the fact, A were set to a. Likewise, let $Y(a, m)$ denote the potential outcome that would be observed if, possibly contrary to the fact, A were set to a and M were set to m. We also make assumptions referred to as the consistency and composition assumptions [7]. The consistency assumption for (A, M) is that amongst the subgroup with the observed treatment $A = a$ and the observed mediator $M = m$, the observed outcome Y is equal to $Y(a, m)$. The consistency assumption for the effect of the treatment on the mediator is that amongst the subgroup with the observed treatment $A = a$, the observed mediator M is equal to $M(a)$. The composition assumption is that $Y(a) = Y(a, M(a))$.

Robins and Greenland [1] and Pearl [2] considered the natural direct effect of treatment A on outcome Y, $\{Y(1, M(0)) - Y(0, M(0))\}$. This natural direct effect compares the potential outcome under treatment and control given the mediator M at its natural level under control $M(0)$, so is also referred as the "pure direct effect" [1]. The natural indirect effect $\{Y(1, M(1)) - Y(1, M(0))\}$ they considered compares the potential outcome that would be observed when the subject is treated and mediator is changed from $M(0)$ to $M(1)$. This natural indirect effect is also referred as the "total indirect effect" [1]. The total effect can then be decomposed into the natural direct and indirect effect as: $Y(1) - Y(0) = Y(1, M(1)) - Y(0, M(0)) = \{Y(1, M(1)) - Y(1, M(0))\} + \{Y(1, M(0)) - Y(0, M(0))\}$. Alternatively, we can also decompose the total effect as: $Y(1) - Y(0) = \{Y(1, M(1)) - Y(0, M(1))\} + \{Y(0, M(1)) - Y(0, M(0))\}$, where $\{Y(1, M(1)) - Y(0, M(1))\}$ is referred as the "total direct effect" and $\{Y(0, M(1)) - Y(0, M(0))\}$ as the "pure indirect effect."

Because we are not able to observe all the potential outcomes for one subject in a real study, the individual level effects cannot be identified. On the other hand, under some assumptions, the population average effects can be identified. Given confounders $C = c$, the population average effects are conditional expectations of the individual level effects $E[Y(1) - Y(0)|c]$, $E[Y(1, M(1)) - Y(1, M(0))|c]$, and $E[Y(1, M(0)) - Y(0, M(0))|c]$. Various assumptions have been proposed for the identification of the population average natural direct and indirect effects. When A and Y have common causes we say that A-Y relation suffers from confounding. Most of the literature first assumes no unmeasured confounding on three relationships.

A1. *No unmeasured confounding of the A-Y relation.*

$$Y(a,m) \coprod A|C \quad for\, all\, (a,m).$$

A2. *No unmeasured confounding of the M-Y relation.*

$$Y(a,m) \coprod M(a)|A = a,C \quad for\, all\, (a,m).$$

A3. *No unmeasured confounding of the A-M relation.*

$$M(a) \coprod A|C \quad \textit{for all } a.$$

These three assumptions imply that after conditioning (i.e. adjusting for) a set of measured confounding factors, association means causation. For example, under consistency and assumptions A1 and A2, $E[Y(a,m)|\ A = a,\ M = m,\ C = c] = E[Y(a,m)|\ C = c]$ holds. It follows that the conditional association between (A, M) and Y given C equals the corresponding population causal effect given C. For instance, $\{E[Y|\ A = 1,\ M = 1,\ C = c] - E[Y|\ A = 0,\ M = 0,\ C = c]\}$ equals $\{E[Y(1,1)|\ C = c] - E[Y(0,0)|\ C = c]\}$. In addition, Pearl [2] made the following assumption for identification:

A4. *A cross-world independence assumption.*

$$Y(a,m) \coprod M(a^*)|C \quad \textit{for all } (a, a^*, m).$$

If we assume that data are generated from Pearl's nonparametric structural equation model (NPSEM) [15], then A4 will hold if there is no mediator-outcome confounder that is affected itself by the treatment. Figure 2b shows a causal diagram that is compatible with assumptions A1–A4 under Pearl's NPSEM.

2.2 *Additional Assumptions for Identification When There Is a Mediator-Outcome Confounder That Is Affected by the Treatment*

If a mediator-outcome confounder L is affected by the treatment (Fig. 2a), then without additional assumptions, natural direct and indirect effects cannot be nonparametrically identified even under Pearl's NPSEM, irrespective of whether such a confounder is measured or not [16]. Instead, we need to assume other strong assumptions for identification in addition to the assumptions of no unmeasured confounders similar to A1–A3 [17]. Robins and Greenland [17] assumed the absence of treatment-mediator interactions at the individual level in the sense that $\{Y(1,m) - Y(0,m)\}$ is a random variable that does not depend on m. Petersen et al. [18] relaxed it to

$$E[Y(1,m) - Y(0,m)|M(0),c] - E[Y(1,m) - Y(0,m)|c] = 0 \quad \textit{for all } m.$$

Robins and Richardson [19] and Tchetgen and VanderWeele [20] proposed additional assumptions for identification within the NPSEM. One of the assumptions proposed by Tchetgen and VanderWeele [20] can be used for any type of (that is, non-binary) L, and is given by:

$$E[Y|a,m,l,c]-E[Y|a,m^*,l,c]-E[Y|a,m,l^*,c]+E[Y|a,m^*,l^*,c]=0,$$

where $m^* \neq m$ and $l^* \neq l$. That is, there is no average additive interaction between L and M. Based on the principal stratification framework, Taguri and Chiba [21] proposed the following assumptions for a binary mediator:

$$E[Y(1,1)-Y(1,0)|A=1,M=1,c]-E[Y(1,1)-Y(1,0)|A=0,M=1,c]=0,$$

for the pure direct effect and total indirect effect, and

$$E[Y(0,1)-Y(0,0)|A=1,M=0,c]-E[Y(0,1)-Y(0,0)|A=0,M=0,c]=0,$$

for the total direct effect and pure indirect effect. Taguri and Chiba [21] showed that their estimator would have small bias in typical situations even if their assumptions were violated by deriving the bounds of the bias terms. They also proposed a simple method of sensitivity analysis.

3 Mediation Analysis for Two Causally Non-ordered Mediators

Now we consider the situation that there are two causally non-ordered mediators M_1 and M_2, meaning that the causal relationship between M_1 and M_2 is absent as in Fig. 1b. For example, a cavity prevention intervention (A) for high risk patients often has an antibacterial component to reduce oral bacteria as well as fluoride therapy to strength the teeth, where the two mediators oral bacteria level (M_1) and fluoride level (M_2) are not causally related [22]. Another example in cancer epidemiology is that obesity (A) may increase the incidence of colorectal cancer (Y) through two different mechanisms: one is that increasing insulin resistance (M_1) and the other is that increasing a low-grade chronic inflammatory state (M_2). With two causally non-ordered mediators involved, there are three path-specific effects from exposure (A) to outcome (Y): the direct pathway ($A \rightarrow Y$), the indirect pathway through M_1 only ($A \rightarrow M_1 \rightarrow Y$), and the indirect pathway through M_2 only ($A \rightarrow M_2 \rightarrow Y$) (Fig. 1b).

3.1 Notation and Assumptions

Let $M_1(a)$, $M_2(a)$, and $Y(a, m_1, m_2)$ be obvious extensions of the potential outcomes defined in Sect. 2.1. We also assume the consistency and composition assumptions for these potential outcomes. The observed outcome Y is equal to $Y(A, M_1(A), M_2(A))$. We assume that the potential mediator $M_2(a, m_1) = M_2(a)$ does not depend on the value of m_1, implying that M_2 is not causally affected by M_1.

We extend Assumptions A1–A4 to B1–B4 for two causally non-ordered mediators M_1 and M_2.

B1. *No unmeasured confounding of the A-Y relation.*

$$Y(a, m_1, m_2) \coprod A|C \quad for\, all (a, m_1, m_2).$$

B2. *No unmeasured confounding of the* (M_1, M_2)*-Y relation.*

$$Y(a, m_1, m_2) \coprod \{M_1(a), M_2(a)\}|A = a, C \quad for\, all\, (a, m_1, m_2).$$

B3. *No unmeasured confounding of the A-*(M_1, M_2) *relation.*

$$M_k(a) \coprod A|C \quad for\, all\, (a, k).$$

B4. *An extended cross-world independence assumption.*

$$\begin{aligned} &Y(a, m_1, m_2) \coprod \{M_1(a^*), M_2(a^{**})\}|C, \\ &M_1(a^*) \coprod M_2(a^{**})|C, \quad for\, all\, (a, a^*, a^{**}, m_1, m_2). \end{aligned}$$

Again, under the NPSEM, B4 will hold if there is no mediator-outcome confounder that is affected by the treatment. See Robins and Richardson for a more detailed discussion on the NPSEM and its relation to other graphical causal models [19]. Assumptions B1–B4 are sufficient to identify $E[Y(a, M_1(a^*), M_2(a^{**}))|c]$ for all (a, a^*, a^{**}) [23].

3.2 A Two-Way Decomposition of the Total Effect into the Joint Natural Direct and Indirect Effects

Under the causal relationshipsin Fig. 1b, one may consider M_1 and M_2 as a joint mediator [24]. According to VaderWeele and Vansteelandt [24], the natural direct and indirect effects with (M_1, M_2) as the mediator is defined by $\{Y(1, M_1(0), M_2(0)) - Y(0, M_1(0), M_2(0))\}$ and $\{Y(1, M_1(1), M_2(1)) - Y(1, M_1(0), M_2(0))\}$, respectively. The joint natural indirect effect here is the treatment effect mediated through M_1 or M_2, and the joint natural direct effect is the effect through neither M_1 nor M_2. Then, the total effect is decomposed into the joint natural direct and indirect effects as follows:

$$\begin{aligned} Y(1) - Y(0) = &\{Y(1, M_1(1), M_2(1)) - Y(1, M_1(0), M_2(0))\} \\ &+ \{Y(1, M_1(0), M_2(0)) - Y(0, M_1(0), M_2(0))\} \end{aligned} \tag{1}$$

The definition is a natural extension of the decomposition of the total effect into the total indirect effect and the pure direct effect to the two mediators setting. Another similar decomposition of the total effect into the joint total direct effect and the joint pure indirect effect is given as: $Y(1) - Y(0) = \{Y(1, M_1(1), M_2(1)) - Y(0, M_1(1), M_2(1))\} + \{Y(0, M_1(1), M_2(1)) - Y(0, M_1(0), M_2(0))\}$.

The differences between the "pure" and "total" direct (indirect) effects are due to the differential inclusion of the interaction between the treatment and the mediators. In a single mediator case, VanderWeele [25] showed that the difference {total natural direct effect − pure natural direct effect} = {total natural indirect effect – pure natural indirect effect} corresponds to a "mediated interaction" between A and M, which is the product of an additive interaction of the treatment and the mediator on the outcome, $\{Y(1,1) - Y(1,0) - Y(0,1) + Y(0,0)\}$, and the effect of the treatment on the mediator, $\{M(1) - M(0)\}$ (see Sect. 2.1 for the notation). This mediated interaction is arguably a part of the mediated effect, in the sense that it requires that the treatment changes the mediator. Thus, we will focus on the decomposition (1) in the remainder of this article for illustration. However, the methods discussed in the paper could be directly applied to the other decomposition. It is important to note that the joint natural direct and indirect effects can be identified even if M_1 and M_2 are causally related [24].

3.3 *Two Three-Way Decompositions of the Joint Natural Indirect Effect into Path-Specific Natural Indirect Effects*

If our aim is to compare the relative importance of M_1 and M_2 as a mediator, then we are interested in three path-specific effects from treatment to outcome; (i) the direct effect around the two mediators ($A \to Y$), (ii) the indirect effect through M_1 only ($A \to M_1 \to Y$), and (iii) the indirect effects through M_2 only ($A \to M_2 \to Y$) (Fig. 1b). Then, the joint natural indirect effect in (1) can be further decomposed into two path-specific effects, as follows:

$$
\begin{aligned}
&Y(1, M_1(1), M_2(1)) - Y(1, M_1(0), M_2(0)) \\
&= \{Y(1, M_1(1), M_2(1)) - Y(1, M_1(0), M_2(1))\} \\
&\quad + \{Y(1, M_1(0), M_2(1)) - Y(1, M_1(0), M_2(0))\}
\end{aligned} \tag{2}
$$

$$
\begin{aligned}
&= \{Y(1, M_1(1), M_2(0)) - Y(1, M_1(0), M_2(0))\} \\
&\quad + \{Y(1, M_1(1), M_2(1)) - Y(1, M_1(1), M_2(0))\},
\end{aligned} \tag{3}
$$

where the first terms in (2) and (3) are indirect effects through M_1, whereas the second terms in (2) and (3) are indirect effects through M_2. Daniel et al. [12] showed that there are six decompositions of the total effect into three path-specific effects. Of these six decompositions, Lange et al. [26] focused on (2) and (3) in conjunction with (1), while Imai and Yamamoto [27] considered other two decompositions. Here we will focus on (2) and (3) because these are only two decompositions such that the sum of the indirect effects through M_1 and through M_2 is equal to the joint total natural indirect effect in (1). For notational convenience, we use $\text{PSE}_1(a) = Y(1, M_1(1), M_2(a)) - Y(1, M_1(0), M_2(a))$ $(a = 0, 1)$ to denote indirect effects through M_1. Likewise, we use $\text{PSE}_2(a) = Y(1, M_1(a), M_2(1)) - Y(1, M_1(a), M_2(0))$ $(a = 0, 1)$ to denote indirect effects through M_2. Using this notation, (2) = $\text{PSE}_1(1) + \text{PSE}_2(0)$ and (3) = $\text{PSE}_1(0) + \text{PSE}_2(1)$.

3.4 *A Three-Way Decomposition of the Joint Natural Indirect into Path-Specific Natural Indirect Effects and an Interactive Effect*

If we are interested in both M_1 and M_2 there would be no clear reason which decomposition is preferred between (2) and (3). However, the decompositions (2) and (3) will not necessarily give the same results when $\text{PSE}_k(1) \neq \text{PSE}_k(0)$ $(k = 1, 2)$. If the analysis results from (2) and (3) diverge in the sense that indirect effects for $M_1(M_2)$ are different between these two decompositions, then there is no clear guidance which decomposition to use. Note also that the total natural indirect effect through M_1 is equal to $\text{PSE}_1(1)$ [24], which is equal to the first term of (2). Likewise, the total natural indirect effect through M_2 only is equal to $\text{PSE}_2(1)$. This indicates that the sum of the two total natural indirect effect through M_1 and M_2 considered separately is not equal to the joint total natural indirect effect in general.

To overcome these problems, Taguri et al. [23] proposed a further three-way decomposition of the joint natural indirect effect (and thus a four-way decomposition of the total effect). They showed that the joint natural indirect effect can be decomposed into the following three components for binary mediators:

$$
\begin{aligned}
& Y(1, M_1(1), M_2(1)) - Y(1, M_1(0), M_2(0)) \\
& = \{Y(1, M_1(1), M_2(0)) - Y(1, M_1(0), M_2(0))\} \\
& \quad + \{Y(1, M_1(0), M_2(1)) - Y(1, M_1(0), M_2(0))\} \\
& \quad + \{Y(1,1,1) - Y(1,1,0) - Y(1,0,1) + Y(1,0,0)\} \\
& \quad \{M_1(1) - M_1(0)\}\{M_2(1) - M_2(0)\}. \\
& = \mathrm{PSE}_1(0) + \mathrm{PSE}_2(0) + \mathrm{MI},
\end{aligned} \tag{4}
$$

The third component in (4) is called as a "mediated interactive effect" or "mediated interaction" (MI) between M_1 and M_2. It is the product of the additive interaction between M_1 and M_2 with $A = 1$, $\{Y(1, 1, 1) - Y(1, 1, 0) - Y(1, 0, 1) + Y(1, 0, 0)\}$, the effect of the treatment on M_1, $\{M_1(1) - M_1(0)\}$, and the effect of the treatment on M_2, $\{M_2(1) - M_2(0)\}$. This mediated interaction is nonzero if and only if the treatment affects both the two mediators and the additive interaction between M_1 and M_2 on Y is nonzero. This three-way decomposition includes the mediated interactive effect so that it can be explicitly evaluated in a study and also resolves the ambiguity concerning the choice between (2) and (3). In addition, by definition, it follows that $\mathrm{MI} = \mathrm{PSE}_1(1) - \mathrm{PSE}_1(0) = \mathrm{PSE}_2(1) - \mathrm{PSE}_2(0)$. Using these equalities, we obtain the following relations: $\mathrm{PSE}_k(1) = \mathrm{PSE}_k(0) + \mathrm{MI}$ ($k = 1,2$). Thus, we can understand that the difference between (2) and (3) are the differential inclusion of the mediated interaction for the indirect effect of M_1 (decomposition (2)) or for the indirect effect of M_2 (decomposition (3)). Thus, the results from (2) and (3) may diverge when there exists a large additive interaction between the two mediators. Furthermore, using decomposition (4), we can understand how much of the joint natural indirect effect is explained by the interactive effect of the mediators, as well as by each separate indirect effect.

Given the individual level decomposition (4), we can obtain a similar decomposition in the population average effect conditional on $C = c$ by using B4, as follows:

$$
\begin{aligned}
& E[Y(1, M_1(1), M_2(1)) - Y(1, M_1(0), M_2(0))|c] \\
& = E[Y(1, M_1(1), M_2(0)) - Y(1, M_1(0), M_2(0))|c] \\
& \quad + E[Y(1, M_1(0), M_2(1)) - Y(1, M_2(0), M_2(0))|c] \\
& \quad + E[Y(1,1,1) - Y(1,1,0) - Y(1,0,1) + Y(1,0,0)|c] \\
& \quad E[M_1(1) - M_2(0)|c]E[M_2(1) - M_2(0)|c].
\end{aligned} \tag{5}
$$

Taguri et al. [23] show the general formula which can be used for any-types (that is, non-binary) of mediators. They also discuss extensions for the cases that there are three mediators and there exists a vector of mediator.

3.5 Identification and Estimation

Under B1–B4, we obtain the following identification formula of $E[Y(a, M_1(a^*), M_2(a^{**}))|c]$ for all (a, a^*, a^{**}):

$$E[Y(a, M_1(a^*), M_2(a^{**}))|c] = \sum_{m_1}\sum_{m_2} E[Y|a, m_1, m_2, c]p(m_1|a^*, c)p(m_2|a^{**}, c). \tag{6}$$

For continuous mediators, we simply replace sums by integrals in (6). Under B1 and B2, we have $E[Y(a, m_1, m_2)|c] = E[Y|a, m_1, m_2, c]$, and $\Pr(M_k(a) = m_k|c) = p(m_k|a, c)$ for $k = (1, 2)$. Then, the all components in (5) as well as the joint natural direct effect can be identified from the observed data by the following formulas which can also be used for non-binary mediators:

$$\begin{aligned}
E[\text{NDE}|c] &= \textstyle\sum_{m_1}\sum_{m_2} \{E[Y|A=1, m_1, m_2, c] - E[Y|A=0, m_1, m_2, c]\}p(m_1|A=0, c) \\
&\quad \times p(m_2|A=0, c), \\
E[\text{PSE}_1(0)|c] &= \textstyle\sum_{m_1}\sum_{m_2} E[Y|A=1, m_1, m_2, c]\{p(m_1|A=1, c) - p(m_1|A=0, c)\}p(m_2|A=0, c), \\
E[\text{PSE}_2(0)|c] &= \textstyle\sum_{m_1}\sum_{m_2} E[Y|A=1, m_1, m_2, c]p(m_1|A=0, c)\{p(m_2|A=1, c) - p(m_2|A=0, c)\}, \\
E[\text{MI}|c] &= \textstyle\sum_{m_1}\sum_{m_2} E[Y|A=1, m_1, m_2, c]\{p(m_1|A=1, c) - p(m_1|A=0, c)\} \\
&\quad \times \{p(m_2|A=1, c) - p(m_2|A=0, c)\},
\end{aligned} \tag{7}$$

In (6) and (7), we considered effects conditional on the level of the covariates $C = c$. To obtain marginal effect estimates, we average these expressions over the marginal distribution of C. If at least one of the mediators is continuous and a linear regression model for Y does not hold, then we cannot generally obtain analytical formulas of (6) and (7) because we have to evaluate the integral on mediators. In such a case, we can use a Monte Carlo approach according to the method described in Imai et al. [27] to obtain marginal effect estimates. Standard errors and confidence intervals can be obtained based on the nonparametric bootstrap.

Another possible approach for the estimation is the inverse probability weighting (IPW) [26]. We can obtain an estimator of $E[Y(a, M_1(a^*), M_2(a^{**}))]$ by taking a weighted average of the outcome Y with the following weight w_i for the individual i:

$$\begin{aligned}
w_i = &\frac{I(A_i = a)}{\Pr(A_i = a|C_i = c_i)} \times \frac{\Pr(M_{1i} = m_{1i}|A_i = a^*, C_i = c_i)}{\Pr(M_{1i} = m_{1i}|A_i = a, C_i = c_i)} \\
&\times \frac{\Pr(M_{2i} = m_{2i}|A_i = a^{**}, C_i = c_i)}{\Pr(M_{2i} = m_{2i}|A_i = a, C_i = c_i)},
\end{aligned}$$

where $I(\cdot)$ denotes the indicator function.

3.6 Application

We apply the methods discussed in Sects. 3.4 and 3.5 to understand the mediation effects in The Caries Management by Risk Assessment (CAMBRA) randomized controlled clinical trial [28]. This trial aimed to assess whether combined antibacterial and fluoride therapy has beneficial effects on preventing new caries over 24 months follow-up. In the study, participants in the control group ($A = 0$) received conventional treatment per usual practices, while participants in the intervention group ($A = 1$) received a combined antibacterial and fluoride therapy. The primary analyses showed that the intervention group had a statistically significantly lower caries risk at follow-up and suggested a lower average caries increment compared with control over 24 months [28]. Our interest in this mediation analysis is whether this overall intervention effect was due mainly to bacteria reduction through antibacterial therapy, fluoride increase through fluoride therapy, or both.

The potential mediators of interest are two salivary oral bacteria (mutans streptococci (MS) and lactobacilli (LB)) levels and salivary fluoride level at 12 months. To make our identification assumptions more plausible, we consider MS and LB levels as a vector of mediators ($\mathbf{M}_1$) and consider fluoride level as the other mediator (M_2), where $\mathbf{M}_1$ and M_2 are assumed to work through independent pathways. The outcome of interest (Y) was the increment from baseline in the number of decayed, missing, and filled permanent surfaces (ΔDMFS) at 24 months. From a total of 231 participants randomized, 101 (intervention group: 51; control group: 50) patients who had completed data on ΔDMFS and relevant covariates were analyzed. Variables that were included in the set of C were: age, sex, race, education, timing of last dental visit, brushed two times or more yesterday, used fluoride toothpaste, fair or poor oral health, drank alcohol in past week, and smoked cigarette within 30 days. We modeled $p(y|\ a, \mathbf{m}_1, m_2, c)$ with a negative binomial regression and the conditional distributions of the three mediators with linear regression models assuming normally distributed errors. In addition to the main effects of all the covariates, we included interaction terms between A and $\mathbf{M}_1$, A and M_2, and $\mathbf{M}_1$ and M_2, in the model for the outcome.

The estimated joint natural direct effect was −0.298 (95% CI −1.894 to 1.805), and the joint natural indirect effect was −0.490 (95% CI −1.652 to 0.172), and thus the total effect was −0.298 + (−0.490) = −0.788 (95% CI −2.108 to 0.847). Applying the three-way decomposition of the joint natural indirect effect, the indirect effect through $\mathbf{M}_1$ only was −0.373 (−1.541 to 0.195), the indirect effect through M_2 only was −0.022 (95% CI −0.366 to 0.789), and the mediated interaction was −0.095 (95% CI −0.807 to 0.171). Thus, of the total effect, −0.298/−0.788 = 37.8% was attributable to the joint natural direct effect, −0.373/−0.788 = 47.3% was attributable to the indirect effect through $\mathbf{M}_1$ only, −0.022/−0.788 = 2.8% was attributable to the indirect effect through M_2 only, and −0.095/−0.788 = 12.1% was attributable to the mediated interaction. The overall proportion mediated was 47.3 + 2.8 + 12.1 = 62.2%. The results indicate that the effect of the intervention (A) on ΔDMFS (Y) was mainly through its effect in decreasing salivary oral bacteria levels ($\mathbf{M}_1$), although the effect is not significant due to the smaller sample size for this analysis compared to the primary analysis. Of the mediated effect, only a small portion of the effect was due to the effect in increasing salivary fluoride levels (M_2). However, the moderated size of the mediated interactive effect of $\mathbf{M}_1$ and M_2 (more than 10%) indicates the effect of increased salivary fluoride level on ΔDMFS through its interaction with decreased oral bacterial level.

4 Discussion

In this chapter, we review methods of mediation analysis in the presence of multiple causal pathways. We discuss the cases that (1) there is a mediator-outcome confounder that is affected by the treatment when we are interested in one mediator and (2) there are causally non-ordered multiple mediators. We have seen that to estimate direct and indirect effects, several strong assumptions are needed about confounding. We assume that there are no unmeasured confounders between the treatment and outcome (B1), the mediators and outcome (B2), and the treatment and mediators (B3). Although Assumptions B1 and B3 usually hold in a randomized trial, Assumption B2 does not necessarily hold even under the randomization of the treatment because the mediator cannot be randomized in a real study. Thus, there will be utility in conducting sensitivity analyses that examine the effect of violations of B2. Further research is needed on this issue in the presence of multiple mediators. Recently, VanderWeele and Tchetgen [29] considered mediation analyses when treatments and mediators vary over time. When longitudinal data on treatments and mediators are obtained, their method can potentially increase power in the direct and mediated effects by utilizing more data for the mediation analysis.

Acknowledgements This work was partially supported by Grant-in-Aid for Scientific Research (No. 15K15951) from the Ministry of Education, Culture, Sports, Science, and Technology of Japan.

References

1. Robins JM, Greenland S. Identifiability and exchangeability for direct and indirect effects. Epidemiology. 1992;3:143–55.
2. Pearl J. Direct and indirect effects. In: Proceedings of the seventeenth conference on uncertainty in artificial intelligence. San Francisco: Morgan Kaufmann; 2001. p. 411–20.
3. van der Laan MJ, Petersen ML. Direct effect models. Int J Biostat. 2008;4:1–27.

4. Kaufman S, Kaufman JS, MacLehose RF. Analytic bounds on causal risk differences in directed acyclic graphs involving three observed binary variables. J Stat Plan Infer. 2009;139:3473–87.
5. Sjölander A. Bounds on natural effects in the presence of confounded intermediate variables. Stat Med. 2009;28:558–71.
6. VanderWeele TJ. Marginal structural models for the estimation of direct and indirect effects. Epidemiology. 2009;20:18–26.
7. VanderWeele TJ, Vansteelandt S. Conceptual issues concerning mediation, interventions and composition. Stat Interface. 2009;2:457–68.
8. Imai K, Keele L, Tingley D. A general approach to causal mediation analysis. Psychol Methods. 2010;15:309–34.
9. Imai K, Keele L, Yamamoto T. Identification, inference and sensitivity analysis for causal mediation effects. Stat Sci. 2010;25:51–71.
10. Daniels MJ, Roy JA, Kim C, Hogan JW, Perri MG. Bayesian inference for the causal effect of mediation. Biometrics. 2012;68:1028–36.
11. Chiba Y, Taguri M. Alternative monotonicity assumptions for improving bounds on natural direct effects. Int J Biostat. 2013;9:235–49.
12. Daniel RM, De Stavola BL, Cousens SN, Vansteelandt S. Causal mediation analysis with multiple mediators. Biometrics. 2015;71:1–14.
13. Neyman J. On the application of probability theory to agricultural experiments: essay on principles, Section 9. Annals of Agricultural Science 1923; Translated in Statistical Science 1990;5:465–72.
14. Rubin DB. Estimating causal effects of treatments in randomized and nonrandomized studies. J Educ Psychol. 1974;66:688–701.
15. Pearl J. Causality: models, reasoning, and inference. 2nd ed. New York: Cambridge Unversity Press;2009.
16. Avin C, Shpitser I, Pearl J. Identifiability of path-specific effects. In: Proceedings of the international joint conference on artificial intelligence; 2005. p. 357–63.
17. Robins JM. Semantics of causal DAG models and the identification of direct and indirect effects. In: Green P, Hjort NL, Richardson N, editors. Highly structured stochastic systems. New York: Oxford University Press; 2003. p. 70–81.
18. Petersen M, Sinisi S, van der Laan M. Estimation of direct causal effects. Epidemiology. 2006;17:276–84.
19. Robins JM, Richardson TS. Alternative graphical causal models and the identification of direct effects. In: Causality and psychopathology: finding the determinants of disorders and their cures. New York: Oxford University Press; 2010. p. 103–58.
20. Tchetgen TEJ, VanderWeele TJ. Identification of natural direct effects when a confounder of the mediator is directly affected by exposure. Epidemiology. 2014;25:282–91.
21. Taguri M, Chiba Y. A principal stratification approach for evaluating natural direct and indirect effects in the presence of treatment-induced intermediate confounding. Stat Med. 2015;34:131–44.
22. Cheng J, Chaffee BW, Cheng NF, Gansky SA, Featherstone JD. Understanding treatment effect mechanisms of the CAMBRA randomized trial in reducing caries increment. J Dent Res. 2015;94:44–51.
23. Taguri M, Featherstone J, Cheng J. Causal mediation analysis with multiple causally non-ordered mediators. Stat Methods Med Res. in press. Article first published online: November 23, 2015. doi:https://doi.org/10.1177/0962280215615899.
24. VanderWeele TJ, Vansteelandt S. Mediation analysis with multiple mediators. Epidemiol Methods. 2013;2:95–115.
25. VanderWeele TJ. A three-way decomposition of a total effect into direct, indirect, and interactive effects. Epidemiology. 2013;24:224–32.
26. Lange T, Rasmussen M, Thygesen LC. Assessing natural direct and indirect effects through multiple pathways. Am J Epidemiol. 2014;179:513–8.

27. Imai K, Yamamoto T. Identification and sensitivity analysis for multiple causal mechanisms: revisiting evidence from framing experiments. Political Anal. 2013;21:141–71.
28. Featherstone JD, White JM, Hoover CI, Rapozo-Hilo M, Weintraub JA, Wilson RS, Zhan L, Gansky SA. A randomized clinical trial of anticaries therapies targeted according to risk assessment (caries management by risk assessment). Caries Res. 2012;46:118–29.
29. VanderWeele TJ, Tchetgen Tchetgen EJ. Mediation analysis with time varying exposures and mediators. J R Stat Soc Ser B. 2017;79:917–38.

Sample Size Calculation for Differential Expression Analysis of RNA-Seq Data

Stephanie Page Hoskins, Derek Shyr and Yu Shyr

Abstract The Holy Grail of precision medicine is the comprehensive integration of patient genotypic with phenotypic data to develop personalized disease prevention and treatment strategies. Next-generation sequencing technologies (NGS) and other types of high-throughput assays have exploded in popularity in recent years, thanks to their ability to produce an enormous volume of data quickly and at relatively low cost compared to more traditional laboratory methods. The ability to generate big data brings us one step closer to the realization of precision medicine; nevertheless, across the life cycle of such data, from experimental design to data capture, management, analysis, and utilization, many challenges remain. In this paper, we reviewed and discussed several statistical methods to estimate sample size based on the Poisson and Negative Binomial distributions for RNAseq experimental design.

Keywords Cancer genomics · Next-generation sequencing · RNA-seq data · Sample size calculation

1 Introduction

Next generation sequencing (NGS) technology has revolutionized genomic and genetic research [1]. Replacing Sanger chain-termination sequencing that achieved a number of significant accomplishments, including the completion of the human genome sequence, NGS is a much faster and more economical application that has shifted the paradigm of genomics to address biological questions on a genome-wide

---

S.P. Hoskins (✉) · Y. Shyr
Center for Quantitative Sciences, Vanderbilt University, Nashville, TN, USA
e-mail: stephanie.p.hoskins@Vanderbilt.Edu

Y. Shyr
e-mail: yu.shyr@Vanderbilt.Edu

D. Shyr
Department of Biostatistics, Harvard T.H. Chan School of Public Health, Boston, MA, USA
e-mail: derek.shyr@mail.harvard.edu

S. Matsui and J. Crowley (eds.), *Frontiers of Biostatistical Methods and Applications in Clinical Oncology*, DOI 10.1007/978-981-10-0126-0_22

scale. Whereas early protocols relied on samples that were harvested outside of the typical clinical pathology workflow, standard formalin-fixed, paraffin-embedded specimens can more regularly be used as starting materials for NGS. Furthermore, protocols for the analysis and interpretation of NGS data, as well as knowledge bases, are being amassed, allowing clinicians to act more easily on genomic information at the point of care for patients.

In parallel, new therapies that target somatically mutated genes identified through clinical NGS are gaining US Food and Drug Administration (FDA) approval, and novel clinical trial designs are emerging in which genetic identifiers are given equal weight to histology. Indeed, the application of NGS, predominantly through whole-genome (WGS) and whole-exome technologies (WES), has produced an explosion in the context and complexity of cancer genomic alterations, including point mutations, small insertions or deletions, copy number alterations and structural variations. By comparing these alterations to matched normal samples, researchers have distinguished two categories of variants: somatic and germ line. The whole transcriptome approach (RNA-seq) can not only quantify

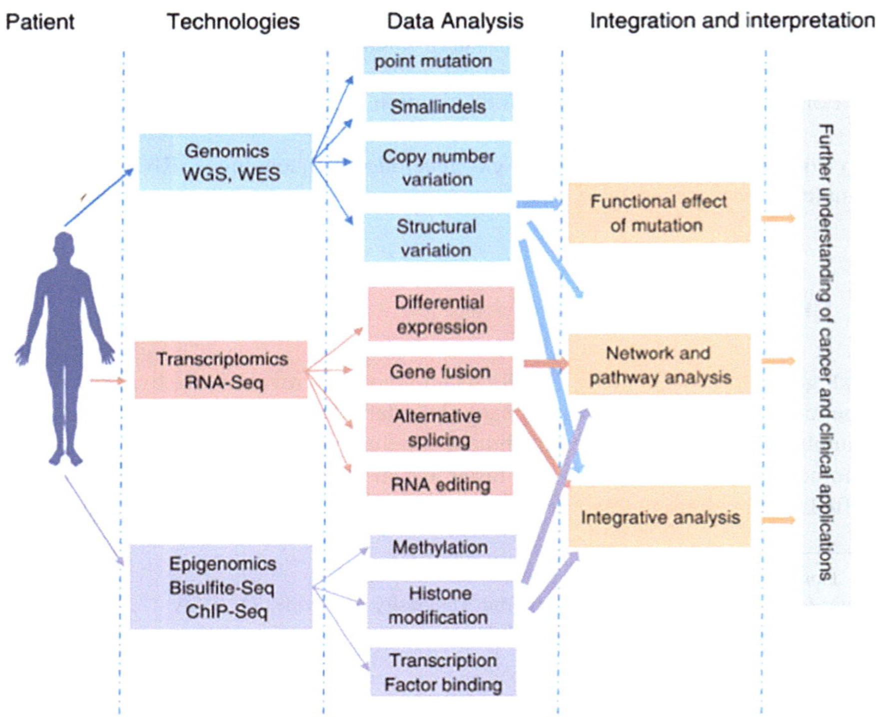

Fig. 1 The workflow of integrating omics data in cancer research and clinical application. NGS technologies detect the genomic, transcriptomic and epigenomic alterations including mutations, copy number variants, structural variants, differentially expressed genes, fusion transcripts, DNA methylation change, etc. Various kind of bioinformatic tools are used to analyze, integrate, and interpret the data to improve our understanding of cancer biology and develop personalized treatment strategy [1]

gene expression, allelic expression, and intragenic expression profiles, but can also detect alternative splicing, RNA editing and fusion transcripts. In addition, epigenetic alterations, DNA methylation changes and histone modifications can be studied using other sequencing approaches including Bifulfite-Seq and ChIP-seq. The combination of these NGS technologies provides a high-resolution and global view of the cancer genome. Using powerful bioinformatic tools, researchers are gaining the capacity to mine huge amounts of data to improve our understanding of cancer biology and develop personalized treatment strategies. Figure 1 illustrates the workflow of integrating omics data in cancer research and clinical application.

2 Application of NGS Technologies in Cancer Genomics

Recent NGS-based studies have focused on the comprehensive molecular characterization of cancers to identify novel genetic alterations contributing to oncogenesis, cancer progression and metastasis, and to study tumor complexity, heterogeneity and evolution. These efforts have yielded significant achievements for breast cancer [2–8], ovarian cancer [9], colorectal cancer [10, 11], lung cancer [12], liver cancer [13], kidney cancer [14], head and neck cancer [15], melanoma [16], acute myeloid leukemia (AML) [17, 18], etc. Table 1 summarizes the recent advances in cancer genomics research applying NGS technologies.

Table 1 Recent NGS based studies in cancer

Cancer	Experiment design	Description	References
Colon cancer	72 WES, 68 RNA-seq, 2 WGS	Identify multiple gene fusions such as RSP02 and RSP03 from RNA-seq that may function in tumorigenesis	[11]
Breast cancer	65 WGS/WES, 80 RNA-seq	36% of the mutations found in the study were expressed. Identify the abundance of clonal frequencies in an epithelial tumor subtype	[7]
Hepatocellular carcinoma	1 WGS, 1 WES	Identify TSC1 nonsense substitution in subpopulation of tumor cells, intra-tumor heterogeneity, several chromosomal rearrangements, and patterns in somatic substitutions	[13]
Breast cancer	510 WES	Identify two novel protein-expression-defined subgroups and novel subtype-associated mutations	[2]
Colon and rectal cancer	224 WES, 97 WGS	24 genes were found to be significantly mutated, in both cancers. Similar patterns in genomic alterations were found in colon and rectum cancers	[10]

(continued)

Table 1 (continued)

Cancer	Experiment design	Description	References
Squamous cell lung cancer	178 WES, 19 WGS, 178 RNA-seq, 158 miRNA-seq	Identify significantly altered pathways including NFE2L2 and KEAP1 potential therapeutic targets	[12]
Ovarian carcinoma	316 WES	Discover that most high-grade serous ovarian cancer contain TP53 mutations and recurrent somatic mutations In 9 genes	[9]
Melanoma	25 WGS	Identify a significantly mutated gene, PREX2 and obtain a comprehensive genomic view of melanoma	[16]
Acute myeloid leukemia	8 WGS	Identify mutations in relapsed genome and compare it to primary tumor. Discover two major clonal evolution patterns	[17]
Breast cancer	24 WGS	Highlights the diversity of somatic rearrangements and analyzes rearrangement patterns related to DNA maintenance	[5]
Breast cancer	31 WES, 46 WGS	Identify eighteen significant mutated genes and correlate clinical features of oestrogen-receptor-postive breast cancer with somatic alterations	[4]
Breast cancer	103 WES, 17 WGS	Identify recurrent mutation in CBFB transciption factor gene and deletion of RUNX1. Also found recurrent MAGI3-AKT3 fusion in triple-negative breast cancer	[3]
Breast cancer	100 WES	Identify somatic copy number changes and mutations in the coding exons. Found new driver mutations in a few cancer genes	[6]
Acute myeloid leukemia	24 WGS	Discover that most mutatons in AML genomes are caused by random events in hematopoietic stem/progenitor cells and not by an initiating mutation	[18]
Breast cancer	21 WGS	Depict the life history of breast cancer using algorithms and sequencing technologies to analyze subclonal diversification	[8]
Head and neck squamous cell carcinoma	32 WES	Identify mutation in NOTCH 1 that may function as an oncogene	[15]
Renal carcinoma	30 WES	Examine intra-tumor heterogeneity reveal branch evolutionary tumor growth	[14]

2.1 Discovery of New Cancer-Related Genes

Cancer is largely caused by the accumulation of genetic alterations, which can be inherited in the germ line or acquired somatically during a cell's life cycle. The effects of these alterations in oncogenes, tumor suppressor genes or DNA repair genes, allows cells to escape growth and regulatory control mechanisms, leading to the development of a tumor [19]. The progeny of the cancer cell may also undergo further mutations, resulting in clonal expression [20]. As clonal expansion pervades, clones eventually invade surrounding tissues and metastasize to distant areas from the primary tumor [21].

The sequencing of cancer genomes has revealed a number of novel cancer-related genes, especially in breast cancer. Six contemporary papers have reported findings on large-scale datasets related to breast cancer: The Cancer Genome Atlas (TCGA) performed exome sequencing on 510 samples from 507 patients [2], Banerji et al. conducted exome sequencing on 103 samples and whole genome sequencing on 17 samples, Ellis et al. did exome sequencing on 31 samples and whole genome sequencing on 46 samples [4], Stephens et al. applied exome sequencing on 100 samples, Shah et al. performed whole genome/exome and RNA sequencing on 65 and 80 samples of triple-negative breast cancers [7], and Nik-Zanial et al. performed whole genome sequencing on 21 tumor/normal pairs [8]. Besides confirming recurrent somatic mutations in TP53, GATA3 and PIK3CA, these studies also discovered novel cancer-related mutations. Although novel mutations occur at low frequency (less than 10%), mutations of specific genes are enriched in the subtype of breast cancers and could be grouped into cancer-related pathways. For example, mutations of MAP3K1 frequently occur in luminal A subtype [2, 4]. Pathways involving p53, chromatin remodeling and ERBB signaling are overrepresented in mutated genes [7]. Furthermore, some mutations indicated therapeutic opportunities such as the mutant GATA3, which might be a positive predictive marker for aromatase inhibitor response [4].

2.2 NGS and Tumor Heterogeneity

What makes cancer a difficult disease to conquer has much to do with the evolution of cancer that results from the selection and genetic instability occurring in each clone, leading to heterogeneity in tumors [21]. This idea was first proposed by Peter Nowell in 1976 as the clonal evolution model of cancer, which attempted to explain the increase in tumor aggressiveness over a period of time. Further work by other researchers in the 1980s supported this theory with studies of metastatic subclones from a mouse sarcoma cell line [21]. NGS studies have demonstrated that tumors typically compromise a founding clone and multiple subclones, and the possible combination of mutations in each tumor clone is enormous, making each tumor genetically unique. Clonal heterogeneity is strongly believed to have a role in cancer progression, relapse, metastasis, and chemo-resistance due to functional differences in genetically unique subclones, and recent therapeutic advances in oncology have been driven by the identification of tumor genotype variations between patients, called interpatient heterogeneity, that predict the response of patients to targeted treatments. Subpopulations of cancer cells with unique genomes in the same patient may exist across different geographical regions of a tumor or evolve over time, called intratumor heterogeneity. NGS technologies can characterize intratumor heterogeneity at diagnosis, monitor clonal dynamics during treatment and identify the emergence of clinical resistance during disease progression. Yet, genetic interpatient and intratumor heterogeneity can pose challenges for the design of clinical trials that use these data.

There has been a dramatic increase in the number of clinical trials using NGS technologies since 2010 [1]. Ranging from WGS to RNA-seq and targeted sequencing, clinical trials are using NGS to find genetic alterations that are the drivers of certain diseases in patients and apply that knowledge into the practice of clinical medicine. The information gained from these studies may help with drug development and explain the resistance of certain treatments.

3 RNA-Seq Data

NGS-based studies of RNA populations from cancer cells have revealed vital mechanisms of transcriptional activity and its role in cancer. A review by Patrick Nana-Sinkam and Carlo Croce [22] discussed the role of microRNAs in gene regulation in cancers. White et al. [23] presented important new descriptions of long non-coding RNAs (lncRNAs) in lung cancers, and Wyatt et al. [24] described transcriptomes in the context of therapy response in high-risk prostate cancers. The method for detecting allele-specific expression contributed by Mayba et al. [25] will also yield important insights into which variants detected by DNA sequencing are actually being expressed in the transcriptome of cancer cells. The role of the epigenome in contributing to the patterning of transcriptomes and the possibility of modulating RNA expression is emphasized in three primary research articles exploring this aspect of tumor heterogeneity (Lund et al. [26], Fleischer et al. [27], and Charlton et al. [28]).

RNA-seq technology has had a revolutionary impact on the field of expression research. RNA-seq refers to the use of NGS technologies to sequence cDNA in order to get information about a sample's RNA content. Compared to microarray technology, the RNA-seq method offers several distinct advantages. First, the detection range of RNA-seq is not limited to a set of predetermined probes, as with microarray technology, so RNA-seq is capable of identifying new genes. Second, the resolution of a microarray is limited to the gene level for most arrays and the exon level for specially designed exon arrays, whereas RNA-seq can detect expression at the gene, exon, transcript, and coding DNA sequence (CDS) levels. Finally and most importantly, RNA-seq can detect structural variants, such as alternative splicing and gene fusion. With the advancement of NGS technologies, the price of RNA-seq is becomingly increasingly comparable to microarrays. The competitive price and additional genomic information make RNA-seq an attractive alternative technology for expression profiling. Recent studies predict the inevitable replacement of microarray by RNA-seq [29, 30]; however, before this replacement can occur, we must understand the differences and similarities of these two technologies.

3.1 *Microarray Versus RNA-Seq*

The Microarray Quality Control (MAQC) project has shown that there is a high level of intra-platform consistency across test sites and inter-platform concordance in terms of genes identified as differentially expressed by microarray methods [31]. Similar to these microarray tests, RNA-seq data has been shown to estimate expression level with high reproducibility [32]. In the largest comparative study between microarray and RNA-seq methods to date using The Cancer Genome Atlas (TCGA) data, Guo et al. [33] found high correlations between expression data obtained from the Affymetrix one-channel microarray and RNA-seq (Spearman correlations coefficients of ~ 0.8) that provides definitive evidence that RNA-seq can indeed replace microarray in terms of expression analysis [33].

This large-scale, comprehensive analysis of RNA-seq and microarray gene expression consistency using human data was the first evaluation of repeatability and concordance of profiling between the two technologies that utilized data from TCGA, a massive, collaborative initiative that has catalogued genomic data for over 20 types of cancers by the National Cancer Institute (NCI), the National Human Genome Research Institute (NHGRI), and 27 institutes and centers of the National Institute of Health (NIH). Because TCGA continuously collects and characterizes various tumor types from genome results from around the world, choosing data sets from here has the potential of showing an accurate estimate of each cancer site's estimated power and samples size. The study tested the consistencies between RNA-seq and microarray data using Spearman's correlation instead of Pearson's correlation for two reasons: (1) The Robust Multi-array Average (RMA) normalization uses log2 transformation for microarray data, which is an impractical log transformation for RNA-seq data given the number of zeros reported in this method. (2) Pearson's correlation is heavily influenced by outliers, and RNA-seq data is heavily skewed. In addition to raw expression correlation, the directionality and agreement of the significantly differentially expressed gene list between the two technologies were also measured [33].

Although RNA-seq outperforms microarray analysis when it comes to expression profiling, microarray technology does still hold several advantages over RNA-seq. The analysis of microarray data is much less complex, where an acceptable normalization method is RMA and a simple *t*-test is used to detect differentially expressed genes. However, more complicated models have been developed to handle RNA-seq's non-expressed genes such as negative binomial: DESeq [34], edgeR [35], baySeq [36], NBPseq [37], and Poisson distribution: TSPM [38], DEGseq [39]; however, a consensus on the best approach for RNA-seq data analysis has not been reached.

3.2 *RNA-Seq Data Analysis*

RNA-seq data analysis generally includes reads alignment, gene expression quantification, differentially expressed genes/isoforms or alternative splicing detection and novel transcripts discovery. RNA-seq data are a set of short RNA reads that are often summarized as discrete counts. There are two major approaches to map RNA-seq reads. One is to align reads to the reference transcriptome using standard DNA-seq reads aligner. The alternative is to map reads to the reference genome allowing for the identification of novel splice junctions using a RNA-seq specific aligner. Having aligned reads, expression values are quantified by aggregating reads into counts and differential expression analysis is performed based on counts (DEseq [34], edgeR [35]) or FPKM/RPKM values (Cufflinks [40, 41]). Estimating isoform-level expression is very difficult since many genes have multiple isoforms and most reads are shared by different isoforms. To deal with read assignment uncertainty, Alex-seq [42] counts only the reads that map uniquely to a single isoform, while Cufflinks [40, 41] and Miso [43] construct a likelihood model that best explains all the reads obtained in the experiment. In addition, fusion transcripts can be detected, and a growing number of pathway-oriented tools is now becoming available.

Alongside the technological innovations that have facilitated the large-scale generation of RNA-seq data, it is important to consider the specific computational and analytical challenges that still must be overcome. For example, RNA-seq is not without computational cost; as compared to microarray analysis, RNA-seq data analysis is much more complicated and difficult, and the discussion of experimental design issues have recently emerged in regards to the relevant principles of randomization, replication, and blocking of the RNA-seq framework [29, 30].

4 RNA-Seq Sample Size

One of the principle questions in designing an RNA-seq experiment is: What is the optimal number of biological replicates to achieve the desired power? (Note: In this chapter, the term "sample size" is used to refer to the number of biological replicates or number of subjects.) Currently, the field is developing and evaluating methods to estimate power and sample size for RNA-seq in complex experimental designs. Since RNA-seq data are counts, the Poisson distribution has been widely used to model the number of reads obtained for each gene in order to identify differential gene expression [31, 32]. Further, published literature has used a Poisson distribution to model RNA-seq data and derive a sample size calculation formula based on the Wald test for a single gene differential expression analysis [30].

4.1 Correction of Error Rates for Multiple Comparisons

Thousands of genes are assessed in a RNA-seq experiment, and differential expression among these genes is tested simultaneously, requiring correction of error rates for multiple comparisons. Several corrective measures have been proposed, such as family-wise error rate (FWER) and false discovery rate (FDR), with many testing circumstances illustrating the benefit of controlling FDR [33], as the Bonferroni correction for FWER is often too conservative [44].

Many control methods of FDR in high-dimensional data have been proposed, with many of the concepts extending to calculate sample size for microarray studies [36, 37]. The sample size calculation methods for microarray studies are developed based on two-sample *t*-test under the Gaussian distribution assumption. However, since RNA-seq count data often have skewed distributions, the *t*-test is inappropriate for count data. Therefore, the sample size calculation method for microarray studies cannot be directly applied to RNA-seq count data.

4.2 Past Methods for Calculating RNA-Seq Sample Size

One of the distributions that have been used to model RNA-seq is the Poisson distribution. For instance, Marioni et al. [32] proposed a Poisson log-linear model and utilized the likelihood ratio test; Wang et al. [39] assumed that log ratios of counts have a normal distribution and utilized z-score; Li et al. [45] proposed a Poisson log-linear model and utilized the score test [31, 32, 38]. It is worth noting that a critical assumption of the Poisson model is that the mean and variance are equal. And, as demonstrated by Li et al. [46], this assumption proves to be problematic due to RNA-seq's over dispersion (variance greater than mean). When the read counts exhibit over-dispersion, the sample size calculation based on the

Poisson model will be underpowered due to underestimation of the variance, and, therefore, a study based on the corresponding sample size will be underpowered. To handle data with over-dispersion, Li et al. [45] suggested using a power transformation to make the data follow a Poisson distribution more closely. For data with over-dispersion then, sample size calculation methods based on transformed data could enable wider applicability.

On the other hand, to model with data with over-dispersion directly, several approaches have been proposed, such as the negative binomial. Unlike Poisson, a special case of negative binomial, this distribution can not only model count data, but also have unequal mean and variance, allowing for over-dispersion. Another important consideration for the design of an RNA-seq experiment is the number of replicates for each biological condition. Ideally, researchers would like to know the optimal number of replicates required to achieve a desired level of statistical power to find differential expression.

4.3 Sample Size Calculation Based on the Exact Test

Specifically in RNA-seq experiments, an exact test is used to measure the statistical significance of change in gene expressions between two conditions A and B. Li et al. [46] developed a model to calculate statistical power and estimate sample size for RNA-seq experiments based on a negative binomial model of variation in counts per gene in each sample, and evaluated an exact test for differential expression that tested for differentially expressed genes between two treatments or conditions [47]. In Li et al.'s [46] comparison between the Poisson and negative binomial distribution for the transcript regulation data set that had significant over-dispersion, the results showed that the latter required a larger sample size than the former. This difference appeared to be more significant as the fold change increased, which, as a result, could signify the negative binomial's flaw in over-powering an experiment's sample size [39].

Proposing a calculation method based on an exact test set forth by Robinson et al. that replaced the hypergeometric probabilities of Fisher's exact test with negative bionomial properties, Li et al. [46] used the edgeR package to analyze the expression values of selected genes from the RNA-seq data by returning the dispersion values and applying the exact test to calculate the fold change values of the samples. After organizing the fold change values based on the set boundaries and randomly selecting them based on the number of genes at the site, the desired sample size, mean, dispersion, and fold change values are in a loop to create a list of important values. These count values are arranged based on the control and treatment groups and then input into particular edgeR functions, which output the *p*-adjusted values. However, studies rarely have enough information to estimate all of these parameters in practice, which leads to a conservative estimate of the required sample size. Since the power increases as fold change and average read count increases and decreases with dispersion, Li et al. [46] presents a sample size calculation method based on the minimum fold change of differentially expressed genes, the minimum average read counts of differentially expressed genes in the control group, and the maximum dispersion of differentially expressed genes under negative binomial models [47]. As expected, such a method would be very conservative.

The paper evaluated sample size requirements in a simulation experiment and by reanalyzing published data for a liver and kidney RNA-seq data set. In this simulation, in which variance among replicates was low ($\phi^* = 0.1$) and $\log_2$-fold change was 2.0 or more, only three to six replicates were required to find all of the differential expression genes with coverage greater than five reads and a FDR less than 5%. Increasing the variance to $\phi^* = 0.5$ triples the number of required replicates, and lowering the $\log_2$-fold change to 1.0 (a twofold change in expression) increases the required number of replicates to 20 [47].

The general conclusion from the evaluation of this sample size calculation method is that it is straightforward but not ideal for pilot data or data with a specified desired minimum fold change, minimum read count, and maximum dispersion; the simulation and application sections showed how published RNA-seq experiments often have very low power, as the calculated minimum sample size required to achieve 80% power was impractically large for present RNA-seq experiments [47]. And with a low study power leading to a decrease in research reproducibility, this study draws attention to a critical issue in RNA-seq experiments: the need to raise the quality of preclinical studies through more rigorous experimental designs. Among fifty-three cancer papers that were published in high-impacting journals and regarded as "landmark" studies, only six of them were reproducible. Among of the six reproducible results, the studies paid attention to bias, controls, randomization, and other important factors that can impact the reliability of the results [48, 49].

4.4 Power Simulation of RNA-Seq Sample Size

As previously outlined, methods of calculating sample size for RNA-seq gene differential expression experiments based on the Poisson distribution and the negative binomial distribution have been developed and evaluated. While the Poisson may seem to be an appropriate model, the issue of the distribution lies with its critical assumption that the mean and variance must be equal, which proves problematic with RNA-seq's over-dispersion. Although the negative binomial distribution can model count data and have unequal mean and variance, allowing for over-dispersion, the distribution requires a substantially larger sample size as fold change increases, which could lead to overpowering an experiment's sample size. In an attempt to devise a method that could handle the variety of RNA-seq data structures and not be limited by any assumption that the Poisson and negative binomial distribution require, Shyr et al. [50] developed an empirical, simulation-based approach to estimate the sample size for RNA-seq gene differential expression experiments [50].

Power simulations generally follow a series of steps. First, a distribution of parameters, such as sequencing depth and fold change, must be established from some data set that could be from published literature or study. From that data, estimates of the model, including the mean, variance-covariance matrix, and other parameters, can be obtained to help calculate the power. Second, count data needs to be randomly generated from the distribution with the parameters estimated from step one. Finally, the count data is used to determine whether the sample has sufficient evidence to reject the null hypothesis and be statistically significant. Once this is done for each sample, the power of the experiment can be calculated for that particular sample size.

Shyr et al. [50] chose data sets from TCGA, selecting RNA-seq data of three cancer organ sites—lung (LUSC), colorectal (COAD), and breast (BRCA)—containing 459, 411, and 1062 samples, respectively. Conducting the simulations with R version 3.0.2, the investigators created two functions, the first function enabling the input of sample size, RNA-seq data, group variables (such as tumor and no tumor; control and treatment), minimum number of reads, FDR cutoff, fold change boundaries, and the number of random samples. The genes with a count value greater than the minimum set for the function were selected from the RNA-seq data, and edgeR was used to analyze their expression values by returning the dispersion values and applying the exact test in order to calculate the fold change values of the samples. Once the fold change values were organized according to the set boundaries and randomly selected based on the number of genes at the site, the desired sample size, mean, dispersion, and fold change values were used in a loop to create a list of important values. Then, the SimCount function was implemented to produce raw counts using the negative binomial distribution based on the input parameters of the loop. Count values were arranged according to control and treatment groups and inserted into specified edgeR functions, which generated *p*-adjusted values. Based on the FDR cutoffs and the group of the samples, the false negatives, false positives, true negatives, and true positives were calculated and stored in the final output list containing the matrix, fold change, dispersion and number of genes (Fig. 2) [50].

In the second function developed, the investigators provided two different methods of calculating power. The first method used the sensitivity formula, which is the number of true positives divided by the sum of the number of true positives and false negatives. The second method took the number of true positives divided by the total number of genes. Both types of power were compiled with corresponding sample size and run time, and a violin plot is generate to capture the details of the dispersion, as demonstrated in Fig. 3 [50].

Similar to the studies previously discussed [46, 51], the three cancer sites of the RNA-seq data from TCGA have dispersion distributions that were heavily skewed to the right. Yet, all three cancer sites had a dispersion value between 2 and 2.5 at the 95th percentile, with a maximum dispersion ranging from 9.686 to 15.88. Therefore, there were relatively few samples in these three cancer sites that had a

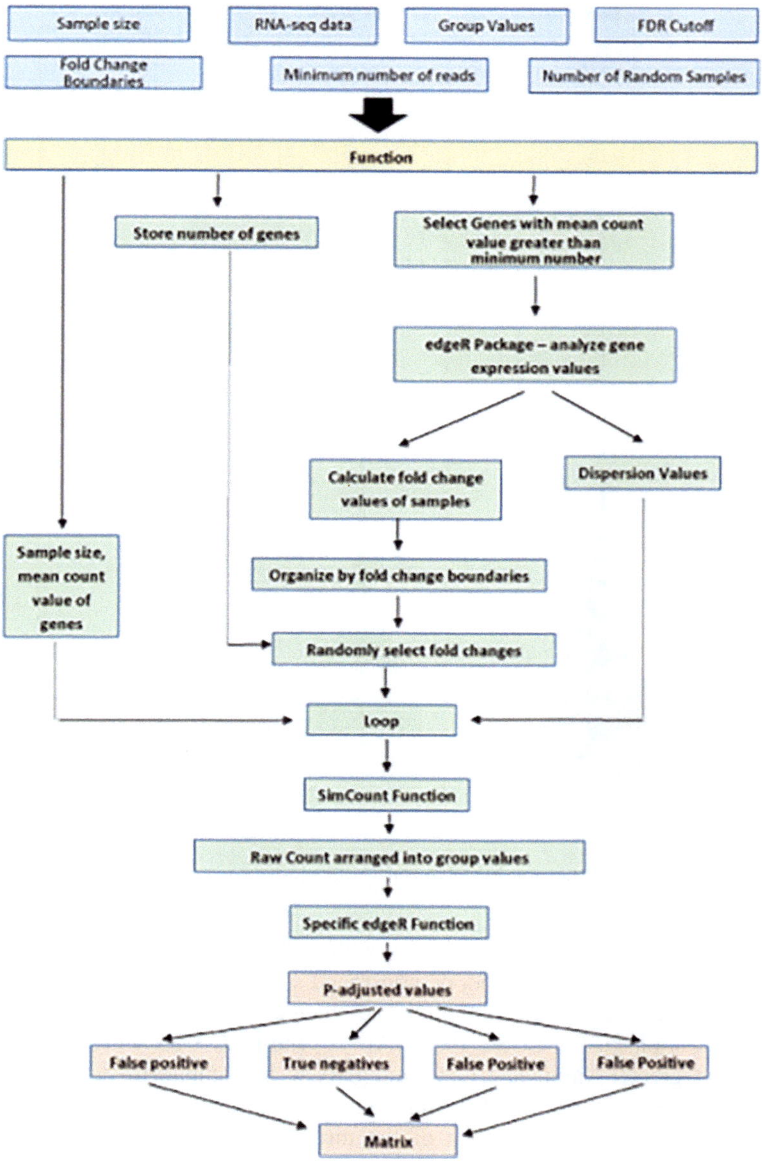

Fig. 2 Flow chart of power simulation function

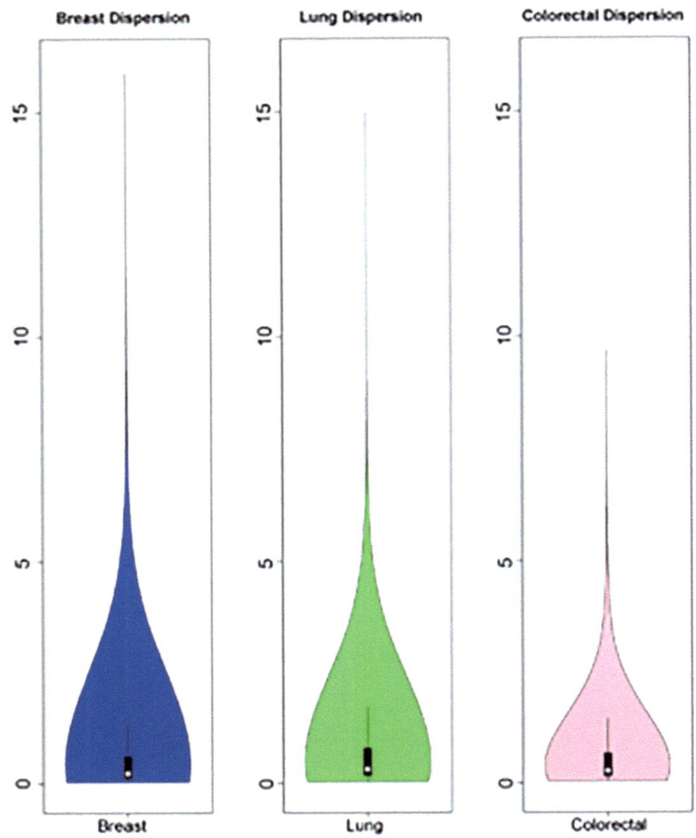

Fig. 3 Violin plots of dispersion for three cancer sites [50]

large dispersion. Running simulations with different parameters for FDR and minimum reads, the investigators demonstrated a relationship between sample size and power when the desired minimum fold change was 2.0. From this, 80% power required a sample size of LUSC 18, COAD 20, and BRCA 25, which appropriately reflects the greater variance LUSC and BRCA in comparison to COAD. This remained true even when the FDR and the minimum number of reads was adjusted, and the results showed that each of the three cancer sites had its own unique dispersion distribution, causing the sample size estimation to vary accordingly.

To evaluate the robustness of this method, Shyr et al. [50] conducted a simulation based on the same kidney data set and transcript regulation data set used by Li et al. [46] in their proposed sample size determination method based on the exact test [51, 50]. Li et al. [46] showed that the kidney dataset required about 15 samples to attain a power of 80% based on the Poisson and negative binomial model, whereas the empirical method proposed by Shyr et al. [50] showed a sample size of 15 reaching a minimum power of 90%, indicating a higher change of detecting the true positives at a reduced experimental design cost. Similarly, for the transcript regulation dataset, Li et al. [46] required a sample size of 79 and 31 for the negative binomial model and Poisson model, respectively [51]. Shyr et al. [50] demonstrated a power of 95 and 90% for the same sample size of 79 and 31, respectively, requiring a much smaller sample size than Poisson and negative binomial models.

The proposed method requires the estimation of hyper-parameters. If a relatively large pilot dataset is available, these parameters can be estimated on the pilot data. Otherwise, it is recommended to conduct a pilot or feasibility study to generate preliminary data for sample size calculation. When researchers construct an experimental design, it's important to have preliminary data on the number of biological replicates needed for their experiment. While researchers criticize power analyses for having too many mathematical assumptions, an empirical method overcomes this issue and simply requires RNA-seq data for power and sample size estimation. The flexibility of such a method also allows users to modify the proposed procedure of the simulation by using different software packages to calculate power or sample size, and it a realistic approach that reveals relationships among parameters relevant to the power analysis.

Due to the complexities of RNA-seq experiments, it is no longer feasible to rely on one simple power versus sample size curve while treating all other factors as fixed input and holding strong assumptions, such as exchangeability between genes and equating nominal error rate as actual error rate. Further, the definition of power itself can vary in RNA-seq experiments: it could be the average marginal power as the proportion of all identified differentially expressed genes, or the targeted power as the proportion or number of differentially expressed genes identified from a subset of genes. Therefore, sample size decisions based on a comprehensive evaluation of statistical power and actual type I error over a range of sample sizes is more ideal. Power simulations enable the user to visualize the relationship between various types of power and sample size, expression level and biological variation, and understand the cost of false discovery in different strata of genes. The power simulation can thus assist the decision on sequencing depth, analysis plan, and ultimately a sample size for an acceptable power.

4.5 Web-Based Tools for RNA-Seq Power and Sample Size Calculation

The rise of next generation sequencing (NGS) technology has been a boon for the field of bioinformatics, since the unprecedented throughputs—along with the diversity of possible applications in research and healthcare—brought forth a new generation of software tools for sequence analysis and interpretation. Yet, the advent of NGS technology has simultaneously created several challenges for analysts. For example, the data storage cost is significantly higher for RNA-seq than microarray, and there is a lack of consensus on the best statistical method for detecting differentially expressed genes, and as outlined in this chapter, the field currently lacks general methods to estimate power and sample size for RNA-seq in complex experimental designs. To date, most methods apply open-source software whose development is based on the sharing and collaborative improvement of the software source code, such as an R code. Open-source software often benefits from regular input from the bioinformatic community, resulting in continued improvement and increased utility, robustness and stability. While open-source tools have many advantages, some of the limitations include a variable level of long term support and maintenance and licensing for solely academic or non-profit institutions, making it difficult for commercial companies to incorporate the software into their platforms.

In recent years, the field has witnessed the onset of interactive web-based applications that assist researchers with devising an experimental design with an appropriate sample size and read depth to satisfy user-defined objectives. For instance, RNAseqPS, a web-based power and sample size calculation tool created by Guo et al. [52], not only addresses the multiple comparisons problem, but also offers a highly interactive and intuitive graphical user interface [52]. Combining the

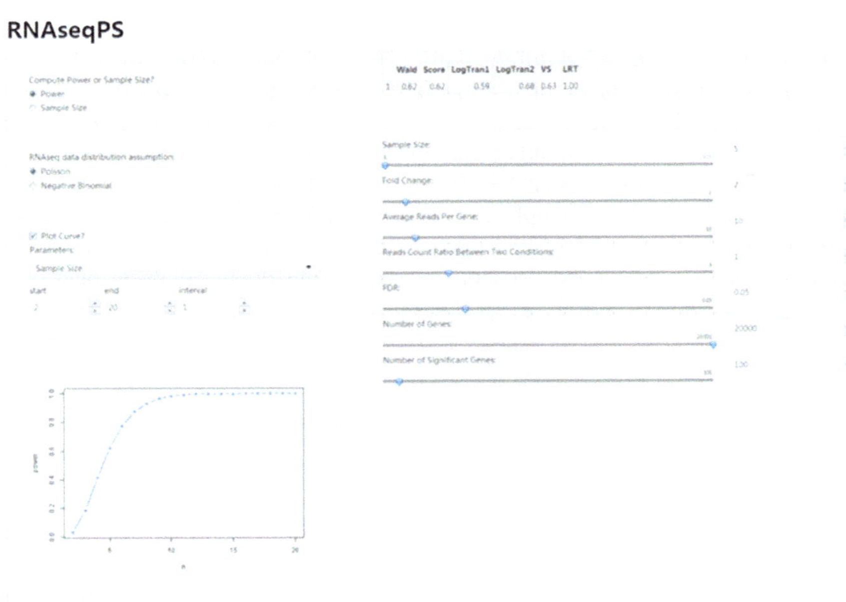

Fig. 4 Example of the graphical interface of RNAseqPS

computation power of R with the interactivity of the modern web, RNAseqPS incorporates applications that automatically react with different input and output parameters, displaying new estimations of sample size and power with every modification. This function enables users without any experience in statistics or programming languages to easily visualize and assess the intrinsic relationship between specified parameters and power [52] (Fig. 4).

5 RNA-Seq in the Era of Precision Medicine

Advances in genomics over the past several years have had a profound impact on our grasp of molecular biology and genetics. In the laboratory, next-generation sequencing (NGS) has been applied to identifying novel genomes for an array of organisms, DNA resequencing, transcriptome sequencing, and epigenetics. Within clinical settings, NGS is gaining prominence as an invaluable diagnostic tool. Specifically, the ability to interpret the genetic mechanisms that underlie variations in human gene expression through the direct analysis of the transcriptome makes RNA-seq an attractive method to clinical diagnosticians. RNA-seq examines the dynamic nature of the cell's transcriptome, the portion of genome that is actively transcribed into RNA molecules. While DNA remains relatively unchanged throughout an individual's lifespan, RNA, in the form of transcriptional elements, can vary dramatically due to influences on epigenetic regulators, alternative spliced variants, or post-transcriptional modifications.

Through the study of transcriptomes, researchers hope to determine when and where genes are turned on or off in a variety of cell types. Methods such as RNA-seq are quantifiable and provide insights to the level of gene activity or expression within a cell. For instance, transcript information could reveal the gene expression profile changes that are associated with cancer. Moreover, careful analysis of the transcriptome may provide a comprehensive snapshot of what genes are active during various stages of development.

Yet, for RNA-seq to transition from a purely analytical research discovery method to a clinically useful tool, scientists and regulatory officials must adopt standard analysis methodology and benchmark datasets for their level of accuracy and reproducibility. Although there have been a number of publications and conferences recently that tackle the topics of assessing sequencing platforms, specific laboratory protocols, and data analysis software, consensus is far from being unanimous. Additionally, recent comparisons of RNA-seq with conventionally employed clinical methodologies for the analysis of differential expression were found to be similar among RNA-seq, qPCR and microarrays. In general, RNA-seq has provided increased detection sensitivity and allowed for new research opportunities in transcriptome analyses, such as the study of gene fusions, allele-specific expression and novel alternative transcripts.

Since RNA-seq has such a wide dynamic range, the clinical pathologies that would benefit from its sequencing capabilities are almost limitless, but most scientists and publications would point to various types of cancers as being atop the list of potential primary candidates for clinical RNA-Seq usage. For example, fusion gene detection is quickly becoming a standard for several types of cancers such as NSCLC (non-small cell lung cancer) and hematological disorders. If the laboratory discovery phase is indicative of the breadth of disease states that RNA-seq could address, then the era of precision medicine should begin to expand exponentially within the next few years. RNA-seq is well positioned to handle the large clinical workload if scientists can institute the appropriate practices and procedures that are essential for precision clinical medicine.

References

1. Shyr D, Liu Q. Next generation sequencing in cancer research and clinical application. Biol Proced Online. 2013;15(1):4.
2. Cancer Genome Atlas Research Network. Comprehensive molecular portraits of human breast tumours. Nature. 2012;490:61–70.
3. Banerji S, Cibulskis K, Rangel-Escareno C, Brown KK, Carter SL, Frederick AM, Lawrence MS, Sivachenko AY, Sougnez C, Zou L, Cortes ML, Fernandez-Lopez JC, Peng S, Ardlie KG, Auclair D, Bautista-Pina V, Duke F, Francis J, Jung J, Maffuz-Aziz A, Onofrio RC, Parkin M, Pho NH, Quintanar-Jurado V, Ramos AH, Rebollar-Vega R, Rodriguez-Cuevas S, Romero-Cordoba SL, Schumacher SE, Stransky N, Thompson KM, Uribe-Figueroa L, Baselga J, Beroukhim R, Polyak K, Sgroi DC, Richardson AL, Jimenez-Sanchez G, Lander ES, Gabriel SB, Garraway LA, Golub TR, Melendez-Zajgla J, Toker A, Getz G, Hidalgo-Miranda A, Meyerson M. Sequence analysis of mutations and translocations across breast cancer subtypes. Nature. 2012;486:405–9.
4. Ellis MJ. Whole-genome analysis informs breast cancer response to aromatase inhibition. Nature. 2012;486:353–60.
5. Stephens PJ. Complex landscapes of somatic rearrangement in human breast cancer genomes. Nature. 2009;462(1):005–1010.
6. Stephens PJ. The landscape of cancer genes and mutational processes in breast cancer. Nature. 2012;486:400–4.
7. Nik-Zainal S. The life history of 21 breast cancers. Cell. 2012;149:994–1007.
8. Shah SP. The clonal and mutational evolution spectrum of primary triple-negative breast cancers. Nature. 2012;486:395–9.
9. Nik-Zainal S. Mutational processes molding the genomes of 21 breast cancers. Cell. 2012;149:979–93.
10. Cancer Genome Atlas Research Network. Integrated genomic analyses of ovarian carcinoma. Nature. 2011;474:609–15.
11. Cancer Genome Atlas Research Network. Comprehensive molecular characterization of human colon and rectal cancer. Nature. 2012;487:330–7.

12. Seshagiri S, Stawiski EW, Durinck S, Modrusan Z, Storm EE, Conboy CB, Chaudhuri S, Guan Y, Janakiraman V, Jaiswal BS, Guillory J, Ha C, Dijkgraaf GJ, Stinson J, Gnad F, Huntley MA, Degenhardt JD, Haverty PM, Bourgon R, Wang W, Koeppen H, Gentleman R, Starr TK, Zhang Z, Largaespada DA, Wu TD, de Sauvage FJ. Recurrent R-spondin fusions in colon cancer. Nature. 2012;488:660–4.
13. Hammerman PS, Hayes DN, Wilkerson MD, Schultz N, Bose R, Chu A, Collisson EA, Cope L, Creighton CJ, Getz G, Herman JG, Johnson BE, Kucherlapati R, Ladanyi M, Maher CA, Robertson G, Sander C, Shen R, Sinha R, Sivachenko A, Thomas RK, Travis WD, Tsao MS, Weinstein JN, Wigle DA, Baylin SB, Govindan R, Meyerson M. Comprehensive genomic characterization of squamous cell lung cancers. Nature. 2012;489:519–25.
14. Totoki Y, Tatsuno K, Yamamoto S, Arai Y, Hosoda F, Ishikawa S, Tsutsumi S, Sonoda K, Totsuka H, Shirakihara T, Sakamoto H, Wang L, Ojima H, Shimada K, Kosuge T, Okusaka T, Kato K, Kusuda J, Yoshida T, Aburatani H, Shibata T. High-resolution characterization of a hepatocellular carcinoma genome. Nat Genet. 2011;43:464–9.
15. Gerlinger M, Rowan AJ, Horswell S, Larkin J, Endesfelder D, Gronroos E, Martinez P, Matthews N, Stewart A, Tarpey P, Varela I, Phillimore B, Begum S, McDonald NQ, Butler A, Jones D, Raine K, Latimer C, Santos CR, Nohadani M, Eklund AC, Spencer-Dene B, Clark G, Pickering L, Stamp G, Gore M, Szallasi Z, Downward J, Futreal PA, Swanton C. Intratumor heterogeneity and branched evolution revealed by multiregion sequencing. N Engl J Med. 2012;366:883–92.
16. Agrawal N, Frederick MJ, Pickering CR, Bettegowda C, Chang K, Li RJ, Fakhry C, Xie TX, Zhang J, Wang J, Zhang N, El-Naggar AK, Jasser SA, Weinstein JN, Trevino L, Drummond JA, Muzny DM, Wu Y, Wood LD, Hruban RH, Westra WH, Koch WM, Califano JA, Gibbs RA, Sidransky D, Vogelstein B, Velculescu VE, Papadopoulos N, Wheeler DA, Kinzler KW, Myers JN. Exome sequencing of head and neck squamous cell carcinoma reveals inactivating mutations in NOTCH1. Science. 2011;333:1154–7.
17. Berger MF. Melanoma genome sequencing reveals frequent PREX2 mutations. Nature. 2012;485:502–6.
18. Ding L. Clonal evolution in relapsed acute myeloid leukaemia revealed by whole-genome sequencing. Nature. 2012;481:506–10.
19. Wong KM, Hudson TJ, McPherson JD. Unraveling the genetics of cancer: genome sequencing and beyond. Annu Rev Genomics Hum Genet. 2011;12:407–30.
20. Cahill DP, Kinzler KW, Vogelstein B, Lengauer C. Genetic instability and Darwinian selection in tumours. Trends Cell Biol. 1999;9:M57–60.
21. Brosnan JA, Iacobuzio-Donahue CA. A new branch on the tree: next-generation sequencing in the study of cancer evolution. Semin Cell Dev Biol. 2012;72:4875–82.
22. Nana-Sinkam SP, Croce CM. MicroRNA regulation of tumorigenesis, cancer progression and interpatient heterogeneity: towards clinical use. Genome Biol. 2014;1(5):445.
23. White NM, Cabanski CR, Fisher-Silva JM, Dang HX, Govindan R, Maher CA. Transcriptome sequencing reveals altered long intergenic non-coding RNAs in lung cancer. Genome Biol. 2014;15:429.
24. Wyatt AW, Mo F, Wang K, McConeghy B, Brahmbhatt S, Jong L, Mitchell DM, Johnston RL, Haegert A, Li E, Liew J, Yeung J, Shrestha R, Lapuk A, McPherson A, Shukin R, Bell RH, Anderson S, Bishop J, Hurtado-Coll A, Xiao H, Chinnaiyan AM, Mehra R, Lin D, Wang Y, Fazli L, Gleave ME, Volik SV, Collins CC. Heterogeneity in the inter-tumor transcriptome of high risk prostate cancer. Genome Biol. 2014;15:426.
25. Mayba O, Gilbert HN, Liu J, Haverty PM, Jhunjhunwala S, Jiang Z, Watanabe C, Zhang Z. MBASED: allele-specific expression detection in cancer tissues and cell lines. Genome Biol. 2014;15:405.
26. Lund K, Cole J, VanderKraats ND, McBryan T, Pchelintsev NA, Clark W, Copland M, Edwards JR, Adams PD. DNMT inhibitors reverse a specific signature of aberrant promoter DNA methylation and associated gene silencing in AML. Genome Biol. 2014;15:406.

27. Fleischer T, Frigessi A, Johnson KC, Edvardsen H, Touleimat N, Klajic J, Riis MLH, Haakensen V, Wärnberg F, Naume B, Helland Å, Børresen-Dale AL, Tost J, Christensen BC, Kristensen VN. Genome-wide DNA methylation profiles in progression to in situ and invasive carcinoma of the breast with impact on gene transcription and prognosis. Genome Biol. 2014;15:435.
28. Charlton J, Williams RD, Weeks M, Sebire NJ, Popov S, Vujanic G, Mifsud W, Alcaide-German M, Butcher LM, Beck S, Pritchard-Jones K. Methylome analysis identifies a Wilms tumor epigenetic biomarker detectable in blood. Genome Biol. 2014;15:434.
29. Wang Z, Gerstein M, Snyder M. RNA-Seq: a revolutionary tool for transcriptomics. Nat Rev Genet. 2009;10:57–63.
30. Shendure J. The beginning of the end for microarrays? Nat Methods. 2008;5:585–7.
31. Shi L, Reid LH, Jones WD, Shippy R, Warrington JA, et al. The MicroArray Quality Control (MAQC) project shows inter- and intraplatform reproducibility of gene expression measurements. Nat Biotechnol. 2006;24:1151–61.
32. Marioni JC, Mason CE, Mane SM, Stephens M, Gilad Y. Rnaseq: an assessment of technical reproducibility and comparison with gene expression arrays. Genome Res. 2008;18(9):1509–17.
33. Guo Y, Sheng Q, Li J, Ye F, Samuels DC, Shyr Y. Large scale comparison of gene expression levels by microarrays and RNAseq using TCGA data. PLoS ONE. 2013;8(8):e71462.
34. Andres S, Huber W. Differential expression analysis for sequence count data. Genome Biol. 2010;11:R106.
35. Robinson MD, McCarthy DJ, Syth GK. edgeR: a Bioconductor package for differential expression analysis of digital gene expression data. Bioinformatics. 2010;26:139–40.
36. Hardcastle TJ, Kelly KA. baySeq: empirical Bayesian methods for identifying differential expression in sequence count data. BMC Bioinform. 2010;11:422.
37. Di YSD, Cumbie JS, Chang JH. The NBP negative binomial model for assessing differential gene expression from RNA-Seq. Stat Appl Genet Mol Biol. 2011;10:1–28.
38. Auer PL, Doerge RW. A two-stage Poisson model for testing RNA-Seq data. Stat Appl Genet Mol Biol. 2011;10:1–26.
39. Wang L, Feng Z, Wang X, Zhang X. DEGseq: an R package for identifying differentially expressed genes from RNA-seq data. Bioinformatics. 2010;26:136–8.
40. Trapnell C, Hendrickson DG, Sauvageau M, Goff L, Rinn JL, Pachter L. Differential analysis of gene regulation at transcript resolution with RNA-seq. Nat Biotechnol. 2012;31:46–53.
41. Trapneel C, Roberts A, Goff L, Pertea G, Kimn D, Kelley DR, Pimentel H, Salzberg SL, Rinn JL, Pachter L. Differential gene and transcript expression analysis of RNA-seq experiments with TopHat and Cufflinks. Nat Protoc. 2012;7:562–78.
42. Griffith M, Griffith OL, Mwenifumbo J, Goya R, Morrissy AS, Morin RD, Corbett R, Tang MJ, Hou YC, Pugh TJ, Robertson G, Chittaranjan S, Ally A, Asano JK, Chan SY, Li HI, McDonald H, Teague K, Zhao Y, Zeng T, Delaney A, Hirst M, Morin GB, Jones SJ, Tai IT, Marra MA. Alternative expression analysis by RNA sequencing. Nat Methods. 2010;7:843–7.
43. Katz Y, Wang ET, Airoldi EM, Burge CB. Analysis and design of RNA sequencing experiments for identifying isoform regulation. Nat Methods. 2010;7:1009–15.
44. Anders S, Huber W. Differential expression analysis for sequence count data. Genome Biol. 2010;11:R106.
45. Li J, Witten DM, Johnstone IM, Tibshirani R. Normalization, testing, and false discovery rate estimation for RNA-sequencing data. Biostatistics. 2011;23(6):493–500.
46. Li CI, Su PF, Guo Y, Shyr Y. Sample size calculation for differential expression analysis of RNA-seq data under Poisson distribution. Int J Comput Biol Drug Des. 2013;6(4):358–75.
47. Fang Z, Cui X. Design and validation issues in RNA-seq experiments. Brief Bioinform. 2011;12(3):280–7.
48. Begley CG, Ellis LM. Drug development: raise standards for preclinical cancer research. Nature. 2012;483:531–3.
49. Problems with scientific research: how science goes wrong. The Economist. 2013.

50. Shyr D, Li CI. Sample size calculation of RNA-sequencing experiment: a simulation-based approach of TCGA data. J Biomet Biostat. 2014;5:3.
51. Li CI, Su PF, Shyr Y. Sample size calculation based on exact test for assessing differential expression analysis in RNA-seq data. BMC Bioinform. 2013;14:357.
52. Guo Y, Zhao S, Li CI, Quanhu S, Shyr Y. RNAseqPS: a web tool for estimating sample size and power for RNAseq experiment. Cancer Inform. 2014;13(S6).

Efficient Study Designs and Semiparametric Inference Methods for Developing Genomic Biomarkers in Cancer Clinical Research

Hisashi Noma

Abstract In the development of genomic biomarkers and molecular diagnostics, clinical studies using high-throughput assays such as DNA microarrays generally require enormous costs and efforts. Several efficient study designs for reducing the costs of such expensive measurements have been developed, mainly in the field of epidemiology. Under these efficient designs, expensive measurements are collected only on selected subsamples based on adequate response-selective sampling schemes, and total measurement costs are effectively reduced. In this study, we discuss the application of these effective designs to genomic analyses in cancer clinical studies, and provide relevant statistical methods such as gene selection (e.g., multiple testing based on the false discovery rate). Efficient semiparametric inference methods using auxiliary clinical information are also discussed.

Keywords Nested case-control study · Case-cohort study · Two-phase designs · Genomic biomarker · Semiparametric inference · Weighted estimating equation · Calibration estimator

1 Introduction

The establishment of high-throughput technologies such as DNA microarrays has enabled the genome-wide investigation of cancer tumor samples to characterize diseases at a molecular level, namely, that of genes. Such genomic studies are potentially useful for elucidating disease biology and aggressiveness, identifying new therapeutic targets, and developing new molecular diagnostics for optimized

H. Noma (✉)
Department of Data Science, The Institute of Statistical Mathematics,
10-3 Midori-cho, Tachikawa, Tokyo 190-8562, Japan
e-mail: noma@ism.ac.jp

S. Matsui and J. Crowley (eds.), *Frontiers of Biostatistical Methods and Applications in Clinical Oncology*, DOI 10.1007/978-981-10-0126-0_23

medicine for individual patients [1–3]. One of the primary objectives of these genome-wide studies is the screening of differentially expressed genes among different phenotypes, such as clinical subtypes and prognostic classes of disease, for further investigation. Because of the large scale of these data, false findings are a serious issue, and thus many researchers are concerned about controlling false positives in the framework of multiple testing, particularly controlling the false discovery rate (FDR) [4, 5]. However, distinguishing relevant genes from thousands of non-interesting genes with null associations generally requires large sample sizes to achieve sufficient statistical power [2, 3].

Furthermore, these genomic studies usually require enormous financial and other resources to collect and/or process the large-scale measurements involved. In particular, it is still expensive to implement biological experiments using high-throughput assays such as microarrays, and clinical researchers often find it burdensome to plan and conduct such studies. Also, in most previous cancer clinical studies using such high-throughput assays, these expensive experiments have been conducted for all samples in the corresponding cohort (e.g., [6–8]). However, this strategy is not necessarily cost-effective.

To resolve such serious practical issues, enormous efforts have been dedicated to develop and apply effective study designs to reduce the costs and efforts of obtaining expensive measurements in epidemiological studies [9]. Although these methods have not been widely discussed in genomic clinical studies, they would also be useful and effective tools to improve cost-effectiveness in this setting. The underlying concept of these designs is to conduct the expensive experiments on selected subsamples from the corresponding cohort based on adequate sampling designs, and to implement valid inference using the observed information of the subsamples while retaining statistical efficiency. For gaining efficiency, the subsample selection scheme is systematically constructed from the outcome statuses of each participant, and is called outcome-dependent sampling or response-selective design [10, 11]. In particular, using recently developed semiparametric inference methods, auxiliary variable information measured on the entire cohort (age, sex, clinical stages, etc.) can be adapted for improving statistical efficiency [12–14].

In this chapter, we discuss efficient study designs and recent semiparametric inference methods in applications to genomic analyses of cancer clinical studies. The chapter is organized as follows: first, we briefly review the study designs and basic statistical methods of the efficient study designs in Sect. 2. After that, we discuss the semiparametric efficient inference methods of these designs in Sect. 3. In Sect. 4, we present simulation studies to assess the utility of these designs in the context of genomic studies. In Sect. 5, we briefly note the applications of these designs to the development of prediction and classification algorithms. Lastly, we provided concluding remarks in Sect. 6.

2 Effective Study Designs

2.1 Setting and Notation

The concrete examples we consider in this chapter are microarray experiments, but our methodology can be applied to other high-throughput measurements, e.g., genome-wide association studies [15]. The gene expression data considered here comprise normalized log ratios from two-color cDNA arrays or normalized log signals from oligonucleotide arrays (e.g., Affymetrix GeneChip). First, we assume a certain cohort that is composed of n participants. In efficient study designs, outcome-dependent sampling is conducted for this cohort and expensive measurements are obtained for the subsamples, e.g., for a situation in which biopsy samples were previously frozen and cryosectioned for all cohort participants, and microarray experiments were implemented for the samples of the selected participants.

For the ith participant, $X_i = (X_{i1}, X_{i2}, \ldots, X_{iq})$ denotes the covariates measured for the entire cohort, and $Z_i = (Z_{i1}, Z_{i2}, \ldots, Z_{ip})$ denotes the gene expression data measured by the microarrays. For the phenotype variable, we typically assume censored time-to-event outcomes (T_i, C_i) ($i = 1, 2, \ldots, n$) as in ordinary cancer clinical studies, where T_i is the time-to-event variable and C_i is the indicator variable of the event. In typical previous studies, the researchers measured gene expression data for the all samples of n participants in the entire cohort, and conducted standard analyses (e.g., Cox regression analyses for assessing associations between gene expression and time-to-event outcomes) with a small degree of control for false findings in terms of the FDR [2, 3, 16].

2.2 Nested Case-Control Design

The nested case-control design [17] is one of the oldest and most widely used designs for these purposes. We consider the proportional hazards regression model,

$$\lambda(t|X_i, Z_i) = \lambda_0(t)\exp(\beta_1 X_i + \beta_2 Z_i)$$

in which our interest is in the regression parameters $\beta = (\beta_1, \beta_2)$. Here $\lambda_0(t)$ is the baseline hazard function. In this situation, the participants whose events are observed during the follow-up period are regarded as cases, and the others as non-cases. The parameter β is validly estimable using the ordinary Cox's partial likelihood method if the covariates are observed for all of the participants. To reduce measurement costs in the nested case-control design, case-control sampling is conducted within the cohort.

Without loss of generality, we denote the times of event occurrences in the cohort as $t_1 < t_2 < \cdots < t_{n1}$ where n_1 is the total number of cases, and denote the corresponding indices of these cases as 1, 2, ..., n_1. We also denote $\mathcal{R}(t_j)$ as the risk-set at time $t_j (j = 1, 2, \ldots, n_1)$ in the entire cohort. In this design, at each event time t_j, k matched controls are sampled from the risk sets $\mathcal{R}(t_j)$, i.e., a small number of controls are sampled from the risk set of the entire cohort whenever an event occurs. This sampling scheme is called risk-set sampling. We denote the index sets of the case and selected controls at t_j as $\mathcal{F}(t_j)$. Expensive covariates Z_i are measured only for the cases and selected controls. Although the covariate data of Z_i are partially observed in the entire cohort, we can validly estimate the regression parameter β regarding the cases and selected controls as a matched case-control dataset stratifying by the event times via the conditional likelihood function [17],

$$\mathcal{L}_{NCC}(\beta) = \prod_{j=1}^{n_1} \left[\frac{\exp(\beta_1 X_j + \beta_2 Z_j)}{\sum_{k \in \mathcal{F}(t_j)} \exp(\beta_1 X_k + \beta_2 Z_k)} \right]$$

Note that, in the random selection of controls from the risk set, a participant randomly selected from the risk set as a control at an early time point can develop an event and serve as a case at a later time point. However, this sampling assures the validity of the inference based on $\mathcal{L}_{NCC}(\beta)$. The asymptotic variance can be consistently estimated by the standard model variance based on $\mathcal{L}_{NCC}(\beta)$.

2.3 Case-Cohort Design

The nested case-control design can effectively reduce the cost of measuring expensive covariates in the study as a whole. However, when there are multiple outcomes of interest as seen in many clinical or epidemiologic studies, controls are sampled for each of the outcomes, resulting in different controls across the outcomes and thus elevating the total cost of the measurement of the covariates. The case-cohort design [18] was developed to circumvent this issue. In this design, controls are selected randomly from the entire cohort without referring to the outcomes. Because a single, common set of controls is sampled for the multiple outcomes, the total cost and effort required for measuring the expensive covariates for multiple outcomes can be markedly reduced compared with the nested case-control design. Since the control set is a representative subset of the entire cohort, it is called a *subcohort* [9]. Note that some case and control samples can be duplicated in this sampling scheme, because the controls are sampled from the entire cohort. However, the measures of effects (e.g., hazard ratio) can be unbiasedly estimated using the methods outlined in the next subsection.

2.3.1 Analysis of Time-To-Event Outcomes

We here use the same notation as in Sect. 2.2, and we consider the proportional hazards model. In this design, although the covariate data of Z_i are also only partially observed in the entire cohort, the regression parameter β is estimable by modifying the Cox's partial likelihood [18–21]. The most popular one is the inverse probability weighting (IPW)-type pseudo-likelihood [20, 22, 23],

$$\mathcal{L}_{IPW}(\beta) = \prod_{j=1}^{n_1} \left[\frac{\exp(\beta_1 X_j + \beta_2 Z_j)}{\sum_{k \in \tilde{\mathcal{R}}(t_j)} \omega_k \exp(\beta_1 X_k + \beta_2 Z_k)} \right]$$

where $\omega_k = 1$ for cases; $\omega_k = (n_0/n)^{-1}$ for non-cases, where n_0 is the size of subcohort; and n_0/n is the sampling proportion of the subcohort from the entire cohort. Also, $\tilde{\mathcal{R}}(t_j)$ means the index set of risk set of time t_j in the cases and selected controls. Through adjusting the partial likelihood function by the sampling probabilities of individual participants, we can obtain a consistent hazard ratio estimator. The standard errors can be evaluated by the robust variance estimators [20, 22].

Note that the sampling probabilities can be varied across certain strata, i.e., the conventional stratified case-control sampling is applicable for the case-cohort design. Stratified sampling enables us to effectively prevent an imbalance of distributions of relevant covariates, and to possibly increase the efficiency of estimation of the regression parameter of the expensive covariate of primary interests (in particular, if there is a strong correlation between the stratification covariates and Z) [21]. For the stratified sampling designs, the hazard ratio can be consistently estimated by adjusting the weights to the inverses of the stratum-specific sampling probabilities of $\mathcal{L}_{IPW}(\beta)$.

Example 2.1 (Desmedt et al. [24])
Although the majority of patients with early breast cancer receive systemic adjuvant therapy that may have serious side effects, it remains a challenge to predict which patients actually require this therapy. To predict patients' prognosis in lymph node–negative primary breast cancer patients, Wang et al. [8] developed a 76-gene prognostic signature based on gene expression data with Affymetrix HG-U133A GeneChips (Affymetrix, Santa Clara, CA; m = 22,283). Desmedt et al. [24] conducted a validation study of the 76-gene profile in 198 patients. For illustrative purposes, we generated simulated case-cohort data from this cohort. We sampled all 41 cases who developed distant metastases during the follow-up period, and randomly selected 99 patients as a subcohort (50% of the entire cohort). The total subsample size was 140 (70.7% of the entire cohort), and the number of duplicated samples was 21. We estimated standardized hazard ratios (increment of hazard ratio per 1 SD of gene expression data for individual probes) by univariate Cox regression with the IPW method. Table 1 presents the comparative results of the entire cohort and the simulated case-cohort data for selected probes of the 76 genes

Table 1 Results of a simulated case-cohort study based on the breast cancer clinical study of Desmedt et al. [24]

Gene (probe id)	Entire cohort			Case-cohort data			Bias	ARE
	β_2	SE	*P*-value	β_2	SE	*P*-value		
204015_s_at	−0.325	0.134	0.016	−0.304	0.157	0.053	−0.020	0.727
217767_at	−0.200	0.138	0.147	−0.238	0.140	0.090	0.038	0.968
201664_at	0.369	0.162	0.022	0.345	0.164	0.035	0.023	0.972
219724_s_at	−0.314	0.124	0.011	−0.289	0.128	0.024	−0.025	0.940
212014_x_at	0.256	0.172	0.150	0.288	0.174	0.099	−0.032	0.969
201288_at	−0.404	0.149	0.007	−0.435	0.160	0.007	0.031	0.863
201068_s_at	0.159	0.160	0.319	0.195	0.174	0.263	−0.036	0.839
214919_s_at	−0.365	0.159	0.022	−0.368	0.174	0.035	0.003	0.838
203306_s_at	−0.386	0.151	0.010	−0.379	0.162	0.019	−0.007	0.868
219510_at	0.277	0.179	0.119	0.278	0.186	0.135	0.000	0.924
216693_x_at	0.155	0.162	0.340	0.178	0.176	0.313	−0.022	0.851
220886_at	0.231	0.173	0.181	0.225	0.178	0.207	0.006	0.940

Estimates for selected genes in the 76 gene prognostic signature of Wang et al. [8] from the entire cohort and the simulated case-cohort data

β_2 is the standardized log hazard ratio (log hazard ratio increment per 1 SD of the corresponding gene expression data)

Bias, ARE (asymptotic relative efficiency): estimated bias and ARE based on the estimate of β_2 of case-cohort data compared with that of the entire cohort data

in the prognostic signature. Using the IPW method, similar hazard ratio estimates can be obtained with the case-cohort subsamples. In addition, although the sample size can be reduced to around 70%, the asymptotic relative efficiency (ARE) could generally be kept over 80%, and was greater than 90% for some probes. In other words, if the cost and effort involved in microarray experiments of 198 samples were available, more efficient statistical inference could be implemented using the efficient study designs from a larger source population.

2.3.2 Analysis of Binary Outcomes

The case-cohort design can be applied to a cohort study with a binary outcome (although the nested case-control design can be also formally adopted, if there is no censoring). For cohort studies with binary outcomes, the sampling scheme of the case-cohort design is quite the same as that of the time-to-event outcome, and the control set is randomly sampled from the entire cohort. Analyses of these data are relatively simple because the sampling scheme of case-cohort designs exactly accord with conventional case-control studies [25]. This indicates that all methodological results for the analyses of case-control studies can be applied to case-cohort designs. Therefore, the odds-ratio in the entire cohort can be estimated by the ordinary prospective logistic regression model [26]. Only the intercept is non-identifiable. Also, standard errors of the other regression coefficients β are consistently estimated by the model variance. The odds-ratio estimator derived by standard logistic regression achieves semiparametric efficiency provided that the distribution of covariates is left unspecified [26, 27].

In addition, using the IPW method, the intercept of the logistic model can also be validly estimated. Risk differences and risk ratios are also estimable by the IPW method using binomial regression models with identity and log link functions [25]. Further, for comparing mean expression levels among cases and non-cases, the *t*-test or Wilcoxon tests between the cases and non-cases in the selected subsamples retain their validities because the sampling scheme of the case-cohort design is equivalent to that of the case-control study.

Example 2.2 (Hatzis et al. [28])
Hatzis et al. [28] conducted a prospective multicenter study at the M.D. Anderson Cancer Center to develop genomic predictors for neoadjuvant chemotherapy for invasive breast cancer. Predictive signatures for response to preoperative neoadjuvant chemotherapy were developed based on gene expression analysis using Affymetrix HG-U133A microarrays (Affymetrix, Santa Clara, CA). We consider here a two-group comparison problem between 86 excellent-response patients with pathologic complete response or minimal residual cancer burden (RCB-I) and 215 lesser-response patients with moderate or extensive residual cancer burden (RCB-II/III). We also simulated the case-cohort data from this cohort; we sampled all 81 RCB-I patients and also 137 subsamples (45.5%) as a subcohort. The number of RCB-II/III patients in the subcohort was 95 (total number of subsamples was 181; 60.1%), and the number of duplicated samples was 42. We could implement logistic regression analyses as noted above, but here, we considered the assessments of differences of mean gene expression levels between the two groups. We estimated standardized mean differences (SMD; mean difference for standardized gene expression data by SD of individual probes) and evaluated the differences between the two groups via Student's *t*-tests. We provide the comparative results of the entire cohort and the simulated case-cohort data for selected probes with the smallest *P*-values in Table 2. The biases of SMD estimates in the case-cohort data from the entire cohort were generally not very large. Also, the sample size was reduced to 60.1%, but the ARE were generally over 70% for all of the probes presented.

Case-cohort designs have several advantages over nested case-control designs. The subcohort samples may allow the estimation of the population frequencies of certain covariates (e.g., genotypes) and permit multiple analyses to be conducted with different time scales (e.g., time-on-study and attained age). Also, unlike nested case-control studies, subcohort sampling is possible even in situations where the case or non-case status of a cohort member is unknown prior to the control sampling to determine the risk set at an event time. Further, as noted above, the case-cohort design is more cost-effective for analyzing multiple outcomes. Owing to these practical advantages, case-cohort designs are becoming more popular in

Table 2 Results of a simulated case-cohort study based on the breast cancer clinical study of Hatzis et al. [28]

Gene (probe id)	Entire cohort				Case-cohort data				Bias	ARE
	SMD	95% CI		*P*-value	SMD	95% CI		*P*-value		
205225_at	−0.872	−1.122	−0.622	<0.001	−0.874	−1.165	−0.583	<0.001	0.002	0.739
203702_s_at	0.866	0.615	1.116	<0.001	0.886	0.594	1.179	<0.001	−0.021	0.732
220624_s_at	0.861	0.611	1.111	<0.001	0.810	0.515	1.104	<0.001	0.052	0.722
206373_at	0.840	0.590	1.090	<0.001	0.832	0.538	1.126	<0.001	0.008	0.725
202134_s_at	0.813	0.563	1.063	<0.001	0.731	0.439	1.022	<0.001	0.082	0.736
219051_x_at	−0.807	−1.057	−0.557	<0.001	−0.812	−1.105	−0.519	<0.001	0.005	0.729
221203_s_at	0.799	0.549	1.049	<0.001	0.705	0.414	0.995	<0.001	0.094	0.742
209644_x_at	0.798	0.547	1.048	<0.001	0.745	0.450	1.039	<0.001	0.053	0.720
221864_at	−0.782	−1.032	−0.532	<0.001	−0.676	−0.966	−0.386	<0.001	−0.106	0.743
209747_at	−0.782	−1.032	−0.531	<0.001	−0.964	−1.155	−0.573	<0.001	0.082	0.738
213699_s_at	0.773	0.523	1.023	<0.001	0.708	0.418	0.997	<0.001	0.065	0.745
214053_at	−0.766	−1.016	−0.516	<0.001	−0.834	−1.126	−0.542	<0.001	0.068	0.733

Estimates for selected genes with the smallest *P*-values from the entire cohort and the simulated case-cohort data

Bias, ARE (asymptotic relative efficiency): estimated bias and ARE based on the estimate of β_2 of case-cohort data compared with that of the entire cohort data epidemiologic research [12]. Also, this design can straightforwardly treat the case of binary outcomes. So, in the remainder of this chapter, we mainly focus on the case-cohort design when explaining various methodologies. However, most of the methodological framework can be similarly adapted to the nested case-control design.

3 Efficient Inference Methods

3.1 Formulation as Two-Phase Sampling Designs

As shown in the previous chapter, the nested case-control and case-cohort designs can effectively reduce the cost and effort of conducting cancer clinical studies with expensive covariate measurements by utilizing conventional inference methods that only use the outcome and covariate information for selected participants. On the other hand, in most studies, data on outcome and other covariates (whose measurements are not necessarily expensive) are available for the other participants *not sampled* from the entire cohort. Recently, several efficient inference methods have been developed by incorporating such auxiliary information from the entire cohort [12–14].

It is convenient to formulate these designs as *two-phase sampling designs* as shown in Fig. 1. First, as a random sample we consider a target population that is actually a source population from which the entire cohort is constructed. This random sampling from the source population is regarded as *phase-1* sampling.

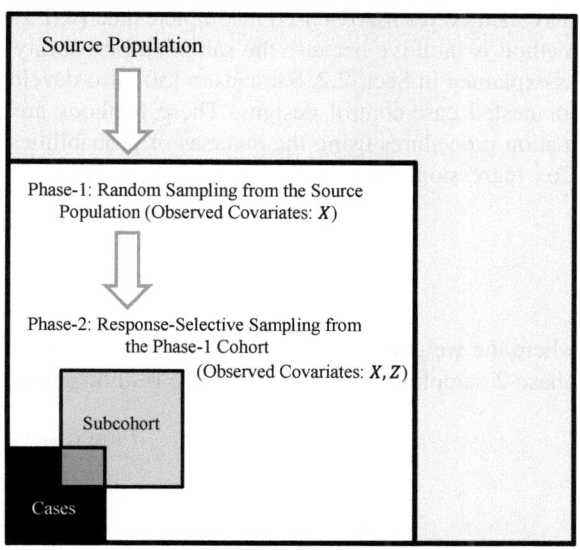

Fig. 1 Conceptual diagram of the two-phase sampling designs (this figure is from Fig. 1 of Kulathinal et al. [23] with modifications)

Second, outcome-dependent sampling (not random sampling) is conducted from the phase-1 entire cohort. This sampling is regarded as *phase-2* sampling. These designs can be completely formulated as two-phase sampling designs from the source population.

We usually have complete outcome variable data Y_i and partial covariates $X_i = (X_{i1}, X_{i2}, \ldots, X_{iq})$ for all of the participants in the phase-1 entire cohort (i = 1, 2, …, n). In addition, the expensive covariates $Z_i = (Z_{i1}, Z_{i2}, \ldots, Z_{ip})$ are measured for the subsamples selected during the phase-2 sampling. In other words, for the not-sampled participants at phase-2, the expensive covariates Z_i are not observed. Thus, considering the phase-1 cohort as the analysis set, we can formally regard the dataset of (Y_i, X_i, Z_i) (i = 1, 2, …, n) as an incomplete dataset from which the covariates Z_i are partially *missing*. Also, whether Z_i is observed or missing is completely discriminated by whether a participant is selected or not at phase-2 sampling. Importantly, this missing mechanism is also completely explained by the observed variables, because the stochastic mechanism of the phase-2 sampling is completely specified by the adopted designs. Therefore, the missing mechanism of Z_i is assured to be *missing at random* (MAR). So, efficient statistical inference can be implemented by applying efficient methods for the missing data analyses under the MAR mechanism.

3.2 Semiparametric Inference Methods

3.2.1 IPW Estimator

One of the most popular approaches of semiparametric inference methods is the IPW method for MAR-based incomplete data [29]. For two-phase designs, the IPW method is intuitive because the sampling probability of each participant is known, as explained in Sect. 2.2. Samuelson [30] also developed an IPW inference method for nested case-control designs. These methods are formulated as weighted estimation procedures using the inverses of probabilities of phase-2 sampling. For the Cox regression, the pseudo-likelihood function is

$$\mathcal{L}_{IPW}(\beta) = \prod_{j=1}^{n_1} \left[\frac{\exp(\beta_1 X_j + \beta_2 Z_j)}{\sum_{k \in \tilde{\mathcal{R}}(t_j)} w_{IPW,k} \exp(\beta_1 X_k + \beta_2 Z_k)} \right]$$

where the weights are $w_{IPW,k} = \pi_k^{-1}$ and are inverses of the known probabilities of phase-2 sampling (π_k). Explicitly, the resulting weighted estimating function

$$U_{IPW}(\beta) = \frac{\partial \log \mathcal{L}_{IPW}(\beta)}{\partial \beta}$$

is unbiased, $E[U_{IPW}(\beta)] = 0$. So, the estimator of regression parameters β has consistency. When the stratified sampling is adopted at phase-2, the weights are changed to the inverses of stratum-specific sampling probabilities. Here we call this weight the "design weight." The standard error can be estimated by the sandwich estimator [29], and the pseudo-Wald test and confidence interval can be constructed in the standard manner.

3.2.2 Improving Efficiency Using Estimated Weights

The IPW estimator provides an (asymptotically) unbiased estimate of β based on the dataset of (Y_i, X_i, Z_i) from the phase-2 samples. However, the auxiliary information of (Y_i, Z_i) are available for all the participants in the phase-1 cohort. Using this auxiliary information to improve the precision of inference on β, the simplest but effective method is by altering the design weights to "estimated weights." In the nested case-control and case-cohort designs, the missing mechanism is completely specified as noted above. Concretely, the models of missing probabilities can be expressed by adequate binomial regression models, e.g., the logistic regression model,

$$\text{logit}\,\Pr(R_i = 1|W_i) = \gamma_0 + \gamma_1 W_{i1} + \cdots + \gamma_l W_{il} \qquad (1)$$

where R_i is the observation/missing indicator of Z_i with a value of 1 when the ith participant is sampled at phase-2, and otherwise, a value of 0. Also, $W_i = (W_{i1}, \ldots, W_{il})$ are the explanatory variables of this logistic regression model, which involve the outcome variables and phase-1 covariates Z_i. In the usual missing data analyses in clinical studies, we cannot know the true values of γ or whether the missing mechanism is MAR or not MAR. However, in these cases, the missing mechanism is necessarily known to be MAR and the true values of γ are completely specified by the sampling designs. As noted above, we can use the true probabilities of sampling at phase-2 based on the true value of γ in the IPW estimation, which correspond to the design weights.

However, Robins et al. [29] and Henmi and Eguchi [31] revealed a paradoxical characteristic of the IPW estimator, namely that the asymptotic variance of this estimator based on the true probabilities of being missing is uniformly improved by altering it to the estimated weight that is based on the estimated probabilities of being missing by the missing data mechanism model (1). Note that the estimated probabilities have errors compared to the true probabilities and they are necessarily misspecified, but it was shown that the resultant IPW estimator retains consistency and gains efficiency [29, 31]. So, we can obtain a more precise estimator of β using the estimated weight obtained by the model (1) into which an adequate estimate of γ is plugged-in (usually, the maximum likelihood estimate). A typical case involving estimated weights uses the sampling fraction of stratified case-cohort sampling in IPW estimation, not the known true probabilities of sampling (the "design weight" noted above). This is well-known as Borgan's type-II estimator in stratified case-cohort designs [21]. Note that the model (1) should be correctly specified for assuring consistency, so all of the covariates related to the sampling mechanism at phase-2 should be involved. However, it is better to model additional covariates unrelated to the model (1) involving interaction terms to improve the fit of the model. The theoretical reasons can be explained by geometric arguments. For readers who are interested, please see Henmi and Eguchi [31].

The asymptotic variance can be consistently estimated by the sandwich estimator [29]. For the IPW estimator with estimated weights, the asymptotic variance estimator becomes more complex because we should consider the joint estimating equation for (β, γ). However, the computational program of the variance estimator for the Cox regression and generalized linear models is available at `R` package `survey` [14, 32]. The `R` package `survey` involves computational tools of the IPW estimation for the two-phase sampling designs explained here. For the details of the package, please see Lumley [32] and Lumley et al. [14].

3.2.3 Semiparametric Efficient Estimator

Under the MAR missing mechanism, although the IPW estimator has consistency, it generally does not have asymptotic efficiency. Therefore, recent methodological studies have explored providing improved estimators to gain efficiency. Robins et al. [29] provided a theoretical general framework involving the IPW estimator to construct the semiparametric efficient estimator that is the most precise estimator within a class of semiparametric estimators. In this case, we consider a semiparametric model that does not provide parametric assumptions for the distribution of Z_i, because there should be required parametric specification of the distribution of Z_i for ordinary inference of the outcome dependent sampling [10]. Robins et al. [29] derived the augmented IPW estimator (it is also known as the doubly robust estimator in incomplete data analyses) as the semiparametric efficient estimator, which has an adequate augmented term to the IPW estimating function. Several researchers have presented practical computational methods to achieve semiparametric efficiency in these designs [33, 34]. For instance, Qi et al. [34] provided a method to construct the augmented IPW estimating function of Cox regression using a kernel smoothing function, and discussed its applications to case-cohort designs. However, the augmented term involves unknown quantities to be estimated, and it has computational difficulties in general [35]. So, some researchers (e.g., Breslow and Wellner [35]) have discussed the fact that this term has never been applied in practice with nested case-control and case-cohort designs. In the near future, more advanced theoretical studies might resolve these problems, but in current practice, we do not have sufficient methods or computational tools for applying efficient methods to these study designs. Thus, recent studies have proposed other efficient strategies that effectively circumvent these issues, as shown in the next subsection.

Note that, for settings of binominal outcome data with only discrete categorical covariates, explicit semiparametric efficient estimators were developed for two-stage case-control designs [11, 36]. Although these estimators can be applied to restrictive settings, under some situations they might be practically useful in clinical research with genomic data. See Noma and Tanaka [25] for the details of their applications to case-cohort designs.

3.2.4 Application of the Calibration Technique in Sample Survey Theory

In sample survey theory, many studies have been dedicated to improving the conventional Horvitz-Thompson estimator [37], which has the same form as the IPW estimator and partially inspired the development of IPW theory. These improved estimators, which include the generalized regression estimator, post-stratification estimator, raking estimator, and others [38], use information on auxiliary variables collected from the source population to improve the efficiency, similar to the two-phase designs in epidemiology. The calibration method, proposed by Deville and Särndal [38], is a general framework that generalizes these estimators. Breslow et al. [12, 13] proposed to apply this calibration technique to improve the IPW estimator in case-cohort designs as a tractable alternative to the semiparametric efficient methods (it can similarly be applied to the nested case-control designs [39]).

Here we first explain the general methodological framework of the calibration method. We use different notational approaches to maximize the clarity of our explanations. As a simple formulation, we consider an estimating problem for the population total $a_{tot} = \sum_{(i,j)\in\Omega} a_{ij}$, of a certain target variable a_{ij} ($i = 1, \ldots, N_j$; $j = 1, \ldots, J$) in the phase-1 samples under stratified sampling (but, we directly use this formulation in the applications to analyses of case-cohort designs), where J is the number of strata, N_j is the sample size of the jth stratum, and Ω is that of phase-1 cohort samples. We denote λ_{ij} ($i = 1, \ldots, N_j$; $j = 1, \ldots, J$) as the sampling probability of each participant from phase-1, and $d_{ij} = \lambda_{ij}^{-1}$ as its corresponding design-based weight. Note that λ_{ij} and d_{ij} are common within each stratum. The well-known Horvitz-Thompson estimator of a_{tot} is the weighted sum of a_{ij} among the phase-2 samples $\hat{a}_{HT} = \sum_{(i,j)\in\Xi} d_{ij}a_{ij}$, where Ξ is the index set of phase-2 samples. Apparently, $\hat{a}_{HT}$ has consistency, but it only uses the observed information of a_{ij} at phase-2. We also assume the availability of some auxiliary variables Q_{ij} ($i = 1, \ldots, N_j$; $j = 1, \ldots, J$) that are measured for all participants in the phase-1 cohort. If the auxiliary variables Q_{ij} strongly correlate to the target variable a_{ij}, then intuitively their information might be effectively used for improving the Horvitz-Thompson estimator, because they have substantial information for unmeasured a_{ij}. In the calibration technique [38], the naïve design weight is calibrated using the auxiliary information to improve the efficiency. To determine the adjusted weight, we consider the following calibration equation:

$$\hat{Q}_{tot} = \sum_{(i,j)\in\Xi} w_{ij} Q_{ij} = \sum_{(i,j)\in\Omega} Q_{ij} = Q_{tot}$$

where there should be certain weights w_{ij} that satisfy the above equation. Intuitively, when the auxiliary variables Q_{ij} have strong correlation with a_{ij}, $\hat{a}_{tot} = \sum_{(i,j)\in\Xi} w_{ij} a_{ij}$ might provide a more accurate estimator than $\hat{a}_{HT}$. For an extreme example, when Cor(a_{ij}, Q_{ij}) = 1, the adjusted Horvitz-Thompson estimator $\hat{a}_{tot}$ exactly equals the estimated parameter a_{tot}. The adjusted weights $w_{ij} = d_{ij}\, g_{ij}$ are the so-called "calibrated weights" [12, 13], where g_{ij} are correction factors. In general, restriction of the calibration equation does not uniquely specify the weights and requires some additional restrictions. Deville and Särndal [38] proposed to set the calibrated weight as near as possible to the design weight d_{ij} based on a measure of distance for quantifying the closeness $G(w, d)$, i.e., the weight that minimizes the sum of the distances $G(w_{ij}, d_{ij})$ over all i, j. Several distance measures have been discussed e.g., $G_1(w, d) = (w - d)^2/2d$ (linear function) and $G_2(w, d) = w \log (w/d) - w + d$ (Poisson deviance). For more distance measures and their properties, see Deville and Särndal [38] and Deville et al. [40]

In case-cohort designs, we want to estimate β with individual score contributions $U_{ij}(\beta)$ and information matrix $I_{ij}(\beta)$. Using the first-order Taylor approximation of the score function around β_0, the true value of β, the weighted estimator with naïve design weight is approximated as

$$\hat{\beta}_{IPW} \approx \beta_0 + \sum_{\Xi} d_{ij} I_{ij}^{-1}(\beta_0) U_{ij}(\beta_0)$$

Because β_0 is a fixed quantity, the calibration technique can be formally applied to the estimation of a population total, a problem discussed above, and we would calibrate the weight with respect to some auxiliary variables correlated with $I_{ij}^{-1}(\beta_0)U_{ij}(\beta_0)$. A natural choice would be the dfbetas

$$Q_{ij} = I_{ij}^{-1}\left(\hat{\beta}\right) U_{ij}\left(\hat{\beta}\right)$$

where $\hat{\beta}$ is the maximum likelihood estimate for complete phase-1 cohort data. However, several phase-2 variables are missing, so in general, $\hat{\beta}$ and the phase-1 dfbetas are unknown. Breslow et al. [12, 13] proposed using approximate dfbetas obtained as follows:

(i) In obtaining the phase-1 cohort estimate $\hat{\beta}$, several phase-2 variables are missing. Breslow et al. [12, 13] proposed imputing a single suitable value to the missing covariates. For predicting the missing covariates, construct a regression model with the fully observed covariates as explanatory variables and establish a prediction model using a weighted estimation.

(ii) Using the imputed phase-1 complete dataset, with the predicted values generated in step (i), conduct a complete data analysis (e.g., a Cox regression). Then, extract the dfbetas from the regression model.

Therefore, using the dfbetas as auxiliary variables to obtain new weights w_{ij}, the calibration method can be implemented. Also, through a weighted regression analysis with the calibrated weights, we can obtain the final estimates. Although this procedure involves complex calculations, these computations are fully feasible using the `survey` package [14, 32] in `R` (R Foundation for Statistical Computing, Vienna, Austria). The variance estimation is also complicated because of the uncertainty of the weight calibration, but this computation can be also implemented by the `survey` package.

4 Simulation Studies for Evaluating Efficiency

To illustrate the uses of these estimators in clinical studies with genomic data, we conducted simulation studies based on the breast cancer clinical study of Hatzis et al. [28] that was adopted in Example 2.2. In Example 2.2, we simulated case-cohort data in which we considered the microarray gene expression data as the phase-2 variables, and applied the IPW method with design weights to detect differentially expressed genes between the excellent-response patients (RCB-I) and the lesser-response patients (RCB-II/III) groups. Here we conducted similar simulation studies to evaluate the semiparametric estimators in Sect. 3.

We supposed the two-group comparison problem here, with the goal of detecting differentially expressed genes between the RCB-I and RCB-II/III groups. To avoid imbalances of relevant covariates in phase-2 sampling, we adopted stratified sampling, with stratification by nodal status, estrogen receptor (ER) status, and the outcome variable. We considered several different scenarios, with sampling probabilities of 50, 60, …, 90%. We generated 400 phase-2 samples from the 301 patients of the original cohort and analyzed these datasets by three IPW estimators with design weights, estimated weights, and calibrated weights.

For the IPW estimator with calibrated weights, we constructed normal regression models using individual gene expression data as the response variables and the following independent variables as predictors: age, grade, ER status, progesterone receptor status, and HER2 status. Also, we used the ranking distance function for calibration. For the IPW estimator with estimated weights, we estimated the weights using a predictive logistic regression model involving the stratum indicator and the dfbeta, which was obtained in the construction process of the calibrated weights. The design weights were set to inverses of the sampling proportions of the corresponding stratum. In computing the three weighted estimators and their standard error, we used the `survey` package of `R` (R Foundation for Statistical Computing, Vienna, Austria) [14, 32]. In addition, as a reference conventional method, we simulated 400 case-cohort data by unstratified sampling with the same sample sizes, and conducted conventional t-tests between the sampled RCB-I and RCB-II/III groups.

As one of the standard analyses, we conducted multiple testing for screening differentially expressed genes that control FDR. Since the obtained P-values for the four methods above are valid, the standard P-value-based FDR controlling procedures can be straightforwardly adopted. Here, we used the Benjamini-Hochberg (BH) procedure [4] with FDR set at 1, 5, and 10%. The results are presented in Table 3. The number of genes detected via the BH procedure increased monotonically with both the proportion of subsamples and their efficiency gains, the latter of which would be reflected in the statistical powers of these tests. Compared with conventional t-tests, the number of significant genes identified by the IPW methods, which use the phase-1 auxiliary information for improving efficiency, were markedly larger. Even the naïve IPW method using the design weights performed well compared with the t-tests. So, the stratified sampling and IPW analyses would be favored compared with the crude t-tests to improve efficiency. The numbers of significant genes were even larger for the IPW estimators with estimated and calibrated weights. Along with the theoretical properties of these estimators explained above, the efficiency would be reflected in the powers of the corresponding

Table 3 Results from 400 simulated case-cohort studies from the breast cancer clinical study of Hatzis et al. [28]

Proportion of total subsamples (%)	FDR	t-test[a]	IPW methods		
			Design weight	Estimated weight	Calibrated weight
50	0.01	27.1	183.0	225.4	233.9
	0.05	234.4	718.4	844.7	863.4
	0.10	596.4	1330.4	1528.8	1553.3
60	0.01	89.2	281.1	318.6	324.5
	0.05	502.2	960.7	1058.6	1071.8
	0.10	1053.0	1677.7	1826.8	1843.4
70	0.01	347.2	562.9	583.7	581.9
	0.05	1300.1	1569.1	1607.0	1602.5
	0.10	2243.6	2484.6	2536.2	2529.9
80	0.01	402.1	759.4	773.4	772.5
	0.05	1439.4	1910.2	1933.4	1931.5
	0.10	2418.2	2884.3	2916.2	2913.9
90	0.01	495.9	935.6	942.9	943.0
	0.05	1606.3	2174.1	2184.5	2184.4
	0.10	2582.7	3185.6	3201.6	3200.0

Means of the numbers of significant genes by the Benjamini-Hochberg procedure with FDR controlled at 1, 5, and 10%

[a]The t-tests were applied to simulated unstratified case-cohort studies with the same sample size as a reference method. The numbers of significant genes for t-tests of the entire (phase-1) cohort data were 979, 2293 and 3264 under FDRs of 0.01, 0.05 and 0.10

statistical tests. In practical gene screening in genomic research, these methods would be useful tools to improve efficiency using phase-1 auxiliary variables.

We also evaluated the concrete efficiency gains for the phase-2 component of the standard errors. In Fig. 2, we provide boxplots of the IPW estimates with calibrated weights for SMD of 50 selected genes (with the largest SMD at the phase-1 cohort data) for 400 simulated case-cohort designs. In general, all the means of the estimates were located around the SMD estimates of the phase-1 cohort, and they generally had small biases due to the phase-1 estimates. Also, the variations of the estimates reflected the phase-2 component of the standard errors of estimates, and they became smaller as the sizes of the total subsamples became larger. These results clearly indicated the concrete efficiency of the calibration estimator. Although the variations of the estimates seemed large when the proportions of

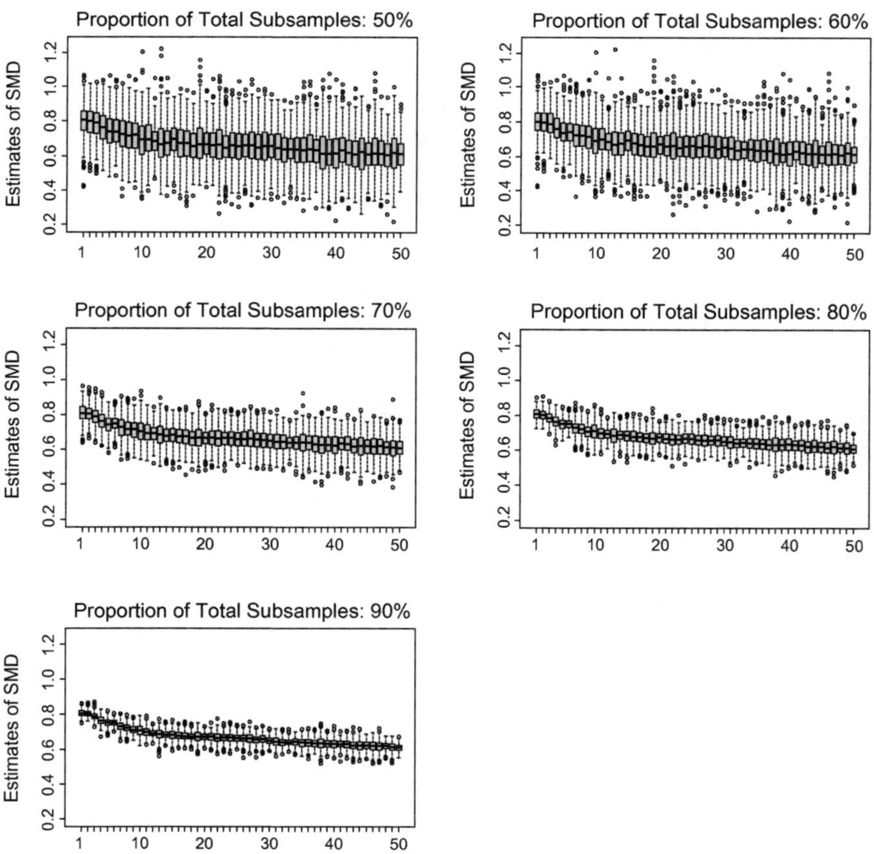

Fig. 2 IPW estimates with calibrated weights for SMD of 50 selected genes (with the largest SMD at phase-1 cohort) for 400 simulated case-cohort studies from the breast cancer clinical study of Hatzis et al. [28]

subsamples were small, they would be controlled via designing adequate sample sizes. This implies that the same levels of efficiency could be achieved by smaller sample sizes when effective study designs are adopted. The efficiency gains would be directly reflected in the powers of multiple testing as shown above.

5 Predication and Classification

Another important goal of genomic analyses in cancer clinical studies is developing prediction and classification algorithms. The effective designs can be also applied for this purpose, because many standard classification algorithms are constructed by plugging in valid estimates to discriminant functions developed by optimal theoretical criteria (e.g., the Bayes rule) [41]. For example, to construct two-group classification algorithms for linear discriminant analysis or diagonal linear discriminant analysis, the mean and variance-covariance parameters are required for constructing the discriminant functions. As shown in Sects. 2 and 3, these parameters can be unbiasedly and efficiently estimated by the IPW estimators. Also, in developing the logistic discriminant function, the IPW estimators of the logistic regression model for the case-cohort designs can be directly applied (remember, the case-cohort sampling scheme is equivalent to the case-control sampling). Also, for survival prediction models, e.g., based on the Cox proportional hazard regression model, the hazard ratio estimators can be validly estimated by the IPW methods as noted in Sect. 3. The baseline hazard function is also unbiasedly estimable via the IPW-adjusted Breslow estimator [13]. For more complex algorithms (e.g., based on the regularized discriminant functions [42] or machine learning methods [43]), methodological research should be undertaken to develop valid and optimal classification algorithms, but these algorithms would be able to be handled by similar principles.

6 Concluding Remarks

Methodological studies of efficient study designs in epidemiology began in 1970s. Many useful methodologies have been developed thus far, and they have been sufficiently established to be used at a practical level. These designs have already been applied in many epidemiological studies, and they will be increasingly important in research in various fields. In this chapter, we discussed their utility in genomic studies of cancer clinical research, specifically for reducing the enormous costs and efforts involved in high-throughput experiments. As shown in the simulation studies and several numerical examples, the effectiveness of these methodologies in genomic studies is expected in practice. In particular, the semiparametric methods should be useful tools to improve efficiency in statistical inference. If these methodologies are used effectively, the costs and efforts of these studies should be effectively reduced while still retaining statistical efficiency.

Acknowledgements This research was supported by the GSK Japan Research Grant, JST-CREST (JPMJCR1412), and a Grant-in-Aid for Scientific Research (15K15954) from the Ministry of Education, Culture, Sports, Science and Technology of Japan.

References

1. Simon R. Genomic clinical trials and predictive medicine. New York: Cambridge University Press; 2013.
2. Crowley J, Hoering A, editors. Handbook of statistics in clinical oncology. 3rd ed. Boca Raton: Chapman Hall/CRC; 2012.
3. Matsui S, Buyse M, Simon D, editors. Design and analysis of clinical trials for predictive medicine. Boca Raton: Chapman Hall/CRC; 2015.
4. Benjamini Y, Hochberg Y. Controlling the false discovery rate—a practical and powerful approach to multiple testing. J R Stat Soc B. 1995;57(1):289–300.
5. Storey JD. A direct approach to false discovery rates. J R Stat Soc B. 2002;64(3):479–98. doi:10.1111/1467-9868.00346.
6. Rosenwald A, Wright G, Chan WC, Connors JM, Campo E, et al. The use of molecular profiling to predict survival after chemotherapy for diffuse large-B-cell lymphoma. N Engl J Med. 2002;346(25):1937–47. doi:10.1056/NEJMoa012914.
7. van de Vijver MJ, He YD, van't Veer LJ, Dai H, Hart AAM, et al. A gene-expression signature as a predictor of survival in breast cancer. N Engl J Med. 2002;347(25):1999–2009. doi:10.1056/NEJMoa021967.
8. Wang Y, Klijn JG, Zhang Y, Sieuwerts AM, Look MP, et al. Gene-expression profiles to predict distant metastasis of lymph-node-negative primary breast cancer. Lancet. 2005;365 (9460):671–9. doi:10.1016/S0140-6736(05)17947-1.
9. Rothman KJ, Greenland G, Lash TL. Modern epidemiology. 3rd ed. Philadelphia: Lippincott Williams & Wilkins; 2008.
10. Lawless JF, Kalbfleisch JD, Wild CJ. Semiparametric methods for response-selective and missing data problems. J R Stat Soc B. 1999;61(2):413–38. doi:10.1111/1467-9868.00185.
11. Breslow NE, McNeney B, Wellner JA. Large sample theory for semiparametric regression models with two-phase, outcome dependent sampling. Ann Stat. 2003;31(4):1110–39. doi:10.1214/aos/1059655907.
12. Breslow NE, Lumley T, Ballantyne CM, Chambless LE, Kulich M. Using the whole cohort in the analysis of case-cohort data. Am J Epidemiol. 2009;169(11):1398–405. doi:10.1093/aje/kwp055.
13. Breslow NE, Lumley T, Ballantyne CM, Chambless LE, Kulich M. Improved Horvitz–Thompson estimation of model parameters from two-phases stratified samples: applications in epidemiology. Stat Biosci. 2009;1(1):32–49. doi:10.1007/s12561-009-9001-6.
14. Lumley T, Shaw PA, Dai JY. Connections between survey calibration estimators and semiparametric models for incomplete data. Int Stat Rev. 2011;79(2):200–20. doi:10.1111/j.1751-5823.2011.00138.x.
15. Laird NM, Lange C. The fundamentals of modern statistical genetics. New York: Springer; 2011.
16. Simon RM, Korn EL, McShane LM, Radmacher MD, Wright GW, et al. Design and analysis of DNA microarray investigations. New York: Springer; 2003.
17. Thomas DC. Addendum to a paper by Liddell FDK, McDolad JC, Thomas DC, and Cunliffe SV. J R Stat Soc Ser A. 1977;140(4):483–5.
18. Prentice RL. A case-cohort design for epidemiologic cohort studies and disease prevention trials. Biometrika. 1986;73:1–11. doi:10.1093/biomet/73.1.1.
19. Self SG, Prentice RL. Asymptotic distribution theory and efficiency results for case-cohort studies. Ann Stat. 1988;16(1):64–81. doi:10.1214/aos/1176350691.

20. Barlow WE, Ichikawa L, Rosner D, Izumi S. Analysis of case-cohort designs. J Clin Epidemiol. 1999;52(12):1165–72.
21. Borgan Ø, Langholz B, Samuelsen SO, Goldstein DR, Pogoda J. Exposure stratified case-cohort designs. Lifetime Data Anal. 2000;6(1):39–58. doi:10.1023/A:1009661900674.
22. Barlow WE. Robust variance estimation for the case-cohort design. Biometrics. 1994;50 (4):1064–72. doi:10.2307/2533444.
23. Kulathinal S, Karvanen J, Saarela O, Kuulasmaa K. Case-cohort design in practice: experiences from the MORGAM Project. Epidemiol Perspect Innov. 2007;4:15. doi:10.1186/ 1742-5573-4-15.
24. Desmedt C, Piette F, Loi S, Wang Y, Lallemand F, et al. Strong time dependence of the 76-gene prognostic signature for node-negative breast cancer patients in the TRANSBIG multicenter independent validation series. Clin Cancer Res. 2007;13(11):3207–14. doi:10. 1158/1078-0432.CCR-06-2765.
25. Noma H, Tanaka S. Analysis of case-cohort designs with binary outcomes: improving the efficiency using whole cohort auxiliary information. Stat Methods Med Res. 2014;. doi:10. 1177/0962280214556175.
26. Prentice RL, Pyke R. Logistic disease incidence models and case-control studies. Biometrika. 1979;66(3):403–11. doi:10.2307/2335158.
27. Breslow NE, Robins JM, Wellner JA. On the semi-parametric efficiency of logistic regression under case-control sampling. Bernoulli. 2000;6(3):447–55.
28. Hatzis C, Pusztai L, Valero V, Booser DJ, Esserman L, et al. A genomic predictor of response and survival following taxane-anthracycline chemotherapy for invasive breast cancer. J Am Med Assoc. 2011;305(18):1873–81. doi:10.1001/jama.2011.593.
29. Robins JM, Rotnitzky A, Zhao LP. Estimation of regression-coefficients when some regressors are not always observed. J Am Stat Assoc. 1994;89(427):846–66. doi:10.2307/2290910.
30. Samuelsen SO. A pseudolikelihood approach to analysis of nested case-control data. Biometrika. 1997;84(2):379–94. doi:10.1093/biomet/84.2.379.
31. Henmi M, Eguchi S. A paradox concerning nuisance parameters and projected estimating functions. Biometrika. 2004;91(4):929–41. doi:10.1093/biomet/91.4.929.
32. Lumley T. Analysis of complex survey samples. J Stat Softw. 2004;. doi:10.18637/jss.v009. i08.
33. Kulich M, Lin DY. Improving the efficiency of relative-risk estimation in case-control studies. J Am Stat Assoc. 2004;99(467):832–44. doi:10.1198/016214504000000584.
34. Qi L, Wang CY, Prentice RL. Weighted estimators for proportional hazards regression with missing covariates. J Am Stat Assoc. 2005;100(472):1250–63. doi:10.1198/01621450 5000000295.
35. Breslow NE, Wellner JA. Weighted likelihood for semiparametric models and two-phase stratified samples, with application to Cox regression. Scand J Stat. 2007;34(1):86–102. doi:10.1111/j.1467-9469.2006.00523.x.
36. Scott AJ, Wild CJ. Fitting regression models to case-control data by maximum likelihood. Biometrika. 1997;84(1):57–71. doi:10.1093/biomet/84.1.57.
37. Horvitz D, Thompson D. A generalization of sampling without replacement from a finite population. J Am Stat Assoc. 1952;47(260):663–85. doi:10.2307/2280784.
38. Deville JC, Särndal C-E. Calibration estimators in survey sampling. J Am Stat Assoc. 1992;87 (418):376–82. doi:10.2307/2290268.
39. Stoer NC, Samuelsen SO. Comparison of estimators in nested case-control studies with multiple outcomes. Lifetime Data Anal. 2012;18(3):261–83. doi:10.1007/s10985-012-9214-8.
40. Deville JC, Särndal C-E, Sautory O. Generalized raking procedures in survey sampling. J Am Stat Assoc. 1993;88(423):1013–20. doi:10.2307/2290793.
41. McLachlan GJ. Discriminant analysis and statistical pattern recognition. Hoboken: Wiley; 2004.
42. Guo Y, Hastie T, Tibshirani R. Regularized linear discriminant analysis and its application in microarrays. Biostatistics. 2007;8(1):86–100. doi:10.1093/biostatistics/kxj035.
43. Hastie T, Tibshirani R, Friedman J. The elements of statistical learning: data mining, inference, and prediction. 2nd ed. New York: Springer; 2009.

Supervised Dimension-Reduction Methods for Brain Tumor Image Data Analysis

Atsushi Kawaguchi

Abstract The purpose of this study was to construct a risk score for glioblastomas based on magnetic resonance imaging (MRI) data. Tumor identification requires multimodal voxel-based imaging data that are highly dimensional, and multivariate models with dimension reduction are desirable for their analysis. We propose a two-step dimension-reduction method using a radial basis function–supervised multi-block sparse principal component analysis (SMS–PCA) method. The method is first implemented through the basis expansion of spatial brain images, and the scores are then reduced through regularized matrix decomposition in order to produce simultaneous data-driven selections of related brain regions supervised by univariate composite scores representing linear combinations of covariates such as age and tumor location. An advantage of the proposed method is that it identifies the associations of brain regions at the voxel level, and supervision is helpful in the interpretation.

Keywords Brain image · Multimodal · Big data · Risk score

1 Introduction

Glioblastoma is a World Health Organization (WHO) grade IV glioma, the most common malignant primary brain tumor in humans and one having a poor prognosis. The first line of treatment is usually surgery followed by radiation therapy or combined with chemotherapy. Biomarkers provide useful information about prognosis, diagnosis, and treatment strategy. Measurements based on magnetic resonance imaging (MRI) are one such biomarker, used mainly for tracking treatment response and tumor recurrence [20]. Image data have also been used in a

A. Kawaguchi (✉)
Center for Comprehensive Community Medicine,
Faculty of Medicine, Saga University, Saga, Japan
e-mail: akawa@cc.saga-u.ac.jp

S. Matsui and J. Crowley (eds.), *Frontiers of Biostatistical Methods and Applications in Clinical Oncology*, DOI 10.1007/978-981-10-0126-0_24

randomized multicenter clinical trial to evaluate recurrence of glioblastoma in patients treated with bevacizumab [7].

A tumor is divided into three major regions: edema, necrotic, and active with two subtypes (enhancing and non-enhancing). In order to identify these, most studies use four types of MR images taken using different parameters. To illustrate, Fig. 1 shows one axial slice of an MR image of a glioblastoma patient; it has been segmented into edema (dark blue), necrotic (green), enhancing active tumor (red), and non-enhancing active tumor (light blue) areas. Also shown are the four MR image types commonly used in this context: T1-weighted, T1-weighted contrast (T1c), T2-weighted, and T2-weighted fluid-attenuated inversion recovery (FLAIR). T1 is often used to look at brain structure. T1c is obtained by injecting gadolinium into the body, causing tumor borders to appear brighter. T2 is the inverse of T1: bright parts in T1 appear dark in T2, and vice versa. FLAIR is very similar to T2 and is helpful in separating the edema region from the cerebrospinal fluid (CSF), because the free water signal is dark. The definition of tumor type based on these MRI types was provided by Porz et al. [22] and Gutman et al. [9]: in short, edema by T1, T2, and FLAIR; necrotic by T2 and FLAIR; enhancing by T1 and T1c; non-enhancing by T1c, T2, and FLAIR. This general technique is called multi-modal imaging and can reveal several disease mechanisms; see Liu [15] for an overview of brain imaging techniques not only for brain tumors but also for anatomical and functional biomarkers.

One of the most used collections of tumor characteristics is the Visually Accessible Rembrandt Image (VASARI) feature set (https://wiki.cancerimagingarchive.net/display/Public/VASARI+Research+Project), developed using multimodal MR images by The Cancer Genome Atlas (TCGA) radiology

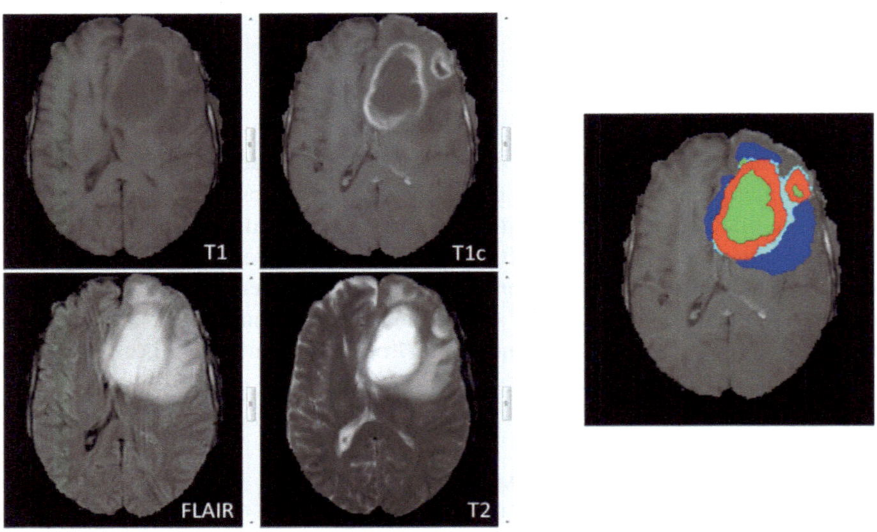

Fig. 1 Multimodal images of brain tumor

working group, which has done extensive work on tumor analysis. They have relied partly on image segmentation, which extracts binary images from the original MR images to represent the tumor type and location, followed by computation of the volume and identification of the tumor location. Such extractions have conventionally been performed manually by trained radiologists; recently, however, fully automated methods have been proposed. Gooya et al. [8] used a computer-based glioma image segmentation and registration segmentation algorithm. Porz et al. [22] provided the fully automatic segmentation software BraTumIA (Brain Tumor Image Analysis), which allows the raw image as input and provided the output given in Fig. 1. Tustison et al. [26] introduced supervised segmentation based on random forests. Recently, deep learning has also been used [14]. These methods can be regarded primarily as clustering analysis techniques that use the intensity to extract the tumor region and evaluate the volume. A number of reviews of these are available in the literature; see, for example, Bauer et al. [2], Liu et al. [16], El-Dahshan et al. [6], and Dupont et al. [5]. The Multimodal Brain Tumor Segmentation (BRATS) challenge has been ongoing since 2012 and has provided benchmark data sets and the results from several methods.

The main goal of the technique described in this chapter is to evaluate a patient's prognosis using tumor information based on MRI data. There have been many studies associating various MRI features with differences in survival time [9, 10, 19, 21]. Rios Velazquez et al. [25] and Wangaryattawanich et al. [27] investigated relationships between MRI features and survival time, and the latter group presented a table giving details of VASARI features. Among researchers applying advanced prediction methods, Cui et al. [4] used the survival LASSO method and Macyszyn et al. [17] used the SVM to predict survival times of less than or greater than 18 months.

In contrast to focusing on MRI features such as tumor volume, in this study we have attempted whole-brain data analysis using all voxel values as input. Brain imaging data consist of the image intensity values for a million voxels in a 3-D array. Each voxel value corresponds to a variable in a statistical term, so the data set is high-dimensional. The voxel values represent the brain structure and tumor, and we should expect to do some exploratory analysis. The strength of the whole-brain approach is that we should be able to obtain additional information about the volume from the segmentation. Because we will convert an image into a template (namely, a common space in which each voxel corresponds to an anatomical division of the brain region), it will be possible to interpret the resulting voxel related to the prognosis by referring to the corresponding brain region. The statistical challenge is that the data set is high-dimensional because of the large number of voxels, and there is a strong correlation among intensities for voxels in the same neighborhood.

In order to overcome these challenges, we used a two-step dimension-reduction method. Its original was proposed by Reiss and Ogden [24], and it was extended by Araki et al. [1], Yoshida et al. [28], and Kawaguchi [11]. In the first step, taking into account correlations based on data structure (namely, voxel neighborhood), dimension is reduced by basis expansion. In the second step, taking into account correlations based on data values, dimension is reduced by supervised multi-block sparse principal component analysis (SMS–PCA), a technique that is proposed in this study.

This chapter is organized as follows: Sect. 2 describes the data to be analyzed; in Sect. 3, the proposed method is given; in Sect. 4, the proposed method is applied to the real data described in Sect. 2; and Sect. 5 summarizes the study, giving a final conclusion.

2 Data and Preprocessing

We assessed the validity of the proposed method by applying it to real data. The data used were obtained from The Cancer Imaging Archive (TCIA) database (http://cancerimagingarchive.net), which is sponsored by the National Cancer Institute (NCI) and is available through download [see Clark et al. [3] and Prior et al. [23] for details]. Since TCGA has already de-identified patients, no Institutional Review Board approval was required.

Our data set is for 86 glioblastoma patients with survival time and covariates [age, gender, Karnofsky performance status (KPS)]. There are 63 events (27% censored). Four images (types T1, T1c, T2, FLAIR) per patient are available. For multimodal images and good performance, preprocessing was required. The first step was to perform intensity homogeneity and resolution corrections by the biasv_correct function with the N4 bias correction from the ANTsR package (https://github.com/stnava/ANTsR). Skull stripping was also implemented using the fslbet_robust function of the fslr package (http://CRAN.R-project.org/package=fslr). All brain images for each modality were registered into the corresponding template based on the SyN algorithm and B–spline interpolation.

The preprocessed images of the four image types were converted into probability maps for four tumor types—edema, necrosis, enhancing tumor, and non-enhancing tumor—to reduce the dependency on the segmentation algorithm and to move away from the binary image type. First, the preprocessed images were segmented into the four tumor types by using BraTumIA, which provides the result as binary images representing one of the tumor types rather than as voxels. Next, we used the random forests model on each resulting binary image and preprocessed the four image types as predictors to compute the voxel-by-voxel classification probabilities for each patient. The resulting four probability maps for non-enhancing tumor, enhancing tumor, necrosis, and edema were used as inputs for the method described in the following section to evaluate a patient's prognosis.

3 Method

In this section, the two-step dimension-reduction method is described. Let the data for n patients be represented by the notation

$$\{(s_{1\alpha}, s_{2\alpha}, s_{3\alpha}, s_{4\alpha}, Z_\alpha); \quad \alpha = 1, \ldots, n\},$$

where the brain imaging data (probability maps for edema, necrosis, enhancing tumor, and non-enhancing tumor) are represented by $s_m = (s_m(\mathbf{v}_1), s_m(\mathbf{v}_2), \ldots, s_m(\mathbf{v}_N))^\top$, $m = 1, 2, 3, 4$ (the vectorized image data), in which $\mathbf{v}_j \in \mathbb{Z}^3$ ($j = 1, 2, \ldots, N$) is the voxel location and N is the number of voxels (assuming the same number among the modalities). $\boldsymbol{Z}$ is the scalar supervising measure, which can be one or a combination of several baseline measurements related to the outcome (survival time). The combination would be formularized using a regression model or by using clinical input.

In the first step, the number of dimensions of the imaging data is reduced by applying the basis expansion taking into account correlations based on data structure (namely, voxel neighborhood). It should be noted that the use of a basis expansion of this nature as a preprocessing procedure for reducing the number of dimensions has been helpful for neuroimaging analysis as in, for example, Reiss and Ogden [24], Araki et al. [1], Yoshida et al. [28], and Kawaguchi [11]. As the dimensions for each mth image are the same, we use the same basis function to reduce the dimension from N to q. $\boldsymbol{X}_m = \mathbf{S}_m\mathbf{B}$ is the $n \times q$ matrix, where $\mathbf{S}_m = \{s_{m\alpha}\}$ is the $n \times N$ matrix and $\mathbf{B} = \{\phi_k(\mathbf{v}_j)\}_{j=1,\ldots,N,k=1,\ldots,q}$ is the $N \times q$ matrix in which each element is the radial B–spline function

$$\phi_k(\mathbf{v}) = \frac{1}{4h^2}\begin{cases} h^3 - 3h^2 d_k(\mathbf{v}) + 3h d_k(\mathbf{v})^2 + 3 d_k(\mathbf{v})^3 & (d_k(\mathbf{v}) \leq 0) \\ (h - d_k(\mathbf{v}))^3 & (0 < d_k(\mathbf{v}) \leq h) \\ 0 & (d_k(\mathbf{v}) > h) \end{cases}$$

where $d_k(\mathbf{v}) = \| \mathbf{v} - \boldsymbol{\kappa}_k \| - h, \boldsymbol{\kappa}_k \in \mathbb{Z}^3 (k = 1, \ldots, q)$ is the pre-specified knot and $h > 0$ is the distance between knots. This basis function reduces the number of parameters from N to q by converting each voxel to a component of the function. The number q of basis functions is determined by the number of voxels and the distance between pre-specified knots. In this study, we used 4–voxel (therefore, $h = \sqrt{3 \times 4^2} = 6.93$) equally spaced knots because our simulation study [28] showed that accuracy increased as the distance between knots became smaller.

Dimension reduction using the basis function is then followed by the use of the SMS–PCA method, taking into account (sample) correlations based on data values; this is the second step. We consider score $\boldsymbol{t}$ for the $n \times q$ matrices $\boldsymbol{X}_m$, where $m = 1, 2, \ldots, M$ ($M = 4$ in this study), with the following multi-block structure:

$$\boldsymbol{t} = \sum_{m=1}^{M} b_m \boldsymbol{X}_m \boldsymbol{w}_m, \tag{1}$$

where $\boldsymbol{w}_m$ is the weight vector for the mth sub-block $\boldsymbol{X}_m$, and b_m is the weight for the super-block. Here it should be noted that the scores in [1] are referred to as the super score, whereas $\boldsymbol{t}_m = \boldsymbol{X}_m \boldsymbol{w}_m$ is referred to as the block score. Thus, the super score, which is used in an application such as construction of a risk score, has a hierarchical structure.

When matrix $\boldsymbol{X}_m$ is normalized by its columns, the weights $\boldsymbol{w} = (\boldsymbol{w}_1, \boldsymbol{w}_2, \ldots, \boldsymbol{w}_M)^\top$ and $\boldsymbol{b} = (b_1, b_2, \ldots, b_M)^\top$ are estimated by maximizing the function

$$\mathrm{L}(\boldsymbol{b}, \boldsymbol{w}) = (1-\mu)\boldsymbol{t}^\top \boldsymbol{t} + \mu \boldsymbol{t}^\top \boldsymbol{Z} - \sum_{m=1}^{M} \mathrm{P}_{\lambda_m}(\boldsymbol{w}_m) \tag{2}$$

subject to $\|\boldsymbol{w}_m\|^2 = 1$ and $\|\boldsymbol{b}\|^2 = 1$, where $\mu \in [0, 1]$ is the proportion of the supervision ($\mu = 0.9$ is used in this study), $\mathrm{P}_\lambda(x)$ is the penalty function [$\mathrm{P}_\lambda(x) = 2\lambda|\boldsymbol{x}|$ is used in this study], and $\lambda > 0$ is the regularized parameter that is used to control the sparsity. The algorithm given in Table 1 is used to estimate the weights in (1) by maximizing L in (2).

The larger value of the regularization parameter λ_m has many nonzero elements in $\boldsymbol{w}_m$, from which its optimal value is selected by minimizing the Bayesian information criterion (BIC):

$$\mathrm{BIC}(\boldsymbol{\lambda}) = \log\left(\frac{\sum_{m=1}^{M}\left\|\widehat{\boldsymbol{X}}_m^{(r)} - \boldsymbol{X}_m\right\|^2}{nMq}\right) + \frac{\log(nMq)}{nMq}\mathrm{df}(\boldsymbol{\lambda}),$$

where $\widehat{\boldsymbol{X}}_m^{(r)} = \boldsymbol{T}_m^{(r)} \boldsymbol{P}_m^{(r)^T}$ with $\boldsymbol{T}_m^{(r)} = \left[\boldsymbol{t}_m^{(1)}, \ldots, \boldsymbol{t}_m^{(r)}\right]$ and $\boldsymbol{P}_m^{(r)} = \left[\boldsymbol{p}_m^{(1)}, \ldots, \boldsymbol{p}_m^{(r)}\right]$ obtained from r deflation steps (the projection of $\boldsymbol{X}_m$ onto the r-dimensional subspace), $\boldsymbol{\lambda} = (\boldsymbol{\lambda}_1, \ldots, \boldsymbol{\lambda}_M)^\top$, and df is the number of effective parameters (nonzero elements in $\boldsymbol{w}_m$), which depends on the value of $\boldsymbol{\lambda}$.

Table 1 Algorithm for SMS–PCA method

1. Initialize $\boldsymbol{t}$ and normalize the super scores $\boldsymbol{t} \leftarrow \boldsymbol{t}/\|\boldsymbol{t}\|_2$.
2. Repeat until convergence 2.1 Set $\tilde{\boldsymbol{w}}_m = h_{\lambda_m}\left(b_m \boldsymbol{X}_m^\top\{(1-\mu)\|\boldsymbol{t}\| + \mu \boldsymbol{Z}\}\right)$, where $h_\lambda(y) = \mathrm{sign}(y)(\lvert y\rvert > \lambda)_+$, and normalize as $\hat{\boldsymbol{w}}_m = \tilde{\boldsymbol{w}}_m / \tilde{\boldsymbol{w}}_2$ $(m = 1, 2, \ldots, M)$ 2.2 Set $\boldsymbol{t}_m = \boldsymbol{X}_m \widehat{\boldsymbol{w}}_m$ and $\tilde{b}_m = \boldsymbol{t}_m^\top\{(1-\mu)\|\boldsymbol{t}\| + \mu\boldsymbol{Z}\}$; then set $\tilde{\boldsymbol{b}} = (\tilde{b}_1, \tilde{b}_2, \ldots, \tilde{b}_M)^\top$ and normalize as $\tilde{\boldsymbol{b}} = \tilde{\boldsymbol{b}}/\tilde{\boldsymbol{b}}_2$ 2.3 Set $\boldsymbol{t} = \sum_{m=1}^{M} \hat{b}_m \boldsymbol{X}_m \hat{\boldsymbol{w}}_m$
3. (Deflation step) Set $\boldsymbol{p}_m = \boldsymbol{X}_m^\top \boldsymbol{t}_m / \boldsymbol{t}_m^\top \boldsymbol{t}_m$ and $\hat{\boldsymbol{X}}_m = \boldsymbol{t}_m \boldsymbol{p}_m^\top$, and $\boldsymbol{X}_m \leftarrow \boldsymbol{X}_m - \widehat{\boldsymbol{X}}_m$

Note that the deflation step yields multiple components and has several alternatives

The R package msma is provided to implement the SMS–PCA method and is available from the Comprehensive R Archive Network (CRAN) at http://CRAN.R-project.org/package=msma.

4 Application

The proposed method was applied to TCGA data after images were preprocessed and converted by the method described in Sect. 2. For the scalar supervising measure Z, we computed the predicted value from a Cox regression model using a dummy variable based on categorized age and tumor location as covariates. The tumor location was identified by using the binary images from BraTumIA that were byproducts of the computation of the probability images along with the standardized atlas coordinate system provided by WFU (Wake Forest University) PickAtlas [18], finding the portion of the tumor represented in the atlas region for each patient. The dummy variable for Z represents three strata defined partly by the age category and partly by the survival tree with the tumor location as predictors: (1) age ≥ 70, or $40 \leq$ age < 70 and enhancing tumor located outside the atlas; (2) $40 \leq$ age < 70 and edema located inside the atlas but not in the superior frontal gyrus; and (3) $40 \leq$ age < 70 and edema located in the superior frontal gyrus, or age <40.

The risk score was computed from the Cox proportional hazards model with the SMS–PCA super score, and in order to take into account the different baseline hazards, the strata were also incorporated into the model as a covariate. The final variables were selected by the BIC based on the partial likelihood from the Cox model. For the purpose of comparison, we also computed the score from the unsupervised version of the method (MS–PCA), which is the case of $\mu = 0$ in (2).

Two components (Components 3 and 10) were selected from ten candidate components for the proposed method. These components were of the forms: $T_3 = 0.54\text{edema} + 0.37\text{necrosis} + 0.49\text{enhancing} + 0.57\text{nonenhancing}$ and $T_{10} = 0.42\text{edema} + 0.62\text{necrosis} + 0.49\text{enhancing} + 0.44\text{nonenhancing}$. In both components, the tumor types were equally associated. Table 2 shows the regression coefficients, its exponential, its standard errors, the test statistics, and the p values from the multivariate Cox model with scores computed using the proposed method, the unsupervised version, the volume with the strata as covariates, and the strata only for comparison. Use of the strata was very effective for this data set; however, the SMS–PCA super scores were also effective in computing the risk score in addition to the strata that are incorporated in the Cox model as a covariate.

In addition, we computed the prediction errors by the Brier score, which is a kind of mean squared error for the bootstrap cross-validation technique:

$$BS(t, \hat{S}) = \frac{1}{n} \sum_{i=1}^{n} \left(Y_i(t) - \hat{S}(t|X_i)\right)^2,$$

Table 2 Results of the Cox model

	Coef.	exp(coef.)	se(coef.)	z	*p* value
Proposed method					
Component 3	−0.03	0.97	0.01	−4.29	<0.0001
Component 10	0.04	1.04	0.02	2.28	0.0228
Strata 2 versus 1	−0.92	0.40	0.30	−3.11	0.0019
Strata 3 versus 1	−2.58	0.08	0.48	−5.40	<0.0001
Unsupervised version					
Component 1	−0.03	0.97	0.01	−2.83	0.0047
Component 2	0.03	1.03	0.01	4.88	<0.0001
Component 5	0.02	1.02	0.01	2.46	0.0139
Component 6	0.02	1.02	0.01	2.28	0.0229
Strata 2 versus 1	−0.77	0.46	0.30	−2.54	0.0111
Strata 3 versus 1	−2.98	0.05	0.55	−5.45	<0.0001
Volume with strata					
Enhancing (2000 units)	0.03	1.03	0.01	2.61	0.0091
Strata 2 versus 1	−0.74	0.48	0.32	−2.32	0.0204
Strata 3 versus 1	−1.86	0.16	0.45	−4.17	<0.0001
Strata only					
Strata 2 versus 1	−0.99	0.37	0.29	−3.47	0.0005
Strata 3 versus 1	−2.10	0.12	0.43	−4.89	<0.0001

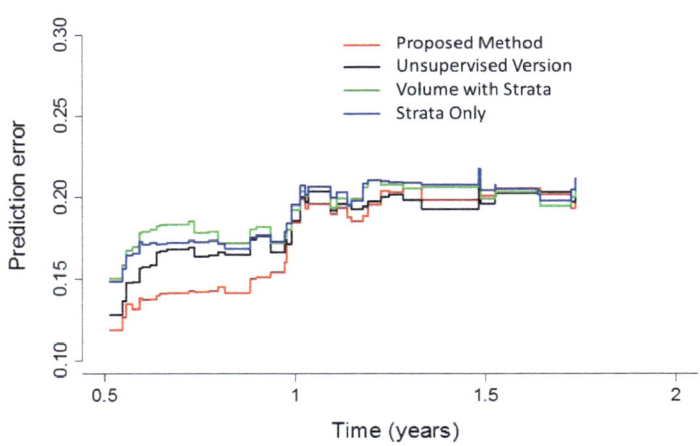

Fig. 2 Prediction error curves

where $Y_i(t) = \mathrm{I}(T_i > t)$ is the observed survival time for patient i in the test set, and $\hat{S}(t|x)$ is the estimated survival function from the Cox model given covariates x in the training set. Figure 2 shows the prediction errors as a function of survival time. Our method (red line) had lower errors for survival times of up to one year.

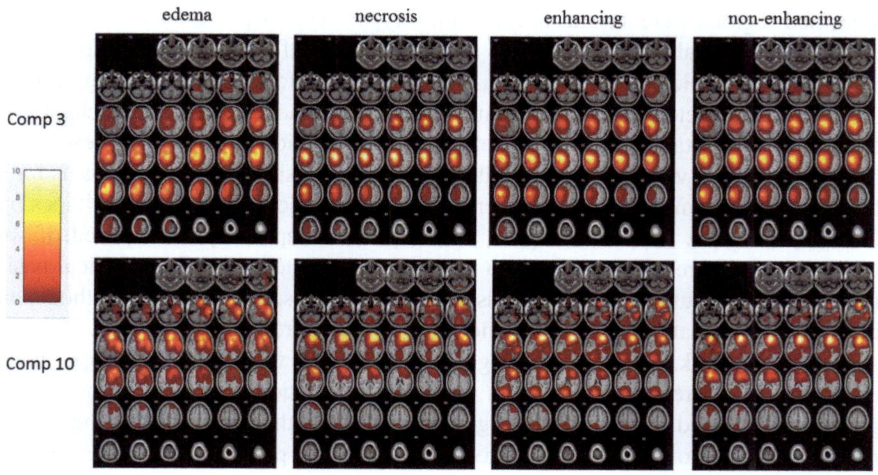

Fig. 3 Result for identified regions

Figure 3 shows the **B***w* values overlaid onto the anatomical space for each tumor tissue type. For Component 3, it can be seen that postcentral and cingulate gyrus, sub-gyral are important and that its super score is negatively associated with survival; that is, as the score increases, the prognosis is worsened. For Component 10, the frontal lobe is important, and its super score is positively associated with survival.

5 Summary

We have proposed a novel approach for multimodal brain tumor image analysis using a two-step dimension-reduction method, taking into account two types of correlation and incorporating a supervised-learning feature, which is a part of our ongoing study [13]. The software has been provided as the R package msma. Our results show that the proposed method can produce a more accurate predictive risk score than either the unsupervised version or the volume data. Although the predictive factors could be obtained from age and tumor location, the SMS–PCA score had a complementary role in improving the accuracy. As an alternative approach, stratified dimension reduction by the strata was considered to focus on the tumor location; however, greater predictive accuracy was not obtained.

We used the BraTumIA software for the segmentation because of its ease of implementation; however, its application is limited to patient sets that include all four required MR modalities: T1, T1c, T2, and FLAIR. Although we converted to probability images to eliminate the dependency on the segmentation algorithm, the application of other algorithms would be worth investigating. On the other hand, identified regions were similar in four tumor types. This is probably because of the usage of the probability map; it may also be because of the spherical shape of the basis function, which yields a wider associated region (for example, the region near the eyes was detected). Since the radius of the basis function used in this chapter is defined by the distance between voxels, the basis function on the higher resolution image (with more voxels) yields smaller spheres even using the same radius as for a lower resolution image. These smaller spheres could allow more flexible shapes by their combination. Thus, although a more optimal shape may be required, if we could use higher resolution images it would be adequate to use the spherical basis function. In this study, although cross-validation was used to evaluate methods, an independent validation data set should also be considered as in Cui et al. [4].

For future work, selection of images by using regularization on the super level could be considered. In addition, a study of associations between imaging and genomics (referred to as "imaging genomics," or "radiogenomics" in the terminology of Ellingson [7]) could be considered using a partial least-squares framework. Only gene expression data for glioblastoma have been analyzed in our previous study [12]. Furthermore, another modality such as PET imaging, which is used in many cancer studies, could be incorporated, and such a study would provide new knowledge about the interaction of different aspects of brain mechanisms.

In conclusion, this method has application in a number of multimodal imaging studies and will be helpful for improving the construction of predictive risk scores.

Acknowledgements This study was supported in part by Intramural Research Grant (27–8) for Neurological and Psychiatric Disorders of NCNP. We used the supercomputer of ACCMS, Kyoto University.

References

1. Araki Y, Kawaguchi A, Yamashita F. Regularized logistic discrimination with basis expansions for the early detection of Alzheimer's disease based on three-dimensional MRI data. Adv Data Anal Classif. 2013;7(1):109–19.
2. Bauer S, Wiest R, Nolte LP, Reyes M. A survey of MRI-based medical image analysis for brain tumor studies. Phys Med Biol. 2013;58(13):R97–129.
3. Clark K, Vendt B, Smith K, et al. The cancer imaging archive (TCIA): maintaining and operating a public information repository. J Digit Imaging. 2013;26(6):1045–57.
4. Cui Y, Tha KK, Terasaka S, et al. Prognostic imaging biomarkers in glioblastoma: development and independent validation on the basis of multiregion and quantitative analysis of MR images. Radiology. 2016;278(2):546–53.
5. Dupont C, Betrouni N, Reyns N, Vermandel M. On image segmentation methods applied to glioblastoma: state of art and new trends. IRBM. 2016;. doi:10.1016/j.irbm.2015.12.004.
6. El-Dahshan ESA, Mohsen HM, Revett K, Salem ABM. Computer-aided diagnosis of human brain tumor through MRI: a survey and a new algorithm. Expert Syst Appl. 2014;41 (11):5526–45.
7. Ellingson BM. Radiogenomics and imaging phenotypes in glioblastoma: novel observations and correlation with molecular characteristics. Curr Neurol Neurosci Rep. 2015;15(1):1–12.

8. Gooya A, Biros G, Davatzikos C. Deformable registration of glioma images using EM algorithm and diffusion reaction modeling. IEEE Trans Med Imaging. 2011;30(2):375–90.
9. Gutman DA, Cooper LA, Hwang SN, et al. MR imaging predictors of molecular profile and survival: multi-institutional study of the TCGA glioblastoma data set. Radiology. 2013;267 (2):560–9.
10. Gutman DA, Dunn WD Jr, Grossmann P, et al. Somatic mutations associated with MRI-derived volumetric features in glioblastoma. Neuroradiology. 2015;57(12):1227–37.
11. Kawaguchi A. Diagnostic probability modeling for longitudinal structural brain MRI data analysis. In: Truong YK, Lewis MM, editors. Statistical techniques for neuroscientists. Boca Raton: CRC Press; 2016. p. 361–74.
12. Kawaguchi A, Yajima N, Tsuchiya N, et al. Gene expression signature-based prognostic risk score in patients with glioblastoma. Cancer Sci. 2013;104(9):1205–10.
13. Kawaguchi A, Yamashita F. Supervised multiblock sparse multivariable analysis with application to multimodal brain imaging genetics. Biostatistics (2017, in press) doi:10.1093/biostatistics/kxx011
14. Kleesiek J, Urban G, Hubert A, et al. Deep MRI brain extraction: a 3D convolutional neural network for skull stripping. Neuroimage. 2016;129:460–9.
15. Liu CH. Anatomical, functional and molecular biomarker applications of magnetic resonance neuroimaging. Future Neurol. 2015;10(1):49–65.
16. Liu J, Li M, Wang J, et al. A survey of MRI-based brain tumor segmentation methods. Tsinghua Sci Technol. 2014;19(6):578–95.
17. Macyszyn L, Akbari H, Pisapia JM, et al. Imaging patterns predict patient survival and molecular subtype in glioblastoma via machine learning techniques. Neuro Oncol. 2016;18 (3):417–25.
18. Maldjian JA, Laurienti PJ, Kraft RA, Burdette JH. An automated method for neuroanatomic and cytoarchitectonic atlas-based interrogation of fMRI data sets. Neuroimage. 2003;19 (3):1233–9.
19. Mazurowski MA, Desjardins A, Malof JM. Imaging descriptors improve the predictive power of survival models for glioblastoma patients. Neuro Oncol. 2013;15(10):1389–94.
20. Nicolaidis S. Biomarkers of glioblastoma multiforme. Metabolism. 2015;64(3 Suppl 1):S22–7.
21. Nicolasjilwan M, Hu Y, Yan C, et al. Addition of MR imaging features and genetic biomarkers strengthens glioblastoma survival prediction in TCGA patients. J Neuroradiol. 2015;42(4):212–21.
22. Porz N, Bauer S, Pica A, et al. Multi-modal glioblastoma segmentation: man versus machine. PLoS ONE. 2014;9(5):e96873. doi:10.1371/journal.pone.0096873.
23. Prior FW, Clark K, Commean P et al. TCIA: an information resource to enable open science. In: Conference proceedings IEEE engineering in medicine and biology society; 2013; Osaka, Japan: Oaska International Convention Center, 3–7 July 2013. p. 1282–285.
24. Reiss PT, Ogden RT. Functional generalized linear models with images as predictors. Biometrics. 2010;66(1):61–9.
25. Rios Velazquez E, Meier R, Dunn WD Jr, et al. Fully automatic GBM segmentation in the TCGA-GBM dataset: prognosis and correlation with VASARI features. Sci Rep. 2015;5:16822. doi:10.1038/srep16822.
26. Tustison NJ, Shrinidhi KL, Wintermark M, et al. Optimal symmetric multimodal templates and concatenated random forests for supervised brain tumor segmentation (simplified) with ANTsR. Neuroinformatics. 2015;13(2):209–25.
27. Wangaryattawanich P, Hatami M, Wang J, et al. Multicenter imaging outcomes study of The Cancer Genome Atlas glioblastoma patient cohort: imaging predictors of overall and progression-free survival. Neuro Oncol. 2015;17(11):1525–37.
28. Yoshida H, Kawaguchi A, Tsuruya K. Radial basis function-sparse partial least squares for application to brain imaging data. Comput Math Methods Med. 2013;2013:591032. doi:10.1155/2013/591032.

An Evaluation of Gene Set Analysis for Biomarker Discovery with Applications to Myeloma Research

Pingping Qu, Erming Tian, Bart Barlogie, Gareth Morgan and John Crowley

Abstract In this paper, we evaluate 15 methods for gene set analysis in microarray classification problems. We employ four datasets from myeloma research and three types of biological gene sets, encompassing a total of 12 scenarios. Taking a two-step approach, we first identify important genes within gene sets to create summary gene set scores, we then construct predictive models using the gene set scores as predictors. We propose two powerful linear methods in addition to the well-known SuperPC method for calculating scores. By comparing the 15 gene set methods with methods used in individual-gene analysis, we conclude that, overall, the gene set analysis approach provided more accurate predictions than the individual-gene analysis.

Keywords Gene set analysis · Individual-gene analysis · Score · Classification · Microarray · Myeloma

P. Qu (✉) · J. Crowley
Cancer Research and Biostatistics, Seattle, WA, USA
e-mail: pingpingq@crab.org

J. Crowley
e-mail: johnc@crab.org

E. Tian · G. Morgan
Myeloma Institute at University of Arkansas for Medical Sciences, Little Rock, AR, USA
e-mail: tianerming@uams.edu

G. Morgan
e-mail: GJMorgan@uams.edu

B. Barlogie
Mt Sinai School of Medicine, New York, NY, USA
e-mail: bart.barlogie@mssm.edu

S. Matsui and J. Crowley (eds.), *Frontiers of Biostatistical Methods and Applications in Clinical Oncology*, DOI 10.1007/978-981-10-0126-0_25

1 Introduction

Gene expression profiling (GEP) via DNA microarrays has been used extensively in cancer research to study disease mechanisms and make predictions of clinical outcomes. A typical microarray data analysis focuses on the selection of individual genes. For example, to identify differentially expressed genes under different conditions, one typically calculates a statistic and p value for each gene, followed by multiple comparison adjustments since normally tens of thousands of genes are measured in a microarray experiment. To select genes for predicting clinical outcomes, one can resort to methods such as semi-supervised principal component analysis (SuperPC) [1], partial least squares [2], Lasso [3], random forest [4], and so on. However, this type of analysis can miss some important genes whose individual contributions to a particular outcome may be moderate but whose combined effects are significant. Another limitation of the individual-gene approach is frequently inconsistent gene findings from similar studies conducted by different institutes [5, 6]. These problems of the individual-gene analysis were discussed in Mootha et al. [7] and Subramanian et al. [8], where they proposed a gene set enrichment analysis (GSEA) idea, incorporating prior biological knowledge into the analysis routine to identify important genes through gene sets. Since then many new statistical methods have been proposed for making inference on associations or predictions at gene set levels instead of individual-gene levels.

A gene set is a group of genes related in certain ways (e.g., they may be from the same pathway or perform similar molecular functions). There are public databases holding such information, for example those with the Gene Ontology (GO) annotations [9] and the Kyoto Encyclopedia of Genes and Genomes (KEGG) pathways [10]. For differential expression analysis, a gene set method aims to determine via hypothesis testing whether a gene set as a whole is associated with an outcome of interest. Examples include the pioneering GSEA algorithm [8], the Global Test [11], ANCOVA Global Test [12], SAM-GS [13], and GSA [14], to name just a few. For biomarker discovery, i.e. finding genes to build models for diagnostic/prognostic purposes, the idea of incorporating gene set information is to improve both performance and interpretability of resulting models. Tai and Pan [15] proposed a modified linear discriminant analysis (LDA) approach for classification by regularizing the covariance matrix and incorporating correlations among the genes within gene sets. With simulated and real datasets plus information from KEGG pathways, they showed that the new approach performed better than not incorporating the correlations within gene sets. Chen and Wang [16] proposed a two-step procedure: first to create a "super gene score" using SuperPC [1] within each a priori gene set obtained from GO and then to use Lasso or SuperPC again to build a final model based on the super gene scores. With two survival microarray data they demonstrated that their gene set-based models enjoyed improved prediction accuracy and generated more biologically interpretable results. Ma et al. [17] also took a two-step approach, where they first divided genes into clusters by k-means, followed by applying Lasso within each cluster to get refined gene clusters, and then they selected important gene clusters with group Lasso [18]. Luan and Li [19] proposed a group additive regression model to incorporate pathway information and the use of gradient descent boosting for model fitting. With both simulations and a real microarray survival dataset, they showed improved accuracy by their method when compared to not using gene group information.

In this paper, we aim to investigate several score methods in conjunction with trees and random forests for gene set analysis and compare with individual-gene analysis in classification problems. In the individual-gene analysis, neither the gene selection nor the prediction process utilizes any biological information. For the gene set analysis, we first identify important genes within a priori gene sets to create summary gene set scores, and we then use the gene set scores as predictors for constructing predictive models. We explore four myeloma microarray datasets and three types of gene sets, and demonstrate that predictive accuracy depends on both the method and the type of gene sets being investigated. In the next section we first introduce our datasets from myeloma research. We then describe the analysis methods in Sect. 3 and show our results from applying the methods to the myeloma datasets in Sect. 4. Finally in Sect. 5, we conclude with a comparison of our results with findings reported by others.

2 Datasets

All GEP datasets used in this investigation were from the Myeloma Institute (MI) at the University of Arkansas for Medical Sciences (UAMS). Multiple myeloma (MM) is a cancer of plasma cells in the bone marrow, with symptoms such as elevated **c**alcium, **r**enal failure, **a**nemia, and **b**one lesions (the so-called CRAB symptoms). Normal plasma cells produce many immunoglobulins (antibodies) that the body needs to identify and fight pathogens such as bacteria and viruses. With MM, abnormal plasma cells from a single clone accumulate and eventually crowd out normal plasma cells, causing the body to produce only one type of immunoglobulin. It is not clear what causes MM, but it is characterized by genetic abnormalities such as gene mutations and translocations. For example, deletions of chromosome 17p and *P53* gene mutations have been linked to poor clinical outcomes in numerous MM studies. Typically prior to developing MM, abnormal plasma cells accumulate in the body and the patient undergoes an asymptomatic phase, comprising monoclonal gammopathy of uncertain significance (MGUS) and smoldering multiple myeloma (SMM). Compared to MGUS, SMM has more abnormal plasma cells in the bone marrow and higher levels of monoclonal immunoglobulin (M-protein) in the serum. Both MGUS and SMM patients lack the CRAB symptoms that define MM. However, MGUS patients have an approximately 1% risk per year of developing MM [20]. Among patients with SMM, about 10% annually will progress to MM within 5 years, and after the 5-year mark the progression rate is similar to MGUS [21].

In previous work, based on an earlier Affymetrix platform with ~12,000 genes, we identified differentially expressed genes that could distinguish in plasma cells between normal and MM and between normal and MGUS [22]. An interesting finding at the time was a lack of ability of the models to discriminate between MGUS and MM at the gene expression level. Based on the newer platform U133Plus2, and more samples, we aimed to do a more refined analysis in this investigation, specifically to identify signature genes and build predictive models to distinguish between (1) normal and MGUS, (2) MGUS and SMM, (3) SMM and MM, and (4) *P53* deletion and no deletion in MM. The MM patients in this study were enrolled in a series of Total Therapy (TT) clinical trials, with the MGUS/SMM patients in two observational clinical trials (SWOG S0120 and MI M0120). *P53* deletion was determined at baseline by interphase fluorescence in situ hybridization (iFISH). For GEP, purified plasma cells (PC) by CD138 expression were obtained from normal healthy subjects and the MM (MGUS/SMM) patients prior to therapy (at registration of the observational trials). Microarray raw intensity values were preprocessed and normalized using the MAS5 algorithm provided by the manufacturer, and the normalized data also went through batch effect checking and corrections [23].

3 Methods

Table 1 gives the sample sizes in each dataset. To ensure data quality, we first implemented the following steps prior to analysis:

1. Use the genes with current annotations from Affymetrix.
2. Take the median if a gene is represented by more than one probe set.
3. Keep only those genes whose raw intensity values are >128 in at least 80% of the samples to avoid any resolution problems that may be encountered by low microarray intensity values.

Table 1 Number of samples used in the training and test sets for each disease comparison

Disease comparison	Group 0	Group 1	# samples in training set (group 0, group 1)	# samples in test set (group 0, group 1)
Normal versus MGUS	Normal	MGUS	(25, 73)	(13, 44)
MGUS versus SMM	MGUS	SMM	(73, 89)	(44, 75)
SMM versus MM	SMM	MM	(89, 174)	(74, 178)
P53 deletion versus no deletion	without *P53* deletion	with *P53* deletion	(377, 45)	(294, 29)

Since applying the above procedure to each GEP dataset separately produced similar sets of genes, for simplicity we applied it to all the data combined to obtain a total of 9624 genes before analysis.

3.1 What Gene Sets to Use?

There are different types and sources of biological gene sets. The Molecular Signatures Database (MSigDB) [24] on the Broad Institute website is one of the largest and most popular repositories. We downloaded three types of gene sets from MSigDB: those associated with the GO biological processes (BP), the hallmark gene sets, and the positional gene sets. Each gene set groups certain genes together that share a particular biological property. GO BP gene sets contain genes associated with biological processes, each of which is made up of many chemical reactions or events leading to chemical transformations. However, the GO BP gene sets are a broad category and do not necessarily comprise co-regulated genes. On the other hand, the hallmark gene sets represent well-defined biological states or processes and contain genes with coordinate expression [25]. The positional gene sets group genes by chromosome and cytogenetic band. Such gene sets are helpful in identifying effects related to chromosome abnormalities.

3.2 Approach for Gene Set Analysis

Our general approach for gene set analysis is a two-step procedure: (1) within each a priori gene set create a summary gene set score after gene selection, and (2) construct a predictive model based on the resulting gene set scores. Both Chen and Wang [16] and Ma et al. [17] pointed out that typically not all members of a gene set will participate in a biological process, or be relevant to the outcome of interest, and not doing gene selection within gene sets could result in inferior prediction accuracy. Thus we carry out variable selection twice, first to select important genes within each gene set to calculate a summary gene set score (step 1), and then to select important gene sets based on the gene set scores and build a final predictive model (step 2).

3.3 Variable Selection and Model Building

We investigated several linear and nonlinear methods for variable selection and model building. The linear methods included the Lasso and three univariate score methods, and the nonlinear methods included decision trees and random forests.

Lasso is a multivariate regression technique [3] that has become popular and essential in genomic data analysis. By shrinking regression coefficients using an L_1

penalty term in the likelihood function for a logistic regression model, the regression coefficients for some genes become exactly zero, thus enabling variable selection. Classification will be done according to the estimated probabilities from the resulting sparse model with the shrunken coefficients. We implemented Lasso via the R package *glmnet* [26].

The idea of univariate score methods is to first rank genes by univariate analysis (e.g., doing a t-test for each gene in a two-class problem) and then create a score by a linear combination of the top ranking genes. There are many variants of this method and we investigated three in this paper. In a two-class problem, let x_i and t_i denote the expression level and the two-sample t-statistic for gene i, respectively. The first score is based on a regularized compound covariate, where the t-statistics are shrunken towards 0 by soft-thresholding. We denote it by ccscore, that is,

$$ccscore = \sum_{i=1}^{p} \text{sign}(t_i)(|t_i| - \Delta)_+ x_i, \tag{1}$$

where p is the total number of genes, $(x)_+ = x$ if $x > 0$ and 0 otherwise, and $0 \le \Delta \le max_i(|t_i|)$ is a tuning parameter to be determined by cross-validation. The non-regularized version of the compound covariate method is also a popular choice for constructing scores, which was originally proposed by Tukey [27] and discussed in Huang and Pan [28] for classification problems with microarray data. The second score is one that, instead of using the t-statistics from univariate analysis, only the signs of the t-statistics are used, followed by dividing by the total number of selected genes. We refer to it as "score", that is,

$$score = \frac{1}{|S|} \sum_{i \in S} \text{sign}(t_i) x_i, \tag{2}$$

where $S = \{i{:}|t_i| \ge \Delta\}$, $|S|$ = number of genes in S, and Δ is a tuning parameter determined by cross-validation. Originally we employed a similar method to develop the robust GEP70 model for risk stratification for MM patients undergoing standard therapy [29]; we then modified it to its current form in (2). The third score is an extension of SuperPC [1], originally developed for time-to-event data and shown to perform well in gene set analysis [16]. It takes the top ranking genes and calculates their first principal component as a score. We denote it here by pcscore, that is,

$$pcscore = \sum_{i \in S} b_i x_i, \tag{3}$$

where $S = \{i{:}|t_i| \ge \Delta\}$, b_i are loadings from the first principal component of the genes selected in S, and Δ is a tuning parameter determined by cross-validation. For all the aforementioned score methods, they were first created as continuous variables, and we then dichotomized them, balancing both sensitivity and specificity to create 2-group classification rules.

There is a rich literature concerning the development of predictive models using decision trees and random forests and their applications in genomic data analysis (e.g., see [4, 30–34]). A decision tree model based on recursive partitioning has the advantage of easy interpretation. In a random forest model, many decision trees are built by utilizing bootstrap samples and results from each tree are aggregated by majority voting to make final predictions. By building each tree to the fullest, the method is able to achieve low bias, and by aggregating results from many trees it can also achieve low variance. Importantly, a random forest considers only a random subset of the variables at each split. Doing so allows it to (1) produce less similar bootstrap samples and trees and therefore low variance at the end, and (2) identify a diverse set of important variables associated with the outcome of interest even when there is multicollinearity in the data. We implemented decision trees and random forests via the R packages *rpart* and *randomForest*.

For the individual-gene analysis, we used methods such as the Lasso, score, ccscore, pcscore, trees, and random forests. For the gene set analysis, to maintain focus we considered only various (instead of all) combinations of the methods from individual-gene analysis. As genes within a biological gene set are more likely to be co-regulated or co-expressed, we restricted to linear methods in step 1 (within gene sets), while in step 2 (between gene sets) we explored both linear and nonlinear methods. There were a total of 15 combinations in the gene set analysis we considered. We denote each combined methodology by using a period between the names of the methods used in the two steps. For example, suppose in step 1 we chose the score method to select genes while in step 2 trees were employed; we would refer to the combined method by score.tree. Tables 2 and 3 list all the methods and their notations for both the gene set and individual-gene analysis.

Table 2 Methods investigated in individual-gene analysis

Classification method	Notation
Lasso	Lasso
score	score
ccscore	ccscore
pcscore	pcscore
decision tree	tree
random forest	rf

Table 3 Methods investigated in gene set analysis

Classification method (within gene sets + between gene sets)	Notation
Lasso + Lasso	lasso.lasso
Lasso + random forest	lasso.rf
Lasso + tree	lasso.tree
score + Lasso	score.lasso
score + score	score.score
score + random forest	score.rf
score + tree	score.tree
pcscore + Lasso	pcscore.lasso
pcscore + pcscore	pcscore.score
pcscore + random forest	pcscore.rf
pcscore + tree	pcscore.tree
ccscore + Lasso	ccscore.lasso
ccscore + ccscore	ccscore.ccscore
ccscore + random forest	ccscore.rf
ccscore + tree	ccscore.tree

3.4 Cross-Validation to Determine Tuning Parameter

For the univariate score methods described above, we employed 10-fold cross-validation to select appropriate values for the tuning parameter Δ and to achieve variable selection. The search range for Δ is normally between 0 and $max_i(|t_i|)$ as suggested in (1–3), which can be a big range. To reduce computational burden, we restricted our search within the range of 1000 most significant genes when doing the cross-validation. For example, if the absolute values of the t statistic in the top 1000 genes vary between 4.5 and 5.6, we would assess each value from 4.5 to 5.6, with an increment of 0.1 in search of an optimal threshold for Δ. We used error rate as the performance measure in the cross-validation.

3.5 Model Comparison

Each of the four datasets was split into training and test sets (Table 1), and we only report error rates from the test sets as a guide to compare performance of the different methods. All model building steps were performed in the training sets, including gene selection or shrinkage parameter estimation with cross-validation.

4 Results

There are currently a total of 825 GO BP, 50 hallmark, and 326 positional gene sets on the Broad website that we downloaded. Due to the fact that we had previously performed a gene filtering step, we were left with fewer numbers of gene sets (736 GO BP, 50 hallmark, and 278 positional) as well as fewer genes within the gene sets when we applied these gene sets to our datasets. We also focused on gene sets containing at least 5 genes. Table 4 gives a summary of the number of genes in the gene sets of our datasets. Both the GO BP and positional categories have a small percent of gene sets with a large number of genes in them. However, if we look at the median number of genes within gene sets, the hallmark gene sets have the largest number (86) followed by the GO BP gene sets (54.76) and the positional gene sets (25.9).

4.1 Methods Comparison

Table 5 shows the test set error rates achieved in the individual-gene analysis for each disease comparison. To compare the methods, we ranked them by their averaged error rates (AER) over all the disease comparisons—lower AER is better. Overall, ccscore and score ranked as the top two classifiers in the individual-gene analysis with AER being 0.16 and 0.17 respectively, followed by Lasso

Table 4 Summary on number of genes within each type of gene sets in our datasets

Type of gene sets	Minimum	1st. quartile	Median	Mean	3rd. quartile	Maximum
GO BP	5	9	16	54.76	47	1110
Hallmark	9	50.5	85.5	86	114	186
Positional	5	10	17	25.9	30	281

Table 5 Test set error rates achieved in the individual-gene analysis (columns 2–5), where D1, D2, D3, D4 denote the four disease comparisons: normal versus MGUS, MGUS versus SMM, SMM versus MM, p53 deletion versus no deletion, respectively

Classification method	D1	D2	D3	D4	Average	Rank by average
ccscore	0.16	0.31	0.10	0.10	0.16	1
score	0.19	0.31	0.08	0.10	0.17	2
lasso	0.25	0.39	0.06	0.07	0.19	3
rf	0.23	0.36	0.12	0.09	0.20	4
pcscore	0.19	0.31	0.15	0.16	0.20	5
tree	0.28	0.32	0.19	0.10	0.22	6

The last two columns have the averaged error rates (average) over 4 disease comparisons and the rankings of the methods by the averaged error rates

(AER = 0.19), random forest (AER = 0.20), and pcscore (AER = 0.20), and the tree method ranked the lowest (AER = 0.22). Note that the AER were rounded to the 2nd decimal point while the rankings were calculated using all decimal points.

For the gene set methods, Table 6 gives the test set error rates for each disease comparison/type of gene sets combination (a total of 12 scenarios). Note that both the method and type of gene sets affected the error rates for each disease comparison. We ranked the methods by their averaged error rates (AER) across all 12 scenarios. It turned out that lasso.lasso and all the methods that employed trees in step 2 of the gene set analysis were low performers. However, Lasso performed well in conjunction with random forests. When not combined with trees in the 2nd step, the ccscore-related methods consistently ranked at the top followed by the pcscore- and score-related methods, although the differences among them were small (≤ 0.02) by the AER measure. More often than not, random forests were good choices when combined with the score methods or Lasso.

4.2 Gene Set Analysis Versus Individual-Gene Analysis

The question is: did the gene set analysis improve prediction accuracy over the individual-gene analysis? We compared the two types of analysis by calculating differences in error rates. For example, suppose in individual-gene analysis we used the Lasso, then we would compare it with those gene set methods that employed Lasso in 2nd step of the gene set analysis such as ccscore.lasso, score.lasso, pcscore.lasso, and lasso.lasso. By doing such comparisons, one can gauge whether step 1 of the gene set analysis is necessary—without step 1 the gene set analysis just reduces to individual-gene analysis. Table 7 lists reductions in error rate by using gene set analysis compared to individual-gene analysis in all such comparisons. Note that each gene set method was applied for each disease comparison three times, each time utilizing a different kind of gene sets (either GO BP, hallmark, or positional), while each individual-gene method was applied only once for each disease comparison. Thus when calculating the differences in error rate, we replicated those error rates of the individual-gene methods three times. We can see in Table 7 that both the method and the type of gene sets affected whether there was any improvement in performance by doing gene set analysis, where improvement was measured by reduction in error rate. We highlighted those scenarios when the reductions in error rate by doing gene set analysis were somewhat meaningful (≥ 0.04), although 0.04 is an arbitrary choice. The fact that there are both positive and negative values in Table 7 indicates that sometimes individual-gene analysis was better than gene set analysis in terms of prediction accuracy. Averaged reductions in error rate were also calculated for each gene set method in comparison to an appropriate individual-gene method (last column of Table 7).

Table 6 Test set error rates achieved in the gene set analysis using 3 types of gene sets (GO BP, hallmark, and positional), where D1, D2, D3, D4 denote the four disease comparisons: normal versus MGUS, MGUS versus SMM, SMM versus MM, p53 deletion versus no deletion, respectively

Classification	GO BP				Hallmark				Positional				Average	Rank by average
Method	D1	D2	D3	D4	D1	D2	D3	D4	D1	D2	D3	D4		
ccscore.ccscore	0.18	0.37	0.06	0.09	0.21	0.30	0.09	0.08	0.18	0.32	0.08	0.07	0.17	2
ccscore.lasso	0.18	0.37	0.06	0.09	0.21	0.30	0.09	0.08	0.18	0.32	0.08	0.07	0.17	2
ccscore.rf	0.18	0.35	0.11	0.09	0.18	0.30	0.09	0.07	0.14	0.31	0.10	0.07	0.16	1
ccscore.tree	0.14	0.31	0.14	0.08	0.23	0.35	0.14	0.07	0.26	0.35	0.13	0.08	0.19	11
score.score	0.21	0.35	0.07	0.09	0.21	0.31	0.09	0.09	0.21	0.32	0.10	0.07	0.18	9
score.lasso	0.21	0.35	0.07	0.09	0.21	0.31	0.09	0.09	0.21	0.32	0.10	0.07	0.18	9
score.rf	0.19	0.32	0.12	0.10	0.18	0.30	0.10	0.07	0.16	0.33	0.12	0.06	0.17	7
score.tree	0.23	0.35	0.12	0.09	0.32	0.35	0.15	0.08	0.18	0.38	0.17	0.08	0.21	14
pcscore.pcscore	0.21	0.36	0.08	0.09	0.19	0.30	0.10	0.08	0.16	0.31	0.09	0.08	0.17	4
pcscore.lasso	0.21	0.36	0.08	0.09	0.19	0.30	0.10	0.08	0.16	0.31	0.09	0.08	0.17	4
pcscore.rf	0.21	0.35	0.11	0.09	0.18	0.31	0.12	0.07	0.12	0.31	0.13	0.07	0.17	8
pcscore.tree	0.23	0.37	0.15	0.09	0.26	0.36	0.15	0.09	0.21	0.39	0.14	0.09	0.21	15
lasso.lasso	0.21	0.37	0.05	0.09	0.26	0.35	0.06	0.10	0.25	0.43	0.10	0.10	0.20	12
lasso.rf	0.16	0.37	0.06	0.08	0.14	0.33	0.05	0.09	0.19	0.42	0.06	0.09	0.17	6
lasso.tree	0.26	0.37	0.06	0.10	0.18	0.44	0.06	0.10	0.19	0.50	0.09	0.08	0.20	13

The last two columns have the averaged error rates (average) over all disease comparisons/types of gene sets and the rankings by the averaged error rates

Table 7 Reductions in test set error rate by doing gene set analysis compared to individual-gene analysis, where D1, D2, D3, D4 denote the four disease comparisons: normal versus MGUS, MGUS versus SMM, SMM versus MM, p53 deletion versus no deletion, respectively

Gene set analysis method	Individual gene analysis method	GO BP				Hallmark				Positional				Average
		D1	D2	D3	D4	D1	D2	D3	D4	D1	D2	D3	D4	
ccscore.ccscore	ccscore	−0.02	−0.07	**0.04**	0.01	−0.05	0.01	0.01	0.01	−0.02	−0.02	0.02	0.03	0.00
score.score	score	−0.02	−0.04	0.01	0.01	−0.02	−0.01	−0.01	0.01	−0.02	−0.02	−0.02	0.03	−0.01
pcscore.pcscore	pcscore	−0.02	−0.05	**0.08**	**0.08**	0	0.01	**0.06**	**0.08**	**0.04**	−0.01	**0.06**	**0.09**	0.03
ccscore.lasso	lasso	**0.07**	0.02	0	−0.02	**0.04**	**0.09**	−0.02	−0.02	**0.07**	**0.07**	−0.02	0	0.02
score.lasso	lasso	**0.04**	**0.04**	−0.01	−0.02	**0.04**	**0.08**	−0.03	−0.02	**0.04**	**0.07**	−0.04	0	0.01
pcscore.lasso	lasso	**0.04**	0.03	−0.01	−0.02	**0.05**	**0.09**	−0.03	−0.02	**0.09**	**0.08**	−0.03	−0.01	0.02
lasso.lasso	lasso	**0.04**	0.02	0.01	−0.02	−0.02	**0.04**	0	−0.03	0	−0.04	−0.04	−0.03	−0.01
ccscore.rf	rf	**0.05**	0.01	0.01	0.01	**0.05**	**0.06**	0.03	0.02	**0.09**	**0.04**	0.02	0.02	0.03
score.rf	rf	**0.04**	0.03	0	0	**0.05**	**0.06**	0.02	0.02	**0.07**	0.03	0	0.03	0.03
pcscore.rf	rf	0.02	0.01	0.01	0.01	**0.05**	**0.05**	0	0.02	**0.11**	**0.04**	−0.01	0.02	0.03
lasso.rf	rf	**0.07**	−0.02	**0.06**	0.02	**0.09**	0.03	**0.07**	0	**0.04**	−0.06	**0.06**	0	0.03
ccscore.tree	tree	**0.14**	0.02	**0.04**	0.01	**0.05**	−0.03	**0.05**	0.02	0.02	−0.03	**0.06**	0.02	0.03
score.tree	tree	**0.05**	−0.03	**0.06**	0	−0.04	−0.03	0.03	0.02	**0.11**	−0.06	0.01	0.01	0.01
pcscore.tree	tree	**0.05**	−0.05	0.03	0.01	0.02	−0.03	0.03	0.01	**0.07**	−0.07	**0.04**	0.01	0.01
lasso.tree	tree	0.02	−0.05	**0.13**	0	**0.11**	−0.12	**0.13**	0	**0.09**	−0.18	**0.1**	0.02	0.02

Values that are ≥ 0.04 are bold-faced. The last column (average) gives the averaged reductions in error rate

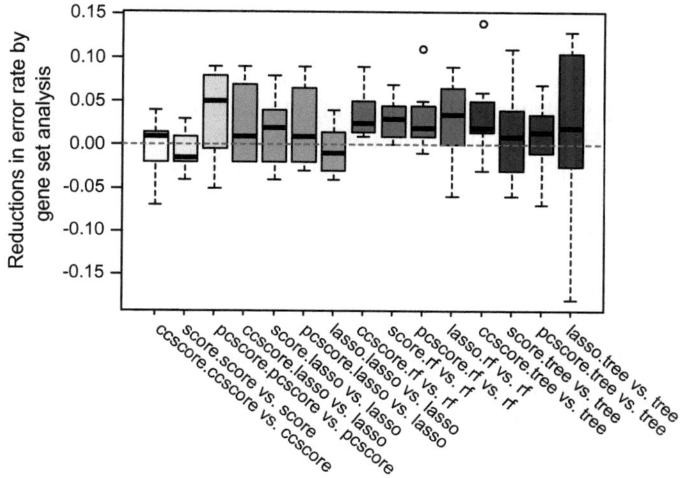

Fig. 1 Boxplots of the reductions in test set error rate (shown in Table 7) by using each of 15 gene set methods compared to corresponding individual-gene methods

By this measure, all 15 gene set methods except two produced more accurate models with reduced error rates. Figure 1 provides a visualization of the reductions in error rate. Despite the variations, overall across all the methods, gene set analysis reduced error rates by 0.02 on average, and 25% of the time by at least 0.05.

4.3 Disease Comparisons

Tables 5 and 6 is also a good summary of the overall prediction error rates for the disease comparisons. To have a focused discussion here, we consider only the ccscore and ccscore.lasso methods in this subsection and the next, as respectively they were among the top methods used in the individual-gene and gene set analysis. It appears that both the individual-gene and gene set methods were able to classify SMM versus MM and *P53* deletion versus no deletion very well with error rates varying between 0.06 and 0.10. Clinically, SMM is characterized by a higher percentage of abnormal plasma cells in the bone marrow and higher levels of M-protein in the serum than MGUS. Thus being able to classify SMM versus MM implies being able to discriminate between MGUS and MM as well. It turned out that our hypothesis was right when we went to verify it—the test set error rate for discriminating between MGUS and MM by an individual-gene analysis with the ccscore was 0.099. This is contradictory to the findings reported in Hardin et al. [22], where all the models failed to classify MGUS versus MM. A couple of factors could be the cause here. First, the newer microarray platform U133Plus2 covers the whole genome more comprehensively than the older platform, so there is a better chance to detect differentiable genes and therefore create more powerful models. Second, we had more MGUS samples in this investigation: 73 compared to 21 in Hardin et al. [22], while the MM samples in both investigations were plenty (174 in ours and 218 in Hardin et al.). Nonetheless, the difficult case for us was to discriminate between MGUS and SMM, as the error rates for this classification were between 0.3 and 0.37 for the individual-gene and gene set analysis. This indicates that at the molecular level MGUS and SMM are different for the most part, yet they share certain genetic features that make them less indistinguishable. Also interesting were the error rates for classifying MGUS versus normal varied between 0.16 and 0.21.

Taken together, these data seem to suggest that in terms of gene expression levels SMM is very different from MM, while MGUS is somewhere between normal and SMM, but more similar to SMM. At this point careful interpretation of the results is warranted. When using CD138 expression to isolate plasma cells (PC) before GEP—a standard procedure routinely performed at the Myeloma Institute, the MGUS/SMM PC samples were infiltrated with normal PC, while the MM PC samples were largely abnormal. Consequently, some of the differentially expressed genes we identified between MGUS/SMM PC and MM PC samples might be due to differences in the amount of normal PC in the samples rather than due to disease differences. This problem was less when comparing normal versus MGUS and MGUS versus SMM PC samples, as they were more comparable in terms of the amount of normal PC in the samples.

4.4 Gene Lists and Gene Selection

We provide a list of genes and gene sets identified for each disease comparison by the ccscore and ccsore.lasso methods from the individual-gene and gene set analysis respectively (for the same reason described in the last subsection) (Tables 8, 9, 10, and 11). For the ccscore.lasso gene set analysis, we chose the gene set that gave the best result for each disease comparison (2nd row in Table 6). Furthermore, we summarized the total number of genes identified by the two types of analysis. In all except the comparison of *P53* deletion versus no deletion, more genes were selected by ccscore.lasso than ccscore, with comparatively few overlapping genes (Table 12).

4.5 Computing Time

We recorded computing time for all the methods in the individual-gene analysis (Table 13). The evaluations were conducted on a laptop using 64-bit Windows 7 and running on a 4-core 3 GHz CPU with 8 GB of memory. For all the methods except Lasso, we started with all 9624 genes. For random forests, however, we

Table 8 Genes and gene sets identified from the classification of normal versus MGUS (the methods used were ccscore and ccscore.lasso for the individual-gene and gene set analysis, respectively)

Disease comparison	Analysis type	Gene set	Genes
Normal versus MGUS	Individual-gene analysis		*AMPD3, APOBEC3B, ARPC5L, ATP6V0E1, CCDC6, CD81, CDKN1A, DHX29, EFHC1, HACD2, HCST, HGF, MOB3B, NDNF, PASK, RTN4, TMEM167A, TMEM38B, TMX1, TPST2*
	Gene set analysis (GO BP)	POSITIVE REGULATION OF RESPONSE TO STIMULUS	*UBE2 N*
		REGULATION OF SECRETION	*PYCARD, DNAJC1*
		SYSTEM DEVELOPMENT	*RTN4, UGT8*
		BIOGENIC AMINE METABOLIC PROCESS	*OAZ2*
		REGULATION OF BIOLOGICAL QUALITY	*CDKN1A, CDKN2C, HIF1A, CD59, GLRX2, UBB, NDUFS1, CLCN3*
		DNA METABOLIC PROCESS	*POLD1, POLE, UBE2 N, GADD45A, CDK2AP1, MMS19, RAD51C, ERCC1, IGF1, DNMT3B, UBE2B, RBMS1, CDC6*
		BIOPOLYMER CATABOLIC PROCESS	*UBE2 N, ERCC1, UBE2B, UBE4A, UBB, GSPT1, UPF2, AMFR, ANAPC4*
		RNA METABOLIC PROCESS	*ESRRG, TCF7, RBFOX2, HIF1A, NR1D2, TROVE2, SOD2, MMS19, RBPJ, MDFIC, RSF1, TCF19, CEBPB, SUPT16H, NR3C1, POU2F2, SMARCA2, TFDP1, HNRNPC, RBMS1, GSPT1, NMI, UPF2*
		PROTEIN OLIGOMERIZATION	*STOM, DGKD*
		DNA REPAIR	*POLD1, POLE, UBE2 N, GADD45A, MMS19, RAD51C, ERCC1, UBE2B*
		POSITIVE REGULATION OF TRANSLATION	*SPN*
		MUSCLE DEVELOPMENT	*TAZ, IGF1, UBB*
		POSITIVE REGULATION OF CELL DIFFERENTIATION	*SOCS5*
		PROTEIN FOLDING	*FKBP5, GLRX2*
		PHOSPHOLIPID BIOSYNTHETIC PROCESS	*CD81*
		NEGATIVE REGULATION OF NUCLEOBASENUCLEOSIDENUCLEOTIDE AND NUCLEIC ACID METABOLIC PROCESS	*RBFOX2, RBPJ, RSF1*
		GLYCEROPHOSPHOLIPID BIOSYNTHETIC PROCESS	*CD81, PIGC*
		NUCLEOBASENUCLEOSIDE AND NUCLEOTIDE METABOLIC PROCESS	*AMPD3, NDUFS1, DCTD, FIGNL1*
		NEGATIVE REGULATION OF CELLULAR METABOLIC PROCESS	*CDKN1A, RBFOX2, CDKN2C, RBPJ, RSF1, ERCC1, SIGIRR, CDC6, DNAJC1*
		PROTEIN AUTOPROCESSING	*KIAA1804*

Table 9 Genes and gene sets identified from the classification of MGUS versus SMM (the methods used were ccscore and ccscore.lasso for the individual-gene and gene set analysis, respectively)

Disease comparison	Analysis type	Gene set	Genes
MGUS versus SMM	Individual-gene analysis		*CTSH, GATA2, GSTA1, IGHD, IGHM, IGK, IGKC, IGLC1, IGLJ3, IGLV1-44, TNFRSF18*
	Gene set analysis (Hallmark)	TNFA SIGNALING VIA NFKB	*BIRC3, TNIP1, ID2, NFAT5, TNFAIP3*
		DNA REPAIR	*SUPT5H, AAAS, POLE4*
		APOPTOSIS	*IGFBP6, BIRC3, CYLD*
		PROTEIN SECRETION	*SEC31A, RAB2A*
		INTERFERON GAMMA RESPONSE	*HIF1A, IL10RA, TNFAIP3*
		COMPLEMENT	*CTSH, CALM1, TNFAIP3, APOBEC3F, PLA2G4A*
		EPITHELIAL MESENCHYMAL TRANSITION	*EFEMP2*
		IL2 STAT5 SIGNALING	*TNFRSF18, CD81, IL10RA, CDC42SE2*

included another filtering step to consider only the top 1500 differentially expressed genes prior to model selection. Our experience is that random forests can be very slow without pre-filtering. As shown in Table 13, computing time increases as sample size increases. The ccscore/score/pcscore finished in decent amounts of time (a couple of minutes) but Lasso was no doubt the fastest algorithm in all cases.

5 Conclusions and Discussion

In this paper, we evaluated 15 methods for gene set analysis in classification problems using four GEP myeloma datasets and three types of biological gene sets, encompassing a total of 12 scenarios. By comparing the 15 methods with individual-gene methods, we conclude that, overall, the gene set analysis provided more accurate models than the individual-gene analysis. Within a biologically defined gene set, genes are more likely to be co-regulated or co-expressed. We propose to use linear methods such as the ccscore, score, and pcscore (an extension of the SuperPC [1]) for calculating gene set scores before constructing final predictive models.

Our overall results after averaging across different datasets/gene sets are comparable to those reported by other authors. For example, Ma et al. [17] proposed

Table 10 Genes and gene sets identified from the classification of SMM versus MM (the methods used were ccscore and ccscore.lasso for the individual-gene and gene set analysis, respectively)

Disease comparison	Analysis type	Gene set	Genes
SMM versus MM	Individual-gene analysis		*ATXN7L3B, C2CD4C, CDC5L, CDT1, DENND2D, FOXO1, GMIP, KIAA1033, KLHDC3, MELK, MTUS1, NCOA1, ND6, RPL37A, RPL38, RRM2, SH3KBP1, STIL, ZWINT*
	Gene set analysis (GO BP)	POSITIVE REGULATION OF PHOSPHATE METABOLIC PROCESS	*GLMN, AKTIP, ANG, IL20, LYN*
		NEGATIVE REGULATION OF CELLULAR METABOLIC PROCESS	*CDT1, ZHX1, GMNN, DRAP1, TIPIN, ZMYND11, PA2G4, GTPBP4, PHB, STAT3*
		REGULATION OF HYDROLASE ACTIVITY	*CASP9, ADAP1, MTCH1, ANG, CDKN2A, FGD2, S1PR4*
		TRNA PROCESSING	*ADAT1, AARS, SARS*
		REGULATION OF BIOLOGICAL QUALITY	*LMAN1, GTPBP4, SLC40A1, GCHFR, ACVR2A, CXCL12, CD59, XRN2, CDKN2C, EIF2B2, EIF2B5, PAIP1, ERP44, SOD1, CALR, BDKRB1, FXN, F7, GPI, CAPRIN2, BARD1, NPC2, NDUFS1, TARBP2, CDKN2A, NOTCH2, CLCN3, FTH1, LYN, FLI1, SLC30A5, CYSLTR1, CDKN1A, FGD2, SERTAD2, AGT, NPTN, CLN3, APTX, DERL2, COG3, NEBL, S1PR4, GCLM, ENO1, SMAD4, LDB1, ARF6, CCDC88C, WAS, CEBPG, RPS19, CAPG, SGMS1*
		DNA METABOLIC PROCESS	*CDT1, PURA, RBBP8, KPNA2, GMNN, POLE3, TIPIN, ATRX, TLK1, CHEK1, GTPBP4, XAB2, FEN1, IGF1, MCM2, PARP3, TINF2, SUPV3L1*
		AMINO SUGAR METABOLIC PROCESS	*CSGALNACT1, NAGK*
		BIOPOLYMER CATABOLIC PROCESS	*UBE2C, ANAPC2, GSPT1, AMFR, STUB1, UBE2G1, UBE2H, ABCE1, FBXO22, XRN2, RNASEH2A, SOD1, ANAPC10, UBE2E1, HNRNPD, CDC23, PSMD14, CDKN2A*
		RNA METABOLIC PROCESS	*FOXO1, PTTG1, ZHX1, TRIP13, EZH2, RBBP8, KLF7, DRAP1, ZNF367, ZMYND11, ASH1L, PA2G4, ATRX, RUVBL1*
		PROTEIN POLYUBIQUITINATION	*AMFR, STUB1*
		PROTEIN OLIGOMERIZATION	*STOM, AMFR, TRPV5, INSR, NOD1, DGKD, CCDC88C, MALT1*
		DNA REPAIR	*RBBP8, ATRX, XAB2, FEN1, PARP3, POLD1, RUVBL2, RAD23B, MSH3, SOD1, MMS19, CSNK1D*

(continued)

Table 10 (continued)

Disease comparison	Analysis type	Gene set	Genes
		POSITIVE REGULATION OF TRANSLATION	*SPN, TLR1, TNFRSF8, GLMN, EIF2B5, TLR6*
		RESPONSE TO VIRUS	*CXCL12, APOBEC3F, ABCE1, RSAD2, BNIP3L, IFNAR1, IFNGR1, TARBP2, IFNAR2, APOBEC3G*
		MUSCLE DEVELOPMENT	*UTRN, IGF1, NOTCH1, SOD1, FKTN, MYBPC3*
		POSITIVE REGULATION OF CELL DIFFERENTIATION	*ACVR2A, SOCS5, IL20, BOC, BTG1*
		MITOTIC CELL CYCLE CHECKPOINT	*ZWINT, CCNA2, BUB1B, MAD2L1, PCBP4*
		ACTIN FILAMENT ORGANIZATION	*KPTN, SORBS3, ARHGEF10L, SHROOM2, NF2*
		PROTEIN FOLDING	*LMAN1, CCT4, HSPE1, PFDN4, STUB1, ERP29, RUVBL2, CCT3, DNAJB2, ERP44, CCT6A, PPIH, DNAJA1, CLN3, UGGT1, PPIA, FKBP5, CLPX*
		REGULATION OF RHO PROTEIN SIGNAL TRANSDUCTION	*RAC1, FGD2, ARF6*
		AXON GUIDANCE	*OPHN1, UBB*
		LIPID CATABOLIC PROCESS	*CPT1A, PLA2G15, SMPD3, ECH1*
		PHOSPHOLIPID BIOSYNTHETIC PROCESS	*ETNK1, PIGO, PIGV, PIK3C2A, AGPAT1, SGMS1, IMPA1*
		NEGATIVE REGULATION OF NUCLEOBASENUCLEOSIDENUCLEOTIDE AND NUCLEIC ACID METABOLIC PROCESS	*CDT1, ZHX1, GMNN, DRAP1, TIPIN, ZMYND11, PA2G4, GTPBP4, PHB, STAT3*
		CYTOKINESIS	*RACGAP1, NUSAP1, PRC1*
		SPLICEOSOME ASSEMBLY	*SCAF11, SF3A2, SRSF1, SRSF5, SF3A1, SNRPD1*
		GLYCEROPHOSPHOLIPID BIOSYNTHETIC PROCESS	*PIGO, PIGV, PIK3C2A, AGPAT1, IMPA1*
		NUCLEOBASENUCLEOSIDE AND NUCLEOTIDE METABOLIC PROCESS	*TYMS, PPAT, ADM, NUDT5, FPGS, NDUFS1*
		NUCLEAR IMPORT	*KPNA2, HNRNPA1, ZFYVE9, RANBP2, PPIH, KPNB1*

Table 11 Genes and gene sets identified from the classification of p53 deletion versus no deletion (the methods used were ccscore and ccscore.lasso for the individual-gene and gene set analysis, respectively)

Disease comparison	Analysis type	Gene set	Genes
P53 deletion versus no deletion	Individual-gene analysis		*ACADVL, ADPRM, ARHGAP19, ASB7, BTBD10, C17orf85, C1QBP, CEP85, CKS2, CRK, CTDNEP1, CTNS, CYB5D1, DHX33, ELK1, ELP5, EZH2, FANCI, FXR2, GABARAP, GEMIN4, GLOD4, GPS2, GTF2E1, HARBI1, HMMR, HPS3, INPP5 K, ITGAE, KIAA0753, KIF18B, LOC101928000, MAD2L1, MED11, MIS12, MPDU1, NAA38, NXT2, OIP5, P2RX1, PCMTD1, PFAS, PITPNA, PITPNA-AS1, PRC1, PRPF8, RABEP1, RANGRF, RBBP8, RNMTL1, SAPCD2, SAT2, SENP3, SHPK, SPAG7, TMEM107, TMEM256, TP53, TPX2, TRAPPC2, UBE2G1, VAMP2, WEE1, ZBTB4, ZNF33B, ZWILCH*
	Gene set analysis (positional)	chr6q13	*SENP6, MYO6*
		chr17p11	*MAP2K4, TTC19*
		chr10q24	*ARHGAP19*
		chr1p34	*NSUN4, HYI, KIF2C*
		chr6q16	*MANEA, FBXL4, UBE2J1*
		chr15q26	*PRC1, ASB7*
		chr3q28	*AP2M1, OPA1*
		chr9q22	*CKS2*
		chr6q23	*CITED2, STX7*
		chr17p13	*SAT2, SPAG7, RABEP1, PRPF8, MED11, PFAS, VAMP2, GABARAP, ZBTB4, RNMTL1, CYB5D1, CTNS, DHX33, SENP3, C1QBP, MIS12, TP53, PITPNA, TMEM107, C17orf85, CRK, ACADVL, ITGAE, MPDU1, P2RX1, GPS2, GEMIN4, KIAA0753, PHF23, SLC25A11, NUP88, LOC728392, WDR81, PAFAH1B1, MYBBP1A, DERL2, TSR1*

Table 12 Number of genes selected and number of overlapping genes in the individual-gene and gene set analysis (the methods used were ccscore and ccscore.lasso for the individual-gene and gene set analysis, respectively)

Disease Comparison	# genes selected in individual-gene analysis	# genes selected in gene set analysis	# overlapping genes
Normal versus MGUS	20	96	4
MGUS versus SMM	11	26	2
SMM versus MM	19	260	3
P53 deletion versus no deletion	66	55	32

Table 13 Computing time (in minutes) for training different models in individual-gene analysis. Note that there were 9624 genes to begin with for the Lasso, score, ccscore, and pcscore methods, and 1500 genes for random forest (rf)

Comparison	Sample size in training set	Lasso	score	ccscore	pcscore	rf
Normal versus MGUS	98	0.04	1.03	1.05	1.08	0.17
MGUS versus SMM	162	0.05	1.25	1.24	1.26	0.27
SMM versus MM	263	0.08	1.71	1.66	1.69	0.39
P53 deletion versus no deletion	422	0.12	2.25	2.25	2.27	0.61

using Lasso within gene clusters to first select important genes before applying group Lasso [18] on the refined gene clusters. In four microarray datasets, they demonstrated either equal or better performance of their method than using regular Lasso in individual-gene analysis. In our study, lasso.lasso, ccscore.lasso, score. lasso, and pcscore.lasso are similar to their approach. Although both are two-step procedures, in their 1st step they created refined gene clusters rather than summary genet set scores. As shown in Tables 5 and 6, when compared to regular Lasso, the ccscore.lasso, score.lasso, and pcscore.lasso each had a reduction in error rate between 0.01 and 0.02, although lasso.lasso had a 0.01 increase in error rate.

Our general approach resembles with that of Chen and Wang [16]. In the 1st step they created "super gene scores" with SuperPC [1], and in the 2nd step they employed either Lasso or again SuperPC using the super gene scores as predictors. With two microarray survival datasets they demonstrated the superiority of their methods when compared to not using gene set information. Our pcscore is essentially an extension of the SuperPC for binary outcomes, and therefore our pcscore. pcscore and pcscore.lasso directly correspond to their methods except that they focused on survival prediction instead of classification. When comparing to only using pcscore or lasso in individual-gene analysis, we saw an averaged reduction of at least 0.02 in error rate for pcscore.pcscore and pcscore.lasso (Tables 5 and 6), confirming comparability of our results with theirs.

Additionally, Tai and Pan [15] proposed a modified LDA approach to incorporate pathway information. With both simulated and real datasets, their method was shown to perform better than not incorporating pathway information (e.g., when compared to PAM [35], which considers genes as independent). Genes are naturally not independent from each other, therefore the improvements by their method were reasonable and expected. Importantly, our ccscore/score/pcscore methods already draw strength by combining correlated genes. As Park et al. [36] have shown, averaging genes within gene clusters can improve prediction accuracy. Our score method is essentially an extension of the averaged gene expression method to account for genes with both positive and negative correlations with the outcome. Although it is beyond the scope of this paper, it would be interesting to apply their approach and PAM on myeloma datasets in future research. Further investigations on the genes identified to examine whether the gene set analysis could provide more coherent biological insights into the myeloma disease mechanisms would be another avenue of research.

References

1. Bair E, Tibshirani R. Semi-supervised methods to predict patient survival from gene expression data. PLoS Biol. 2004;2(4):e108.
2. Nguyen DV, Rocke DM. Tumor classification by partial least squares using microarray gene expression data. Bioinformatics. 2002;18(1):39–50.
3. Tibshirani R. Regression shrinkage and selection via the lasso. J R Stat Soc Ser B (Methodol). 1996;1:267–88.
4. Díaz-Uriarte R, De Andres SA. Gene selection and classification of microarray data using random forest. BMC Bioinform. 2006;7(1):1.
5. Ein-Dor L, Kela I, Getz G, Givol D, Domany E. Outcome signature genes in breast cancer: is there a unique set? Bioinformatics. 2005;21(2):171–8.
6. Solé X, Bonifaci N, López-Bigas N, Berenguer A, Hernández P, Reina O, Maxwell CA, Aguilar H, Urruticoechea A, de Sanjosé S, Comellas F. Biological convergence of cancer signatures. PLoS ONE. 2009;4(2):e4544.
7. Mootha VK, Lindgren CM, Eriksson KF, Subramanian A, Sihag S, Lehar J, Puigserver P, Carlsson E, Ridderstråle M, Laurila E, Houstis N. PGC-1α-responsive genes involved in oxidative phosphorylation are coordinately downregulated in human diabetes. Nat Genet. 2003;34(3):267–73.
8. Subramanian A, Tamayo P, Mootha VK, Mukherjee S, Ebert BL, Gillette MA, Paulovich A, Pomeroy SL, Golub TR, Lander ES, Mesirov JP. Gene set enrichment analysis: a knowledge-based approach for interpreting genome-wide expression profiles. Proc Natl Acad Sci. 2005;102(43):15545–50.
9. Ashburner M, Ball CA, Blake JA, Botstein D, Butler H, Cherry JM, Davis AP, Dolinski K, Dwight SS, Eppig JT, Harris MA. Gene ontology: tool for the unification of biology. Nat Genet. 2000;25(1):25–9.
10. Kanehisa M, Goto S, Furumichi M, Tanabe M, Hirakawa M. for representation and analysis of molecular networks involving diseases and drugs. Nucleic Acids Res. 2010;38(suppl 1): D355–60.
11. Goeman JJ, Van De Geer SA, De Kort F, Van Houwelingen HC. A global test for groups of genes: testing association with a clinical outcome. Bioinformatics. 2004;20(1):93–9.
12. Mansmann U, Meister R. Testing differential gene expression in functional groups Goeman's global test versus an ANCOVA approach. Methods Inf Med. 2005;44(3):449–53.

13. Dinu I, Potter JD, Mueller T, Liu Q, Adewale AJ, Jhangri GS, Einecke G, Famulski KS, Halloran P, Yasui Y. Improving GSEA for analysis of biologic pathways for differential gene expression across a binary phenotype. COBRA Prepr Ser. 2007; 16.
14. Efron B, Tibshirani R. On testing the significance of sets of genes. Ann Appl Stat. 2007;1:107–29.
15. Tai F, Pan W. Incorporating prior knowledge of gene functional groups into regularized discriminant analysis of microarray data. Bioinformatics. 2007;23(23):3170–7.
16. Chen X, Wang L. Integrating biological knowledge with gene expression profiles for survival prediction of cancer. J Comput Biol. 2009;16(2):265–78.
17. Ma S, Song X, Huang J. Supervised group Lasso with applications to microarray data analysis. BMC Bioinform. 2007;8(1):1.
18. Meier L, Van De Geer S, Bühlmann P. The group lasso for logistic regression. J R Stat Soc Ser B (Stat Methodol). 2008;70(1):53–71.
19. Luan Y, Li H. Group additive regression models for genomic data analysis. Biostatistics. 2008;9(1):100–13.
20. Kyle RA, Therneau TM, Rajkumar SV, Offord JR, Larson DR, Plevak MF, Melton LJ III. A long-term study of prognosis in monoclonal gammopathy of undetermined significance. N Engl J Med. 2002;346(8):564–9.
21. Kyle RA, Remstein ED, Therneau TM, Dispenzieri A, Kurtin PJ, Hodnefield JM, Larson DR, Plevak MF, Jelinek DF, Fonseca R, Melton LJ III. Clinical course and prognosis of smoldering (asymptomatic) multiple myeloma. N Engl J Med. 2007;356(25):2582–90.
22. Hardin J, Waddell M, Page CD, Zhan F, Barlogie B, Shaughnessy J, Crowley JJ. Evaluation of multiple models to distinguish closely related forms of disease using DNA microarray data: an application to multiple myeloma. Stat Appl Genet Mol Biol. 2004;3(1):1–21.
23. Stein CK, Qu P, Epstein J, Buros A, Rosenthal A, Crowley J, Morgan G, Barlogie B. Removing batch effects from purified plasma cell gene expression microarrays with modified ComBat. BMC Bioinform. 2015;16(1):1.
24. Liberzo A, Subramanian A, Pinchback R, Thorvaldsdóttir H, Tamayo P, Mesirov JP. Molecular signatures database (MSigDB) 3.0. Bioinformatics. 2011;27(12):1739–40.
25. Liberzon A, Birger C, Thorvaldsdóttir H, Ghandi M, Mesirov JP, Tamayo P. The molecular signatures database hallmark gene set collection. Cell Syst. 2015;1(6):417–25.
26. Glmnet vignette. http://www.stanford.edu/~hastie/glmnet/glmnet_alpha.html.
27. Tukey JW. Tightening the clinical trial. Control Clin Trials. 1993;14(4):266–85.
28. Huang X, Pan W. Linear regression and two-class classification with gene expression data. Bioinformatics. 2003;19(16):2072–8.
29. Shaughnessy JD, Zhan F, Burington BE, Huang Y, Colla S, Hanamura I, Stewart JP, Kordsmeier B, Randolph C, Williams DR, Xiao Y. A validated gene expression model of high-risk multiple myeloma is defined by deregulated expression of genes mapping to chromosome 1. Blood. 2007;109(6):2276–84.
30. Breiman L, Friedman J, Stone CJ, Olshen RA. Classification and regression trees. Boca Raton: CRC Press; 1984.
31. Breiman L. Random forests. Mach Learn. 2001;45(1):5–32.
32. Cutler A, Cutler DR, Stevens JR. Random forest. In: Machine learning. 2011. http://www.researchgate.net/publication/236952762.
33. Hastie T, Tibshirani R, Friedman J. The elements of statistical learning: data mining, inference, and prediction. 2nd ed. Springer series in statistics. 2011.
34. Boulesteix AL, Janitza S, Kruppa J, König IR. Overview of random forest methodology and practical guidance with emphasis on computational biology and bioinformatics. Wiley Interdiscip Rev Data Min Knowl Discov. 2012;2(6):493–507.
35. Tibshirani R, Hastie T, Narasimhan B, Chu G. Class prediction by nearest shrunken centroids, with applications to DNA microarrays. Stat Sci. 2003;1:104–17.
36. Park MY, Hastie T, Tibshirani R. Averaged gene expressions for regression. Biostatistics. 2007;8(2):212–27.

Index

S. Matsui and J. Crowley (eds.), *Frontiers of Biostatistical Methods and Applications in Clinical Oncology*, DOI 10.1007/978-981-10-0126-0

MIX
Papier aus verantwortungsvollen Quellen
Paper from responsible sources
FSC® C105338

If you have any concerns about our products,
you can contact us on
ProductSafety@springernature.com

In case Publisher is established outside the EU,
the EU authorized representative is:
Springer Nature Customer Service Center GmbH
Europaplatz 3, 69115 Heidelberg, Germany

Printed by Libri Plureos GmbH
in Hamburg, Germany